Gerontological Nursing Care

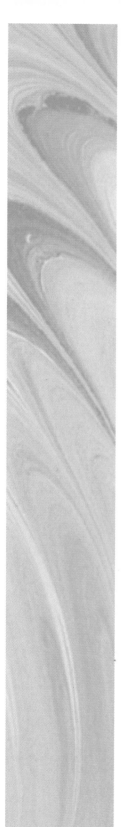

Shirley Rose Tyson, RN, MA, EdD

Nurse, Teacher, Consultant, Psychotherapist

Professor Emerita
Department of Nursing
New York City Technical College
City University of New York
New York, New York

Geriatric Education Associate
Mt. Sinai/Hunter College
Geriatric Education Center
City University of New York
New York, New York

Gerontological Nursing Care

W.B. SAUNDERS COMPANY
A Division of Harcourt Brace & Company
Philadelphia • London • Toronto • Montreal • Sydney • Tokyo

W.B. SAUNDERS COMPANY

A Division of Harcourt Brace & Company

The Curtis Center
Independence Square West
Philadelphia, Pennsylvania 19106

Library of Congress Cataloging-in-Publication Data

Tyson, Shirley Rose.

　　Gerontological nursing care / Shirley Rose Tyson.—1st ed.

　　　p. cm.

　　ISBN 0–7216–5009–0

　　1. Geriatric nursing.　I. Title.
　　[DNLM:　1. Geriatric Nursing.　2. Aging—physiology nurses'
instruction. WY 152 T994g 1999]

RC954.T97 1999　　　　　610.73976—dc21

DNLM/DLC　　　　　　　　　　　　　　　　　　98–7041

ISBN 0–7216–5009–0

Printed in the United States of America.

Last digit is the print number:　9　8　7　6　5　4　3　2　1

This book is dedicated with love to:

The memory of my dear husband John, in grateful remembrance of his constant love, support and vision which guided me through the writing of this book.

Our son Sydney, our joy, who lovingly cares for others in his daily work.

My mother Olga Rose, a dynamic nonagenarian, and the memory of my father, Sydney Rose.

Merle Rose Facey and Shelton Rose, my siblings, who are so proud of my accomplishments.

Reviewers

Ardelina Albano Baldonado, PhD, RN, CTN
Loyola University of Chicago
Niehoff School of Nursing, Chicago, Illinois

Mary Bliesmer, DNS, RN, MPH
Mankato State University
School of Nursing, Mankato, Minneapolis

Louvenia Carter, PhD, RN, CNA, CNS
Northwestern State University of Louisiana
School of Nursing, Shreveport, Louisiana

Linda Dune, MSN, RN, CEN
Wharton County Junior College
School of Nursing, Wharton, Texas

Kristen L. Easton, RN, MS, CCRN, CS
Valparaiso University
School of Nursing, Valparaiso, Indiana

Carol A. Goff, MSN, RN
Warren County Area Vocational–Technical
  School
Practical Nursing Program, Warren,
  Pennsylvania

Mary Ann Haeuser, MSN, RN-C, FNP
Dominican College
School of Nursing, San Rafael, California

Judith Wright Harmer, MSN, RN, CNS-G
Golden West College
School of Nursing, Huntington Beach,
  California

Maureen A. Harris, RN, MS
Veterans Administration Medical Center
Wilkes-Barre, Pennsylvania

Beulah A. Hofmann, MSN, RN
IVY Technical State College
School of Nursing, Terre Haute, Indiana

Tomasita R. Jacubowitz, MSN, RN, CS
University of North Carolina at Greensboro
School of Nursing, Greensboro, North Carolina

Bernice C. Johnson, RN, BS
Memorial Hospital,
Bedford County School of Nursing, Bedford,
  Virginia

Sharon Elaine Melberg, RN, BA, MPA
University of California, Davis
School of Nursing, Sacramento, California

Patricia Ann O'Leary, DSN, RN
Middle Tennessee State University
School of Nursing, Murfreesboro, Tennessee

Netha O'Meara, MSN, RN, CNS
Wharton County Junior College
School of Nursing, Wharton, Texas

Joyce Ott, MSN, RN
University of Pittsburgh Medical Center,
  Beaver Valley, Rochester, Pennsylvania

Linda R. Pierce, MSN, RNCS, ARNP, CNP
Bryan Memorial Hospital
School of Nursing, Lincoln, Nebraska

Helen L. Sloan, MSN, RN, CS
University of Southwestern Louisiana
School of Nursing, Lafayette, Louisiana

Joy Suhrheinrich, MSN, RN
Indiana University, East Campus
School of Nursing, Richmond, Indiana

June Vincent, EdD, RN
Indiana University, East Campus
School of Nursing, Richmond, Indiana

Marilyn J. Vontz, PhD, MSN, RN, MA, BS
Bryan Memorial Hospital
School of Nursing, Lincoln, Nebraska

Wanda May Webb, MSN, RN, CS
Hickory House Nursing Home, Inc., Honey
  Brook, Pennsylvania

Emily C. Zabrocki, PhD, MSN, RN
Joliet Junior College
School of Nursing, Joliet, Illinois

Contributors

Lovely Abraham, MSN, RNCS, GNP
Affiliate Faculty, Vanderbilt University School
of Nursing; Geriatric Nurse Practitioner,
VA Medical Center, Nashville, Tennessee
*Maintaining Wellness of the Lungs and
Respiration*

Barbara Diebold Ahlheit, MSN, RNCS
Adjunct Faculty, Vanderbilt School of Nursing;
Family Nurse Practitioner, VA Medical
Center, Nashville, Tennessee
*Maintaining Wellness of the Lungs and
Respiration*

Martha A. Badger, MSN, RNCS, GNP
Geriatric Nurse Practitioner, Brentwood,
Tennessee
*Maintaining Wellness of the Lungs and
Respiration*

Annette Bairan, PhD, RNCS, FNP
Professor of Nursing (Teacher of graduates in
Primary Care Nursing Program), Kennesaw
State University, Kennesaw, Georgia
*Community Health Care: Health Promotion and
Community Living; Acute Health Care*

Vergie M. Brannon, MSN, RN-C
Gerontological Nurse Practitioner, Baylor
Hospital: Senior Health Services, Dallas, Texas
Maintaining Wellness of the Brain and Nerves

Vanessa Jones Briscoe, RN, MSN
Assistant Professor, Tennessee State University,
Nashville, Tennessee
*Maintaining Wellness of the Lungs and
Respiration; Maintaining Wellness of the
Metabolic System*

Carol Dennis, DSN, RN
Assistant Professor of Nursing, Faculty Practice
Position, Kennesaw State University,
Kennesaw; Health Resource Manager,
Atherton Place, Marietta, Georgia
*Assessing the Older Adult: The Nursing Process;
Maintaining Wellness of the Bones and
Muscles; Maintaining Wellness of the Skin*

Paula Fishman, EdD, RD
Retired Assistant Professor, Hunter College,
City University of New York; Faculty
Member, Mt. Sinai/Hunter Geriatric
Education Center, New York, New York
Nutritional Needs

Clari Gilbert, RN, BSN, MA
Senior Vice President of Operations, Center
for Nursing and Rehabilitation Healthcare
Network, Brooklyn, New York
*Long-Term Care; Choices in Gerontological
Nursing*

Carol Sue Holtz, RN, BSN, MN, PhD
Associate Professor of Nursing, Kennesaw
State University, Kennesaw, Georgia
*Acknowledging the Whole Person: Culture,
Ethnicity, and Religion; Personal Safety:
Pharmacologic, Physical, Social;
Maintaining Wellness of the Immune System*

Paula Hudgins, MS, RNCS
Clinical Nurse Specialist–Mental Health
Nursing, North Texas Veterans Affairs
Medical Center, Dallas, Texas
Maintaining Wellness of the Brain and Nerves

Mary Kipple, RN, MSN
Professor of Nursing, New Mexico Junior
College, Hobbs, New Mexico
*Maintaining Wellness of the Heart and
Circulation*

Joyce Lusan, RN, BA, MS
Formerly Coordinator/Instructor, Interfaith
Medical Center School of Nursing;
Assistant Director of Nursing for Staff
Development and Infection Control,
Center for Nursing and Rehabilitation;
Coordinator for Infection Control and
Nursing Rehabilitation, Wartburg Lutheran
Home for the Aged and Wartburg Nursing,
Inc., Brooklyn, New York
*Maintaining Wellness of the Stomach and
Gastrointestinal Tract*

Vimala Philipose, RN, BSN, MSN, PhD
Formerly Assistant Professor, Howard
   University College of Nursing, Washington,
   DC. Gerontological Nurse Practitioner,
   Suburban Hospital, Bethesda, Maryland
   *Legal Aspects of Older Adult Care; Addressing
   Cognitive Issues*

Suzanne S. Resner, RN, DNSc
Program Analyst, United States Department of
   Health and Human Services, Health Resources
   and Services Administration, Rockville, Maryland
   *Alterations in Lifelong Capabilities: Social,
   Physical, Sexual*

Jacklen Swopes Robinson, MSN, RNCS
Family Nurse Practitioner, VA Medical Center,
   Nashville, Tennessee
   *Maintaining Wellness of the Lungs and
   Respiration*

Ellen Shipes, RN, MN, CETN
Adjunct Associate Professor, Vanderbilt
   University School of Nursing; Clinical
   Nurse Specialist—Wound Management

Service, Vanderbilt University Medical
Center, Nashville, Tennessee
*Maintaining Wellness of the Geritourinary
   System*

Shirley Rose Tyson, RN, MA, EdD
Professor Emerita, Department of Nursing,
   New York City Technical College, City
   University of New York
Geriatric Education Associate, Mt.
   Sinai/Hunter College, Geriatric Education
   Center, City University of New York, New
   York, New York
   *Nursing for the Aging Population; Ethical Issues
   Arising with Age; Alterations in Lifelong
   Capabilities: Social, Physical, Sexual; The
   Five Senses: Sensation and Perception;
   Activity, Rest, and Sleep; Supporting
   Mental Health; Death and Dying*

Sydney L. Tyson, MD, MPH
Associate Surgeon, Wills Eye Hospital,
   Philadelphia, Pennsylvania
   The Five Senses: Sensation and Perception

This new text, *Gerontological Nursing Care,* evolved to meet the learning needs of nursing students. It is also designed to assist nurses in any clinical setting who care for older adults. Written by leaders in the gerontological nursing community, this easy-to-read text addresses care of older adults in a positive, caring, humanistic manner and offers a clear introduction to gerontological nursing care, including its role, purpose, and some future trends.

The book is structured on a caring and wellness framework, with short caring and wellness quotes emphasizing these themes in each chapter. Because promotion of health is the responsibility of every nurse, especially in an era when the world's population is living longer, it is imperative that older adults embrace wellness and maintain healthy lifestyles. Consequently, nurses are encouraged throughout each chapter of the text to maintain that focus in learning, teaching, and practice.

Both nursing students and practicing nurses will benefit from this concise yet comprehensive, up-to-date resource that is applicable to each nurse's individual practice and learning needs. As a nursing instructor for many years, with the relatively recent responsibility of revising a curriculum to include gerontological nursing, I have worked with students, faculty, and nurses in gerontological settings to achieve this goal. Accordingly, this textbook consists of seven major units.

Unit I, *Nursing and the Older Adult,* provides background information for the geriatric nurse. **Chapter 1,** *Nursing for the Aging Population,* presents a basic overview of aging, theories of aging, concepts of caring and wellness, and contemporary issues associated with aging. **Chapter 2,** *Assessing the Older Adult,* presents the nursing process in depth. **Chapter 3,** *Ethical Issues Arising with Age,* and **Chapter 4,** *Legal Aspects of Older Adult Care,* cover ethical and legal issues pertaining to older adults and the role of the nurse who cares for them.

Unit II, *Psychosocial Health in Maturity,* addresses a variety of issues that impact on the lives of older adults. **Chapter 5,** *Acknowledging the Whole Person,* emphasizes the importance of the cultural, ethnic, and religious aspects of the older adult client. **Chapter 6,** *Alterations in Lifelong Capabilities,* addresses the social, physical, and sexual challenges of aging, with emphasis on wellness.

Unit III, *Physiological Health in Aging,* looks at the physical components of health related to older adults. **Chapter 7,** *Nutritional Needs,* is a comprehensive view of sustenance from requirements to assisted eating. **Chapter 8,** *The Five Senses,* delineates the modifying sensory perceptions of aging adults. **Chapter 9,** *Activity, Rest, and Sleep,* addresses the daily rhythms of healthy individuals and notes some interventions for those experiencing difficulties in these areas. **Chapter 10,** *Personal Safety,* covers issues of pharmacological, physical, and social safety, and expands on the avoidance of falls, a topic first introduced in the preceding chapter.

Unit IV, *Supporting Wellness in Diverse Settings,* again underscores the many older adults who are maintaining health and vigor throughout the life span. **Chapter 11,** *Community Health Care,* addresses the growing trend toward caring for older adults in their homes and in community clinics rather than in inpatient settings. **Chapter 12,** *Acute Health Care,* focuses on the temporary need for acute care and how it is delivered. **Chapter 13,** *Long-Term Care,* looks at the contemporary ways of providing long-term care for older adults with disabling conditions.

Unit V, *Physiological Challenges of Aging,* presents nine chapters devoted to maintaining wellness of the body systems. **Chapters 14** through **22** are each written on a continuum from wellness to common disorders, beginning with health teaching for the maintenance of wellness.

Unit VI, *Cognitive Challenges of Aging,* moves

into the area of cognition, memory, mental health, and preparation for dying. **Chapter 23,** *Addressing Cognitive Issues,* takes a general look at cognition and dementia, then focuses in on the identification of and interventions for Alzheimer's disease. **Chapter 24,** *Supporting Mental Health,* is a general review of mental health issues apart from dementia. **Chapter 25,** *Death and Dying,* is a look at the issues that nurses can address with patients who are dealing with the end of life.

Unit VII, *The Professional Gerontological Nurse,* provides an overview of this area of nursing. **Chapter 26,** *Choices in Gerontological Nursing,* encourages consideration of this growing specialty for nurse professionals.

Special chapter features include:

- Learning Objectives
- Key Terms (boldfaced in text)
- Caring and Wellness Highlights
- Critical Thinking Exercises
- Resources

- References (and sometimes Further Readings)

Finally, a Glossary at the end of the book includes all Key Terms.

An **Instructor's Manual** is available to adopters of the textbook. It contains multiple-choice test questions and suggestions for assignments to provide experiences that encourage respect for older adults. These assignments also can foster insight into how nurses can enhance quality of life for older adults.

I am hopeful that this text will provide nursing faculty, students and professional nurses with a positive view of gerontological nursing. My experience has been that, with appropriate role models in teaching and nursing practice, students can be educationally fortified to embark on a journey of caring as they gain confidence and acquire the needed skills that promote wellness and equip them for a career that includes this nursing specialty.

SHIRLEY ROSE TYSON

Acknowledgments

I wish to thank:

The contributing authors for their hard work and for sharing their expertise with others.

Ethel M. Madison, my friend and typist, whose constant support was so encouraging.

Marie Thomas of W.B. Saunders, for her cheerful voice on the telephone and for her never-ending assistance whenever I called.

The many older adults, nurses, and nursing students for whom this book has evolved.

Contents

UNIT V

PHYSIOLOGICAL CHALLENGES OF AGING   271

UNIT VI

COGNITIVE CHALLENGES OF AGING   435

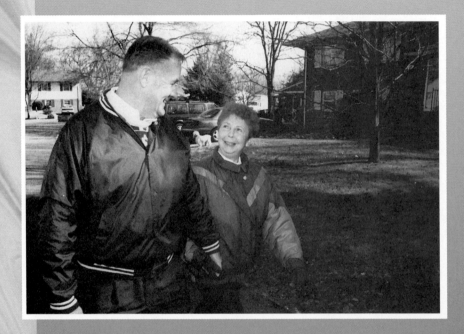

Nursing and the Older Adult

The greatest happiness usually comes not in youth but in old age. Men generally are happiest during their mid-sixties, women during their seventies.

GAIL SHEEHY, PATHFINDERS

The Navaho Nation, in the benediction of their prayers, still ask that they may "grow old in harmony and die naturally of old age."

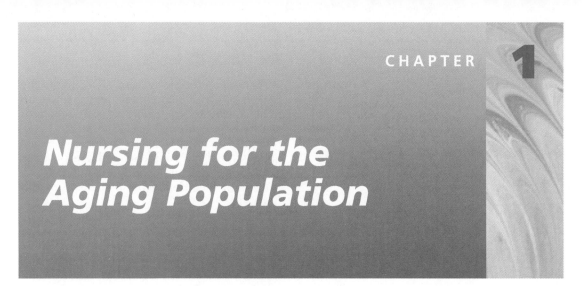

CHAPTER 1

Nursing for the Aging Population

Shirley Rose Tyson, RN, MA, EdD

CHAPTER OUTLINE

OBJECTIVES

After completing this chapter, the reader should be able to:

1. Explain how professional standards define nursing practice.
2. Describe the changing demographics of the United States and their effect on the health care system.
3. Describe the relevance to nursing practice of the presented theories of aging.
4. Conduct life reviews with older adult clients.
5. Discuss how physical, mental, and social health and activity contribute to successful aging.
6. Explain how economics and politics impact aging.
7. Discuss the nurse's role in health promotion and health protection within an aging society.

KEY TERMS

activity theory
caring
continuity theory
disengagement theory
gerontological nursing
life review (reminiscence)
middle old
old old
wellness
young old

A global phenomenon of aging is upon us. Populations everywhere continue to increase in the number and proportion of their older adults; as a corollary, older adults are also increasing in age. For the first time, humanity as a whole is growing older. This phenomenon has arisen both from scientific breakthroughs that modified the rate of aging and from the eradication of many childhood diseases. During the 4500 years from the Bronze Age to 1900, human life expectancy is estimated to have increased only 27 years; then, in the 80 years from 1900 to 1980, it increased another 27 years. Thus, of all the people in the history of humankind who ever lived to be 65 years of age, half of them are alive today (Rowe, 1993).

The middle of the 20th century (after World War II) was distinguished by a rise in the birth rate that is popularly called the "baby boom." As the numerous baby boomers grow older, the average age of the population will increase much faster than it has so far. To have lived to be 65 years of age is a great accomplishment. Older adults show that they have stamina, resilience, survivor skills, and varying degrees of physical and emotional health. *The great majority of older adults are well and will continue to be well.*

The term *older* is often broken down into three stages:

- **Young old**—65 to 74 years
- **Middle old**—75 to 84 years
- **Old old**—85 years and older

The fastest growing number of older adults is in the old-old age group.

WELLNESS

Wellness is a process involving all aspects of the person—physical, emotional, mental, and spiritual. **Wellness** is a feeling of satisfaction or well-being about one's health or physical condition; it involves a balance between internal and external environments and the physical, emotional, spiritual, social, and cultural process of life. Wellness is the theme of this book.

Nurses can help people to maintain wellness, even into old-old age, through health teaching and preventive services that guide them to take responsibility for their health maintenance. For as long as the longevity trend continues, medical and nursing interventions must take an approach to the care of older adults that is increasingly focused on health promotion and disease prevention.

Wellness is the key to successful aging. Each chapter of this book incorporates a wellness theme. Psychosocial health in maturity and physiological health in aging grow out of a series of adjustments by each individual. Nurses are finding that some older adults are manifesting alterations in capabilities, whereas others may simply require health teaching to meet nutritional, safety, and exercise needs. Wellness for older adults is supported by nurses in many diverse settings, including an array of community agencies.

As the aging and wellness trends intersect, emphasis moves toward taking individual responsibility for living a healthy lifestyle. Access to and need for health care must be correlated to a wide range of individual lifestyles. Issues that have an impact on the health and wellness of older adults include the following:

1. Promoting health and wellness among all Americans through individual responsibility and healthy lifestyle choices.
2. Ensuring a high quality of health care that is affordable and accessible to all.
3. Formulating a plan that will identify intelligent approaches to preventing or resolving health care problems; here, time is of the essence because of the increased numbers of older adults.
4. Educating and keeping people informed about various therapeutic modalities and preventive interventions, including nutrition, exercise, and recreation.

5. Practicing preventive nursing, medical, and mental health services.

Newly defined health care approaches are emerging as we enter a new century and a new era. Many exciting advances in nursing and health care practice have occurred in response to the perceived demands of the coming years. A more positive view of aging is emerging as attitudes toward older adults are modified to address the demands of a much larger and more diverse older population.

EXAMPLE

On August 4, 1997, a woman thought to be the oldest living person in the world died in France at the age of 122 years. She rode a bicycle until she was 100 years of age, smoked occasionally until she reached 120, and attributed her longevity to olive oil, port wine, and chocolate. She maintained social contacts, had the use of all five senses, and remarked humorously on one recent birthday that maybe God had forgotten about her. Her life demonstrated physical and emotional health and wellness.

Consumers are increasingly participating in their own health care. This ranges from self-diagnosis through information gleaned from the Internet and diagnostic kits available at drug stores to alternative care and nonphysical approaches to healing and wellness.

W e l l n e s s

"*Wellness is a feeling of satisfaction or well-being about one's health or physial condition.***"**

A lifestyle of wellness is practiced in countries with large populations such as China and India through emphasis on the mind–body connection, holism, and nature. In the Chinese culture, *chi* (life force, energy, vitality) incorporates the belief that everything a person does, feels or thinks can have an impact on health; this is also referred to as the *balance of chi*.

A balance is needed to achieve wellness and health. For example, a college student may need more exercise, a farmer may need more rest, and a physician may need more relaxation to have balance and the right amount of *chi* in life. In several cultures, focus on balance, harmony, and nature contribute to a lifestyle of wellness and health. People need to be made aware of their own health, wellness, and natural healing powers; this reinforces self-care activities and overall self-responsibility for health.

Healthier ways of living, preventive services, and therapeutic interventions allow people to live longer while maintaining wellness. Healthy ways of living can prevent or delay the onset or progression of disease or debility.

EXAMPLE

Many older adults are helpful neighbors who look out for and help each other. Mr. Black, age 79, a retired musician, and Mrs. Brown, 92, a retired nurse, are residents of a large co-op that has come to house hundreds of older adults. They represent a current phenomenon—one called "aging in place." Many residents of the co-op have lived in the complex since their mid-20s and 30s and have chosen to remain there. Managers now face new issues of making the complex "older-adult friendly." Ramps, handle bars, and other safety items are provided. Most older adults are healthy and well, live on their own, and enjoy the company of long-time neighbors and friends.

The passage of Social Security legislation, national economic growth, and a healthier group approaching age 65 have brightened the picture for older adults. Conditions for older adults have improved. For the first time ever, there is an adult population for whom neither work nor illness is a defining feature, because the majority of older adults are healthy and well.

EXAMPLE

Students of acting at New York University have met with an ensemble of senior actors, some of whom are in their 90s, for weekly improvisation workshops. Their group is called Roots and Branches. It is an intergenerational theater company that has been studying and performing on stage for 6 years. Their chosen name acknowledges that long-living roots and new branches are all part of the same tree. Some of these older adults are also college students.

Older adults are now "retiring" to a life that

is often as active and diversified as that enjoyed before retirement. Many never had the freedom, opportunity, or time to enjoy activities of choice. Recreational activities now tend to be fast paced and health oriented. Aerobics, water skiing, ballet, and square dancing are in great contrast to the shuffleboard, crocheting, arts and crafts, and group singing of a generation ago.

EXAMPLES

Sixteen older adults are doing a Zen exercise, envisioning themselves as one. They are a senior team preparing for the dragon boat races. A 78-year-old team member who enjoys square dancing and racquetball says that the ancient Chinese sport is her favorite activity and that, in her opinion, outdoor people are generally happy.

Tom Amberry took up shooting baskets as a hobby when he retired at age 70. Eighteen months later he made 2750 consecutive free-throws in 12 hours and entered the Guinness Book of Records. This accomplishment led to television appearances and a book and video now used by coaches nationwide.

Through nursing practice of accurate assessment, health teaching, counseling, and advocacy, older adults are being empowered to realize their potential for decision-making and action concerning maintenance of their health and wellness.

EXAMPLES

Mrs. Brown, age 92, has a 70-year-old daughter who lives in another state and wants her mother to come to live with her. Mrs. Brown says that she is too independent to live with others but enjoys visiting her daughter frequently. Mrs. Brown feels needed (helping her neighbor Mr. Black, 79, when he needs a hand), being active with the senior group, and participating in the community. She enjoys being healthy, active, and well.

Many physicians, nurses, dentists, and psychotherapists have continued the work they love and enjoy into retirement through volunteering their professional services to the needy and uninsured. One such group, headed by a retired neurologist in South Carolina, arranges 10,000 health care contacts yearly by 132 volunteer health care professionals to those in dire need of such care.

A successful adjustment to old age requires an integration of mind, body, and spirit. Ideally, it is advantageous to remain open and receptive to growth and development throughout the life span.

EXAMPLE

Mr. Caz, RN, is employed by a housing complex for older adults that has a senior center and an adult daycare center. One of the older adults, Mrs. Ames, has a diagnosis of hypertension. She has been following her physician's orders for prescribed medications and appropriate diet. However, after a recent upper respiratory tract infection she stated that she felt weak; often she did not receive adequate nutrition, being unable to prepare her own meals. After nursing assessment, Mr. Caz and Mrs. Ames discuss the situation in light of her health status. Both decide on the most immediate course to be taken. She is empowered to action. Meals on Wheels is contacted and informed of her nutritional needs. Mrs. Ames is motivated to keep to her routine of daily medications, exercise, and adequate rest. She is in daily contact with the nurse, who answers any questions and is available for guidance and counseling. Mrs. Ames states that she is feeling stronger, her appetite has improved, and she is "back to normal" after following this plan for 7 days.

It is unfortunate when older adults have not acquired the essential tools for aging, such as knowledge of proper exercise and good nutrition, peer support, and coping mechanisms to deal with physical and psychological changes. In their wellness practice, nurses can teach and encourage the use of a variety of complementary healing therapeutics for body, mind, and spirit as they care for older adults. Things to consider include the following:

1. Once empowered by the nurse, individuals have control over their own behavior and lifestyles. Individuals have strengths that are renewable and expandable.
2. Client-centered collaboration allows health teaching, counseling, knowledge, and clarification. The nurse can be a resource person, advocate, and consultant who addresses the client's immediate needs. Nurses and clients maintain a dialogue to learn what is in the client's interest.
3. Nursing intervention assists older adults to identify problems and issues of concern.

Nurses and clients then plan and act on strategies to prevent or minimize effects of illness.

4. The results of action/interaction/reciprocity between client and nurse can include gained or renewed confidence, gained knowledge, access to community resources, and success in collaborative efforts of caring.

5. Capacity for change and self-motivation contributes to healthy lifestyles as the client moves from unhealthy to healthy behaviors.

6. Strengths of the client and family determine the course in attaining an optimal level of functioning. These strengths allow a focus on attainable health care goals and reinforce patient empowerment.

Wellness and health promotion models of health care are influencing both the number and type of services offered by nurses. The development in the United States of nurse-managed clinics, nursing centers, and individual nurses in private practice settings is a significant step toward creating and testing new, unique health care models.

CARING

The roots of care and **caring** in American nursing trace back to nursing's early history. In the late 19th century, Florence Nightingale thought that medical therapeutics and "curing" were of *less* importance to patient outcome and thus willingly left this realm to the physician. Caring, the arena Nightingale considered of greatest importance, she assigned to the nurse (Reverby, 1987).

Nursing has moved from the medical model of cure to nursing models of care. To meet the needs of the increasing older population, a general shift in focus from cure to care is required. Nursing's primary role is caring for those who need to be nurtured in relation to their health status—wherever, as long as, and as frequently as they need nurturing.

> ### Caring
> **"Nursing has moved from medical models of cure to nursing models of care."**

Although the terms *care* and *caring* have been used throughout nursing history, before the mid-1970s nurses rarely studied the phenomenon of caring (Leininger, 1981). What is caring? How is caring practiced?

Caring has been defined, described, characterized, and identified by nurse educators, theorists, authors, clinicians, and administrators (Bevis, 1981; Kelly, 1988; Kurtz and Wang, 1991; Leininger, 1981; Watson, 1988) as the following:

- A humanizing force required for working with others
- A fundamental value of the nursing profession
- Knowledge; discovering creative approaches in nursing practice
- Healing; a curative component, transmitting positive energy
- Comfort, warmth, gentleness
- Commitment, respect, protection
- A moral focus, ethical awareness
- Nurturing
- Acceptance, empathy, genuineness
- The art and science of nursing
- A key to empowerment
- "High touch" that counterbalances "high tech"
- An interactive process
- Providing an environment for service to culturally diverse racial and ethnic individuals and groups of all ages

These caring behaviors constitute the practice of nursing. The creation of a nursing model of caring specifically for older adults is fairly new because older adults are a new population to be served. How best to serve older adults who will continue to require services is a question that only recently has been addressed.

> ### Caring
> **"Caring behaviors constitute the practice of nursing."**

Cassel and Neugarten (1994) propose an integration of heroic, humanistic, technological, and psychological approaches to health, in which the welfare of the individual patient is the measure by which any intervention must be assessed. A health care professional who cares for a patient engages in a deliberate and ongoing activity of responding to the patient's needs. Caring shows a relationship between the nurse and the patient. Nurses' knowledge and skill (science and art) lead to identification of the patient's particular condition and needs, enabling appropriate nursing interventions.

The collaborative caring and mutual trust between nurses and patients empower patients to be responsible for their own health. In a setting of warmth, comfort, and respect, patients are encouraged to maintain their healthy status or nurtured back to health.

■ GERONTOLOGICAL NURSING ROLES

Gerontological nursing has always been concerned with promoting the health and function of older adults. The nurse as health promoter must continually review and examine new approaches that will assist individuals to achieve and maintain balance and satisfaction in their lives. Gerontological nurses practice in a variety of roles and functions:

1. *Healers.* Gerontological nurses in the healer role use "hands-on" care, therapeutic touch, and holism to restore balance in the physical, emotional, spiritual, social, and cultural processes. Older adults are taught self-care healing approaches and encouraged to practice alternative healing methods such as therapeutic massage, stress management, yoga, meditation, exercise, relaxation response, nutrition, acupuncture, and the use of herbs. They are taught, aided, and empowered to maintain a healthy lifestyle as active participants in their own health care and health maintenance.
2. *Visionaries.* Gerontological nursing requires futurists who will examine new approaches and trends in health care; those who conceive and conceptualize new ideas and creative ways of practicing must be allowed the flexibility to implement their visions.
3. *Clinicians.* Gerontological nurse practitioners are expert in the clinical knowledge and skills required by older adults. This practitioner role encompasses a great responsibility for quality, for evaluating others, and for maintaining expert clinical skills. The clinician should be on the cutting edge of gerontological nursing practice.
4. *Educators.* Gerontological nursing is taught in classroom and clinical settings; then prac-

ticing nurses take on an informal educational role in health teaching of patients and families. The educator's role is twofold: to educate others and to maintain his or her own expertise.
5. *Advocates.* Older adults are assisted in decision-making processes pertaining to their health care. Individuals are educated concerning their rights, and these rights are upheld by the gerontological nurse advocate.
6. *Reimbursement and budgetary experts.* In today's health care market, experienced persons are needed to acquire and allocate funds, design budgets, manage finances, set controls, and record and report information pertaining to reimbursement of federal, state, city, and private funding.
7. *Regulatory specialists.* Institutional policies are keenly overseen by gerontological nurses for compliance with regulations. These regulations are created by federal, state, and city agencies to assess and evaluate quality of care planned for and given to older adults.

Accurate assessment, health teaching, counseling, and advocacy of individuals by the nurse empower older adults. These nursing interventions can enable older adults to realize their potential for decision-making and action concerning their own physical, emotional, mental, and spiritual wellness.

What will gerontological nursing be like in the 21st century? One thing is certain. As the population ages, the need for gerontological nurses increases. Changing health care demands in an aging society, with the emergence of special populations in long-term, community, and home health care, create further challenges. There are exciting new advances in society, nursing, and health care practice (for more detail, see Chapter 26).

A broad array of social policy issues is being brought to the table in future planning for older adults, both nationally and internationally. Global aging will have an impact on global health care. Nurses who network through international collaboration at conferences, seminars, and presentations will be best prepared to provide culturally competent care.

Decisions made in U.S. public policy arenas define the philosophy and structure of the health care delivery system and define the roles of nurses in this system. Generally, greater consumption of health care services by older per-

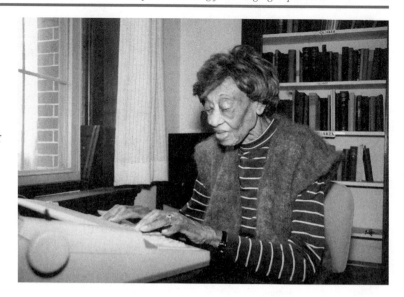

Today's older adults are continuing to express creativity throughout their life span.

sons is a reality. Access to services, health care utilization, and health status are of concern to health care providers, especially nurses.

Some of the issues that impact the health and well-being of older adults are listed below:

- Lifestyle choices and individual responsibility for health maintenance
- The availability of home- and community-based services to maximize independence
- Alternative/complementary therapies
- Housing and home modifications to accommodate the physical changes of aging
- Affordable and accessible transportation when older adults can no longer operate their own vehicles
- Preventive nursing and medical care
- Available mental health services
- The caregiving crisis that overburdens many family and informal caregivers

Input from those working with older adults will be essential as future plans are formulated and implemented in practice.

Gerontological nursing practice focuses on assessing the health and functional status of older adults, planning and providing appropriate nursing and other health care services, and evaluating the effectiveness of care. Emphasis is placed on (1) maximizing functional ability in the activities of daily living; (2) promoting, maintaining, and restoring health, including mental health; (3) preventing and minimizing the disabilities of acute and chronic illness; and (4) maintaining life in dignity and comfort until death (ANA, 1987).

Gerontological nursing requires the following:

1. A good knowledge base of nursing with special emphasis placed on nursing care of older adults and a desire to expand and improve on that knowledge base
2. Alert, caring, responsive practitioners with positive attitudes about aging and toward aging individuals
3. Patience, compassion, sensitivity toward older adults and their families, and a desire to work with this age group
4. Excellent communication, observation, and nursing skills necessary for working with older adults, some of whom may experience sensory deficits
5. The ability to work with an interdisciplinary health care team and practice within a framework of holism and caring
6. Awareness of an individual's ethnicity and culture and how these impact age-related changes, illness, and health care needs

Wellness

"Wellness involves a balance between internal and external environments and the physical, emotional, spiritual, social, and cultural processes of life."

Gerontological nurses should

- Assess the functional ability of the older adult for independent living.
- Encourage self-care ability and independent decision-making in clients.
- Increase the older adult's capacity to adapt to chronic illness.
- Teach older adult clients skills that will help them manage chronic illness.
- Help older adult clients to adapt to aging changes that are normal, such as sensory changes of sight, hearing, taste, smell, and touch.
- Incorporate knowledge and clinical assessment skills in the planning, treatment, and implementation of nursing care specific to aging responses.
- Offer lifestyle counseling with a focus on wellness, even in the presence of chronic illness or substantial impairment.
- Provide emotional, physical, and spiritual support through dying and death while maintaining the dignity of the client and the client's family.
- Practice within the guidelines of the American Nurses' Association Standards of Gerontological Nursing (Box 1–1).

■ OVERVIEW OF AGING

Aging involves biological, psychological, social, and spiritual changes in individuals, who vary in their rate of change. Gender, race, social class, and religious preferences create a complex interaction that contributes to the way in which aging occurs for each individual.

The majority of older adults in America are relatively healthy, relatively independent, vibrant, and alert. What is aging? Why do we age? How do we age? Aging is a process that begins at conception and is a normal part of growth and development; it is a reduced capacity to replace worn-out cells. Aging involves many factors and occurs across the life span. Aging processes can be divided into three general categories—genetic, biochemical, and physiological. Genetic endowment influences longevity and determines the degree of susceptibility to specific health problems. Biochemical processes are influenced by life experiences and related to the changes that take place in the body throughout the life span. Physiological processes are characteristic of promoting normal healthy functioning of the body and are associated with healthy lifestyles.

More rapid and noticeable changes take place in our later years. Why aging occurs is unknown; however, several theories of aging are described later in this chapter. Factors that contribute to healthy aging include

- Physical and mental health
- Heredity
- Personality
- Nutrition
- Life experiences
- Learned coping strategies
- Availability of support systems and resources
- Personal philosophy on life.

Demographics of Aging

Demography is the science of population dynamics. *Demographics of aging* refers to a population that is 65 years of age and older (Figure 1–1). It has become traditional in the United States to define age 65 as the beginning of "old age" for demographical and gerontological studies because that is the age established by Congress earlier in this century at which retirement benefits become available through the Social Security system.

As the population lives longer, the traditional age of retirement benefits will inevitably increase beyond age 65. During the 20th century, the number of persons in the United States who comprise the elderly has ballooned, from 3.1 million in 1900 to 33.2 million in 1994. The elderly U.S. population will more than double between now and the year 2050 (to 80 million). Most of this growth should occur between 2010 and 2030, when the baby-boom generation enters their older adult years (U.S. Bureau of the Census, 1997) (Figure 1–2). Currently, the fastest growing population in the United States is composed of persons older than the age of 85, those often referred to as the "old old."

Diversity and *growth* are two terms that describe the elderly population of the United States. Each age, gender, race, and ethnic group has distinctive characteristics, and the experience of aging is different among the demographic groups. The older population of

Box 1-1   STANDARDS OF GERONTOLOGICAL NURSING PRACTICE

Standard I Organization of Gerontological Nursing Service

All gerontological nursing services are planned, organized, and directed by a nurse executive. The nurse executive has baccalaureate or master's preparation and experience in gerontological nursing plus administration of long-term or acute care services for older adults.

Standard II Theory

The nurse participates in the generation and testing of theory as a basis for clinical decisions. The nurse uses theoretical concepts to guide the effective practice of gerontological nursing.

Standard III Data Collection

The health status of the older person is regularly assessed in a comprehensive, accurate, and systematic manner. The information obtained during the health assessment is accessible to and shared with appropriate members of the interdisciplinary health care team, including the older person and family.

Standard IV Nursing Diagnosis

The nurse uses health assessment data to determine nursing diagnoses.

Standard V Planning and Continuity of Care

The nurse develops the plan of care in conjunction with the older person and appropriate others. Mutual goals, priorities, nursing approaches, and measures in the care plan address the therapeutic, preventive, restorative, and rehabilitative needs of the older person. The care plan helps the older person attain and maintain the highest level of health, well being, and quality of life achievable, as well as a peaceful death. The plan of care facilitates continuity of care over time as the client moves to various care settings and is revised as necessary.

Standard VI Intervention

The nurse, guided by the plan of care, intervenes to provide care to restore the older person's functional capabilities and to prevent complications and unwarranted disability. Nursing interventions are derived from nursing diagnoses and are based on gerontological nursing theory.

Standard VII Evaluation

The nurse continually evaluates the client's and family's responses to interventions in order to determine progress toward goal attainment and to revise the database, nursing diagnoses, and plan of care.

Standard VIII Interdisciplinary Collaboration

The nurse collaborates with other members of the health care team in the various settings in which care is given to the older person. The team meets regularly to evaluate the effectiveness of the care plan for the client and family and to adjust the plan of care to accommodate to the changing needs of the patient.

Standard IX Research

The nurse participates in research designed to generate an organized body of gerontological nursing knowledge, disseminates research findings, and uses them in practice.

Box continued on following page

Box 1-1   STANDARDS OF GERONTOLOGICAL NURSING PRACTICE, *Continued*

Standard X Ethics
The nurse uses the code for nurses established by the American Nurses' Association as a guide for ethical decision-making in practice.

Standard XI Professional Development
The nurse assumes responsibility for professional development and contributes to the professional growth of interdisciplinary team members. The nurse participates in peer review and other means of evaluation to ensure the quality of nursing practice.

From American Nurses' Association. (1987). Standards and Scope of Gerontological Nursing, p 3. Kansas City, MO: American Nurses' Association.

people of color has grown more rapidly than the white population (Espino, 1995). The needs and problems of ethnic minority older adults were first brought to the nation's attention at the 1971 White House Conference on Aging. Since that time, so-called minority aging has had greater visibility.

"Ethnic" older adults, including African Americans, Asian/Pacific Islanders, Hispanics, and Native Americans, are the fastest growing subgroup older than 65 years of age. In 1990, this group constituted 10% of the aged population; it is expected to increase to 15% by the year 2025 (Espino, 1995). Many health care issues confront these "ethnic" elderly. They include

- Language barriers and translation problems
- Use of folk or nontraditional forms of medical care
- Problems in understanding U.S. models of ethical decision-making
- Unfamiliarity with U.S. customs of medical care

The stunning growth of the "old old" throughout the world has various health and economic implications for individuals, families, and governments. The old old, ages 85 and older, often have severe and persistent health problems. In this group, the female majority continues to increase. Women in the United States have a life expectancy of 78.2 years compared with 71.2 years for men (Butler, 1989). Implications for gerontological nursing care of older women include the following:

1. Female majority is concentrated in the upper age range.
2. Older females often live alone.
3. Older females are often in poorer health than men.
4. Older females are often living close to poverty. Many are widows with little financial support.
5. The probability of multiple chronic illnesses with functional limitations increases the likelihood of their living in a nursing home as chronological age increases.

In an increasingly interdependent and aging world, demographic changes will create compelling social, economic, and ethical choices in the 21st century. This phenomenon will also affect health care projections, the education of health care personnel, and health care practice concerning older adults.

Theories of Aging

Searching for the capacity to extend life has intrigued many scientists. Because the study of gerontology is relatively new, exploring this territory generates much excitement. Most gerontologists agree that no single theory can account for all the changes that occur in aging. Growing older is viewed as many different processes. These processes include physical and behavioral changes that occur under normal environmental conditions as an individual advances in age. Scientists who study aging say the secret of longevity probably lies in a combination of heredity, environment, and lifestyle.

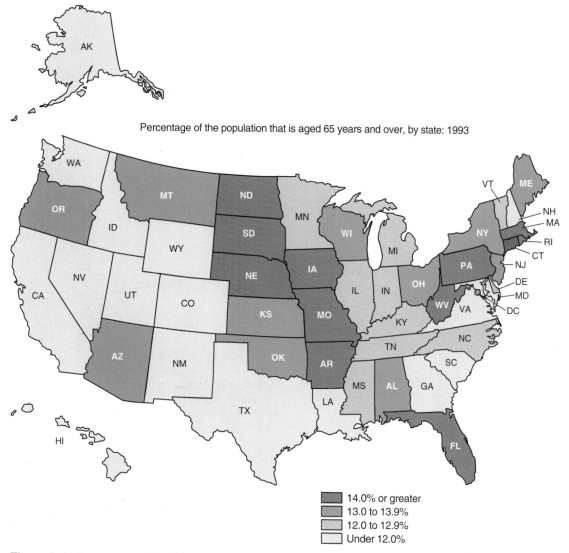

Figure 1–1. Percentage of the U.S. population aged 65 and older, by state. (From U.S. Census Bureau, 1993.)

An understanding of the various theories of aging can help gerontological nurses as they assist their clients to live and function at optimal levels.

BIOLOGICAL THEORIES

There are two major groups of biological theories, one emphasizing internal biological clocks or "programs," and the other external or environmental forces that damage cells or organs until they can no longer function adequately (National Institute on Aging, 1993).

The present theories of aging are not mutually exclusive. Aging is now viewed as a combination of many processes—interactive and interdependent—that determine life span and health on an individual basis.

Internal Etiologies

Genetic Theory: Programmed Senescence. Aging is the result of sequential switching on and

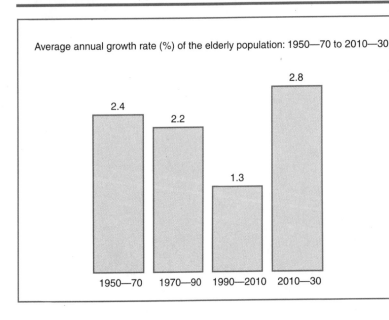

Average annual growth rate (%) of the elderly population: 1950—70 to 2010—30

Figure 1–2. Average annual growth rate (%) of the elderly U.S. population: 1950–1970 to 2010–2030. (From U.S. Census Bureau, 1997.)

off of certain genes, with senescence (old age) defined as the time when age-associated deficits are manifested.

Endocrine Theory. Biological clocks act through hormones to control the pace of aging.

Immunological Theory. In aging, there is greater frequency of precipitating attacks on various tissues through autoaggression or immunodeficiencies. This programmed decline in function of the immune system leads to an increased vulnerability to infections, disorders (e.g., diabetes mellitus, rheumatic heart disease, arthritis), and death. Immunoengineering (selective alteration and replenishment of the immune system) is an emerging retardant.

Error Catastrophe Theory. Damage to mechanisms that synthesize proteins results in faulty proteins, which accumulate to a level that causes catastrophic damage to cells, tissues, and organs.

Somatic Mutation Theory. Genetic mutations occur and accumulate with increasing age, causing cells to deteriorate and malfunction. DNA failure or replication, transcription, or translation between cells may be responsible for aging.

Cells are basic components of all living things. Cells contain various organelles, each with its own function. The organelle called the nucleus holds chromosomes. Chromosomes are made up of DNA and protein. When a cell divides, its chromosomes also divide. The forms and functions of all living things are coded in their DNA. DNA is a large double-stranded molecule with hundreds of thousands of subnets called nucleotides. A gene is a string of DNA bases arranged in a certain sequence, sometimes called *genetic code*. Genes determine the characteristics of species, including maximum life span.

Wear and Tear Theory. Cells and tissues have vital parts that wear out, are overused, or have repeated injuries.

Crosslinking Theory. An accumulation of crosslinked proteins, such as collagen, elastin and DNA molecules, damage cells and tissues, slowing down physiological processes. Aging of the skin with loss of elasticity is an example of crosslinking.

Free Radical Theory. Accumulation of age pigments in tissues choke off oxygen and nutrients causing degeneration, decrease in function, and eventually death of tissue. Vision-related disorders associated with aging have been linked to oxidation.

Stress-Adaptation Theory. Effects from the residual damages of stress accumulate, and the body no longer is able to resist stress and dies.

Internal and external stressors are physical, psychological, social, and environmental.

Lipofuscin Theory. Lipofuscin is the aging process that produces "age pigments," a lipoprotein byproduct of metabolism. Because it is associated with oxidation of unsaturated lipids, it is believed to be similar to the free radical theory. There is a correlation between the amount of lipofuscin in a person's body and the person's age.

External Etiologies

Environment Theory. Many theories emphasize environmental assaults to our systems that gradually cause things to go wrong. External (environmental) forces damage cells and organs until they can no longer function adequately. Some of these are polluted air and water or use of insecticides and other pollutants that cause harm to our bodies.

Nutrition Theory. The link between nutrition and aging is not well understood, although it has been researched for many years. One theory states that restricted diets of fewer calories can increase the life span; undernutrition without malnutrition extends life span in laboratory animals (National Institute on Aging, 1993). In humans, vitamin and mineral supplements in adequate amounts have been known to promote health.

Disease. Organisms such as viruses, bacteria, and fungi contribute to ill health. The relationship of pathogens to the body's decline is not conclusive; however, it is known that when the body's systems are no longer able to fight pathogens, death can occur.

PSYCHOSOCIAL THEORIES

Many theories have been expounded in an attempt to describe attitudes or behavioral approaches to later life and successful aging. Although each theory views the process of aging differently and identifies differing correlates of aging, the individual who reaches an advanced age is unique, having had experiences and adopted lifestyles, attitudes, and behaviors different from everyone else.

Developmental tasks are the challenges that must be met and adjustments must be made to achieve successful aging. Erikson (1963) de-

scribed the developmental tasks of old age as ego integrity versus despair.

Psychosocial theories of aging emphasize behavioral changes, attitudinal changes, and changing roles and situations that occur as one ages. Psychosocial theories include activity theory, disengagement theory, and continuity theory.

Activity Theory. First identified by Havighurst (1952), **activity theory** states that to age successfully the individual must retain active roles, or at least find suitable replacements for roles that must be abandoned. It is important for older adults to be active in a wide variety of pursuits. The number and quality of activities are important, with those involving close personal contact of special value to the individual.

Caring

"Collaborative caring and mutual trust between nurses and clients empower clients to be responsible for their own health."

Disengagement Theory. Proposed by Cumming and Henry (1961), **disengagement theory** suggests a gradual, mutual withdrawal between the older adult and society. This mutual separation benefits both—freeing the older adult from constraining roles and expectations and providing younger people with the opportunity to take their place in society. Much controversy surrounds this theory. As the life span increases, many older adults in all walks of life continue productive lives well into their 80s and 90s.

Continuity Theory. Proposed by Neugarten (1966), **continuity theory** holds that individuals will try to sustain current patterns of activity and interaction as they age. The adjustment to aging is optimized by maintaining and continuing the same level of social activity achieved in younger adulthood. Basic personality traits are said to remain unchanged as one ages.

Life Review, or Reminiscence. Although not a psychosocial theory, **life review** is an intervention often used in the treatment of the older adult. Butler (1963) states that the purpose of life review is to provide for the successful inte-

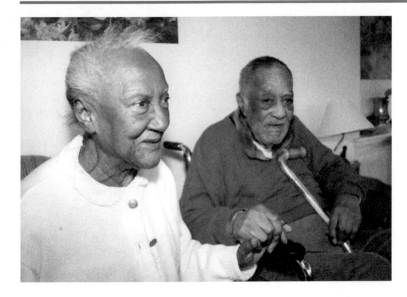

The bonds of affection continue to deepen in later years.

gration of experiences that offer new significance to an individual's life. **Reminiscence** is a reassessment of life that can bring forth depression, acceptance, or satisfaction in final years. Because it is the return of past experiences to the conscious level, with possible reintegration of unresolved conflicts, it is inherently a psychotherapeutic process of insight and self-understanding that may be accompanied by cognitive, affective, and behavioral changes.

As the years pass, people often seek a new perspective in facing the challenges of aging. They begin to face their own mortality and inquire what it means to complete their life. This is a time when they can let down their guard, embrace life, and reach out to others or withdraw, hide from their feelings, and fixate on the past. A successful adjustment to old age requires an integration of mind, body, and spirit. Ideally, an individual needs to remain open and receptive to growth and development throughout the life span.

It is important for nurses to be familiar with the theories of aging so that they have a context within which to assist older adults in meeting the psychosocial challenges associated with aging. Theories of aging may be applied to the following:

- Coping with losses, especially the loss of a spouse, child, or close friend
- Adjusting to transitions such as retirement, moving, and establishing new life patterns

- Living with health changes
- Developing a sense of satisfaction with life, past and present

Psychosocial theories, along with the internal biological and external environmental forces presented earlier, offer a context within which nurses can come to understand the changes that occur with age and how these changes are manifested.

HEALTHY AGING: A LIFE SPAN PERSPECTIVE

The ultimate goal of working with and caring for older adults is to prevent or delay the onset of physical, functional, and social deficits. Nurses have the responsibility to teach older adults how to practice health promotion activities and enhance healthy living. One way to do this would be by incorporating the goals of "Healthy People 2000" (1990), which is part of a national health promotion project of the United States Department of Health and Human Services (USDHHS). The project seeks to

- Increase the span of healthy life for Americans
- Reduce health disparities among Americans
- Achieve access to preventive services for all Americans

Although there is nothing that will reverse,

retard, or prevent aging, there are certain behaviors that can promote healthy aging. Health *promotion* behaviors are activities that enhance wellness, maintain health, and maximize an individual's potential while minimizing the effects of aging. Health *protection* behaviors are activities directed toward reducing the individual's risk of developing a specific illness (Table 1–1). Some of these behaviors can be viewed as both health promotion and protection. An individual's personal attitudes toward life, aging, and healthy choices in individual lifestyle can contribute to healthy aging.

Economics of Aging

The economics of aging affects a large number of older individuals. Poverty is a real issue. Although the challenge of living on a drastically reduced income is encountered by many, it becomes a problem even more severe for minority older adults.

Gerontologists Butler and Lewis (1982) state that our historical gifts to minority citizens have been poverty, poor housing, and lack of medical care and education. The aged poor require services in nutrition, health counseling, transportation, and housing. When their income cannot be stretched sufficiently to meet all these needs, psychological needs (e.g., recreation) are sacrificed. Economic status is a factor that influences the type and quality of health care for all older people.

Changes in health care financing (such as regulatory criteria at state and federal levels, national health insurance, health care reform, and managed care) will broaden the nurse's roles and responsibilities in caring for older adults. Older adults who need ongoing treat-

ment and rehabilitation are being discharged early from hospitals to nursing homes and home health agencies as a result of economic changes in health care.

Gerontological nurses must possess the skills needed to care for older adults through acute stages of illness and for long-term or terminally ill older patients, as this reform in health care and health care financing continues. Additionally, health care personnel must become knowledgeable about the health care system and available resources to assist older adults in gaining access to the health care they require.

W e l l n e s s

Wellness for older adults is supported by nurses in many diverse settings, including an array of community agencies.

Most Medicare beneficiaries—19 million of 32 million, or nearly 60%—are women. Many single or widowed women are in the Medicare population, and many of them are poor and highly vulnerable to increases in Medicare premiums, deductibles, and co-insurances (Butler, 1995). Because women live longer than men, with the possibility of chronic illness for a longer time interval, and one fifth of older women are living below the official poverty line, the economics of aging becomes an issue that transcends age, gender, race, ethnicity, and health.

Politics of Aging

It is hoped that the relationship between aging and politics will bring about continuing posi-

TABLE 1–1. Health Promotion and Health Protection	
Health *Promotion* Activities	**Health *Protection* Activities**
Effective management of stress	Adequate well-balanced nutrition
Social interaction and activity	Appropriate amounts of exercise, rest, and sleep
Intergenerational friendships or contacts	Safeguarding against infections and disease
New career (if desired), hobbies, interests	Prompt intervention when medical care and treatment are required
Maintenance of adequate physical, mental, emotional, and spiritual wellness	Avoidance of known cancer-causing agents
Regular physical and dental examinations	

tive changes at all levels of society. Today's older adults are discovering and exploring new territories as they create new ways of adjusting to aging.

Public policy is composed of the laws and ordinances and their interpretation by courts and public agencies. The ability to promote health for individuals is largely determined by the actions of policymakers, and the roles of health care personnel are based on decisions made by policymakers.

Demographical changes in society have impacted political leadership, including national and local organizations. Some societal and political factors influenced by age-consciousness are:

- Establishment of a National Institute on Aging
- Dramatic growth in gerontology courses, textbooks, departments, and programs
- Evolution of multimillion-member organizations of older persons, such as the American Association of Retired Persons (AARP)
- Establishment of permanent committees on aging in both the Senate and House of Representatives
- Extension of antidiscrimination laws to older age groups
- Private pension reform
- Creation of Medicare and the Older Americans Act
- Cost-of-living increases in Social Security and public pensions

The growth of these societal and political programs reflects a society increasingly aware of, and in most cases positively sensitive to, a growing older population.

■ DELIVERING CARE IN AN AGING SOCIETY

One of the challenges in meeting the health care needs of an aging society is to gain a better understanding of the relationship between age and health. Global aging is a reality. In many countries, aging is seen as the most natural thing in the world and problems are identified only with special groups of the elderly: the disabled, the poor, the frail, and those in institutional care (Tokarski, 1993).

The intersection of the aging trend with the health care system affects the world. What stands out as a primary health goal in an aging society is the control of chronic illness and its consequences among older adults. As life expectancy continues to increase globally, quality-of-life issues for older people will be confronted repeatedly. The number of years of good health in relation to the number of years with chronic illness must be addressed. More long-term illness, disability, and dependency can be expected, with implications for the effective management of chronic illness an issue for gerontological nurses. There is a need for an increase in "high-tech" home health care as patients are discharged earlier from intensive care and other settings to home or nursing home still needing subacute care.

Federal funding largely financed the growth and development of gerontological nursing. Medicare, Medicaid, and the Older Americans Act of 1965 have made a tremendous impact on the shape of health care for older adults in the United States. The Omnibus Reconciliation Act (OBRA) of 1987 modified home health benefits under Medicare. When revisions were made in the Medicare and Medicaid statutory requirements, they caused a surge in community health nursing needs for older adults and expanded the demand for gerontological nurse practitioners.

There are several models of care that have implications for gerontological nursing. The delivery of nursing care in an aging society must demonstrate the following:

- Empowerment of the older adult
- Teaching healthy lifestyles to achieve and maintain wellness
- Caring in nurse/client/family relationships
- Competence in providing quality, cost-effective nursing care

Gueldner and Brent (1995) state that emphasis must be placed on more natural treatments (e.g., nutritional interventions, environmental manipulation, and activity) and there needs to be a reduced reliance on pharmaceuticals. Older adults are being empowered to reach their optimum level of functioning.

The constructs of health, person, environment, nurse, and nursing are used in various settings, including acute, long-term, home health, and community health care. Maintenance of health is viewed as the personal responsibility of the individual, whereas the actions of identifying, managing, and seeking out help can be applied to the client, family, aggregate, or total community.

■ HEALTH CARE PROJECTIONS: PROFILE OF AN AGING SOCIETY

The World Health Organization reported in 1972 that the number-one priority for the future should be care of the aging. The intervening years have seen the United States reluctantly begin to address this monumental challenge. It is now widely understood that the United States will be an older nation during the first half of the 21st century than it is now. Older adults are a heterogeneous group, and this diversity will continue. There will be a larger proportion of older adults who are relatively healthy and vibrant and a growing old-old population (85 years and older) who may not be as physically and socially advantaged.

It is impossible to comprehend the full impact or predict the health care needs associated with illness and its effects on an aging population; at present it is a challenging issue in providing financial support, health care, and housing.

How skilled are we in understanding the economics of health care reform, restructuring, and consolidation as driving forces for health care change? The movement of health care from institution to community is the cornerstone of health care restructuring as the 21st century approaches. Proposals for universal health care have been put forth by politicians, legislators, and professional organizations. There has been debate over possible health care reform concerning consumer plans for health care, universal health care, and changes in health care treatment.

A health care crisis exists. As the population ages, preventive and self-care practices throughout the life span make both physical and fiscal sense. Many individuals are choosing to take more personal responsibility for their health by exploring a variety of self-regulatory, mind/body, and wellness practices, independent of physicians' input and/or knowledge. Attitudes, stress, and feelings of hopelessness, anger, and loss of control all influence an individual's health, behavior, and ability to cope with the potential frailties of aging.

Barrett (1993) states that complementary or alternative care refers to those practices that often come from older, cross-cultural perspectives of health and healing, which focus on lifestyle reevaluation and the mind/body interaction that by their very nature are preventive in intention. Evidence suggests that stress impairs the immune response, which is responsible for protecting against cancer, infections, and autoimmune diseases. Older people frequently undergo life changes that make them more vulnerable to the effects of uncontrollable stress, immune system depression, psychological depression, and increase in chronic illness.

Stress reduction, stress management, and self-care strategies provide opportunities for choice and control that have positive effects on the health and well-being of older adults. The nurse who understands different ways of looking at health and healing in older adults may assist the older client to choose appropriate care—care that addresses the more holistic view of body, mind, and spiritual issues, and helps create a greater sense of control so important to healthy aging.

W e l l n e s s

"In their wellness practice, nurses can teach and encourage the use of a variety of complementary healing therapeutics for body, mind, and spirit."

As the numbers of frail elderly increase, so, too, will the challenge and need for innovative nursing care (Figure 1–3). Mobility problems, memory impairments, and incontinence are necessary geriatric research priorities. Basic research needs to be continued in an effort to understand aging both in individuals and in the aging population. Research in geriatric rehabilitation will demonstrate cost savings and reduction in number of hours of care.

Will future health care consider the control of diseases, promote more healthful living, and foster a more active, independent lifestyle and quality of life for all? It is not possible to make

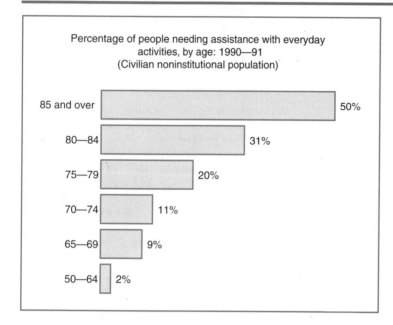

Figure 1–3. Percentage of the U.S. population needing assistance with everyday activities, by age. (From U.S. Census Bureau, 1990–1991.)

health care predictions that will accurately identify the possible outcomes of research affecting health, gerontology, and nursing. However, nurses will have multidimensional roles in providing innovative care.

Trends in care include the following:

1. Gerontological nursing research in clinical practice and in education of nurses will be actively pursued.
2. Retraining or cross-training of gerontological nurses in acute care, subacute care, community health, and rehabilitation nursing skills will be needed to meet the needs of a diverse older population that requires a wide range of care.
3. Managed care revolution will include the management of health care being undertaken by private corporations.
4. Health care reform will continue to be an issue.
5. More scrutiny will be given to prescribed medications with scrupulous assessment of each older adult patient and computer technology to assist in the process.
6. Ethical issues will continue to be debated regarding medical care for the old-old adults. Changes in the insurance industry may further fuel this debate.
7. The older population will continue to be composed of fewer men than women

(whose increased longevity places many among the elderly poor). Because economic status is also a factor in the type and quality of care older women receive, Jorgensen (1993) predicts that women will assert their special concerns and take action to control their health care and improve their health.

8. Increase in numbers of an ethnically diverse older population will require health care professionals who are culturally sensitive to the special needs of a pluralistic older nation.
9. Redesign or revision of nursing education curricula will be needed to prepare students for a community-based practice world.
10. Model relationships will be developed between schools of nursing and regulatory bodies, advancing educational models most appropriate for emerging health care needs and services (National League for Nursing, 1995).

Summary

Health care delivery in America is in transition. Gerontological nursing, which requires patience, compassion, and caring, presents one of the greatest challenges for nurses. The growing population of individuals age 65 and older guarantees that the challenge will continue well into the 21st century.

The concept of *old* has changed drastically over the past years. As the 66 million baby boomers reach their 65th birthdays in the 21st century, greater emphasis is being placed on the needs of an aging population, with concomitant social policy changes.

Caring

"A nurse who cares for a patient engages in a deliberate and ongoing activity of responding to the patient's needs."

Individuals experience physical and psychological changes as they age. Nurses are responsible for ensuring that the older adult's basic needs are met. A plan of care for older adults includes assessment of physical and psychological status, client education, enhancement of client self-care, and helping clients (within the limits of their capability) to become as productive and as active as they desire.

REFERENCES

American Nurses' Association. (1987). A Statement on the Scope of Gerontological Nursing Practice. Kansas City: American Nurses' Association.

Barrett S. (1993). Complementary self-care strategies for healthy aging. Generations 17(3):49–52.

Bevis E. (1981) Caring: A life force. In Leininger M, ed. Caring: An Essential Human Need: Proceedings of Three Caring Conferences, pp 49–59. Thorofare, NJ: Slack.

Butler RN. (1963). Life review: An interpretation of reminiscence in the aged. Psychiatry 26:65.

Butler RN. (1989). Psychosocial aspects of aging. In Sadavoy J, ed. Comprehensive Textbook of Psychiatry. Washington, DC: American Psychiatric Press.

Butler RN. (1995). The women's stake in Medicare's future. Int Longevity News 3 (Sept/Oct):1–2.

Butler RN, Lewis MT. (1982). Aging and Mental Health: Positive Psychosocial Approaches. 3rd ed. St. Louis: CV Mosby.

Cassell, C, Neugarten B. (1994). The goals of medicine in an aging society. In Beauchamp T, Walters K, eds. Contemporary Issues in Bioethics. Belmont, CA: Wadsworth.

Cumming E, Henry NE. (1961). Growing Old: The Process of Disengagement. New York: Basic Books.

Erikson E. (1963). Childhood and Society. 2nd ed. New York: WW Norton.

Espino, D. (1995). Ethnogeriatrics. In Espino, D, ed. Clinics in Geriatric Medicine 2(1).

Gueldner S, Brent B. (1995). Gerontological nursing issues and demands beyond the year 2005 (guest editorial). J Gerontol Nurs 21(6).

Havighurst RJ. (1952). Development Tasks of Later Maturity. New York: David McKay.

Jorgensen LB. (1993). Public policy, health care and older women. J Women Aging 5(3–4):201–220.

Kelly, L. (1988). The ethic of caring: Has it been discarded? Nurs Outlook 36(1):17.

Kurtz RT, Wang J. (1991). The caring ethic: More than kindness, the core of nursing science. Nurs Forum 26(1):4–8.

Leininger M, ed. (1981). Caring: An Essential Human Need. Proceedings of Three National Caring Conferences. Thorofare, NJ: Slack

National Institute on Aging (1993). In Search of the Secrets of Aging. U.S. Department of Health and Human Services publication #93-2756, Washington, DC: U.S. Government Printing Office.

National League for Nursing. (Fall 1995). Vision, Goals, and Mission Statement (Newsletter). New York: National League for Nursing.

Neugarten BL. (1966). Adult personality: A developmental view. Hum Dev 9:61–73.

Reverby S. (1987). Ordered to care: The Dilemma of American Nursing. New York: Cambridge University Press.

Rowe, J. (1993). Summer Lecture Series on "Prevention of Disability and Aging," Mt. Sinai School of Medicine, New York, N.Y.

Tokarski W. (1993). Later life activity from European perspectives. In Kelly JR, ed. Activity and Aging. Los Angeles: Sage.

U.S. Bureau of the Census. (1997). Sixty-Five Plus in America: Current Population Reports, Special Studies, No. P23–178. Washington, DC: U.S. Government Printing Office.

U.S. Department of Health and Human Services. (1990). Healthy People 2000. U.S. Department of Health and Human Services publication #PHS 91-50212. Washington, DC: U.S. Government Printing Office.

Watson J. (1988). Nursing: "Human Science and Human Care—A Theory of Nursing. New York: National League for Nursing.

CRITICAL THINKING EXERCISES

1. In your own words tell your classmates what "aging" means to you. Enter into a discussion with another classmate who views aging differently.
2. What key points would you include in a teaching program that will empower older adults to be responsible for their own health?
3. Lead a discussion with your peers on the effects of racism, sexism, ageism, and poverty on present and future health care trends.

CRITICAL THINKING EXERCISES, Continued

4. Describe the demographics of minority aging and how this phenomenon can be expected to affect the health care of minorities in the 21st century.

5. List the various theories of aging and their implications for nursing.

CHAPTER 2

Assessing the Older Adult:
The Nursing Process

Carol Dennis, DSN, RN

CHAPTER OUTLINE

OBJECTIVES

After completing this chapter, the reader should be able to:

1. Teach a classmate methods of gathering assessment data from older adults.
2. Compare and contrast effectiveness of communication techniques used in assessing an older adult.
3. Distinguish the expected changes of aging from pathophysiological disease states.
4. Describe and distinguish among at least five measurement tools for assessing an older adult.
5. Write a teaching plan for an older client who has several functional limitations and is moving into an assisted living facility.

The older adult population is the most rapidly growing population in America (Skipwith, 1992), and it is increasing more rapidly than the population as a whole. It is expected that this rapid increase of the older adult population will continue into the next century (U.S. Bureau of the Census, 1997). Thus, health care into the year 2000 and beyond will have a major focus within gerontological nursing. Accurate assessment is essential to the continuing health and function of every older client seen by a nurse, and because the older adult population experiences more chronic illness than other age **cohorts** (groups with a common characteristic that are under observation), accurate assessment of the older adult's health status is a priority for nursing and the health care system as a whole. Accurate assessment skills and appropriate use of the nursing process are tools that are—and will continue to be—a necessity for the gerontological nurse.

The **nursing process** is the organizing framework through which nurses determine the care needed to manage health problems and how necessary care can best be implemented. The goal of the nursing process is to maintain maximum functional ability, thus preventing deterioration and dependency. *Assessment* is the first step in this process, but the process also includes *diagnosing, planning, implementation,* and *evaluation.* It is vital to the nursing process that the assessment remain clearly nursing focused, both as a foundation for all the ensuing steps of the process and to provide suitable nursing care. When nursing focus is maintained, care can be provided in an appropriate and individualized manner.

ASSESSMENT OF THE OLDER ADULT

Nursing assessment of an older individual can be a complex and challenging task (Lueckenotte, 1998). Recognition of physical and psychosocial variables is important to the assessment of all individuals, but it is critical to the assessment of older adults. These variables may be seen in older adults who maintain a healthy and active lifestyle, yet older adults are at risk for functional loss from factors over which they have no control. Miller (1995) comments that the normal aging process is characterized by physiological changes that are generally seen by society as physical decline; as that perception is challenged by the number of older adults who are still healthy and active, it is hoped that society will come to view aging in a more positive way. For the purposes of this chapter, we will be looking at the variables that can put older adults at risk for functional loss.

Older adults exhibit decreased efficacy of homeostatic mechanisms, resulting in decreased response to stress; when a physical or emotional stressor is experienced, older adults require a longer period of time to return to prestress levels of functioning. Although older adults do experience more chronic illnesses than younger people, disability does not necessarily ensue. The nurse assessor must look for clues that account for the effects of disease on the individual's functional status. Older adults present different symptoms of illness than younger people (Kresevic and Lincoln, 1995). The determination that a health problem exists in an older individual is often difficult because presentation is so different from the overall norms for health and illness, and the norms for this age cohort have not yet been established.

Confusion, which may be very frightening to the individual, is often an early indication that an older adult is ill. Nursing support provided in a gentle, caring manner is crucial to ease the client's fears during periods of confusion. Often the reassurance that the nurse is available is enough to allay fears.

The assessment process involves gathering data that include three sources of information: primary, secondary, and tertiary. The **primary source** of information is provided by the person who is being assessed. **Secondary sources** include information from medical and nursing records, significant others, and multidisciplinary health care professionals knowledgeable about the individual. **Tertiary source** information is obtained from literary sources, professional journals, or textbooks (Potter and Perry, 1996).

Methods of Gathering Data

There are five techniques generally used to gather data relevant to the assessment process (Potter and Perry, 1996). The *interview* is designed to gather information from the client relating to the health history. The other four techniques, *observation, palpation, percussion,* and *auscultation,* are physical assessment tools.

Observation is a visual skill and is used to inspect the body to identify normal states or deviations from the normal. This method is conducted in a deliberate, organized, and focused way. The nurse assessor must be qualified to make comparisons between the known characteristics and the traits of the section of the body being observed (Kresevic and Lincoln, 1995). For example, most 25-year-old clients have good vision without the assistance of glasses. Poor vision in this age group signals a problem and indicates a need for further investigation into the health status of the individual. In a person older than age 40, decreased visual acuity represents a normal change of aging and most often indicates the need for glasses.

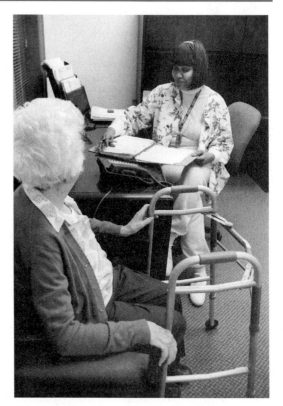

The history is an integral part of the assessment process.

on the external surface of the body, frequently the assessor is attempting to palpate the internal organs. Touch is, therefore, an important aspect of the physical examination.

Percussion is another form of assessing through the use of touch. The fingers of one hand are placed on an external surface of the body and the fingers of the other hand are used to, lightly but sharply, tap the fingers on the body. This method of assessment assists in determining the position, size, and consistency of underlying structures. Also, use of percussion can determine if there is fluid in a body cavity. Abnormalities are determined by the assessor feeling for alterations in vibrations produced by the tapping and listening for alterations in the pitch and resonance of the sound emitted. The assessor must also determine if there is resistance encountered during this process.

Auscultation is the process of listening to sounds within the body and determining if

---

C a r i n g

❝*The caring nurse allows enough assessment time for older adults to reminisce as they provide their health history.***❞**

Palpation is accomplished by using the fingers or hands to feel for abnormalities or evidence of disease. Some examples are placing the fingers over the radial artery to palpate for a pulse or placing the hand gently over an enlarged knee joint to palpate for the presence of local heat. Even though the hands are placed there are alterations by comparing the sound heard to what would normally be expected. Auscultation is usually accomplished with the use of a stethoscope. Common areas of the body assessed with auscultation are the heart, the lungs, and the intestines. It is important when auscultating large organs such as the lungs to auscultate many areas, front and back, and to compare the sides with each other (Seidel et al., 1995). For example, abdominal assessment is accomplished by visually dividing the abdomen into quadrants and inspecting and auscultating each quadrant of the abdomen for abnormalities. Each of the quadrants should be auscultated for at least 1 minute. When assessing the abdomen, palpation is used after auscultation to determine areas of tenderness, distention, masses, and fluid (Seidel et al., 1995).

Nursing Health History

The nursing health history should be completed first in the health assessment of the older adult. The purpose of obtaining a history is to gather both subjective and objective data that will assist in identifying nursing problems related to the client's health status. The focus of the health history is not only on physical processes but also includes information relating to psychosocial, cultural, and spiritual areas of the individual's development. It is important to note in the history whether the client is providing the information (primary) or whether a family member or other sponsor is providing the data (secondary). The reliability of the informant should be noted; this provides an idea of how accurate the information is likely to be. The health history should include information related to both the client's past and current health status. Biographical and demographical data are the first sought (Box 2–1) when completing a health history (Potter and Perry, 1996).

When all the data have been solicited about the current health concern, the nurse gathers information about earlier health problems. What hospitalizations have occurred related to major illnesses or surgeries in the client's life, especially within the past 5 years? What medications are being taken by the individual? Are allergies a problem? What is the immunization status of the client? A family health history is

| **Box 2-1** | **HEALTH HISTORY INFORMATION: BIOGRAPHICAL AND DEMOGRAPHICAL DATA** |

Name _____
Address _____
Telephone number _____
Age/date of birth _____
Gender _____
Ethnic group _____
Religion _____
Marital status _____
Children (names, addresses) or other support system _____
_____
Work status (previous occupation if retired) _____
Educational level _____
Living arrangements (alone or with someone and relationship to person) or
    main contact person _____
Income (adequate, marginal, or inadequate) _____
Hobbies/interests _____
Physician (telephone, address) _____
Smoker _____ consumer of alcohol _____ use of OTC drugs _____
Advance directive in place _____

Box 2-2   **HEALTH HISTORY (CC THROUGH REVIEW OF THE SYSTEMS)**

Current complaint (CC, duration, description)
Current chronic health problems
Childhood illnesses
Earlier health problems (hospitalizations, major illnesses, surgeries)
Medications (dosages, frequencies, site of administration)
Allergies (medication, food, or clothing)
Immunizations (tetanus, influenza, Pneumovax)
Family health history

General

Review of systems
   Integumentary
   Hematopoietic
   Head and neck (eyes, ears, nose, mouth, throat)
   Breasts
   Respiratory
   Cardiovascular
   Gastrointestinal
   Genitourinary
   Musculoskeletal
   Nervous
   Endocrine
   Psychosocial
   Fatigue, weakness, malaise
   Current weight (weight change in past year, loss or gain)
   Appetite change
   Usual sleeping patterns (change, difficulty)
   Night sweats
   Frequent colds, infections

Data from Lueckenotte A. (1998). Pocket Guide to Gerontologic Assessment. 3rd ed. St. Louis: CV Mosby.

necessary to provide insight into the client's health status and the development of possible health problems. A review of systems (ROS) is an important part of the health history to identify any problems or symptoms related to the current complaint (CC) or history that may not already have been discussed. Each system of the body is reviewed by asking specific questions about that system with the intent to elicit additional information not previously mentioned (Potter and Perry, 1996) (Box 2–2).

Communication Techniques

Communication is the act of sending messages from one individual to another. Communicat-ing involves both perception and cultural values (Kneisl, 1996; Townsend, 1996). *Perception* is the individual's understanding of an interaction. An individual's values are what the person deems desirable. Cultural values, learned from a very early age, provide the person with the meaning of the world and its structure. Cultural values impact on personal interpretations of communication; thus, relationships with others can be greatly impacted by an individual's perceptions and cultural interpretation of a message. In general, communication is bound both by an individual's culture (e.g., American) and subculture (e.g., Jewish). Verbal and nonverbal communication components are essential aspects to the message sent. Communication involves not only words spoken but also body language—such as gestures, facial expressions, touch, grooming (including clothing neatness and cleanliness, makeup application, neatness of hair, and facial shaving for men) (Fontaine, 1995; Stuart, 1995).

In interpreting a communication, it is important to determine whether the nonverbal message is congruent with the verbal message; that is, does the nonverbal cue support the verbal statement or does the nonverbal communication refute the verbal message? Nonverbal messages often provide more information than verbal messages. For example, if an individual is discussing a happy moment in life but sounds depressed or is shedding tears, this nonverbal message is more powerful than the statement about the happy event. Important cues to observe for during an interaction are direct eye contact, bodily gestures and hand movements, breathing patterns, speech patterns, and vocal tones (Townsend, 1996).

The nurse who wants to facilitate effective communication with a client must use a nonjudgmental approach. There are several intrinsic factors necessary to maintaining a nonjudgmental attitude. Responding to the client with empathy is one component. **Empathy** means communicating a feeling of compassion. Even if the responder has not experienced the same feelings as the communicator, it is important to let the communicator know that the responder is trying to feel and understand, on an emotional level, the message being sent. *Respect* is also an essential component of the communicative process. Responding to the client with respect allows the communicator to feel valued as being able to solve problems. *Genuineness* is a necessary component to open communication.

It is possible to be genuine while giving the client only that information that is necessary at the time. When the client is capable of accepting more responsibility for information, then more information may be shared.

Both empathy and respect are supported by an attitude of *caring* and *warmth*. Nurses express caring nonverbally by facial expression, by smiling, or by leaning forward and establishing eye contact with the client. A friendly tone conveys caring and allows the client to feel accepted. Allowing the client to have space also demonstrates empathy and respect.

If the nurse is recognized to be *trustworthy,* the communication process will be more effective. With the client's right to confidentiality in mind, the nurse can reassure the client that the information shared with him or her may need to be shared with other members of the health team, when appropriate, but will not be shared with anyone else (Fontaine, 1995; Kneisl, 1996; Schwecke, 1995).

Active listening, giving total attention to what the client is saying and doing, tells the client that the communication is important to the nurse. Both verbal and nonverbal cues of encouragement indicate that the nurse is actively listening. When the nurse is focused on how to respond next, then active listening cannot occur and the client gets the nonverbal message that the nurse's attention is elsewhere. For active listening to be possible, there must be total and explicit focus on what the client is doing and saying (Stuart, 1995; Townsend, 1996).

When used correctly, *silence* is a very effective communication technique. When the nurse remains silent, the client is allowed time to consider what has already been discussed, collect thoughts on an issue, and make alternative plans. However, if the silence is uncomfortable, then it should be broken. Uncomfortable silences can increase the client's anxiety and hinder the communication process. Student nurses, and other nurses new to the profession, need to be careful when using silence as a therapeutic technique. Often, the nurse becomes uncomfortable with silence, even silences of only a few seconds, and may break the silence, thereby interrupting the client's thought process (Kneisl, 1996).

Open-ended questions or broad comments are used to allow clients to address areas of personal concern. The use of this technique lets the client realize that personal interests are important to the nurse. However, overuse of this technique may cause the relationship to remain superficial (Fontaine, 1995).

Giving recognition is acknowledging that something is occurring at present for the client. Although use of this technique is a somewhat superficial level of communication, it stresses to the client that the nurse cares about him or her (Townsend, 1996).

Reflecting is a repetition of the client's verbal or nonverbal message and is done to benefit the client. Content of a message may be reflected or the implied feeling tone of a message may be verbalized back to the client. The client then has the opportunity to think about what has been reflected (Stuart, 1995).

Wellness

"*The older adult is often faced simultaneously with a number of psychosocial stressors while maintaining wellness, and a caring nurse conveys understanding and allows the client to interpret change as loss and to grieve when necessary.***"**

Clarifying is done to help the nurse understand the basic nature of the client's message. If the nurse is confused about the client's thoughts or feelings, it is appropriate for the nurse to say so and to ask the client to rephrase what was said. The nurse may also ask the client to give an example to clarify the meaning of a message (Fontaine, 1995).

Paraphrasing is done when the nurse restates what the client has said. Paraphrasing allows the nurse to ensure understanding the message that the client is communicating (Kneisl, 1996).

Restatement may be used instead of paraphrasing. This technique restates the cognitive component of the client's message using different and fewer words. Restating allows an opportunity for reinforcement of what the client has said. Facts may be explored through use of restating (Townsend, 1996).

Validating perceptions involves telling the client what the nurse is hearing. In this way, confusion about misperceptions can be corrected. The nurse should share perceptions about the client's behaviors, thoughts, and feelings and give the client the opportunity to validate the nurse's perceptions (Kneisl, 1996).

Questioning is a direct method of seeking information from the client. This technique is helpful when soliciting specific kinds of statements. Be careful to limit yes/no (closed-ended) responses so that as much information as possible can be obtained (Kneisl, 1996; Stuart, 1995; Townsend, 1996). Table 2–1 provides examples of the techniques discussed in this section.

Ineffective Communicating

The nurse naturally desires to communicate effectively in all client-focused situations. There are some pitfalls to be avoided so that this goal is achieved. Familiarity with useful techniques is necessary so the nurse is not thinking about what to say next. The nurse should listen to the client carefully while trying to understand what is being communicated and should gently confront any underlying feelings the client may have. When the communication process remains on a superficial level, the communication will be ineffective. Among other ineffective techniques, a judgmental attitude or the offering of advice will block effective communication (Townsend, 1996).

It is important to be rather formal in communications with a new client unless the client indicates otherwise. Using a title in addressing the older adult (Mr. King, Mrs. Brown, Miss Smith) is a way of showing respect and building rapport. Cultural differences between the older adult and the nurse must be integrated into the communication process. Making stereotypical comments to a client demonstrates an uncaring and superficial attitude and tends to reinforce negative myths and attitudes already held by some older adults. Ethnocentric values demonstrated by the nurse are offensive and may not even make sense to a person of a different cultural background from the nurse.

Parroting simply repeats the words the client has spoken to the nurse. It can be interpreted

TABLE 2–1. Effective Communication Techniques

Technique	Example
Active listening	The nurse focuses undivided attention on the client. Decrease environmental stimuli. Don't take notes. Give the client verbal and nonverbal attention.
Silence	Remain silent unless the silence is uncomfortable.
Open-ended question (broad opening)	"Tell me about your current health status." "Tell me something good about your health."
Giving recognition	"That is a really pretty sweater that you are wearing." "Purple is a nice color for you."
Reflecting	"You sound as though you feel that your health is pretty good." "You seem to be uncomfortable about answering these health questions."
Clarifying	"I'm confused about the sequence of occurrence of your health problems. Could you please repeat that part of your history?"
Paraphrasing	"In other words, you exercise for 15 minutes three times a week." "Are you saying that you walk a mile each day and you're 96 years old?"
Restatement	*Client:* "Do you think taking care of myself as a diabetic will be difficult?" *Nurse:* "How difficult do you think that will be?"
Validating perceptions	"I heard you say . . . . Is that correct?" "It sounds as though you are uncertain about living independently. Is that correct?"
Questioning	"What are your concerns about the possibility of having to live with your son?" "What are your thoughts about increasing your nutritional intake?"

as condescending by the client; therefore, any needed clarification cannot take place and the interaction is blocked.

The nurse who introduces new topics at an inappropriate time during the conversation is guilty of changing the subject. Sometimes this is done unintentionally when the nurse becomes uncomfortable with what the client is communicating. Sometimes the client who is uncomfortable with the topic will change the subject. If the nurse changes the topic excessively during a conversation, the client will get the impression that personal messages are not important and rapport will be lost (Fontaine, 1995).

When the nurse disagrees with clients, they are prevented from owning their true thoughts and emotions. Clients believe that disagreement denies them the right to how they feel and think; therefore, they will close the conversation. Challenging the client is likewise a blocker to the communication process. When challenged, clients believe they must give reasons for their underlying thoughts, feelings, and behaviors.

The word *why* can be a detriment to communicating with the client. Requesting an explanation compels clients to believe that they are inappropriate in behavior and feeling. False reassurance and belittling the client's expressed feelings overlook the client's concerns and distress; this is often experienced as "being talked down to." Use of both these styles detracts from the importance of the client's problems.

Probing communicates to clients that the nurse thinks they are not divulging true thoughts or feelings. Probing does not respect the client's right to privacy. Probing may, however, be appropriate when a life-threatening issue exists. It is best if the nurse does not ask more than one question at a time. Double or multiple questions may cause the client to feel confused. Too many questions at one time can bewilder the client about where to begin responding, especially if dementia is a current problem.

The nurse must not tell clients what to do. Advising takes the responsibility of decision-making away from the client. Clients need the opportunity to explore all options and to come to their own conclusions (Fontaine, 1995; Kneisl, 1996; Stuart, 1995; Townsend, 1996).

Use of the previously listed techniques will close a conversation. The client will not wish to communicate with a nurse who continually demonstrates lack of caring through the use of these inappropriate techniques.

Caring

"Even a nurse who is inexperienced with verbal techniques can help the older adult client feel comfortable by demonstrating a nonjudgmental approach, empathy, caring, warmth, and trustworthiness."

TYPES OF ASSESSMENT

Physical Assessment

Accurate assessment of older adults is critical to providing effective nursing care. There are several formats that can be incorporated into the assessment process. Functional ability is frequently assessed as part of the physical assessment. Functional ability includes both **activities of daily living (ADLs)** (Katz et al., 1963), which include self-care activities, and **instrumental activities of daily living (IADLs)** (Lawton and Broody, 1969), which include performance of more complex activities. Functional ability in the older adult is a valuable health indicator (Kresevic and Lincoln, 1995). Many assessments of older adults also include information relating to occupation, recreation, and leisure-time activities (Ebersole and Hess, 1998), most of which are based on choice in the older adult cohort. Older adults often see illness or injury as a threat to their independence and may not provide in-depth discussion about such problems. Older adults may fear that, once their independence is lost, institutionalization is not far away.

One assessment tool that is used with older adults is the FANCAPES (Ebersole and Hess, 1998), an instrument that is based on a survival-needs framework. Areas assessed using this approach include *f*luids, *a*eration, *n*utrition, *c*ommunication, *a*ctivity, *p*ain, *e*limination,

socialization, and *s*ocial skills; this provides a picture of the individual's ability to meet the self's needs and provides a focus for assistance.

The OARS (multidimensional functional assessment of the Older Americans Resources and Services) is also used for the assessment of older adults (Fillenbaum, 1988). This scale, too, collects data about an individual's abilities and disabilities and provides direction for needed assistance.

Another instrument (Dellasega, 1995) to assess self-care ability is the Self-Care of Older Persons Evaluation (SCORE). This tool was developed specifically for assessment of older adults who may exhibit rehabilitation needs and is expected to work well for those older adults in extended care, acute care, or rehabilitation care. Many facilities develop their own assessment tools. No matter which tool is used for older adult assessment purposes, some of the same components will be used to collect data.

The approach the nurse takes to get the assessment completed is open to discretion. However, the process needs to be organized. Generally, a head-to-toe approach maintains organization and allows the assessment to proceed in a systematic, deliberate manner. The nurse needs to develop an assessment approach that is personally comfortable and appropriate to the setting. In preparation for the physical assessment, all necessary equipment needs to be gathered and ready for use and the hands should be washed. The nurse must make sure that the client is comfortable.

Older adults are sensitive to temperature changes, so the individual should be allowed to remain clothed, only removing clothing when it is necessary to examine an area of the body. Adequate lighting without glare is essential. Because older adults are likely to tire easily, to conserve the client's energy the nurse needs to group assessment activities so that few position changes are necessitated. Warmth and caring are displayed by being gentle and explaining the process to the client as the examination progresses.

PHYSICAL EXAMINATION AND NORMAL FINDINGS

A healthy older adult is one who is able to maintain health and an active lifestyle with

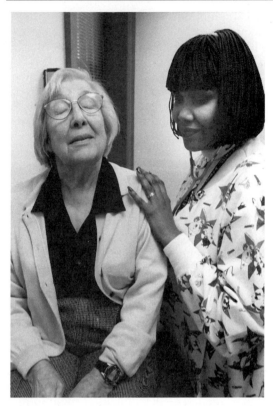

The physical examination always includes palpation, percussion, and auscultation.

some modifications for many years. More and more older adults in the United States are maintaining themselves in this way.

When illness does occur, it often has a unique presentation in the older adult (Ebersole and Hess, 1998; Kresevic and Lincoln, 1995). Illness presents with manifestations not seen in younger adults who have the same problem. Older adults have to adjust to the normal changes of aging; in addition, some must deal with both multiplicity and chronicity of disorders. Confusion may be the first response to an illness. There is an age-related decline in the functioning of the immune system that causes less rapid and less effective response to infections. This alteration in immune system functioning is thought to be responsible for a higher incidence of autoimmune problems as well as for some malignancies. Stress of any type has a more prolonged effect on the older adult than it does on younger people. Older adults require more time for readjustment from stress than younger people.

Complex functioning that requires more than one system to accomplish exhibits the most noticeable decline with normal aging. Any noticed decline in health or functional ability needs careful and thorough evaluation. Some common chronic illnesses of older adults are heart disease, cancer, diabetes, arthritis, vascular problems, renal disease, emphysema, hearing problems, and macular degeneration (Matteson et al., 1997).

COMMON FINDINGS

Skin, Hair, and Nails. With aging the skin loses strength and elasticity, perhaps sagging or appearing wrinkled in texture owing to a decrease in collagen, subcutaneous fat, glutamic acid, and lysine, all of which are necessary to form elastin. There is a loss of sebaceous and sweat glands from the outer layer of skin, leading to dehydration and the problem of dry skin (*xerosis*) with scaliness and itching. Both men and women experience thinning of the skin, beginning with a decrease in gonadal hormones and continuing with advancing age until the skin may appear transparent. The skin is easily damaged and tears readily. Itching and scratching must be controlled to prevent trauma to the skin. The very old have pallor secondary to a loss of melanocytes, which are irregularly deposited. This also may cause dark skin to lighten or to have "white freckles" (small areas of pigment loss). *Lentigo senilis* (liver spots) appear in light-skinned people when melanocytes increase at the dermal-epidermal junction.

Aging skin may develop lesions. There is no known cause, but it is suspected that sun exposure may trigger DNA changes in the cell. *Xanthelasmas* are soft yellowish spots on the eyelids that may be related to hyperlipidemia. *Acrochordons* are peduncles of skin (skin tags) that occur primarily on the neck, axillary area, and eyelids. *Actinic keratoses* are precancerous, normal aging growths occurring especially in fair-skinned people. They appear on exposed areas such as the lips, cheeks, ears, nose, upper extremities, and balding scalp as callous skin plaques ranging from pinkish tan to light brown. *Seborrheic keratoses* (benign skin lesions) can be seen on the neck, chest, and back and at the hair line, are light tan to black in color, and are wart-like, scaly, or greasy. *Cherry an-*

giomas (senile ectasias or vascular lesions) appear as papular lesions on the upper chest and extremities, are ruby red to purplish, and range in size from 1 to 5 mm. *Senile purpura,* a more serious vascular lesion, occurs spontaneously or can appear with mild trauma in older individuals because of fragile blood vessels. Beginning as small red to purple petechiae, senile purpura meet to form larger purple to brown spots. Older skin is susceptible to cancer (basal cell carcinoma, squamous cell carcinoma, and malignant melanoma) caused by exposure to the sun, especially in fair-skinned individuals.

With aging, the most noticeable changes in hair are apparent in color and distribution. Loss of melanocytes is the cause of graying hair; the color can range from a dull gray or white to yellow or yellowish green. In men, hair follicles have decreased by about one third at 50 years of age and continue this decline into old age; women may experience hair loss to a lesser degree. Older women may develop hair growth over the upper lip and lower face related to a decrease in estrogen production. Testosterone levels decrease as age increases, leading to a decline in hair in the axillary and pubic areas. Both sexes tend to develop hair in the ears and nares, men more than women, and men develop coarse, longer hair in the eyebrows.

W e l l n e s s

"Aging does not affect intelligence, abstract thinking, problem solving, or creativity. In fact, experience enhances these things."

Nails decrease in growth rate. Toenails become thick, yellowish, and grooved (Ebersole and Hess, 1998; Murray et al., 1997; Sims et al., 1995). In some individuals, nails may become ridged or develop a tendency to split.

Head and Neck. A loss of collagen tissue and subcutaneous fat causes the bones to appear to be more prominent and the hollow areas to appear deeper. This loss of tissue also contributes to wrinkling of skin. The "Adam's apple" is more visible, especially in men. A shortening of the platysma muscle, which extends from the

neck to the jaw and includes the muscles around the mouth on both sides of the face, causes the neck to look wrinkled and the jaw to look depressed (Sims et al., 1995). Because of the loss of subcutaneous fat, the eyes may appear sunken and the lids may droop, which can account for a sleepy appearance. The skin under the eyes becomes very thin, so that the underlying veins give a bluish color (dark circles) under the eyes. Fluid may collect under the eyes, causing puffiness. If the individual has experienced excessive exposure to the elements, the nose may enlarge and become bulbous. Lips become thinner and are subject to dryness, soreness, and cracking (Ebersole and Hess, 1998; Murray et al., 1997; Sims et al., 1995).

Senses. The presence of *arcus senilis,* a gray opaque line above the limbus (junction of the cornea and sclera), may be seen in adults older than 50 years of age. Peripheral vision declines, as does lens accommodation. *Presbyopia,* which begins around the age of 40 years, is the inability to obtain clear visual focus for near vision and necessitates wearing corrective (magnifying) lenses. Cataracts (opacities of the lens) may develop, so that an increased amount of light, which increases sensitivity to glare, is needed to be able to see.

The color of the iris tends to fade with the aging process. Macular degeneration, in which vision progressively worsens and blindness may result, is a major untreatable stressor of older adults. The conjunctiva becomes thin and yellowish. The eyes experience lessened tearing lubrication, along with increased irritation and infection. The retina exhibits observable vascular changes, impacting the rods and cones and altering color vision. Depth perception is also on the decline. All of these changes combined have implications for the older adult to give up driving, which is a major stressor for the individual (Ebersole and Hess, 1998; Luckmann, 1997; Murray et al., 1997; Sims et al., 1995).

Presbycusis, a decrease in hearing acuity, especially of high-frequency tones, is secondary to loss of hair cells in the inner ear's organ of Corti. The outer auditory canal narrows and may collapse with aging, and this structural change affects the hearing of high-frequency sounds. This may cause the individual to have difficulty understanding language and to appear to be confused; thought processes tend to become more rigid in response to this problem. There may also be a conductive hearing loss related to wax (cerumen) accumulation. Wax accumulation is related to the growth of longer and thicker hair that normally lines the outer auditory canal, especially in men, causing thinning and drying of the tissue lining the canal, more keratin, and a decline in sweat-gland activity. The older adult often has trouble differentiating consonants, which are the high-pitched sounds in English. When there are other distracting noises present in the environment, the older adult has an even greater problem with hearing. As adults move into their older years, they are sometimes slower to process language and may need to ask for repetition in conversations (Ebersole and Hess, 1998; Murray et al., 1997; Sims et al., 1995). For more on sensory changes, see Chapter 8.

Mouth, Nose, and Throat. The senses of smell and taste decline secondary to a decrease in olfactory fibers, atrophy of taste buds, and decreased salivation. With increasing age, bones and tissues in the mouth shrink, which can result in the loss of teeth, necessitating use of dentures or other dental prostheses. Continuing tissue shrinkage may interfere with properly fitting dentures, adversely affecting the individual's nutritional status (Murray et al., 1997).

Cardiovascular Changes. Arterial circulation is affected by decreased vessel compliance and increased peripheral resistance, usually arising from general or local arteriosclerosis or atherosclerosis. Fatty streaks (precursors to plaque) begin to develop in the teen years or by the early 20s. The development of atherosclerosis is related to genetic factors, gender, and lifestyle. Many older adults have cardiovascular changes that affect their psychomotor functioning. The heart muscle loses its efficiency and contractile strength by about 1% per year, decreasing cardiac output in relation to increased demand. Increased peripheral resistance raises systolic blood pressure significantly and diastolic blood pressure slightly. Pulse pressure is widened in an older adult. Diastolic murmurs can be heard in approximately half of the older adult population, with the most common being heard at the base of the heart and arising from sclerotic changes on the aortic valves.

Secondary to arteriosclerosis and incompetence of venous valves, circulation to the lower extremities is decreased, especially at the arteriole level. Diabetes mellitus, varicose veins, and decreased gonadal hormones compromise circulation and cause the skin to become thinner; there is also decreased hair growth on the arms and legs.

Peripheral pulses are usually easy to palpate because of narrowing of the arterial wall and the loss of connective tissue. On palpation, the vessels may feel tortuous and rigid. Pedal pulses may not be as easily palpated owing to arteriosclerotic changes. Feet and hands may be cold and feet may have a mottled appearance, especially at night. Toenails may develop a yellowish appearance and thicken as the result of many years of shoe pressure and poor circulation.

Older adults may experience orthostatic hypotension related to altered sensitivity in baroreceptors. This problem is often complicated by the medications prescribed for the individual (Ebersole and Hess, 1998; Luckmann, 1997; Sims et al., 1995), as well as by decreased fluid intake.

Kyphoscoliosis may change the location of the apex of the heart so that the point of maximal impulse is changed, which has implications of diagnostic significance. Older adults tire more easily, but most have enough energy to maintain ADLs (Ebersole and Hess, 1998; Luckmann, 1997; Sims et al., 1995). For more on cardiovascular changes, see Chapter 14.

Pulmonary Changes. The ribs and vertebrae become osteoporotic, with calcification of the costal cartilage and weakening of the respiratory muscles that causes structural changes such as kyphosis, shortened and stiffened chest wall, and increased anteroposterior chest diameter. All these age-related changes interfere with respiratory efficiency, requiring older adults to expend more energy to breathe efficiently. As compensation for these changes, older people use accessory muscles, especially the diaphragm, for respiration and are thus very sensitive to changes in intraabdominal pressure.

The lungs become smaller, losing about one fifth of their weight. The surface area of the lungs is decreased, blood flow is decreased in the pulmonary capillary system, and the mucosal bed (where diffusion occurs) becomes thickened, leading to less gas exchange during breathing. Elastic recoil diminishes, creating senile emphysema, which most older adults develop by the age of 80 years. Because of decreased gas exchange, the older adult is less able to respond to stress. The individual may be capable of maintaining a daily routine at home but unable to cope with stressors outside the home. For more on pulmonary changes, see Chapter 15.

Gastrointestinal Changes. The basal metabolic rate is decreased in older adults, creating the need for less caloric intake. Older adults are at risk for developing problems related to poor nutrition for several reasons. If an older adult lives alone, that person may not wish to prepare a complete meal. For some older adults, monetary resources are limited, dictating the types of food purchased. Chronic illness is often a problem that requires a special diet, which the older adult may not wish to recognize. Chewing is inefficient when there are problems with the teeth or if dentures do not fit properly. Smell and taste are often impaired in older adults so that food is just not appealing. Malnutrition is a serious health problem among the older adult population.

Older adults may take in less water than younger people do because of decline in the thirst mechanism. Nocturia and incontinence are also reasons why some individuals intentionally limit their water intake. Hydrochloric acid, pepsin, and pancreatic enzyme production are decreased, affecting digestion. Because fat absorption is delayed, the absorption of the fat-soluble vitamins (A, D, E, and K) is affected. Gastric emptying is delayed because of slower gastrointestinal motility and may cause heartburn. A complicating factor for heartburn is a relaxed gastroesophageal sphincter, which results in reflux (Ebersole and Hess, 1998; Murray et al., 1997; Sims et al., 1995).

Constipation is a problem in older adults because of decreased gastrointestinal motility and may be related to less water intake, less physical activity, and inadequate fiber in the diet. This may lead to indiscriminate laxative use. Laxative abuse among older adults is relatively common and may worsen the problem of constipation. Older adults have a high incidence of hiatal hernia, and many experience accompanying gaseous distention, which affects nutritional intake (Ebersole and Hess, 1998; Kresevic and Lincoln, 1995; Sims et al., 1995). For more on gastrointestinal changes, see Chapter 21.

Genitourinary Changes. As an individual approaches 75 to 80 years of age, the nephrons (the functional units in the kidneys) have decreased by about 50%, which decreases the glomerular filtration rate and has implications for drug toxicity. Atherosclerotic renal arteries reduce renal blood flow. Atrophy of the kidneys occurs, making them less efficient. The less-efficient kidney, decreased cardiac output, and decreased glomerular filtration rate together create the possibility of subsequent protein loss from the kidneys. Concentration of urine is ineffective because of decreased tubular functioning; the maximum specific gravity for the older adult is 1.024.

Urination patterns may be altered in men, who are at risk for developing benign prostatic hypertrophy. Ninety-five percent of men older than 85 have benign prostatic hypertrophy, which causes increased urinary frequency and possible urinary retention. A loss of perineal muscle tone, decrease in bladder elasticity and capacity, and loss of sphincter control lead to the development of frequency, urgency, and stress incontinence in women. Nevertheless, incontinence is not normal in older adults. Both men and women experience increased episodes of nocturia. Decreased urinary volumes may be related to less fluid intake as well as a decrease in bladder size.

Men maintain the physical ability for erection and ejaculation but have an increased refractory period. Testosterone production is decreased in men. The testes atrophy and produce less sperm, with a lessened viscosity of the seminal fluid (Ebersole and Hess, 1998; Sims et al., 1995). Libido and sexual satisfaction do not change, but frequency of intercourse is decreased (Murray et al., 1997).

In women, estrogen production is reduced after menopause. The epithelial lining of the vagina atrophies, and the vaginal canal narrows and shortens. Vaginal secretions are decreased, and there is atrophy of the cervix, uterine tubes, and ovaries. The uterus decreases in size and may not be palpable, mucous membrane secretions eventually cease, and there is the possibility that uterine prolapse may occur as a result of weakened musculature. Breast tissue also diminishes (Ebersole and Hess, 1998; Sims et al., 1995; Townsend, 1996). Frequently, these conditions are treated with postmenopausal hormone replacement therapy. Women continue to experience orgasm through these changes. For more on genitourinary changes, see Chapter 22.

Musculoskeletal Changes. Both muscle mass and bone mass decrease with aging. The amount of loss depends on the amount that was present when the individual was young, the amount of exercise the individual gets, and the use of hormone replacement therapy for postmenopausal women. Men experience less muscle loss than women because men usually have greater muscle mass and bone density. Individuals with small, bony frames are at greater risk for loss and also at greater risk for developing pathological fractures of the femur and vertebrae. Because muscle mass is lost, many older adults have bony prominences.

Intervertebral disks become dry and flatten, causing the trunk to shorten and a degree of kyphosis to develop. Those older than age 65 years lose inches from their height. Joints become stiff, have less mobility, and may become larger because of degenerative changes. Body water and protein decrease in proportion to the decrease in metabolic rate, causing a total decrease in body size. Body fat increases in the trunk but decreases in the arms and legs.

Older adults are at risk for falls related to orthostatic hypotension and a changed sense of balance. When older people fall, they fall sideways and fracture hips (unlike younger people, who fall forward, fracturing wrists).

The loss of muscle mass and subcutaneous fat may contribute to a lean, bony, even haggard appearance in the older adult. Older adults are not well insulated, experience decreased sweating, and have an alteration in the hypothalamus affecting sensitivity to temperature. An older adult may choose to wear a heavy sweater even on a hot day. For more on musculoskeletal changes, see Chapter 16.

Neurological Changes. By the age of 25 years, an individual begins to lose neurons at the rate of several thousand each day. The brain decreases in size, and by age 90 weighs about 10% less than it did at its maximum. A 75-year-old, nondiseased brain receives about 90% of the blood flow of a 30-year-old brain. Voluntary as well as autonomic reflexes slow down, so that reaction time is slower. Multiple stimuli may be too much for an older adult to handle. Although older adults are perfectly capable of learning new things, they may be slower in the process. Short-term memory is less than that of younger adults. Aging does not affect intelligence, abstract thinking, problem solving, or creativity. In fact, experience enhances these things.

Older adults generally stay in bed longer than younger people but do not sleep as much. Insomnia, which should be evaluated, may be a problem owing to less stage 4 (deep) sleeping. Older adults spend more time in stages 1 and 2 (lighter) sleep and less time in stages 3 and 4 (deeper) sleep. Stage 4 may even be absent (Clark and Walsh, 1997). Older adults wake up frequently at night, possibly because of pain or nocturia; they may feel that they have not slept at all if there has been less deep-stage sleeping. Alzheimer's disease and arteriosclerosis are the major causes of mental deterioration, but mental deterioration should be evaluated, because many physical problems can influence mentation (Ebersole and Hess, 1998; Luckmann, 1997; Sims et al., 1995).

Medication Assessment

Polypharmacy is of major concern in the older adult age group (Ebersole and Hess, 1998; Haller, 1996). Because medications are the most common method of treating chronic illnesses, often drugs are overused and misused (Kresevic and Lincoln, 1995). All too frequently older adults are treated by more than one physician, to whom they do not report medications prescribed for them by other physicians (Ebersole and Hess, 1998). It should be the goal of the gerontological nurse to determine, through medication assessment, that older adult clients are experiencing intended benefits from their medication regimen rather than experiencing adverse reactions.

Although older adults currently constitute 12% of the total population, they are prescribed a disproportionate one third (25% to 31%) of over-the-counter (OTC) and prescription drugs in the United States (Haller, 1996; Whitney and Rolfes, 1997). Ebersole and Hess (1998) stated that 16% of the U.S. population older than the age of 60 years are taking 40% of prescription drugs. There are very few older adults who do not take at least one medication daily, whereas many take more than one. Because of some of the normal changes that occur with aging, medications react differently in the body of an older adult. Absorption, distribution, metabolism, and excretion of medications may be affected by these normal changes (Haller, 1996; Kresevic and Lincoln, 1995; Matteson et al., 1997). For example, there is an increase in body fat, often accompanied by decreased water intake, allowing for more of a medication to be absorbed and stored in fatty tissue for later release into the system (Luckmann, 1997). Older adults also take a larger number of OTC drugs than other age groups. To minimize adverse reactions and interactions, medications should be prescribed in the lowest possible effective dose for an older adult (Matteson et al., 1997). The medication assessment must include use of OTC drugs as well as prescription drugs. Older adults should carry (brown-bag) all medications currently being used to the scheduled appointment for the physician's scrutiny. This allows the physician to be aware of the medications the older adult is taking and decreases polypharmacy.

Nutrient interactions with medications may occur. Whereas medications may alter absorption, metabolism, and excretion of nutrients, food may likewise alter the same properties for medications (Whitney and Rolfes, 1997). Box 2–3 contains topics for medication assessment. For more on pharmaceutical issues, see Chapter 10.

■ EXAMPLE

Very few older adults who live in one particular retirement community are aware of the medications they are taking or the rationale underlying their need to take them. Individuals seeking an apartment in this community must have a health appraisal (a functional assessment and the Mini-Mental State Exam) completed by the nurse before being accepted as a resident. Individuals seeking this independent living accommodation rarely are able to relate all the information pertinent to the medications they are taking regularly; rarely do these individuals carry a written list of their medications. They may know the color of the "pill" but not the reason for taking the medication, or they may know the rationale for taking the prescription but nothing else about the medica-

---

Box 2-3   **MEDICATION ASSESSMENT**

Medication history
  Prescribed
  Over-the-counter
  Name, amount, frequency, route
Knowledge level of any medication being taken
Have prescription medications been discontinued? For what reason?
Are medications being taken that were prescribed for someone else?
Do you share your medications with anyone?
How are medications obtained and paid for?
Do you manage your own medications?
What age-related changes impact the client's ability to self-manage
  medication therapy (motor dexterity, vision, memory, judgment)?
Can nonmedication interventions solve or control the problem?

Data from Haller G. (1996). Drug therapy in the elderly client. In Pinnell N, ed. Nursing Pharmacology, pp 123–133. Philadelphia: WB Saunders.

tion. Frequently, incomplete and confusing information is provided to the nurse related to medications being taken.

LABORATORY VALUES

Because many older adults exhibit atypical symptoms of illness, the gerontological nurse must often rely on laboratory test results to diagnose an illness. However, even these objective data are not always totally reliable because there are no established values as norms for the older adult population. For the older adult, some laboratory values may be increased or decreased secondary to the presence of chronic medical conditions (Ebersole and Hess, 1998). When a laboratory value seems to be out of the ordinary, the best approach is attempting to distinguish if the cause is related to normal changes of aging or to a medical problem.

ADVANCE DIRECTIVES

Advance directives for health care are a way for individuals to make known their wishes regarding health care during an episode of acute illness or when dying (Ebersole and Hess, 1998). Determining if an older adult has established advance directives ensures that the individual's rights are protected. However, it must be remembered that this legal issue is relatively new to the health care arena, and therefore older adults may require teaching related to the topic of advance directives (Fiesta, 1997). For more about advance directives, see Chapters 3 and 4.

Psychosocial Assessment

Psychosocial assessment gathers data relating to cognition and to social skills and social involvement (Miller, 1995; Potter and Perry, 1996). The many physical changes that occur during the aging process can create psychosocial challenges with which the elderly individual is forced to cope. Other psychosocial problems are generated by life events and are inevitable. The psychosocial changes in the older person's life are often more demanding of energy than the physical changes and chronic illnesses experienced (Miller, 1995).

Many older adults adjust well to the changes they face because they have developed sufficient coping strategies over their lifetime. Thus, many of the following challenges may be averted or seen as opportunities by psychologically healthy elders.

Life events faced by older adults may be different from those experienced earlier; they can be perceived by older adults as losses rather than gains, and frequency of occurrence may diminish personal adjustment time (Miller, 1995). Life events that challenge older adults include death of a spouse, retirement, income changes, relocation, physical changes, possible chronic illness, possible functional impairment, and death of friends. Death of a spouse may necessitate the most profound adjustment.

Retirement affects income, role identity, status and authority, schedule structure, purpose in life, and peer contacts. Retired older adults may experience perplexity about what to do with so much time. At first, they may feel at loose ends without the routine of a daily schedule.

Many older adults relocate to be near their children, and relocation may mean moving to a new state or a new part of the country. With long-distance relocation, both friends and the comfort of familiarity are lost. Relocation could involve movement into a retirement community where the older adult may have less space in which to live and less privacy. In one retirement community that houses approximately 220 residents, 50% of them have come from outside the state, 30% have come from outside the county, and only 20% of the residents have come from the same county.

More stressful than moving to a retirement community is relocation into a nursing home. Based on inquiry in this same retirement community, older adults do not fear death as much as the loss of independence. Residents view a relocation within the same retirement community, from an independent living apartment to an assisted living apartment, as one of the worst things that could happen to them. A move of this sort is equated with a loss of independence. It is rare for residents to make the decision for this move on their own. Usually, after completing a functional assessment and administration of the Mini-Mental State Exam on a resident, the nurse on staff explains to the resident why the move is necessary. Even with the assessment data to support the decision, the resident often does not agree.

Chronic illness can mean immobility, sensory loss, additional medications with new side effects, the risk of increased dependency, and increased expense for health care (Ebersole and Hess, 1998). In the retirement community, residents are allowed the use of assistive devices, such as wheelchairs and scooters, but must be able to move about with the device independently or with the assistance of a spouse. When chronic illness leads to immobility, the older adult fears institutionalization in a nursing home (Matthiesen, 1995).

For older adults, the greater the number of chronic illness diagnoses, the greater the risk of becoming dependent, and the greater the requirement for increased amounts of money to pay for health care. When there is not enough money to cover the high costs of health care, some problems may go untreated (Miller, 1995).

The death of friends results in a loss of companionship and causes older adults to see their own vulnerability (Miller, 1995). The lost companions may decrease the individual's socialization. Even when there are 220 people residing in the same facility, sharing the same daily activities, such as meals and programs, and other opportunities for socialization, loneliness is a major observable problem.

One other major psychosocial stressor for the older adult is the loss of being able to drive a car. Many states currently require a test to be taken before reissuing a driver's license to those 70 years and older (Ebersole and Hess, 1998). Children of older adults often have difficulty in helping the older person to make the right choice when driving is the issue.

The psychosocial issues of older adulthood necessitate a support system. The nurse needs to have knowledge about the availability and type of social support system on which the older adult depends. A good support system can boost the individual's coping ability and enhance decision-making processes (Potter and Perry, 1996). Assessment tools that include a psychosocial component are the Multidimensional Functional Assessment of Older Adults, the Duke Older Americans Resources

and Services Procedures (OARS) (Fillenbaum, 1988), and the Sickness Impact Profile (SIP) (Bergner et al., 1976).

Caring

“Confusion, which is often an early indication of illness, can be very frightening to the individual. A gentle, caring manner and assurance of availability is critical to ease such fears.”

All these psychosocial stressors can be overwhelming to an older adult, especially when several occur at once (e.g., relocation to a new city, giving up one's acquaintances and longtime friends, giving up some household possessions if moving to a smaller living accommodation). The nurse should let the older adult know that he or she understands how difficult these changes are. Older adults should be allowed to interpret a change as a loss and to grieve. For more about psychosocial issues, consult Chapters 5 and 6.

Mental Health Assessment

The mental health assessment is sometimes included as part of the psychosocial assessment. However, the two are separated here because there are some psychiatric mental health disorders common to the older adult.

Psychopathology in the older adult is most often related to a dementing disorder. There are a number of causative factors related to the dementias. However, dementia of the Alzheimer's type accounts for about 50% of the dementing disorders among older adults. This disorder occurs insidiously and continues as a progressive cognitive debility (Townsend, 1996). The Mini-Mental State Exam (Folstein et al., 1975) is a useful tool for screening cognition of older adults. It is easy to use and provides the nurse assessor with pertinent information about the client's state of cognition.

Older adults are particularly at risk for developing depression related to the many psychosocial, physical, cognitive, functional, and emotional losses that are likely to occur and to alter self-concept in this age group (Townsend, 1996). The more losses that are perceived by older adults, the greater will be their feelings of loss of control and helplessness, which may create a state of depression. It is estimated that depression affects 15% of the older adult population and that percentage rises in those older adults who are institutionalized (Baldwin et al., 1995; Matthiesen, 1995; Townsend, 1996). For the older adult, depression may manifest as cognitive impairment or dementia, which requires a thorough dementia evaluation, preferably by a multidisciplinary health care team led by a psychiatric geriatrician, to differentiate between physiological and cognitive causes of symptomatology.

A high rate of suicide exists among depressed older adults. Some suicides go unreported when it appears to be a passive indirect (or an "accidental") attempt, such as starvation or ingesting too much medication (Kuhlman, 1996). Moody (1994) reported that the rate of suicide among older adults accounts for 17% of all suicides. McBride and Burgener (1994) state that older adults comprise 21% of the reported suicide cases, and McIntosh (1992) reported the suicide rate to be 20.9% among older adults. Box 2–4 presents certain characteristics that increase the risk of suicide for the older adult.

■ CASE STUDY

Larry Smith, a 92-year-old man, lives alone in an apartment. His apartment is located in a subsidized residential community of older adults. Larry was diagnosed with macular degeneration 20 years ago and is legally blind. With the use of a powerful, lighted magnifying glass, and by holding reading material close to his eyes, he is able to read short items. On a recent visit to the ophthalmologist's office, Larry was told that he would be completely blind in the near future. This news caused him to become despondent. Larry concluded that because he was very old, was soon to be totally blind, was having difficulty hearing, and had several other troubling chronic illnesses, he did not wish to live any longer. However, Larry was not a violent individual and could not commit suicide by a means that was immediate and final. Thus, Larry decided that he would fast until he became weak and unconscious. Then his living will would not allow for lifesaving intervention to be implemented

and his problems would be over. Larry did achieve his goal of becoming weak and was then admitted to the local hospital's mental health unit, where antidepressant treatment was begun. After this hospitalization, Larry returned to his apartment, stating that he would attempt suicide again, in the same manner.

Although some older adults do abuse alcohol and/or drugs, the actual extent of this problem is undocumented because many more use or abuse them than are reported. Older adults who have used alcohol all their lives are at greater risk for use in late life than those who have not been alcohol users. Because older individuals are less able to detoxify and excrete alcohol and other substances, they are more vulnerable to the effects of these substances (Kuhlman, 1996). The combination of substance abuse, polypharmacy, and OTC drug use contributes greatly to falls and other accidents among older adults. For more on mental health, see Chapter 24.

Nutritional Assessment

Older adults require increased amounts of calcium and vitamins A and C in their diets but otherwise have the same minimal nutritional needs as younger adults. With aging the metabolic rate decreases, as does thyroid activity; thus, the requirements for calories and iodine are reduced (Potter and Perry, 1996).

Many variables affect nutritional intake for older adults. Fixed income, which usually occurs with retirement, may decrease the amount of money available for food. Physical symptoms related to health status may interfere with the desire to eat (Sizer and Whitney, 1997). Therapeutic diets are often dictated by an individual's health status and, for those who need to comply with a therapeutic diet, quality of life may be impaired. Older adults in this situation may choose to improve their immediate quality of life by eating foods they desire as opposed to foods dictated by dietary restrictions. Making the choice of favored foods will, of course, negatively impact quality of life over time.

■ CASE STUDY

Emma Green, 88, had been a known diabetic for the past 25 years. When first diagnosed, Emma attended special diabetic classes at the

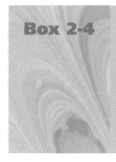

Box 2-4   SUICIDE RISK

High-Risk Older Adult

Gender:	male
Marital status:	divorced or widowed
Ethnic group:	Caucasian
Socioeconomic background:	lower
Medical disorders:	chronic pain, terminal illness, alcohol abuse

local clinic. She learned all the appropriate dietary rules and was very careful to follow them. Living alone at the age of 88, she no longer felt the need to be so careful. Emma did not enjoy preparing three meals a day and she felt cheated because she could not enjoy some of her favorite foods, such as ice cream and cake. Emma stopped avoiding the foods she had been taught not to eat and began to get more immediate satisfaction out of life.

Wearing dentures and having missing or decayed teeth can be deterrents to nutritional intake, especially if the dentures fit poorly. The socialization factor is absent when one has to eat alone, making meals less appealing to some individuals; this can lead to skipped meals. Health status disability and lack of transportation likewise have the potential for impacting nutritional status negatively (Potter and Perry, 1996).

Decreased acuity of the sense of taste due to decreased zinc levels and decreased acuity of smell often interfere with the desire to eat (Potter and Perry, 1996). The taste buds for bitter and sour remain intact longer than those for sweet and salt; frequently experiencing bitter and sour taste sensations may cause a decline in nutritional intake. Also, wearing dentures increases the bitter and sour taste. Less efficient digestion is experienced in older adulthood as a result of a decline in gastric secretions. Other variables that may affect the older adult's nutritional status include adverse drug–nutrient interactions, alcohol abuse, and depression, among many others. Existing chronic medical states may be worsened by poor nutritional intake, and a vicious cycle may ensue. Accurate nutritional assessment is significant for all Americans, but especially so for older adults.

Clinical signs important to the nutritional assessment are listed in Box 2–5. For more on nutritional issues, see Chapter 7.

Cultural Assessment

Culture is defined as a particular way of life for a group of people (Potter and Perry, 1996). Culture encompasses such characteristics as shared patterns of belief, attitudes, feelings, and values that are passed from one generation to the next (Murray et al., 1997). The socialization learned from family is another aspect of culture. Giger and Davidhizar (1995) have identified six cultural phenomena—environmental control, biological variation, social organization, communication, space, and time—that differ from one culture to another. Cultural assessment can include gathering information about each of these six phenomena. For a more complete look at cultural issues, please refer to Chapter 5.

When performing a cultural assessment, the nurse must bear in mind that the client is an individual identified with a cultural group who, as an individual, may not embrace all the beliefs of that culture. Thus, when assessing health problems, it is best to determine what the problem means to the client. The individual can describe the problem for which aid is sought. Having this knowledge allows the nurse to assist the client toward solutions to the problem (Ebersole and Hess, 1998). Hayes (1996) stated that cultural assessment alone is not enough, but often cross-cultural comparisons are needed to increase one's knowledge about those things that are universal to all cultures.

Box 2-5	NUTRITIONAL ASSESSMENT

Important Clinical Signs
General appearance
Weight
Height
Posture
Functioning of all body systems
Energy
Hair
Anthropometry
    Wrist circumference
    Mid and upper arm circumference
    Triceps skin fold

Spiritual Assessment

Spirituality is that aspect of an individual in which the individual seeks to discover the meaning to life as well as the answers to questions about health, illness, and death (Potter and Perry, 1996). Spirituality includes one's beliefs and values system. Many psychosocial issues, such as physical disability and the prospect of death, cause older adults to rely on spiritual beliefs and practices for effective coping. Conflicts between an older adult's beliefs (Why me?) and the reality of an event result in spiritual distress. When experiencing spiritual distress, older adults may question their purpose and the meaning of their life. Supporting the older adult's beliefs and values helps the individual to cope with challenges encountered as an older adult (Miller, 1995). For more detail, please refer to Chapter 5.

Functional Assessment

Functional assessment tools identify what activities an individual is capable of performing and assist in determining the level of independence. These tools are usually capable of identifying areas in which the individual will need extra support to remain independent. By identifying functional areas of need, appropriate interventions can be implemented to enhance the individual's functional capability and to preserve the quality of life for the older adult. Functional assessment is usually inclusive of

ADLs (Katz et al., 1963) and IADLs (Lawton and Broody, 1969). ADLs include self-care areas of functional ability such as bathing, dressing, grooming, eating, toileting, and mobility. Functional assessment is sometimes used as the basis for determining placement for older adults (i.e., nursing home placement vs. assisted living placement vs. an independent retirement community or remaining in one's own home). Expectations of the level of functional ability differ for these various settings. Assessment based on the mentioned areas of function is readily adaptable; each of the functional areas can be expanded. For example, the area of grooming can be further categorized into oral hygiene, hair care, neatness and cleanliness of clothing, and makeup application for women and shaving for men. Then, each of these areas can be assessed according to the amount of assistance the individual needs to complete each task.

IADLs (Lawton and Broody, 1969) are generally part of the functional assessment and include such categories as meal preparation, laundry, transportation, housekeeping, financial management, medication management, grocery shopping, and the ability to use a telephone. Each category is assessed for the amount of assistance the individual needs to accomplish the task. Assessment of IADLs is necessary so that support can be obtained for older adults to allow them to remain independent in their communities as long as possible.

When family or other personal caregivers are not available, community resources may be available. For example, Meals on Wheels may be appropriate for the older adult experiencing difficulty with shopping or meal preparation. Many grocery stores are willing to make home deliveries, which is a resource for the older adult who lacks transportation. There are many reputable businesses available to older adults that offer assistance with financial management (Miller, 1995). Older adults are at risk for experiencing varying degrees of limitations to their functional abilities. The nurse needs to focus on the abilities of the older client, providing positive reinforcement rather than making an issue of limitations.

W e l l n e s s

"The nurse needs to focus on the abilities of the older adult, providing positive reinforcement rather than making an issue of limitations."

The Functional Dementia Scale (Moore, 1983) was developed to be used as an objective monitoring device for the disease course of dementia and for the evaluation of treatment. Caregivers of the Alzheimer's client may complete the scale in their stead. Items included in this scale correspond to the major problems evidenced in a client with dementia.

Fall Risk Assessment

An estimated one third of all people aged 65 years and older who live at home fall each year (National Institute on Aging, 1990). Approximately half of this one third experience more than one fall per year. Falls are a serious and frequent problem related to the aging process. Broken hips occur with falls among older adults and greatly contribute to nursing home admissions (40%) each year (Ebersole and Hess, 1998). Falls are a predominant problem for the old old, those 85 years of age and older. The leading cause of accidental death among the old old can be attributed to falls (Lowenstein and Hunt, 1990; Urton, 1991). Research

conducted using long-term care residents found the most prevalent causes of falling to be stroke, Parkinson's disease, blindness, drug-related hypotension, and arthritis (Lipsitz et al., 1991).

Women fall more often than men. Characteristics of those who fall include more individuals who are functionally impaired, taking more medications, experiencing more difficulty getting out of a chair, experiencing difficulty turning 360 degrees, experiencing impaired positional sense, and using more antidepressant medications. Many changes of the normal aging process (e.g., visual, neurological, musculoskeletal, and cardiovascular changes) increase the risk of falling (Luckmann, 1997), and associated risk factors of visual acuity disturbances, postural hypotension, and cardiac arrhythmias increase proportionately to age.

The physical assessment provides valuable information related to fall risk. Identifying how the normal aging processes have affected the individual will give a basis for overall fall risk assessment. One pertinent question is "Have you ever fallen before?" Those who have fallen previously are at greater risk to fall again (Ebersole and Hess, 1998). The nurse should evaluate the client's visual acuity, gait and balance, muscle control, response/reaction time, short-term memory, mood alterations and/or confusion, presence of postural hypotension, urinary frequency, use of medications (including number and interactions), wearing of appropriate clothing, medical conditions that increase the risk of falling, and environmental hazards (Luckmann, 1997). Assessment tools for the risk of a fall include the Berg Balance Scale (Berg et al., 1992) and the Tinetti Fall Assessment (Tinetti, 1986).

Older adults may develop a fear of falling that leads to a restriction of their activities after having fallen. This can have serious consequences if the individual avoids all activity seen as unnecessary and creates an even more sedentary lifestyle. The immobility associated with restricted activity can lead to many harmful physiological consequences, such as constipation, contractures, and pneumonia (Ebersole and Hess, 1998). The one consequence older adults seem to dread most is loss of independence, and restricted activity certainly leads to that loss. For more about the risk of falls, please refer to Chapter 9.

Pain Assessment

Older adults tend to experience chronic pain more often than acute pain. *Chronic pain* is not limited to a relatively short time span, as is acute pain, but is characterized as persistent (Seidel et al., 1995) and as a state of being. However, pain is not a normal process of aging, and it should neither be overlooked nor accepted. An older adult who complains of pain should undergo a thorough evaluation for the pain, as should an individual of any age group. Because pain is the most common symptom of disease (Ebersole and Hess, 1998), accurate assessment is essential. This can be a difficult process with older adults because pain, as with many other symptoms, may occur in a manner that is atypical. Pain is a subjective perception; thus, many questions must be asked and many descriptors of the pain experience (synonyms for pain) need to be used. Because individuals respond to pain at various thresholds of tolerance, skill of observation is essential. The nurse must be observant of nonverbal cues related to pain because they frequently provide as much information as verbal cues. Observation for these cues to pain is crucial because the older adult, depending on cultural background, may not report it.

Assessment of pain should include its history, determining the impact of the pain on the individual's functional ability, and evaluating pain intensity and quality. There are several scales that assist in the evaluation of a client's perception of pain intensity and quality. Often,

clients are asked to evaluate their pain on a scale of zero to 10, with zero being equivalent to no pain and 10 being equivalent to the most intense pain. For older adults who are cognitively impaired, the pain scale of zero to 10 may be too confusing; these individuals may respond more appropriately if the scale is limited (e.g., zero to 5). A pain scale often used is the Faces Rating Scale (Whaley and Wong, 1993). The full smiling face represents no pain, whereas the full frowning face with tears represents the worst pain. There are four faces between these two extremes, representing various degrees of happiness or sadness that are used to qualify the individual's pain. Box 2–6 provides guidelines to the components of the assessment of pain.

◼ NURSING DIAGNOSIS

After the assessment data are systematically collected, nursing diagnoses can be appropriately identified. Because health states of older adults change frequently, a series of assessments may be necessary; in addition, it is essential to remain aware that some older adults have multiple problems that must be prioritized. Nursing diagnoses are categorized as actual or potential, depending on whether the client actually has the problem or is at risk for developing a problem. Related factors may be different for the same problem. For example, poor nutrition may be related to lack of appetite or poor dentition, which dictates the nursing interventions to be implemented.

The older client's perception of health status, strengths, and limitations must be re-

---

Box 2-6   ASSESSMENT OF PAIN

Location
Duration
Quality
What alleviates the pain?
What makes the pain better?
What exacerbates it?
Does the pain affect your functional status and if so, how?

spected before nursing interventions are implemented. As with any care plan, that for an older adult must be individualized.

For the older adult, it is especially important to foster independence through intervention. Nurses must allow clients to perform as much of their ADLs as possible. One aspect of intervention not to be overlooked is that done with families or significant others. Support groups are especially helpful in providing these intimates with support and with problem-solving skills and education about specific disease processes (Townsend, 1996).

Some common nursing diagnoses for older adults that result from age-related changes include, but are not limited to, the following (Kresevic and Lincoln, 1995; Sims et al., 1995; Doenges et al., 1997):

1. *Cognitive-perceptual problems*
   - Thought processes, altered, related to acute confusional states, stress, or reduced gas exchange
   - Sensory/perceptual alterations related to age-related changes
   - Health maintenance, altered, related to memory deficits or slower learning of new information
2. *Gastrointestinal system changes*
   - Nutrition, altered, less than body requirements related to loss of taste or smell, dentures that do not fit well, or being edentulous
   - Constipation, related to poor nutritional intake, lack of exercise, or dehydration
3. *Genitourinary system changes*
   - Urinary elimination, altered, frequency and urgency related to sensory, cognitive, mobility deficits, or functional incontinence
4. *Musculoskeletal system changes*
   - Activity intolerance, related to muscle weakness, lack of energy, poor nutritional intake, fatigue, or immobility
   - Mobility, impaired, related to age-related respiratory and cardiovascular system changes, osteoporosis, or arthritis
   - Self-care deficit, related to decreased functional ability (same as above)
   - Injury, risk for, related to impaired physical mobility, poor muscle strength in the lower extremities, or poor vision

5. *Cardiopulmonary system changes*
   - Breathing pattern, ineffective, related to age-related respiratory system changes
   - Cardiac output, decreased, related to age-related cardiovascular changes, fluid volume deficit, stress, or increased urinary elimination
6. *Integumentary system changes*
   - Skin integrity, impaired, related to poor circulation, dehydration, immobility, or incontinence
7. *Changes in comfort*
   - Pain, related to pathophysiological processes, indigestion, constipation, immobility, muscle cramps, or skin breakdown

PLANNING

The planning phase of the nursing process involves developing the nursing care plan (Table 2–2). Whenever possible, the older adult should be involved in this phase of the process where priorities of care are established, goals are set, and appropriate interventions are established (Potter and Perry, 1996). Older adults sometimes do not see their needs the same as those identified by the professional.

EXAMPLE

A retirement community was initially developed to meet the needs of independent older adults in their sixth or seventh decade and of those needing assisted living in the same age group. However, over the next few years the average age of the residents increased to 85 and more support was necessary to help them maintain an independent status; thus, a new level of care was developed (supported living) to provide independence.

This level of care provided for those residents who needed assistance with medication management and who exhibited needs in the functional areas of bathing, dressing, and grooming. The residents themselves, however, identified their areas of need as requiring more support in housekeeping functions, such as making the bed (pulling up the covers), taking out the trash, preparing a "light meal," doing the laundry and ironing, and running errands in general. These residents were not pleased to learn that the support being offered was in the form of personal care.

TABLE 2–2. Sample Care Plan for the Older Adult

Expected Outcomes	Interventions	Rationale
Nursing Diagnosis: *Altered Nutrition, Less than Body Requirements*		
The client will maintain or regain weight.	Provide appealing high-protein, high-calorie foods.	The older adult is more likely to eat foods that are appealing to him or her and high-protein, high-calorie foods will meet metabolic demands.
	Have the client eat as many meals as possible with someone else.	Eating alone can produce a negative impact on the older adult. Eating with someone allows for socialization, which is likely to produce a positive impact on the individual's appetite.
	Weigh the client weekly.	It is important to determine if the client is making progress toward the expected outcome.
	Encourage exercise based on the client's capability, unless contraindicated.	Exercise uses calories and increases one's appetite.
Nursing Diagnosis: *Altered Mobility, Impaired Physical*		
Maintains joint mobility by performing range-of-motion (ROM) exercises.	Assess client's capability to perform ROM exercises independently.	Client may need assistance to perform ROM exercises to preserve joint mobility.
	Have the client perform ROM exercises four times each day.	Performing ROM exercises preserves joint mobility.
	Have client walk, or assist if necessary, in the hall three times a day.	Ambulation increases strength and endurance.
	Have client dangle for 1 minute before ambulation.	Dangling helps to prevent postural hypotension, thereby preventing falls.

Appropriate interventions, individualized for each older adult, can be determined after nursing diagnoses are identified. The entire plan of care must be acceptable to the older adult if goals are to be achieved. Including older individuals in the care-planning process enhances independence, promotes well-being, and improves the possibility of compliance with the care plan. For potential problems, planning consists of identifying nursing interventions that will prevent the problem from developing. For already-existing problems, planning consists of developing nursing interventions that will improve, reduce, or eliminate the problem (Potter and Perry, 1996).

IMPLEMENTATION

The implementation phase of the nursing process is begun when nursing interventions are established. Interventions should support independence in functional abilities and assist the individual in adaptation, recovery, or maintenance of the current level of functioning. Care needs to be accomplished when there is plenty of time, because older adults may be slower to respond and can experience an increase in number of existing problems. Families and significant others must be included in the support process relating to the care needs of the older adult (Potter and Perry, 1996).

EVALUATION: EXPECTED OUTCOMES

Evaluation determines if the care plan is achieving the client's expected outcomes. Were the interventions effective? Because change in the older adult is often slow and therefore difficult to detect, evaluation is completely individualized. Should the established interventions be found ineffective, other interventions can be implemented. Through evaluation, new goals can be developed or old ones eliminated.

Sometimes, the frequency of evaluation is established by the type of care plan itself (Potter and Perry, 1996). For instance, in the example care plans, interventions and progress toward the expected outcome for altered nutritional status, less than body requirements, should be evaluated at least weekly. However, for altered mobility, impaired physical, evaluation of joint mobility and interventions should be completed daily (Potter and Perry, 1996).

Summary

Many older adults continue to lead healthy, active lives. The purpose of gerontological nursing assessment is to determine whether the older adult's level of function is satisfactory. Norms for this age cohort are still to be established, so the process of assessment must be done with a view to the expected changes that have been observed to occur with the process of aging. Assessment is only one part of the nursing process, which also includes nursing diagnosis, planning, implementation, and evaluation of expected outcomes.

There is an established system for assessment that dictates the methods of gathering data, the taking of a personal and medical history, appropriate communication techniques, and the ability to discern what is unique about the individual being assessed. Types of assessments include physical, psychosocial, mental, nutritional, cultural, and spiritual. Physical assessment proceeds from head to toe and should include both pain and fall risk.

Older adults face many changes that may not be welcome, including loss of friends and acquaintances, decreases in physical and sometimes mental function, and possible loss of independence, especially when it includes relocating to a new home where privacy may not be possible. The gerontological nurse is able to empathize with the feelings and thoughts these changes inevitably engender in older adults and to introduce adjustments designed to support the highest function and greatest satisfaction possible for them at every age.

REFERENCES

Baldwin B, Stevens G, Friedman S. (1995). Geriatric psychiatric nursing. In Stuart G, Sundeen S, eds. Principles and Practice of Psychiatric Nursing. 5th ed. St. Louis: CV Mosby.

Berg KO, Wood-Dauphine S, Williams JL, Gayton D. (1992). Measuring balance in the elderly: Preliminary development of an instrument. Physio Can 41:304–311.

Bergner M, Bobbit RA, Kressel S, et al. (1976). The sickness impact profile: Conceptual formulation and methodology for the development of a health status measure. Int J Health Serv 6:393–415.

Clark HM, Walsh MB. (1997). Sleep. In Burke MM, Walsh MB, eds. Gerontological Nursing: Wholistic Care of the Older Adult. 2nd ed. St. Louis: CV Mosby.

Dellasega C. (1995). A practical method for assessing the self-care status of elderly persons. Rehabil Nurs Res 4(4):128–135.

Doenges ME, Moorhouse MF, Geissler AC. (1997). Nursing Care Plans: Guidelines for Individualizing Patient Care. 4th ed. Philadelphia: FA Davis.

Ebersole P, Hess P. (1998). Toward Healthy Aging. 5th ed. St. Louis: CV Mosby.

Fiesta J. (1997). Legal Implications in Long-Term Care. Albany, NY: Delmar.

Fillenbaum G. (1988). Multidimensional Functional Assessment of Older Adults: The Duke Older Americans Resources and Services Procedures. Hillsdale, NJ: Laurence Erlbaum Associates. (This is the resource for the OARS Assessment Tool.)

Folstein MS, Folstein SE, McHugh PR. (1975). Mini-Mental State: A practical method for grading cognitive state of patients for the clinician. J Psychiatr Res 12:189–198.

Fontaine K. (1995). Communicating and teaching. In Fontaine K, Fletcher J, eds. Essentials of Mental Health Nursing. 3rd ed. Redwood City, CA: Benjamin/Cummings.

Giger J, Davidhizar R, eds. (1995). Transcultural Nursing: Assessment and Intervention. 2nd ed. St. Louis: CV Mosby.

Haller G. (1996). Drug therapy in the elderly client. In Pinnell N, ed. Nursing Pharmacology, pp 123–133. Philadelphia: WB Saunders.

Hayes J. (1996). Cross-cultural and cultural-specific tools. Reflections 22(4):11–12.

Katz S, Ford AB, Moskowitz RW, et al. (1963). Studies of illness in the aged: The index of ADL. JAMA 185:914. (This is the resource for the ADL tool.)

Kneisl CR. (1996). Therapeutic communication. In Wilson HS, Kneisl CR, eds. Psychiatric Nursing. 5th ed. Menlo Park, CA: Benjamin/Cummings.

Kresevic D, Lincoln R. (1995). Nursing practice with elders. In Phipps W, Cassmeyer V, Sands J, et al., eds. Medical-Surgical Nursing Concepts and Clinical Practice. 5th ed. St. Louis: CV Mosby.

Kuhlman G. (1996). Applying the nursing process with the elderly. In Wilson H, Kneisl C, eds. Psychiatric Nursing. 5th ed. Menlo Park, CA: Benjamin/Cummings.

Lawton MP, Broody EM. (1969). Assessment of older people: Self-maintaining and instrumental activities of daily living. Geriatrics 44(6):29–35. (This is a resource for ADLs.)

Lipsitz L, Jonsson P, Kelly J. (1991). Causes and correlates of recurrent falls in ambulatory frail elderly. J Gerontol 46(4):114.

Lowenstein SR, Hunt D. (1990). Injury prevention in primary care (editorial). Ann Intern Med 113:261.

Luckmann J, ed. (1997). Saunders Manual of Nursing Care. Philadelphia: WB Saunders.

Lueckenotte A. (1998). Pocket Guide to Gerontologic Assessment. 3rd ed. St. Louis: CV Mosby.

Matteson MA, McConnell ES, Linton AD. (1997). Gerontological Nursing Concepts and Practice. 2nd ed. Philadelphia: WB Saunders.

Matthiesen V. (1995). Disorders of older adults. In Fontaine K, Fletcher J, eds. Essentials of Mental Health Nursing. 3rd ed. Redwood City, CA: Benjamin/Cummings.

McBride AB, Burgener S. (1994). Strategies to implement geropsychiatric nursing curricula content. J Psychosoc Nurs Ment Health Serv 32(4):13–18.

McIntosh JL. (1992). Epidemiology of suicide in the elderly. Suicide Life Threat Behav 22(1):15.

Miller C. (1995). Nursing Care of Older Adults. Glenview, IL: Scott, Foresman.

Moody HR. (1994). Aging: Concepts and Controversies. Thousand Oaks, CA: Pine Forge Press.

Moore JT. (1983). A functional dementia scale. J Fam Pract 16:499.

Murray RB, Zentner JP, Pinnell NN, Boland MH. (1997). Health Assessment Promotion Strategies Through the Life Span. 6th ed. Stamford, CT: Appleton & Lange.

National Institute on Aging. (1990). Special Report on Aging, p 4. Washington, DC: U.S. Department of Health and Human Services, Public Health Service.

Potter P, Perry A. (1996). Fundamentals of Nursing Concepts: Process and Practice. St. Louis: CV Mosby.

Schwecke LH. (1995). Communication. In Keltner L. Schwecke LH, Bostrom CE, eds. Psychiatric Nursing. 2nd ed. St. Louis: CV Mosby.

Seidel H, Ball J, Dains J. (1995). Mosby's Guide to Physical Examination. 3rd ed. St. Louis: CV Mosby.

Sims L, D'Amico D, Stiesmeyer J. (1995). Health Assessment in Nursing. Redwood City, CA: Benjamin/Cummings.

Sizer FS, Whitney EN. (1997). Nutrition Concepts and Controversies. 7th ed. Belmont, CA: West/Wadsworth.

Skipwith DH. (1992). The older adult. In Stanhope M, et al., eds. Community Health Nursing: Process and Practice for Promoting Health. St. Louis: CV Mosby.

Stuart G. (1995). Therapeutic nurse-patient relationship. In Stuart G, Sundeen S, eds. Principles and Practice of Psychiatric Nursing. 5th ed. St. Louis: CV Mosby.

Tinetti ME. (1986). Performance-oriented assessment of mobility problems in elderly patients. JAGS 34(2): 119–126.

Townsend M. (1996). Psychiatric and Mental Health Nursing: Concepts of Care. 2nd ed. Philadelphia: FA Davis.

Urton MN. (1991). A community home inspection approach to preventing falls among the elderly. Public Health Rep106(2):192.

U.S. Bureau of the Census. (1997). Sixty-Five Plus in America. Current Population Reports, Special Studies No. P23–178. Washington, DC: U.S. Government Printing Office.

Whaley L, Wong D. (1993). Essentials of Pediatric Nursing. 4th ed. St. Louis: CV Mosby.

Whitney EN, Rolfes SR. (1997). Understanding Nutrition. 7th ed. Minneapolis/St. Paul: West.

CRITICAL THINKING EXERCISES

Jane Smith, age 94, lived alone in a retirement community where she had been living for the past 12 years. In fact, Jane moved in when the building first opened. She knew all the residents in the building as well as all the staff. She felt as if all of them were her family, since she had no living relatives of her own. Her support system was very limited. She had one friend with whom she had attended high school, but who lived in another state, and one friend who lived nearby, but who was often busy with her own children, grandchildren, and great-grandchildren. The nurse had concerns about Jane because frequently her clothes had food spots and other dirty spots on them. Nutrition was a concern, because it was Jane's responsibility to prepare most of her own meals. Safety became an issue as Jane aged and her eyesight was failing. Flammable items were found on the stove in Jane's apartment several times. When an assessment was completed on Jane, she scored in the mildly cognitively impaired range on the Mini-Mental State Exam. The functional assessment revealed that Jane needed assistance with meal preparation, laundry, housekeeping, and safety issues. Jane's management of her blood pressure medication was in question, as was her ability to use the telephone (dialing). Jane was a good candidate for an assisted living apartment. Jane does not want to move and is extremely resistant to moving to an assisted living apartment, stating "There is nothing wrong with me. I'm just exactly like I was when I moved in!"

CRITICAL THINKING EXERCISES, Continued

1. In three to four paragraphs, explain how you would convince Jane to move. Which communication techniques would be best to use and why? How could you demonstrate caring when she is so resistant?
2. From the case study, identify at least three nursing diagnoses and develop a mini care plan for Jane, including nursing interventions and expected outcomes.
3. Which age-related changes could be responsible for the nursing diagnoses identified for Jane?
4. How will these age-related changes impact Jane's life?

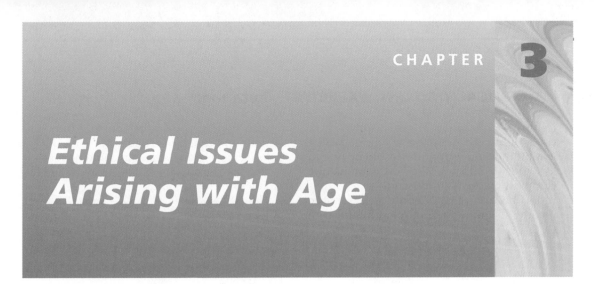

CHAPTER **3**

Ethical Issues Arising with Age

Shirley Rose Tyson, RN, MA, EdD

CHAPTER OUTLINE

OBJECTIVES

After completing this chapter, the reader should be able to:

1. Differentiate among ethics, morals, values, and rights.
2. Compare and contrast ethical theories, including utilitarianism, naturalism, ethical egoism, and deontology.
3. Teach a classmate the ethical principles of autonomy, beneficence, nonmaleficence, justice, and fidelity.
4. Formulate three ethical issues in gerontological nursing and role play solutions with classmates.
5. Create an example of an ethical dilemma and reason through one or more solutions.
6. Specify the staffing and functions of an ethics committee.

KEY TERMS

advance directives
beneficence
bioethics
deontology
duty
ethical dilemma
ethical egoism
ethics
informed consent
morals
natural law
nonmaleficence
rights
utilitarianism
values

Ethical issues regarding the care and treatment of older adults arise for gerontological nurses almost every day. As the population continues to age, the frequency, urgency, and complexities of ethical questions about the older adult will continue to increase. Health care of older adults raises a number of important ethical issues. These issues have evolved as a result of two major occurrences:

1. Global population aging, combined with increasing technological advances, creates an environment where health care professionals have the responsibility to uphold individuals' rights while protecting them from harm.
2. Never before in the history of health care in the United States has there been so much attention focused on the subject of ethics, ethical dilemmas, and ethical decision-making.

We cannot assume that all elderly people are unhealthy and suffer significant physical and mental disabilities. As noted in, Chapter 1 older adults are now separated for convenience into groups according to chronological age: the "young old" are 65 to 74, the "middle old" are 75 to 84, and the "old old" are 85 and over. Even the old old can—and do—enjoy good health and retain an ability to function without assistance from others. However, as people grow older they do face an increased likelihood of ill health, mental and physical impairment, and diminished functional capacity.

We can assume that more than 50% of older adults are experiencing good health, because only 10.2% of people age 65 and older are unable to carry on a major activity such as housekeeping or a job outside the home, and only 37.5% have some limitations of activity caused by chronic conditions (U.S. Department of Health and Human Services, 1991). Nursing professionals have an obligation to help healthy older adults maintain wellness and to address the needs of those who are facing health challenges. Are older adults in our society receiving both preventive health services and necessary health care? Many ethical issues surround the maintenance of good health for older adults, and social policy is beginning to give some attention to this area. (One example of this is the Medicare controversy over financing annual mammography diagnostic services for older female adults.) In addition, print and television media increasingly assist in the education of older adults about their health and its maintenance. Sociopolitical groups such as the American Association of Retired Persons (AARP) focus primarily on older adults, providing information concerning their welfare.

The advances in biomedical technology that have enabled increased numbers of individuals to reach old age often confront us with inescapable decisions that are the basis for the emergence of the contemporary field of **bioethics** (health care ethics, or medical ethics). Dubler (1994) states that we are all responsible for each other in this nation; how all of us are treated and whether all of us have access to care should be as important in bioethics as individual rights. Gerontological nurses, who by virtue of their profession have the responsibility to uphold their patient's rights, face complex real-life situations arising from different circumstances that do not have readily identifiable solutions.

CASE STUDY

An 87-year-old woman, once a dignified college president, is now a frail nursing home resident in the early stages of dementia. Holding on to her last shred of dignity, she refuses to wear any arm or body restraints while seated in a chair in the recreation room. This causes much anxiety for the staff and family, who have witnessed previous falls. They believe that restraints will avert the possibility of a hip fracture. The question arises as to whose rights should be upheld.

Ethical issues in gerontological nursing surrounding patient care include the following:

1. How is "doing good" determined?
2. Who makes the "good" decisions?
3. Who decides to restrain or not to restrain?
4. Who advocates for the resident's autonomy?
5. What are the residents' rights?
6. What are the rights of the staff and nursing home?
7. What are the rights of the family?
8. Is the patient and/or family aware of the risks and benefits of using restraints?

Knowledge about the ethical principles, theories, and concepts that guide professional practice must undergird nursing practice. Nurses bring to the nurse/client relationship their own personal value system combined with their own life experience, which must be acknowledged but not be the basis of client-centered decision-making. This personal value system arises over time and is influenced by family, religious beliefs, teachers, and peers and is usually a significant part of the overall picture when the nurse is implementing patient care or interacting with other health care professionals.

■ HISTORICAL PERSPECTIVE

The discipline of *bioethics*, also known as health care or medical ethics, is a relatively recent development that began in the late 1960s and early 1970s. Although there was interest in the topic, no organized group or literature supported the interest until recently (Beauchamp and Walters, 1994). Over the years, professional codes were formulated:

- Hippocratic oath (revived)
- Nightingale pledge (Box 3–1)
- World Medical Association Declaration at Geneva in 1948
- International Council for Nurses Code of Nursing Ethics in 1953 (a document discussing rights and responsibilities of nurses around the world, Box 3–2)
- American Nurses' Association (ANA) Code for Nurses in 1950 (revised in 1985, Box 3–3). As early as 1897 the ANA (actually, its

forerunner association) had expressed the need for a code of ethics, which was finally adopted in 1950.

Ethics, also known as *moral philosophy*, is derived from the Greek word *ethos* meaning "custom" or "character." **Ethics** are patterns or codes of conduct adopted by a group of people pertaining to the rightness or wrongness of certain behavior or actions. Box 3–4 presents some basic definitions of ethical terms. Principles of ethics that are applied to patient care assist the nurse in clinical practice. Many groups have developed statements that express their positions on equity, truth, and justice for individuals. It is particularly important that those serving the frail older population be conversant with current standards of professional behavior to advocate for them when they are unable to do so for themselves.

■ THEORETICAL PERSPECTIVES

Ethical Theories

A theory is a systematic statement of principles involved. *Ethical theory* is a study about the principles involved in right behavior. Many ethical theories have been proposed and developed by philosophers over the years. Because ethics assist caregivers in determining right or wrong conduct in everyday situations, ethical theories have eminently practical application. Even so, in the United States medical and nursing ethics as formal disciplines are fairly new. Professional obligations have long been recognized in codes of ethics, but only recently has much systematic thought been given to the moral and legal rights of patients (Beauchamp and Walters, 1994).

In the following brief presentation of four ethical theories, you will see that no two theories agree.

1. Utilitarianism. A *utilitarian* is concerned primarily with the usefulness of an action's consequences. **Utilitarianism** holds that the greatest human thought, action, and happiness should be achieved in each situation. Benefits should be maximized, and harm or danger should be minimized. This is often expressed as "the greatest good for the greatest number of people."

Box 3-1   THE NIGHTINGALE PLEDGE (1893)

I solemnly pledge myself before God, and in the presence of this assembly,
To pass my life in purity and to practice my profession faithfully.
I will abstain from whatever is deleterious and mischievous, and will not
    take or knowingly administer any harmful drug.
I will do all in my power to maintain and elevate the standard of my
    profession, and will hold in confidence all personal matters committed to
    my keeping and all family affairs coming to my knowledge in the practice
    of my profession.
With loyalty will I endeavor to aid the physician in his work, and devote
    myself to the welfare of those committed to my care.

2. Deontology. A *deontologist* holds that the highest good is to fulfill obligations. The word **deontology** is derived from the Greek word *deon*, or "duty." Deontologists believe that duty, laws, and rules are based on prior agreements—fundamental or essential facts. Without concern for outcome, ethical decisions are to be made out of respect for moral law—what one *ought* to do—with no exceptions. *Moral law* is what the tradition of a particular society says it is.

3. **Natural law**. A *naturalist* holds the belief that there is a law of nature that humans are born with the ability to reason and to choose good over evil, and evil acts are never condoned, even in the most unusual situations. It is necessary to "do good and avoid evil." The Declaration of Independence cites natural law as its basis.

4. Ethical egoism. An *egoist* (one who subscribes to **ethical egoism**) holds the belief that whatever is best for the individual making the decision is morally "good" or "right." This point of view was expressed in Henry David Thoreau's *On the Duty of Civil Disobedience* and was very popular during the 1970s in the United States.

To explore how caregivers from these differing theoretical perspectives would respond to an ethical situation requiring a decision, consider the matter of a kidney transplant, which involves scarce resources and growing demand as the population ages:

1. The *utilitarian* approach would be that older people should be considered for transplants if they have a chance for a positive outcome. However, scarce resources should be allocated across all age groups for the greatest benefit to all, and thus older adults would be considered *after* other age groups because they would benefit for the shortest amount of time. For strict utilitarians, it would not matter who the patients are or how they had lived their lives, as long as the greatest good or least evil is produced for the majority.

2. The *deontological* approach would be that caregivers have a duty to provide the transplant, so it should be done; society has a duty to protect its citizens and laws should reflect this duty.

3. The *naturalist* approach would be that society, through government, should allocate resources (in this case, kidneys) and provide transplants equally to all, including the oldest members of the population. Not to do this would be evil.

4. The *egoist* approach would be that whatever the decision-maker decides about who is to receive the kidney will be morally right for the decision-maker. Thus, the surgeon who selects a favorite patient over others is making the "right" decision for the surgeon (and, presumably, for the favored patient).

Note that all four ethical systems would favor the transplant, for differing reasons, and that none really addresses the problem of resource allocation. Let us take a look at resource allocation. An aging society and advances in medical technology ensure that the allocation problem will be with us for as far as we can see into the future.

There are various ways in which chronological age might be used as an allocation crite-

Text continued on page 60

Box 3-2   INTERNATIONAL CODE OF NURSING ETHICS (ADOPTED BY THE INTERNATIONAL COUNCIL OF NURSES IN JULY 1953)

Professional nurses minister to the sick, assume responsibility for creating a physical, social and spiritual environment which will be conducive to recovery, and stress the prevention of illness and promotion of health by teaching and example. They render health service to the individual, the family, and the community and coordinate their services with members of other health professions.

Service to mankind is the primary function of nurses and the reason for the existence of the nursing profession. Need for nursing service is universal. Professional nursing service is therefore unrestricted by considerations of nationality, race, creed, color, politics, or social status.

Inherent in the code is the fundamental concept that the nurse believes in the essential freedoms of mankind and in the preservation of human life.

The profession recognizes that an international code cannot cover in detail all the activities and relationships of nurses, some of which are conditioned by personal philosophies and beliefs.

1. The fundamental responsibility of the nurse is threefold: to conserve life, to alleviate suffering, and to promote health.
2. The nurse must maintain at all times the highest standards of nursing care and of professional conduct.
3. The nurse must not only be well prepared to practice but must maintain her knowledge and skill at a consistently high level.
4. The religious beliefs of a patient must be respected.
5. Nurses hold in confidence all personal information entrusted to them.
6. A nurse recognizes not only the responsibilities but the limitations of her or his professional functions, recommends or gives medical treatment without medical orders only in emergencies, and reports such action to a physician at the earliest possible moment.
7. The nurse is under an obligation to carry out the physician's orders intelligently and loyally and to refuse to participate in unethical procedures.
8. The nurse sustains confidence in the physician and other members of the health team; incompetence or unethical conduct of associates should be exposed, but only to the proper authority.
9. A nurse is entitled to just remuneration and accepts only such compensation as the contract, actual or implied, provides.
10. Nurses do not permit their names to be used in connection with the advertisement of products or with any other forms of self-advertisement.
11. The nurse cooperates with and maintains harmonious relationships with members of other professions and with her or his nursing colleagues.
12. The nurse in private life adheres to standards of personal ethics which reflect credit upon the profession.
13. In personal conduct nurses should not knowingly disregard the accepted patterns of behavior of the community in which they live and work.
14. A nurse should participate and share responsibility with other citizens and other health professions in promoting efforts to meet the health needs of the public—local, state, national, and international.

Adopted by the International Council of Nurses, July 1953; printed in American Journal of Nursing 53:1070, 1953.

Box 3-3

1

The nurse provides services with respect for human dignity and the uniqueness of the client, unrestricted by considerations of social or economic status, personal attributes, or the nature of health problems.

1.1 Respect for Human Dignity

The fundamental principle of nursing practice is respect for the inherent dignity and worth of every client. Nurses are morally obligated to respect human existence and the individuality of all persons who are the recipients of nursing actions. Nurses therefore must take all reasonable means to protect and preserve human life when there is hope of recovery or reasonable hope of benefit from life-prolonging treatment.

Truth telling and the process of reaching informed choice underlie the exercise of self-determination, which is basic to respect for persons. Clients should be as fully involved as possible in the planning and implementation of their own health care. Clients have the moral right to determine what will be done with their own person; to be given accurate information, and all the information necessary for making informed judgments; to be assisted with weighing the benefits and burdens of options in their treatment; to accept, refuse, or terminate treatment without coercion; and to be given necessary emotional support. Each nurse has an obligation to be knowledgeable about the moral and legal rights of all clients and to protect and support those rights. In situations in which the client lacks the capacity to make a decision, a surrogate decision maker should be designated.

Individuals are interdependent members of the community. Taking into account both individual rights and the interdependence of persons in decision making, the nurse recognizes those situations in which individual rights to autonomy in health care may temporarily be overridden to preserve the life of the human community, for example, when a disaster demands triage or when an individual presents a direct danger to others. The many variables involved make it imperative that each case be considered with full awareness of the need to preserve the rights and responsibilities of clients and the demands of justice. The suspension of individual rights must always be considered a deviation to be tolerated as briefly as possible.

1.2 Status and Attributes of Clients

The need for health care is universal, transcending all national, ethnic, racial, religious, cultural, political, educational, economic, developmental, personality, role, and sexual differences. Nursing care is delivered without prejudicial behavior. Individual value systems and life-styles should be considered in the planning of health care with and for each client. Attributes of clients influence nursing practice to the extent that they represent factors the nurse must understand, consider, and respect in tailoring care to personal needs and in maintaining the individual's self-respect and dignity.

1.3 The Nature of Health Problems

The nurse's respect for the worth and dignity of the individual human being applies, irrespective of the nature of the health problem. It is reflected in care given the person who is disabled as well as one without disability, the

Box continued on following page

Box 3-3   ANA CODE FOR NURSES, *Continued*

patient with long term illness as well as with acute illness, the recovering patient as well as one in the last phase of life. This respect extends to all who require the services of the nurse for the promotion of health, the prevention of illness, the restoration of health, the alleviation of suffering, and the provision of supportive care of the dying.

The nurse does not act deliberately to terminate the life of any person.

The nurse's concern for human dignity and for the provision of high quality nursing care is not limited by personal attitudes or beliefs. If ethically opposed to interventions in a particular case because of the procedures to be used, the nurse is justified in refusing to participate. Such refusal should be made known in advance and in time for other appropriate arrangements to be made for the client's nursing care. If the nurse becomes involved in such a case and the client's life is in jeopardy, the nurse is obliged to provide for the client's safety, to avoid abandonment, and to withdraw only when assured that alternative sources of nursing care are available to the client.

The measures nurses take to care for the dying client and the client's family emphasize human contact. They enable the client to live with as much physical, emotional, and spiritual comfort as possible, and they maximize the values the client has treasured in life. Nursing care is directed toward the prevention and relief of the suffering commonly associated with the dying process. The nurse may provide interventions to relieve symptoms in the dying client even when the interventions entail substantial risks of hastening death.

1.4 The Setting for Health Care

The nurse adheres to the principle of nondiscriminatory, nonprejudicial care in every situation and endeavors to promote its acceptance by others. The setting shall not determine the nurse's readiness to respect clients and to render or obtain needed services.

2

The nurse safeguards the client's right to privacy by judiciously protecting information of a confidential nature.

2.1 The Client's Right to Privacy

The right to privacy is an inalienable human right. The client trusts the nurse to hold all information in confidence. This trust could be destroyed and the client's welfare jeopardized by injudicious disclosure of information provided in confidence. The duty of confidentiality, however, is not absolute when innocent parties are in direct jeopardy.

2.2 Protection of Information

The rights, well-being, and safety of the individual client should be the determining factors in arriving at any professional judgment concerning the disposition of confidential information received from the client relevant to his or her treatment. The standards of nursing practice and the nursing responsibility to provide high quality health services require that relevant data be shared with members of the health team. Only information pertinent to a client's treatment and welfare is disclosed, and it is disclosed only to those directly concerned with the client's care.

Information documenting the appropriateness, necessity, and quality of care required for the purposes of peer review, third-party payment, and

Box 3-3   ANA CODE FOR NURSES, *Continued*

other quality assurance mechanisms must be disclosed only under defined policies, mandates, or protocols. These written guidelines must assure that the rights, well-being, and safety of the client are maintained.

2.3 Access to Records

If in the course of providing care there is a need for the nurse to have access to the records of persons not under the nurse's care, the persons affected should be notified and, whenever possible, permission should be obtained first. Although records belong to the agency where the data are collected, the individual maintains the right of control over the information in the record. Similarly, professionals may exercise the right of control over information they have generated in the course of health care.

   If the nurse wishes to use a client's treatment record for research or nonclinical purposes in which anonymity cannot be guaranteed, the client's consent must be obtained first. Ethically, this ensures the client's right to privacy; legally, it protects the client against unlawful invasion of privacy.

3

The nurse acts to safeguard the client and the public when health care and safety are affected by incompetent, unethical, or illegal practice by any person.

3.1 Safeguarding the Health and Safety of the Client

The nurse's primary commitment is to the health, welfare, and safety of the client. As an advocate for the client, the nurse must be alert to and take appropriate action regarding any instances of incompetent, unethical, or illegal practice by any member of the health care team or the health care system, or any action on the part of others that places the rights or best interests of the client in jeopardy. To function effectively in this role, nurses must be aware of the employing institution's policies and procedures, nursing standards of practice, the Code for Nurses, and laws governing nursing and health care practice with regard to incompetent, unethical, or illegal practice.

3.2 Acting on Questionable Practice

When the nurse is aware of inappropriate or questionable practice in the provision of health care, concern should be expressed to the person carrying out the questionable practice and attention called to the possible detrimental effect upon the client's welfare. When factors in the health care delivery system threaten the welfare of the client, similar action should be directed to the responsible administrative person. If indicated, the practice should then be reported to the appropriate authority within the institution, agency, or larger system.

   There should be an established process for the reporting and handling of incompetent, unethical, or illegal practice within the employment setting so that such reporting can go through official channels without causing fear of reprisal. The nurse should be knowledgeable about the process and be prepared to use it if necessary. When questions are raised about the practices of individual practitioners or of health care systems, written documentation of the observed practices or behaviors must be available to the appropriate authorities. State nurses' associations should be prepared to provide assistance and support in the development and evaluation of such processes and in reporting procedures.

Box continued on following page

Box 3-3   ANA CODE FOR NURSES, *Continued*

When incompetent, unethical, or illegal practice on the part of anyone concerned with the client's care is not corrected within the employment setting and continues to jeopardize the client's welfare and safety, the problem should be reported to other appropriate authorities such as practice committees of the pertinent professional organizations or the legally constituted bodies concerned with licensing of specific categories of health workers or professional practitioners. Some situations may warrant the concern and involvement of all such groups. Accurate reporting and documentation undergird all actions.

3.3 Review Mechanisms

The nurse should participate in the planning, establishment, implementation, and evaluation of review mechanisms that serve to safeguard clients, such as duly constituted peer review processes or committees, and ethics committees. Such ongoing review mechanisms are based on established criteria, have stated purposes, include a process for making recommendations, and facilitate improved delivery of nursing and other health services to clients wherever nursing services are provided.

4

The nurse assumes responsibility and accountability for individual nursing judgments and actions.

5

The nurse maintains competence in nursing.

6

The nurse exercises informed judgment and uses individual competency and qualifications as criteria in seeking consultation, accepting responsibilities, and delegating nursing activities.

7

The nurse participates in activities that contribute to the ongoing development of the profession's body of knowledge.

7.1 The Nature and Development of Knowledge

Every profession must engage in scholarly inquiry to identify, verify, and continually enlarge the body of knowledge that forms the foundation for its practice. A unique body of verified knowledge provides both framework and direction for the profession in all of its activities and for the practitioner in the provision of nursing care. The accrual of scientific and humanistic knowledge promotes the advancement of practice and the well-being of the profession's clients. Ongoing scholarly activity such as research and the development of theory is indispensable to the full discharge of a profession's obligations to society. Each nurse has a role in this area of professional activity, whether as an investigator in furthering knowledge, as a participant in research, or as a user of theoretical and empirical knowledge.

7.2 Protection of Rights of Human Participants in Research

Individual rights valued by society and by the nursing profession that have particular application in research include the right of adequately informed consent, the right to freedom from risk of injury, and the right of privacy and preservation of dignity. Inherent in these rights is respect for each

Box 3-3 ANA CODE FOR NURSES, *Continued*

individual's rights to exercise self-determination, to choose to participate or not, to have full information, and to terminate participation in research without penalty.

It is the duty of the nurse functioning in any research role to maintain vigilance in protecting the life, health, and privacy of human subjects from both anticipated and unanticipated risks and in assuring informed consent. Subjects' integrity, privacy, and rights must be especially safeguarded if the subjects are unable to protect themselves because of incapacity or because they are in a dependent relationship to the investigator. The investigation should be discontinued if its continuance might be harmful to the subject.

7.3 General Guidelines for Participating in Research

Before participating in research conducted by others, the nurse has an obligation to (a) obtain information about the intent and the nature of the research and (b) ascertain that the study proposal is approved by the appropriate bodies, such as institutional review boards.

Research should be conducted and directed by qualified persons. The nurse who participates in research in any capacity should be fully informed about both the nurse's and the client's rights and obligations.

8

The nurse participates in the profession's efforts to implement and improve standards of nursing.

9

The nurse participates in the profession's efforts to establish and maintain conditions of employment conducive to high quality nursing care.

10

The nurse participates in the profession's effort to protect the public from misinformation and misrepresentation and to maintain the integrity of nursing.

11

The nurse collaborates with members of the health professions and other citizens in promoting community and national efforts to meet the health needs of the public.

11.1 Collaboration with Others to Meet Health Needs

The availability and accessibility of high quality health services to all people require collaborative planning at the local, state, national, and international levels that respects the interdependence of health professionals and clients in health care systems. Nursing care is an integral part of high quality health care, and nurses have an obligation to promote equitable access to nursing and health care for all people.

11.2 Responsibility to the Public

The nursing profession is committed to promoting the welfare and safety of all people. The goals and values of nursing are essential to effective delivery of health services. For the benefit of the individual client and the public at large, nursing's goals and commitments need adequate representation. Nurses should ensure this representation by active participation in decision making in institutional and political arenas to assure a just distribution of health care and nursing resources.

Box continued on following page

Box 3-3   ANA CODE FOR NURSES, *Continued*

11.3 Relationships with Other Disciplines

The complexity of health care delivery systems requires a multidisciplinary approach to delivery of services that has the strong support and active participation of all the health professions. Nurses should actively promote the collaborative planning required to ensure the availability and accessibility of high quality health services to all persons whose health needs are unmet.

Reprinted with permission from Code for Nurses with Interpretative Statements. © 1985, American Nurses' Association, Washington, D.C.

rion. An *overt* use would be seen in the practice of putting elderly Eskimos out on the ice floe to die in isolation (cultural). A *covert* use is the British policy on kidney dialysis, which has never been publicly proclaimed. (In the British National Health Service, long-term dialysis is generally not offered to patients older than 65 years of age, and access to other life-extending measures by elderly patients is also restricted [Wicclair, 1993]). Aaron and Schwartz (1984) observe that there is no official age-rationing policy under the British National Health Service, but that when physicians fail to offer dialysis and other life-extending measures to elderly patients, they are unlikely to characterize

their action as either "rationing" or "age rationing." Poor overall health status is a more likely rationale for failing to offer treatment to patients over a certain age. Aaron and Schwartz further construe the practice of denying or restricting the elderly access to certain life-extending measures as rationing in response to budget constraints (1984). It is also unusual in the United States for an older adult to receive a transplanted organ unless from another older adult. Organ banks usually designate young organs to young people, because this is considered to be more beneficial.

A *direct* use would be a policy of no heart transplants for patients older than age 75. An

Box 3-4   COMMONLY USED TERMS

- **Ethics** are codes of conduct adopted by a group of people relating to the rightness and wrongness of certain actions or behaviors.
- **Bioethics** (*health care ethics or medical ethics*) is the study of ethical problems arising from scientific advances, especially in biology and medicine.
- **Duty** is the moral or legal obligation to follow a certain line of conduct.
- **Values** are personal beliefs used as criteria for justification in action taken. Value systems are introjected beliefs that help a person choose between difficult alternatives.
- **Morals** are established rules that provide standards of behavior and guide the behavior of an individual or social group.
- **Rights** are those things to which an individual is entitled by society and formalized into law. The American Nurses' Association, National League for Nursing, and American Hospital Association have established guidelines for Nurses' Rights and Patients' Rights. The U.S. Constitution makes provision for individual rights as equality in life, liberty, and the pursuit of happiness.

indirect use is not including an intensive-care unit in a nursing home (Moody, 1992), thus necessitating patient transfer to acute care hospitals whenever a health crisis occurs.

The dilemmas of bioethics have been of great concern to nurses, physicians, social workers, and other professionals, whereas questions of social policy and social ethics in an aging society have become more broadly intertwined with debates about the allocation of resources and the role of government. An example of the role of government is the American version of national health insurance for the aged alone, in the form of Medicare (to which most older adults contribute during their working years through payroll deductions).

Major Ethical Principles

There are a number of ethical principles that are commonly applied to problems in health care; thus, they serve as guides for health care professionals. Notable among these bioethical concepts are the following:

1. *Autonomy*—To respect the older adult's rights to make health care decisions, including the right to refuse care, medications, and treatments. *Example:* A 70-year-old woman newly diagnosed with cancer refuses invasive treatment and elects to have alternative therapies of acupuncture, acupressure, and natural remedies. She is utilizing her rights of autonomy.
2. *Beneficence*—To do good and benefit patients. Health care professionals must actively pursue good and benefit the patients in their care. *Example:* In a life-threatening emergency, in which the patient may be unconscious (e.g., victim of a car accident), surgery may be performed *before* consent can be obtained. Thus, beneficence is practiced by saving the life; in other words, the patient could die while the staff is awaiting a consent to perform surgery.
3. *Paternalism*—To interfere with a person's liberty of action. In this principle, health care professionals justify their actions by reasons referring exclusively to the welfare, good, happiness, needs, interests, or values of the patient in their care who is possibly being coerced. *Example:* A 75-year-old male patient is told by his physician that he should have surgery. It may be quite possi-

ble that the surgery should be performed, but the patient has not been given any options nor given an opportunity for second opinions or discussion with others. *Paternal* means "fatherly," and a paternalistic attitude was used in this example. To justify paternalism there must be *strong* cause. It is the overriding of beneficence.
4. *Veracity*—To be truthful in all caregiving situations. *Example:* An 87-year-old woman in the surgical intensive-care unit asks the nurse "Am I going to die?" The nurse responds "You are very ill. That is a possibility. Is there something you would like me to do for you?" The patient asks the nurse to phone her nephew because she needs to talk to him.

Caring

"The caring nurse keeps promises made to patients and respects patient confidences."

5. *Fidelity*—To keep promises made to patients and to respect the patient's confidences. *Example:* There are times when patients may ask the nurse to bring some item (newspaper, deck of cards, Bible) to them. The nurse always agrees to try. If for some reason the nurse forgets to keep the promise, the nurse/patient relationship may be jeopardized.
6. *Justice*—To treat all, including older adults, with dignity and respect. Equal and fair treatment is given for all. *Example:* Society has a moral obligation to ensure that everyone has access to adequate care without being subject to excessive burdens (President's Commission for the Study of Ethical Problems in Medicine and Biomedical and Behavioral Research, 1983).
7. *Distributive justice*—To distribute equally resources and benefits to all, with equal treatment for all. *Example:* A 67-year-old man who is awaiting a kidney transplant should receive the next available kidney if his name is next on the waiting list. His age should not be a deterrent to receiving this valuable resource that is needed to save his life. He has been on the list for 5 years.

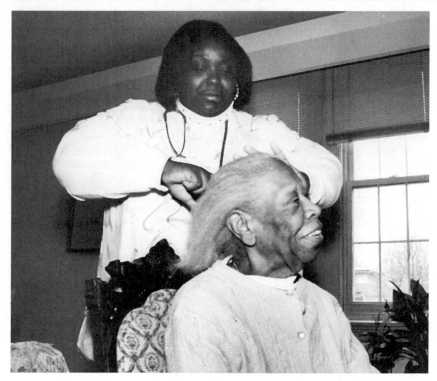

Any information shared by a patient must be kept in strictest confidence.

8. *Nonmaleficence*—To abstain from doing any harm to those older adults in our care. *Example:* A health care professional would abstain from leaving a frail older adult patient unattended in a bathtub during morning care for however short a period of time.

Ethical Concerns

The new field of bioethics has addressed several topics that are intrinsic to health care. Among these are confidentiality, informed consent, disclosure, and invasion of privacy.

Confidentiality means respect for all privileged information about the patient. *Privileged* means that information a patient shares with a member of the health team is kept in strictest confidence. To receive such personal information from another person is a privilege, and the information gained must not be repeated or shared with others, unless not sharing the information would or could be detrimental to the patient's well-being (e.g., "Do not tell my doctor that I don't take my digoxin at home").

▨ EXAMPLE

Nursing students are constantly reminded by their instructors not to discuss their patients while riding on the elevator or sitting in the hospital cafeteria or lobby, because no one knows who might overhear the conversation, thus causing a problem of breach of confidentiality.

Although confidentiality is almost always considered to be good, there are situations in which the greatest good for the greatest number (utilitarian approach) may outweigh the value of keeping a confidence.

▨ EXAMPLE

In the AIDS epidemic, which has been both a medical and social occurrence, confidentiality has been broken to warn others of the danger of infection. Health care professionals argue that if this had been done in the early stages of the public health problem instead of waiting for legislation freeing physicians from liability, AIDS may not have reached its present epidemic proportions.

Informed consent is based on the autonomy of the individual and means that, as long as the patient is able to comprehend information given, all procedures must be completely explained and cannot be implemented without the patient's expressed or written consent. Nurses are often requested to witness patient signatures on documents for consent to medical and surgical procedures. Nurses may explain procedures again to the patient for reinforcement.

▆ EXAMPLE

No surgical procedure can take place without informed consent (otherwise, the surgeon will be liable for damages) except in the event of a life-threatening emergency, when the individual may be unconscious and it is necessary to intervene before consent can be obtained (beneficence).

Disclosure is providing adequate understandable information so that patients will be able to make health care decisions (autonomy).

▆ EXAMPLE

Physicians inform an 80-year-old woman that she has breast cancer. Literature is supplied to assist in the description of this health problem. A decision has to be made by the patient concerning which treatment or intervention modalities she will choose or whether she will choose no treatment if the options are not expected to prolong her life or alleviate the symptoms.

Some ethical concerns are listed below:

1. Is disclosure part of self-determination/autonomy?
2. Should the patient's family be included in disclosure?
3. What is the family's role in this health care decision?
4. Should the health care team influence the patient in any way? (paternalism)

Invasion of privacy is the act of intruding into a patient's private affairs, belongings, or personhood. These actions can cause the patient feelings of discomfort or humiliation (loss of autonomy) if done without the patient's implicit consent. Examples include

- Health care personnel searching through an older individual's belongings
- Taking, removing, or misplacing the individual's belongings without permission
- Requiring the individual to wear institutional clothing rather than personal clothing
- Publicizing the individual's private affairs and clinical information, verbally or in writing

▆ NURSING ETHICS

Care of older people is an ethical problem for western society to face now (Matteson et al., 1997). The field of ethics includes the study of morality and the ethics of care. The ethics of care is a relatively new body of moral reflection. *Ethics of care* focuses on a set of character traits that virtually all people deeply value in close personal relationships: empathy, compassion, fidelity, love, and intimacy. The care perspective is especially important in the roles of nurse, physician, and family members (Beauchamp and Walters, 1994).

Moral choices are made by the nurse as the individual who is "caring" (advocate). The nurse assists the patient working through a morally demanding situation by being a caring individual and building a reciprocal relationship in which the patient and nurse learn to trust each other. This relationship helps the patient and the nurse to identify together what is best, in accordance with the patient's values, beliefs, feelings, and goals in the specific situation.

C a r i n g

❝*The nurse assists the patient working through a morally demanding situation by being a caring individual and building a reciprocal relationship in which the patient and nurse learn to trust each other.*❞

The ANA Code for Nurses with Interpretive Statements (1985) provides guidelines primarily based on ethical principles. The eleven statements in the code may be roughly divided into those that pertain to

- Clients' rights and safety
- Professional obligations and responsibilities
- Obligations to society and the nursing profession

Ethical responsibilities of nurses to their clients include competence and knowledge. For nurses to function more effectively as ethical agents, changes must take place in nursing education and public policy (e.g., curriculum changes, legislation). Inherent ethical responsibilities of nurses include

- Patient advocacy
- Accountability
- Peer reporting

Advocacy is the act of informing and supporting individuals so they can make the best decisions possible for themselves. After the decision is made, the advocate supports the individual in the decision. What are the ethical implications involved in assuming the advocate role? They include confidentiality, disclosure, veracity, fidelity, and autonomy.

Accountability is the demonstration of a willingness by the health care professional to assume responsibility for care given to older adults. Nurses, as licensed health care professionals, are accountable to the older adult for the care they give. Accountability is also required by health care institutions, state boards of nursing, and society. In conjunction with accountability is *peer reporting*. This is a conflictual situation in which behavior or actions by a professional peer may be harmful to a patient, health care professionals, or others; thus, it bears reporting. Health care professionals should not feel intimidated or coerced, but as part of ethical considerations influencing patient care they have a responsibility to report any behavior by another health care professional that is deemed harmful or dangerous to the older adult.

In addition to the codes already discussed, the ANA's *Ethics in Nursing: Position* Statements and Guidelines *(1984–1988) provides the ANA's position on the following issues:*

- Withdrawing or withholding food and fluids (1988)

- Professional risk versus moral responsibility in providing nursing care (1988)
- The ethics of safeguarding client health and safety (1986)
- Mechanism by which state nurses' associations can consider ethical issues and concerns (1985)
- Statements on the nonnegotiable nature of the ANA Code for Nurses, nurses' participation in capital punishment, and nurses' participation on institutional ethics committees (1984, 1988, 1983)

These guidelines were prepared by the ANA Committee on Ethics in Nursing (1984–1988). This document should be used in conjunction with the policies of the geriatric setting or institution. It is the nurse's responsibility to be aware of updated information and policies.

Allocation of scarce services, chronic illness, terminal illness, patients' rights, use of life-support measures, and orders to discontinue feedings are issues impacting nursing ethics. Conflicts may emerge from the nurse's dual responsibilities as a patient advocate and as an employee responsible for carrying out the physician's order and/or the institution's policies.

Ethical Issues in Gerontological Nursing

Autonomy is a central value in U.S. society. Health care ethics has been dominated by the issue of personal autonomy during the past two decades (Hofland, 1994), challenging the paternalism of medicine and fostering an emphasis on the patient as decision maker. Focus on autonomy as the essential ethical force shaping codes of patients' rights led to specific legislation in the 1991 Patient Self-Determination Act (Mezey et al., 1994). What, then, is the ethical responsibility of the gerontological nurse related to patient autonomy?

An evolution has taken place from strong medical paternalism to strong patient autonomy. In the 1960s, physicians began to see their power challenged by patients who wanted to take charge of, or at least participate in, medical decisions (Schneiderman, 1994). Often, just by virtue of their advancing age, older adults are placed in vulnerable and dependent positions. Moody (1992) asked whether autonomy can be upheld for patients at a time when their dependency on others makes autonomy least attainable, and when other needs for care and respect are more pressing.

The ethics involved in these gerontological nursing dilemmas prompts the development of ethics committees whose responsibility it is to address these issues in a manner that is fair and equitable. Older adult patients may have representation on ethics committees. This ensures that patients' rights will be acknowledged. Patients have a right to make decisions, and nurses have an obligation to uphold those rights.

Many specialty groups have developed published lists of rights for patients. With chronically ill patients, ethical issues are becoming increasingly complex. Ethical problems (dilemmas) are often shaped by issues of race, class, gender, ethnicity, education, power, personal history, emotional availability, and the effects of medical staff scheduling (Dubler, 1994).

EXAMPLE

A 63-year-old male Chinese immigrant is admitted to the surgical intensive care unit (SICU) with a diagnosis of hemorrhagic peritonitis and renal failure. He is visited daily by his wife. Neither of them speaks much English. They are overwhelmed by the constant rotation of medical and nursing personnel, some of whom do not even try to communicate with them. Rules in the SICU permit visits at specific time intervals. None of the staff has exclusive and primary responsibility for the patient. Staff are of several ethnic groups, none of them Chinese. The patient's condition becomes worse. Staff meet with the wife and suggest transferring the patient to another unit to ensure comfort measures while he awaits death. The wife, through an interpreter, states that she has no one else and requests all possible interventions. Culturally, to talk about dying and death is taboo, so this situation is frightening for the wife. Additionally, to contradict a physician is seen as causing dishonor or embarrassment and this causes discomfort for the wife.

One bioethical concept arising in the preceding example is paternalism, while issues abound of race, ethnicity, class, gender, education, power, ineffective communication techniques, and inconsistencies in medical staff scheduling and rotation.

Caring

"Protecting the patient's rights should be among the goals that gerontological nurses aspire to achieve for the older adults in their care."

EXAMPLE

How do gerontological nurses tell elderly Chinese, Mexican, Korean, or Italian patients that in the United States the law requires "informed consent" from the patient, and thus the patient must be given all information about his of her condition (disclosure)? Should strategies be devised whereby cultural differences can be accommodated, with the understanding that being respectful involves recognizing patients for their uniqueness, including their cultural context? What about family members who do not want their elderly relative to know the diagnosis?

EXAMPLE

A difficult problem occurs when family members want to keep a poor prognosis from the patient and the patient does not speak English. If a family member serves as interpreter the patient will probably not be told the truth. More serious is the fact that the health care professionals will have no way of knowing whether the patient wants truthful information about the condition (veracity) and the right to make their own decisions about health care and treatment (autonomy). It cannot be assumed that because the individual comes from a culture in which patients generally are not told the truth, and the patient's family does not want the truth told, that this particular patient does not want to know the truth. When a patient's family insists on withholding information from the patient or shielding the patient from information, health care professionals are forced to confront a conflict in the concept of patient autonomy. These are compelling ethical issues.

In the United States, bioethics and the law adopt the view that respect for patient autonomy requires that patients be told everything about their condition and that each patient is the only legitimate decision-maker about treatment or nontreatment (Michel, 1994). Nurses face a multiplicity of ethical problems. They must be familiar with the issues involved in their practice. Ethical issues, conflicts, and problems lead to ethical dilemmas.

Ethical Dilemmas

An **ethical dilemma** is a perplexing situation necessitating a choice between unpleasant alternatives. Ethical dilemmas abound in all geriatric care settings. They arise when there are conflicts (ethical issues) of values, obligations, and loyalties among and within various groups. They generally create an emotionally charged situation. Ethical dilemmas frequently facing health care professionals who work with older adult patients arise in the following areas:

- Death and assisted suicide
- Competency of the individual to process information and make decisions
- Disclosure of health information. Is family included?
- Distribution of scarce resources. There is someone on the transplant list for 5 years who is now 63 years old. Should he receive the next available organ? How are resources allocated?

An ethical dilemma exists when

- A specific ethical conflict arises
- Information, evidence, assessment presented by all involved are not conclusive as to what is morally right and morally wrong
- The health care professional believes that the situation requires imminent action

Some ethical dilemmas facing nurses are listed below:

1. Informed consent for the use of life-sustaining treatment. How much information is understood by the patient and the patient's family *before* they consent to the treatment?
2. Use of restraints and patient autonomy. The patient has a right to refuse. Staff and family can uphold the patient's rights while expressing fear of injury to the patient with repercussions to staff and institution. What are the risks and benefits? What would you do if the patient's care plan included use of restraints?

3. Safety of the patient and the environment. Is the nurse responsible to the patient or to the employing institution in the use of restraints?
4. Nutritional support (which can be a requirement of the courts and seen as an act of beneficence) to a patient who may be comatose and dying.
5. Mechanical ventilation can be interpreted as an act of beneficence.
6. Resuscitation is usually implemented routinely unless there is a do-not-resuscitate (DNR) order. Can this be justified at all times? For example, what about someone with multiple injuries or systems failure who does not have a DNR order?
7. Advance directives are usually required on admission. These documents state a patient's wishes for treatment before a crisis occurs. What is the nurse's responsibility should a patient not want to prepare an advance directive?
8. Withdrawal of/or withholding treatment. If a nurse participates in this act, is it practicing against the principle of nonmaleficence?
9. "Right to die" versus ethics of terminal care. Is this a situation of patient autonomy? If the nurse believes in the patient's right to die, can nonmaleficence be explained? Can palliative care be an alternative?

How can nurses intervene within the complexity of ethical dilemmas? For gerontological nurses to function more effectively as ethical agents, and to manage or reduce their stress, it is suggested that enhanced social support networks, counseling, and help from support groups be sought.

In an ethical dilemma every choice has both risks and benefits. Ethical dilemmas do not have prescribed answers. It is helpful to discuss the critical elements, summarize the processes, and analyze the situation before a resolution can occur through ethical decision-making by an ethics committee. The nurse has a responsibility to protect the rights of older adults (advocacy) while mediating between professional obligations and the rights and interests of society (ANA Code for Nurses, 1985).

The role of the family is another potential factor in the development of an ethical problem. The President's Commission (1983) has identified the family as an important source of information and declared that it plays a significant role in the health care decision-making process for the following reasons. The family

- Is generally most concerned about the good of the patient
- Will usually be most knowledgeable about the patient's goals, preferences, and values
- Deserves recognition as an important social unit
- Is a responsible decision-maker in matters that ultimately affect its members

Health care personnel should be aware that families express fear of reprisal when the family has chosen not to follow the recommended plan of care. Families can experience fear, anger, frustration, fatigue, guilt, grief, and financial strain, which compound the difficult decisions that must be made regarding an older adult relative.

One element that may assist in resolving an ethical problem is the presence of an advance directive or the appointment of a substitute decision-maker for the older adult patient. **Advance directives** are legal documents that specify the individual's wishes for treatment before a crisis occurs. Common advance directives include the living will, the health care proxy, the durable power of attorney for health care, and the do-not-resuscitate order (which may be a choice listed on a living will). For more about these, see Chapter 4.

An advance directive can be revoked or canceled by the person who executed it or by contacting the primary care provider. If the individual moves to another state, the laws of that state should be checked to see if the advance directive is honored in the new state (Uniform Rights of the Terminally Ill Act, 1987).

These advance directives provide a means of extending personal autonomy into situations where the individual is not capable of participating actively in the treatment decision. The presence of an advance directive does not, however, necessarily simplify an ethical dilemma, for the following reasons:

1. It may have been signed years before the event occurred.
2. Patient and family may fear that the directive could be prematurely used.
3. Dilemmas affect the patient, the family, and the staff.
4. The language used in the document may be vague.

5. The directives may be in opposition to the family's beliefs.
6. There may be new treatments since the document was signed.

Most older adults have been contributing to society all their lives in various ways, including working in paying jobs, homemaking, becoming parents, and raising children who are now productive. Their contribution may be different now from when they were younger, but they can continue to contribute their knowledge, wisdom, and experience to others in their roles as grandparents, volunteers, consultants, mentors, and church members. Some groups believe that older adults are therefore due their share of societal goods and services according to their needs to maintain their health and autonomy (Moody, 1992).

W e l l n e s s

❝Most older adults have been contributing to society all their lives in various ways, including working in paying jobs, homemaking, becoming parents, and raising children who are now productive.**❞**

Some provocative questions that present ethical concerns for health care personnel, social ethicists, and legislators are listed below:

1. Can Americans afford to grow old?
2. What is "fair and equitable" distribution of public resources among age groups (distributive justice)?
3. Who appoints the decision-makers (ethics committee) for the ethical decision-making?
4. What should be the ages of the ethics committee members who will make decisions affecting the lives of older adults?
5. Can penicillin for treatment of pneumonia, for example, be withheld from an otherwise healthy 90 year old (rationing resources on the basis of chronological age)?
6. Indeed, can health care be rationed on the grounds of age (resource allocation)? Rationing is sometimes proposed as a means to increase access to some health care services without requiring a corresponding increase in overall health care spending.

An example is the rationing plan in the Oregon Basic Health Services Act of 1989, which was designated in part to provide access to "basic" health care for *uninsured* Oregonians (Klevit, 1991).

7. Should people have the right to end their own lives (autonomy "right to die")?
8. Should families provide for their own members (a standard in many parts of the world)?

Caring

" *Caring includes respecting the older adult's rights to make health care decisions—including the right to refuse care, medications, and treatments.* "

Ethics Committees

Ethics committees have arisen in response to new dilemmas in health care. Before technological advances, dilemmas rarely arose. The main role of an ethics committee is to use the ethical principles of beneficence and justice in solving ethical dilemmas. An ethics committee consists of multidisciplinary professionals who are uninvolved with the patient whose case is brought before the committee. This allows for objectivity, insight, and support in conflict resolution. The composition of the committee can include nurses, physicians, administrators, social workers, clergy, trustees, attorneys, ethicists, patient advocates, community representatives, and competent older adult patients.

Committee members should have at least basic ethical knowledge. Such knowledge includes

- Moral beliefs and a value system (i.e., the individual's morals and values)
- Professional codes of conduct (e.g., ANA Code for Nurses)
- Institutional/governmental policies (e.g., hospital policies, federal and state policies) and legal implications if these policies are not adhered to
- Concepts of beneficence, autonomy or self-

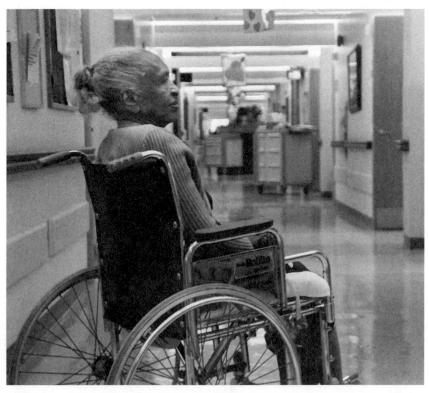

Entering a residential facility inevitably raises issues of autonomy that must be addressed with the utmost respect and sensitivity.

determination, truthfulness or veracity, confidentiality, justice (i.e., ethical principles as taught in the nursing curriculum)

Patients' rights committees are established by institutions that have populations at risk, such as chronically ill older adults (e.g., patients' rights committees and residents' councils found in nursing homes). Ethics committees help to protect the rights of individuals who may be unable to speak for themselves and who may not have advance directives. The committee also protects the rights of nurses who may have divided feelings about the benefit of treatments ordered for the patient or nontreatment.

Hospital administrators are cautioned to pay careful attention to the make-up of interdisciplinary teams. The following are some concerns:

1. Do the committee members have the ability to talk and work together?
2. Do the committee members possess the basic ethical knowledge required?
3. How do the committee members view aging and older adults?

Ethics committees serve several functions, including

- Resolving ethical dilemmas
- Providing a forum for discussion of ethical issues
- Serving as a resource to assist health care professionals with ethical decision-making

Ethical Decision-Making

Steps taken in the decision-making process to resolve an ethical dilemma include the following:

1. Gathering information, identifying the problem/situation/dilemma
2. Discussing the dilemma with others. Several individuals and points of view are involved. Opposing sides present rational arguments.
3. Recognizing the ethical issue or issues; defining the value conflict
4. Analyzing the facts. Who has the right to make the decision?
5. Weighing the alternatives and deciding which action is fair
6. Incorporating an ethic of care that includes compassion, discernment of the patients' wishes, and the patients' best interests

7. Implementing the decided course of action; offering support and reassurance to the patient, family, and staff
8. Evaluating the results

An ethical decision leads to action that is morally right. The foremost objectives must be the very best standard for patient care. Inclusion of patients whenever possible and of families when patients are not competent is of importance in the decision-making process. The solution is based on what is the best outcome for the patient, not on what is "best" for the patient. Special respect should be given to religious perspectives of the older adult.

▨ THE EXPANDED ROLE OF NURSES

Older adult patients are frequent care recipients and use most of the services in acute-care facilities; long-term care facilities; public health, home health, and ambulatory-care settings; critical care units; psychiatric inpatient units; and community mental health centers. Virtually all nurses in the United States spend some time in caring for older adults.

W e l l n e s s

"Patients want to know more about health care and to participate more fully in decisions concerning their health and welfare."

Knowledge of nursing ethics concerning health care needs is essential. The expanded role of the nurse has increased the number and diversity of ethical dilemmas to be encountered in practice. Patients want to know more about health care and to participate more fully in decisions concerning their health and welfare, including assisted suicide and the "right to die." Society is becoming more informed regarding state laws such as the California Natural Death Act (1976), the New York State Do Not Resuscitate Law (1988), the report provided by the President's Commission for the Study of Ethical Problems in Medicine and Biomedical and Behavioral Research (1982), and the 1991 Refusal of Treatment legislation and Update for 1991. The federal Patient Self-Determination Act requires all hospitals and nursing homes that receive federal funds to inform their patients of their legal right to prepare advance directives. This is the first federal statute to focus on advance directives and the rights of adults to refuse life-sustaining treatment (Wolfe, 1994).

In the 1960s and 1970s the respirator (or ventilator) and the kidney dialysis machine were the major foci of ethical debate. These therapies are usually implemented by nurses. In the late 1980s and early l990s, new modes of providing long-term nutrition and hydration to unconscious patients provoked intense discussion in hospitals, nursing homes, academic circles, and the courts (Beauchamp and Walters, 1994). These are also therapies administered by nurses in any setting, including the home and the workplace.

An intervention in which nurses *cannot* participate has to do with euthanasia. Any such action, including making a decision to perform euthanasia or administering a lethal drug, is forbidden to nurses (Nightingale pledge, 1893; ANA Code for Nurses, 1985).

Euthanasia is derived from a Greek term meaning "the good death." Central to most arguments for euthanasia is the principle of autonomy or self-determination; however, Callahan (1992) states that euthanasia is also a matter of social decision between two people, the one to be killed and the other to do the killing.

In 1989 in New York City, the Society for the Right to Die convened a special panel of 12 prominent doctors that proclaimed that it is ethical for doctors to help terminal patients commit suicide (Kevorkian, 1991). Nurses caught on the front line of daily care and having close involvement with patients, and being valuable sources of information and experience, should be involved in the process of decision-making about euthanasia. However, they should not be asked to decide or participate in the act.

The nurse must consider whether the patient is acting under free will (autonomy) or being pressured by anyone and whether the patient has carefully considered the situation and knows the options. If there is any question, it is the duty of the nurse to bring the situation to the attention of the medical team (Humphry, 1991).

Voluntary euthanasia, the process by which the physician must provide both the means and the actual conduct of the final act, greatly amplifies the physician's power over the patient and increases the risk of error, coercion, or abuse (Humphry, 1991).

Passive euthanasia is the process of allowing the patient to die by disconnection of the life support system (this is legally permissible [Uniform Durable Power of Attorney Act, 1983]) (Humphry, 1991).

Active euthanasia is the process of helping a person to die by administrating a lethal drug. (This might be a borderline criminal action until the law forbidding assistance in suicide is changed [Humphry, 1991].)

Assisted suicide is the process of getting some assistance from another person in taking one's own life.

In 1994, legislation was passed in Oregon permitting physicians to "aid in dying to qualified citizens requesting such assistance." The law has yet to be enacted (National League for Nursing, 1995), owing to legal challenges, providing a window of opportunity for study of its potential effect on all health care providers including nurses.

Because other states are considering similar legislation, the National League for Nursing, in 1995, established a task force on "Decision about Assisted Suicide for Terminally Ill Patients." The task force will work to ensure that "nurses are able to assert their right to act on moral choices and have those choices honored without recrimination" (NLN Update, 1995).

In 1997, the Supreme Court of the United States settled one of the most contentious ethical, moral, and legal questions of recent decades, deciding that states may ban doctor-assisted suicide (Greenhouse L., June 27, 1997, N.Y. Times). But the ruling did not settle one of the most pressing crises in modern medicine: inadequate care of patients at the end of life.

While ethicists and lawyers have been debating the right to die, physicians have been busy examining their practices. One physician said "The public is demanding assisted suicide because they are afraid of the quality of end-of-life care. There is a demand for palliative care" (Stolberg, 1997).

Palliative care of the dying has been ignored by most American physicians, not been taught in medical schools, and not been recognized as a specialty in the United States, although it is a specialty in Great Britain and Australia. However, palliative care teams have emerged on the scene. In New York, the United Hospital Fund is financing a $1.1 million effort to install palliative care in five city hospitals (Stolberg, 1997).

Gerontological nurses face many ethical problems as the population ages. They have always included palliative care in their nursing practice, and it is hoped they will continue to do so as part of their professional role (ANA Code for Nurses, 1985); they are the experts in palliative care and are able to teach other health care team members.

The 21st century is approaching rapidly, and projected numbers of older adults and the ethical issues pertaining to them will be challenging, and perhaps sometimes overwhelming. Ethical issues will be ever-evolving, and the health care worker has been thrown into the decision-making process either as a participant, an advocate, or an implementor of the decision made.

W e l l n e s s

❝*It is important to remember that currently more than half of older adults in our society are maintaining their good health.*❞

Summary

The role of ethics in the care of older adults is challenging and needs to be explored in detail. Ethical dilemmas require attention by ethicists, health care professionals, family members, and older adult patients. Educated consumers, better informed health care professionals, legislation, and professional codes of ethics contribute to the making of crucial ethical decisions.

The sophistication of health care today has expanded and complicated the ethical dilemma nurses face. Moral rights and responsibilities of health care professionals, their patients, and the patients' families are upheld through the process of ethical decision-making.

In this chapter, ethical principles were presented in relation to the ethical decisions that nurses must make when working with older adult patients. It is important to maintain the individual's potential throughout the life span, improving quality of life, enhancing positive mental and physical health, and bringing fulfillment to lives. This is accomplished through caring actions, based on nursing knowledge. Additionally, protecting the patient's rights should be among the goals that gerontological nurses aspire to achieve for the older adults in their care.

REFERENCES

Aaron H, Schwartz W. (1984). The Painful Prescription: Rationing Hospital Care. Washington, DC: Brookings Institution.

American Nurses' Association. (1984–1988). Ethics in Nursing: Position Statements and Guidelines. Kansas City, MO: American Nurses' Association.

American Nurses' Association. (1985). Code for Nurses with Interpretive Statements, p 1. Kansas City, MO: American Nurses' Association.

Beauchamp T, Walters L, eds. (1994). Contemporary Issues in Bioethics. 4th ed. Belmont, CA: Wadsworth.

Callahan D. (May/April 1992). When self-determination runs amok. Hastings Center Rep 22(2):52–55.

Dubler N. (Winter 1994). Editorial. Generations 18(4).

Greenhouse L. (June 27, 1997). Court 90 upholds state laws prohibiting assisted suicide. The New York Times.

Hofland B. (Winter 1994). When capacity fades and autonomy is constricted: A client-centered approach to residential care. Generations 18(4):31–35.

Humphry D. (1991). Final exit: The practicalities of self-deliverance and assisted suicide for the dying. New York: The Hemlock Society, Carol Publishing.

International Council for Nurses. (September 1953). International code of nursing ethics. Am J Nurs 53:1070.

International Council for Nurses. (1973). Code for Nurses. Geneva, Switzerland: International Council for Nurses.

Kevorkian J. (1991). Prescription: Medicide, The Goodness of Planned Death: New York: Prometheus.

Klevit H. (1991). Prioritization of health care services: A progress report by the Oregon Health Services Commission. Arch Intern Med 151:912–916.

Matteson M, McConnell E, Linton A. (1997). Gerontological Nursing Concepts and Practice., 2nd ed. Philadelphia: WB Saunders.

Mezey M, Ramsey G, Mitty E. (Winter 1994). Making the patient self-determination act work for the elderly. Generations 18(4):13–18.

Michel V. (Winter 1994). Factoring ethnic and racial differences into bioethics decision making. Generation 18(4):23–26.

Moody H. (1992). Ethics in an aging society. Baltimore: Johns Hopkins University Press.

National League for Nursing. (October 1995). Update: Connecting members of the National League for Nursing. New York: National League for Nursing.

President's Commission for the Study of Ethical Problems in Medicare and Biomedical and Behavioral Research. (1981). Defining Death. Washington, DC: U.S. Government Printing Office.

President's Commission for the Study of Ethical Problems in Medicare and Biomedical and Behavioral Research. (1983). Deciding to Forgo Life-Sustaining Treatment:

Ethical, Medical, and Legal Issues in Treatment Decision. Washington, DC: U.S. Government Printing Office.

Schneiderman L. (Winter 1994). Medical futility and aging: Ethical implications. Generations 18(4):61–65.

Stolberg S. (June 30, 1997). Cries of the dying awaken doctors to a new approach. The New York Times.

U.S. Department of Health and Human Services. (December 1991). Vital and health statistics: Current estimates for the National Health Survey Series 10: Data from the National Health Survey, No. 181, p 106. Hyattsville, MD: DHHS, publication No. 92–1509.

Uniform Durable Power of Attorney Act. (1983). Uniform Durable Power of Attorney Act 8A, U.L.A.

Uniform Rights of the Terminally Ill Act. (1987). Uniform Rights of the Terminally Ill Act 9B, U.L.A.

Wicclair M. (1993). Ethics and the Elderly. New York: Oxford University Press.

Wolfe S. (1994). Sources of concern about the Patient Self-Determination Act. In Beauchamp T, Walters L, eds.

Contemporary Issues in Bioethics. 4th ed. Belmont, CA: Wadsworth.

SUGGESTED READINGS AND RESOURCES

Ethical Dilemmas. (March 1995). Am J Nurs 95(3):656.

Ethical Dilemmas. (March 1996). Am J Nurs 96(3):62–64.

Ethical Dilemmas. (May 1996). Am J Nurs 96(5):66–67.

Murphy P, Price D. (1995). ACT: Taking a positive approach to end-of-life care. Am J Nurs 95(3):42–43.

Oldaker S. (May/June 1996). Legal and ethical issues: Flexibility and faithfulness. J Prof Nurs 2(3):129.

If you have a question on professional or clinical ethics, write to Ethical Dilemmas, American Journal of Nursing, 555 West 57th Street, New York, NY 10019-2961.

CRITICAL THINKING EXERCISES

Mr. Stone is a 76-year-old man with a below-the-knee amputation. He is alert, oriented, and uses a wheelchair for mobility. Mrs. Rose is 79 years of age with dementia that results in periods of confusion and disorientation. Both residents live on the same unit. Mr. Stone has a private room, whereas Mrs. Rose shares a room with another woman. Mrs. Rose frequently visits Mr. Stone in his room. One day a nurse found Mrs. Rose and Mr. Stone in his bed and engaging in sexual activity. The nurse returned Mrs. Rose to her own room.

Mrs. Rose's son visits often and would sometimes meet his mother in Mr. Stone's room. However, one day another resident told him that his mother was "carrying on with the man." The son was upset that he had not been told, and stated strongly that staff should restrict his mother's visits to Mr. Stone.

1. As the nurse in this facility, should you have removed Mrs. Rose to her own room? How should you have made this decision?

2. Despite some disabilities, do these residents have a right to privacy in expressing their sexuality?

3. Under what guidelines would the nursing staff be obliged to inform Mrs. Rose's son? Is there more than one source for determining this obligation?

4. Does her son have the right to restrict Mrs. Rose's visits to Mr. Stone? State the source(s) of your opinion.

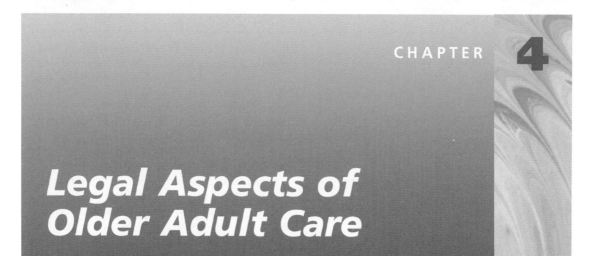

CHAPTER 4

Legal Aspects of Older Adult Care

Vimala Philipose, RN, BSN, MSN, PhD

CHAPTER OUTLINE

OBJECTIVES

After studying this chapter, the reader should be able to:

1. Apply the principle of informed consent to the situation of an 88-year-old woman with dementia who is living in a residential care facility.
2. Formulate a plan for assessing the competency of a 68-year-old patient exhibiting confusion who is refusing treatment for colon cancer. Who should carry out this plan?
3. Differentiate between the living will and the durable power of attorney for health care.
4. Conduct a class discussion of euthanasia and bring the latest controversial issues into the debate.
5. Write a teaching plan for nurses to assess and formulate therapeutic interventions for elder abuse.
6. Develop a module on prevention of elder abuse.
7. Discuss alternatives to the uses of physical and chemical restraints and prioritize their appropriateness.

KEY TERMS

advance directives
competency
do-not-resuscitate (DNR) order
durable power of attorney for health care (DPAHC)
elder abuse
euthanasia
informed consent
living will

Since the 1980s there has been an effort in the United States to address legal issues that are specific to older adults. This effort has resulted, for example, in protection against elder abuse through legislation and policy decisions. In the mid 1980s, both state and federal governments focused on legal and ethical issues, including patients' rights and end-of-life decisions. Although these issues are of concern to all age groups in a just society, the problems to be addressed in this chapter impact older adults directly and profoundly. Today's nurses and other health care professionals are challenged by the increasing attention being paid to legal issues facing older adults.

As has been noted earlier, many older adults continue to maintain health throughout old age. But, because people are living so much longer (see Chapter 1), an increase can be anticipated in the number and incidence of disorders and disabilities that may seriously incapacitate some older adults, negatively affecting their quality of life and their coping mechanisms. When older adults are faced with serious illness or other incapacity, they may react with confusion and dismay, which leaves them vulnerable to others and to the environment. Therefore it is important that these individuals have support and advocacy from nurses and other caregivers as well as adequate recourse under the law. In addition, legal issues arising at the end of life often require the involvement of nurses because so many individuals die in hospitals and other health care settings.

The focus in this chapter is on the topics of informed consent, autonomy, advance directives (including durable powers of attorney and living wills), patients' rights, elder abuse, and the use of restraints. Also addressed are the ways in which nurses can be patient advocates in legal and ethical issues. Many older adults lack information about their rights or the nature of the lifesaving procedures available to them and thus need an advocate for protection and information. The nurse is uniquely positioned and qualified to be this advocate.

Modern medical technology and increased emphasis on cost containment have resulted in new trends in health care delivery and raised issues related to patient autonomy. This frequently becomes an issue for the frail elderly when mental competency becomes questionable. Physicians, nurses, other health care professionals, and the public are facing new challenges raised by these issues. Professionals may experience difficulty in resolving ethical dilemmas and making decisions in these emotionally charged issues. Ethical dilemmas and situations in which legal and ethical issues are in conflict further complicate nurses' decision-making processes as they try to advocate for their patients. An example of such a dilemma is the situation in which a patient who is not terminally ill refuses treatment for a treatable problem. A conflict then arises between the principle of beneficence (doing good, and no harm, to the patient) and the principle of autonomy (respecting the patient's right to decide). Currently, a mentally competent person may refuse lifesaving treatment.

It is important that older adults be made aware of their rights and the need to take responsibility to ensure that their wishes regarding both health decisions and end-of-life issues will be carried out if they are no longer able to make these wishes known. In their advocacy role, nurses responsible for the care of older adults should see that the individuals' wishes are documented in their personal medical records; furthermore, nurses have a duty to make such directives known to other health care professionals involved in the patient's care.

The patient's physician is obligated to inform the patient of rights regarding options for treatment and to ensure that the person is freely consenting of his or her own volition (Goldstein, 1992). However, nurses must also participate by ensuring that the person fully understands the physician's explanation of the nature of the problem and treatment options. It is prudent that there be a balance between the patient's autonomy and the physician's beneficence. In the United States, greater attention is paid to the principle of autonomy than in some other countries. Respect for a patient's autonomy implies that the individual is free to make decisions based on values and beliefs deemed valid by the individual, which may or may not be shared by the health care professional. It is imperative that the older adult's belief system be respected and adhered to in every health care setting.

■ INFORMED CONSENT

The principle of **informed consent** requires that a physician or other health care provider disclose to patients the information necessary for them to make informed choices about their own health care. Historically, informed consent for medical purposes came into being after the Nuremberg trials of war criminals following World War II. The military tribunal that conducted the trial stated that the voluntary consent of each subject is essential; that is, the court found that the subjects of "medical experiments" should have had personal and legal capacity to give consent. Since then, informed consent has included three important elements: (1) the patient must understand the description of the medical procedure, including its risks, benefits, and alternatives; (2) the patient's consent must be voluntary; and (3) the patient must be mentally competent to give the consent (Janofsky, 1990). If the necessary information in the consent is not completely disclosed, there is a potential case of liability for negligence (Guido, 1997).

The patient must be free from coercion by health care professionals and others. However, in an emergency situation, the patient's preferences may be unobtainable because the patient is unconscious or the prognosis is unknown. In such an instance, the physician and other health care professionals generally would decide to preserve the patient's life but would also respect the patient's right to choose medical care, insofar as possible.

The nurse has a responsibility to communicate effectively with the patient in explaining the procedure; however, a patient's refusal of procedures in spite of the health care professional's explanation must be honored. The patient's refusal should be clearly documented in the chart. When the informed consent is signed by the patient in the presence of the health care provider, a witness should be present. Although the physician who prescribes the procedures (e.g., surgery, diagnostic tests) should personally obtain the signatures of the patient, in many instances nurses or other health care providers become surrogates in obtaining written consent. It is critical that the nurse execute that responsibility diligently.

W e l l n e s s

"*Friends and family are best served when healthy adults choose a surrogate or proxy for health care while they remain healthy.*"

Because the American population is becoming more culturally diverse, informed consent forms often need to be available in languages other than English (e.g., many institutions in communities having a significant Hispanic American population provide consent forms in Spanish). Because the old-old population (85 years of age and older) is increasing phenomenally, additional consideration should be given to consent within this group. In this oldest cohort there is a higher risk of cognitive impairment and an increased incidence of multiple chronic illnesses. These older adults may lack the competence to make decisions pertaining to their own health care. The patient must be assessed as to competency (discussed in the next section), and the consent should be read clearly, slowly, and distinctly.

There are those who argue that the very fact the patient is willing to undergo a medical procedure by his own volition indicates informed consent. However, this may not be validated in a court of law if there is a malpractice suit (Guido, 1997).

■ AUTONOMY

The principle of *autonomy* applies to all individuals who enter our health care system (see Chapter 3). However, it is particularly important that it be honored in dealing with older adults, who may experience periods of time when their coping mechanisms are stressed and their ability to care for self is compromised. In addition, each individual has specific preferences about issues surrounding death, and these should be spelled out in advance so that they may be honored. Autonomy encompasses the areas of self-determination, competency, and guardianship. (For definitions related to autonomy, see Box 4–1).

Patient Self-Determination Act (PSDA)

In the past decade, serious efforts have been made to address the legal and ethical issues concerning the elderly, especially in the health care arena (Drugay and Gallagher, 1993). In 1990, Congress passed the Patient Self-Determination Act (PSDA), which went into effect in 1991. This federal legislation mandates that health care institutions (e.g., hospitals, nursing homes, hospices, home health care agencies) receiving Medicare and Medicaid payments must explain to all patients on admission that they have the right to make decisions regarding their own medical care, including whether to accept or refuse treatment and the need to specify advance directives in writing (Swonger and Burbank, 1995). In addition to the federal guidelines, each state has legislated on issues of patient protection. In 1992 the American Nurses' Association (ANA) stated that nurses should be familiar with the laws of the states in which they practice. Health care professionals, including physicians, nurses, social workers,

---

Box 4-1   DEFINITIONS RELATED TO AUTONOMY

Competency. The capacity or ability to perform the task at hand and the ability to handle one's affairs in an adequate manner.

Durable power of attorney for health care (DPAHC). A person designated by a patient to make medical decisions in the event that the patient becomes mentally incompetent. The person could be a family member, lawyer, or friend. DPAHC differs from durable power of attorney, which may cover business or financial matters only.

Financial and property exploitation. An older adult's deprivation of money, property, or other valuables accomplished by stealth or converted to the use of another person by force or threats or by taking advantage of the older adult's trust. Such takeover activities may even include actual violence.

Guardianship. A method of legally appointing a substitute decision-maker. A guardian may make decisions beyond those that are exclusively health related.

Living will. A document stating in advance a person's wishes regarding a "natural" death and covering treatment choices including but not limited to blood products, antibiotics, hemodialysis, artificial hydration, and tube feeding, as well as withdrawal of life support.

Proxy or surrogate. A substitute to make health care decisions for another who is no longer able to express personal choices.

Risk. The probability or chance that harm, injury, danger, or loss will occur unless some action is taken.

Self-determination Act. Legislation in 1991 giving terminally ill patients the right to make their own health care choices. Every patient admitted to a hospital should be advised of this information for him or her to make an informed decision.

Verbal or psychological abuse. Includes threats of violence, name-calling, and threats of isolation and abandonment, causing fear, humiliation, or feeling of helplessness in the elderly. It can be a sudden outburst or a continual or prolonged process of abuse by the caregiver.

and others, should be familiar with the relevant laws and regulations specific to their state because the professional will need to counsel patients and their significant others regarding advance directives.

Competency

The legal concept of **competency** is the ability to handle one's own affairs in an adequate manner (Guido, 1997). When mental competency is in question, there must be a legal determination that requires a psychiatric evaluation and a competency hearing in a court of law. The patient's competence needs to be assessed both clinically and legally. The status of *competency at law* means that "the court has not declared the person incompetent, and the person is able to understand the consequences of his or her actions" (Guido, 1997). There are two exceptions to the legal adult's right to agree or refuse to give informed consent. These exceptions are when the patient has a court-appointed guardian or when the patient has granted another person a valid written power of attorney.

W e l l n e s s

❝ *The best time to prepare advance directives is while you are still in a state of mental and physical wellness.* ❞

Guardianship

If the court rules that an individual is *incompetent*, a guardian may be appointed as a surrogate decision-maker. The court-appointed guardian takes over the function of giving informed consent and can also function in aspects of the individual's life beyond health care issues. All documents should be reviewed to ensure that medical decisions are included in surrogate designations.

But the legal guardianship process is usually expensive, complex, and restrictive. Thus, some states have adopted a system to appoint a substitute decision-maker specifically for medical decision, with the court's involvement. For instance, two physicians (not the patient's primary care providers) give their opinions regarding the patient's competency. If, after their medical evaluation, they declare that the patient is disabled and incompetent, then the next of kin may be asked to make the decision(s) on the patient's behalf.

Guardians are usually selected or chosen from family members, because the law holds that family member(s) generally have the best interests of the patient at heart and also know the patient's wishes most accurately. However, this may not be true in all instances. The order of selection of family surrogates is usually the spouse, followed by the adult children or grandchildren, if available, followed by other relatives. The nurse or other health care provider should verify state laws regarding these judicial decisions because in some states family consent may not be valid. Problems may arise when there are disagreements or conflicts about the consent among family members regarding decisions made about the patient's treatments. This is especially true in the case of the older adult. There may be one adult child who is the caregiver (most often a daughter), and the rest of the siblings may live some distance away. These siblings may occasionally visit the parent but not be aware of or sensitive to the day-to-day problems of their parent, yet they are eager to offer solutions to problems. This is when conflict arises and the need for a single guardian or surrogate becomes important.

■ ADVANCE DIRECTIVES

When the patient is mentally competent, the court prefers a written statement from the patient detailing the patient's personal wishes. Such a statement is known as an *advance directive*, and laws regarding them are in place in 40 states. **Advance directives** are legally binding documents that allow *presently competent* patients to set forth in writing what medical procedures they would or would not want to have done if they were to become mentally incompetent in the future. This avoids the need for guardianship, and the guardian's need to make health care decisions based on inadequate information. The two most important types of advance directives are the living will and the durable power of attorney for health care (DPAHC). For an example of an advance directive that includes both a durable power of attorney for health care and a living will, see Box 4–2.

Living Will

The **living will** is a legal document that spells out the patient's right to a natural death. For example, the individual may have specified the use of pain medication only and directed caregivers not to use "heroic or extraordinary measures" to keep the patient alive. In most states, this document must be witnessed by two disinterested people and must also be notarized (Matteson, McConnell and Linton, 1997). If the document seems to be a valid expression of the patient's intent while the patient was competent, the living will is considered significant in any ruling by a court (Coordinating Council on Life-Sustaining Medical Treatment, 1991). Copies of the living will document should be given to the surrogate (sometimes called "proxy") and the physician, and a copy should be part of the patient's medical record if the patient is hospitalized (Steinbrook and Lo, 1984). Some states do not recognize this type of document (living-will legislation is specific to each state) but health care providers may choose to honor it.

Living wills should be very specific to be accurately implemented. One of the major problems at the present time is that the instructions are not specific enough. Nurses can play a very critical role in overseeing that the document is complete, clear, and specific enough to be implemented if and when indicated. Older adults and their families are encouraged to discuss their wishes regarding specific medical treatments and withholding of life-preserving measures when the patient has a terminal illness.

A **do-not-resuscitate (DNR) order** may be part of a living will. The DNR states that the in-

---

Box 4-2   ADVANCE DIRECTIVES

My Durable Power of Attorney for Health Care, Living Will, and Other Wishes
I, _____, write this document as a directive regarding my medical care.
Put the initials of your name by the choices you want.

Part I. My Durable Power of Attorney for Health Care.
_____ I appoint this person to make decisions about my medical care if there ever comes a time when I cannot make these decisions myself:
Name _____ Home phone _____ Work phone _____
Address _____
If the person above cannot or will not make decisions for me, appoint this person:
Name _____ Home phone _____ Work phone _____
Address _____
_____ I have not appointed anyone to make health care decisions for me in any other document.
_____ I want the person I have appointed, my doctors, my family, and others to be guided by the decisions I have made on the following pages.

Part II. My Living Will.
These are my wishes for my future medical care if there ever comes a time when I cannot make these decisions for myself.

A. These Are My Wishes If I Have a Terminal Condition:
LIFE-SUSTAINING TREATMENTS
_____ I do not want life-sustaining treatments (including CPR) started. If life-sustaining treatments are started, I want them stopped.
_____ I want life-sustaining treatments that my doctors think are best for me.
_____ Other wishes: _____

Box 4-2   ADVANCE DIRECTIVES, *Continued*

ARTIFICIAL NUTRITION AND HYDRATION

_____ I do not want artificial nutrition and hydration started if it would be the main treatment keeping me alive. If artificial nutrition and hydration is started, I want it stopped.
_____ Other wishes: _____

COMFORT CARE

_____ I want to be kept as comfortable and free of pain as possible, even if such care prolongs my dying or shortens my life.
_____ Other wishes: _____

B. These Are My Wishes If I Am Ever In a Persistent Vegetative State:

LIFE-SUSTAINING TREATMENTS

_____ I do not want life-sustaining treatments (including CPR) started. If life-sustaining treatments are started, I want them stopped.
_____ I want life-sustaining treatments that my doctors think are best for me.
_____ Other wishes: _____

ARTIFICIAL NUTRITION AND HYDRATION

_____ I do not want artificial nutrition and hydration started if it would be the main treatment keeping me alive. If artificial nutrition and hydration is started, I want it stopped.
_____ Other wishes: _____

COMFORT CARE

_____ I want to be kept as comfortable and free of pain as possible, even if such care prolongs my dying or shortens my life.
_____ Other wishes: _____

C. Other Directions

You have the right to be involved in all decisions about your medical care, even those not dealing with terminal conditions or persistent vegetative states. If you have wishes not covered in other parts of this document, please indicate them here.

_____

_____

_____

Part III. Other Wishes.

A. Organ Donation

_____ I do not wish to donate any of my organs or tissues.
_____ I want to donate all of my organs and tissues.
_____ I want to donate only these organs and tissues: _____
_____ Other wishes: _____

B. Autopsy

_____ I do not want an autopsy
_____ I agree to an autopsy if my doctors wish it.
_____ Other wishes: _____

Box continued on following page

Box 4-2   ADVANCE DIRECTIVES, *Continued*

If you wish to say more about any of the above choices, or if you have any other statements to make about your medical care, you may do so on a separate sheet of paper. If you do so, put here the number of pages you are adding: _____

PART IV. SIGNATURES.
You and two witness must sign this document for it to be legal.

A. Your Signature
By my signature below I show that I understand the purpose and the effect of this document.

Signature: _____ Date _____
Address: _____

B. Your Witnesses' Signatures
I believe the person who has signed this advance directive to be of sound mind, that he/she signed or acknowledged this advance directive in my presence, and that he/she appears not to be acting under pressure, duress, fraud, or undue influence. I am not related to the person making this advance directive by blood, marriage, or adoption, nor, to the best of my knowledge, am I named in his/her will. I am not the person appointed in this advance directive. I am not a health care provider or an employee of a health care provider who is now, or has been in the past, responsible or the care of the person making this advance directive.

Witness #1   Witness #2
Signature: _____ Date ____ Signature: _____ Date ____
Address: _____   Address: _____

---

dividual does not want to be revived by cardiopulmonary resuscitation (CPR), should breathing cease and the heart stop beating. DNR orders are usually written for terminally ill patients in a hospital or nursing home, but some states allow them to be used by people who want to ensure that they will not be revived if their breathing and heartbeats cease even though they may not be in a hospital or other health care setting.

The physician should review the older person's general health status and discuss the possible outcomes of resuscitation with the patient and family members. Although it is almost impossible to discuss all the possible outcomes with the patient, it is critical that the physician and patient have clear communication so that all decisions are made collaboratively with mutual consent. Older adults unable to make decisions for themselves should have given written consent or no consent for resuscitation and should appoint individuals as proxies to make decisions for them.

Durable Power of Attorney for Health Care

Individuals who are terminally ill or comatose may have, when they were competent, named a person to act on their behalf through a **durable power of attorney for health care (DPHAC)**. This written document authorizes one person to act in the place of, or on behalf of, another person (Uniform Durable Power of Attorney Act, 1983). It specifically applies to situations in which the person who conferred the power has become incapacitated or disabled, and in many states it is applicable to health treatment decisions. The surrogate should know the patient well, having paid particular attention to understanding the patient's values, philosophy, and preferences regarding end-of-life treatment decisions (Matteson, McConnell and Linton, 1997).

Surrogate, or proxy, appointments are made under the general durable power of attorney laws that are in place in all states. The document requires the signature of two witnesses to be valid. After a DPAHC is designated and when the patient is unable to make decisions, it is the physician's responsibility to obtain informed consent from the designated person. The DPAHC should be strongly encouraged to do what the patient would done; that is, the proxy must function in the best interest of the patient.

CPR and DNR Directives

In the absence of a living will, individuals may choose separate CPR or DNR documents that can be readily accessible for emergency care providers. Some experts recommend that this information be on the patient's Medic-Alert bracelet or included in some other form of identification on the person. This will equip the emergency care provider with a directive to not initiate CPR efforts. In most instances, the CPR directive (unlike the living will) is valid only when it is signed and dated by a physician (Goldstein, 1992). It is critical that the primary care physician explicitly convey the patient's wishes to the entire team of health care professionals who are responsible for the care of the patient.

> ### W e l l n e s s
>
> **"***Competent older adults have a right to make decisions about their own life and death. When a thoughtful decision is made by the patient, it should be honored.***"**

In situations in which a patient has written a blanket directive, some procedures can be either withheld or withdrawn. These include (1) closed-chest cardiac massage; (2) endotracheal intubation or other advanced airway management; (3) artificial ventilation; (4) defibrillation; and (5) cardiac resuscitation, drug therapy, or other resuscitation-related procedures. Comfort measures should be provided by the nurse according to the needs of the patient. These may include an open airway and nasal oxygen for easy breathing, frequent mouth care, change of position, medication to relieve pain, and emotional support for the patient and the family.

■ PATIENTS' RIGHTS

Patients' rights in all types of institutions are mandated by the U.S. Constitution and by state and federal laws. Legal rights might vary depending on the setting and the individual's competency. In 1972, the American Hospital Association spelled out its Patient's Bill of Rights (Box 4–3). Institutions are required to post the rights of patients where they are visible; they should be reviewed with the patient on admission. In spite of the existing mandates, there are some institutions that may not abide by these guidelines.

Specific guidelines protect the rights of impaired older adults. The facility's Resident Bill of Rights should be reviewed on admission with patient (if competent), guardian or surrogate, and the family. The setting should establish provision for legal documents regarding competency, guardianship, living will, and durable power of attorney for health care. It should determine the older resident's lifestyle preferences, should apply Standards of Gerontological Nursing Practice and the ANA code of ethics, and should demonstrate respect for the older adult's privacy and dignity (Ebersole and Hess, 1998).

At present, physicians have the primary responsibility for carrying out the patient's living will. However, nurses have historically been patients' advocates and they need to remember that their primary obligation is to the patient (and only secondarily to the family or other health care professionals). The nurse needs to find out what is most valued, meaningful, and significant to the older adult patient.

Competent older adults have a right to make decisions about their own life and death. As caring professionals, we may be uncomfortable in accepting a patient's refusal of treatment if we see it as threatening the person's life. We need to evaluate each patient individually, acknowledging that the refusal of treat-

Box 4-3   YOUR RIGHTS AS A HOSPITAL PATIENT

We consider you a partner in your hospital care. When you are well informed, participate in treatment decisions, and communicate openly with your doctor and other health professionals, you help make your care as effective as possible. This hospital encourages respect for the personal preferences and values of each individual.

While you are a patient in the hospital, your rights include the following:

- You have the right to considerate and respectful care.
- You have the right to be well informed about your illness, possible treatments, and likely outcome and to discuss this information with your doctor. You have the right to know the names and roles of people treating you.
- You have the right to consent to or refuse a treatment, as permitted by law, throughout your hospital stay. If you refuse a recommended treatment, you will receive other needed and available care.
- You have the right to have an advance directive, such as a living will or health care proxy. These documents express your choices about your future care or name someone to decide if you cannot speak for yourself. If you have a written advance directive, you should provide a copy to the hospital, your family, and your doctor.
- You have the right to privacy. The hospital, your doctor, and others caring for you will protect your privacy as much as possible.
- You have the right to expect that treatment records are confidential unless you have given permission to release information or reporting is required or permitted by law. When the hospital releases records to others, such as insurers, it emphasizes that the records are confidential.
- You have the right to review your medical records and to have the information explained, except when restricted by law.
- You have the right to expect that the hospital will give you necessary health services to the best of its ability. Treatment, referral, or transfer may be recommended. If transfer is recommended or requested, you will be informed of risks, benefits, and alternatives. You will not be transferred until the other institution agrees to accept you.
- You have the right to know if this hospital has relationships with outside parties that may influence your treatment and care. These relationships may be with educational institutions, other health care providers, or insurers.
- You have the right to consent or decline to take part in research affecting your care. If you choose not to take part, you will receive the most effective care the hospital otherwise provides.
- You have the right to be told of realistic care alternatives when hospital care is no longer appropriate.
- You have the right to know about hospital rules that affect you and your treatment and about charges and payment methods. You have the right to know about hospital resources, such as patient representatives or ethics committees, that can help you resolve problems and questions about your hospital stay and care.
- You have responsibilities as a patient. You are responsible for providing information about your health, including past illnesses, hospital stays, and use of medicine. You are responsible for asking questions when you do not understand information or instructions. If you believe you can't follow through with your treatment, you are responsible for telling your doctor.

Box 4-3   YOUR RIGHTS AS A HOSPITAL PATIENT, *Continued*

This hospital works to provide care efficiently and fairly to all patients and the community. You and your visitors are responsible for being considerate of the needs of other patients, staff, and the hospital. You are responsible for providing information for insurance and for working with the hospital to arrange payment, when needed.

Your health is dependent not just on your hospital care but, in the long term, on the decisions you make in your daily life. You are responsible for recognizing the effect of lifestyle on your personal health.

A hospital serves many purposes. Hospitals work to improve people's health; treat people with injury and disease; educate doctors, health professionals, patients, and community members; and improve understanding of health and disease. In carrying out these activities, this institution works to respect your values and dignity.

Reprinted with permission of the American Hospital Association, copyright 1992.

---

ment may be due to psychological, physical, socioeconomic, or even spiritual reasons of which we are unaware. We must respect the competent patient's desire for nontreatment. The patient should be offered an opportunity to reason and deliberate within a personal frame of reference. When a thoughtful decision is made by the patient, it should be honored.

Euthanasia

Euthanasia, meaning "good death" and defined as the deliberate ending of the life of a person suffering from an incurable and painful disease (*Dorland's Medical Dictionary,* 1988), is referred to briefly in this chapter only because it is currently a highly controversial and sensitive issue with moral, ethical, emotional, and legal implications. Sometimes known as "mercy killing," euthanasia is considered by some to be an easy and painless end to life when suffering is present and there is no hope of recovery. Those who advocate the "right to die" ignite vehement charges that they might bring about a public policy of subtle genocide aimed at the disabled, poor, elderly, mentally handicapped, minorities, or anyone having a condition that might cause society to devalue that individual's life (Foster, 1991). It is our responsibility to protect the most vulnerable of our citizens, including older adults, from involuntary eu-

thanasia. Despite significant opposition, there is a growing movement in the United States to legalize active euthanasia, in which a physician can assist patients to die; the Hemlock Society is an organization in the forefront of this movement. It is beyond the scope of this chapter to discuss further this crucial, sensitive, and emotional issue.

ELDER ABUSE

Elder abuse is increasing at an alarming rate and is becoming a major societal problem in the United States. Although the occurrence of elder abuse is vastly underreported, it is prevalent both in the community and in institutional settings (Council of Scientific Affairs, 1987). According to some estimates, only one in seven incidents of elder abuse is reported to authorities (Bates, 1993; Taormina, 1996). The House Select Committee on Aging brought the problem of elder abuse to public attention. Annually there are almost 2.5 million older people who are abused in the United States (Bates, 1993).

C a r i n g

❝*The caring nurse is continually alert to signs of elder abuse.*❞

Elder abuse may be defined as an act of omission or comission that leads to harm or threatened harm to the health and welfare of an older person. Generally, elder abuse is classified into six categories; among them, five are inflicted by others and the other is self-inflicted. The categories of elder abuse include

- Physical
- Psychological or emotional
- Sexual
- Financial or material exploitation
- Neglect by the caregiver
- Self-inflected abuse

Most states recognize these types of elder abuse and collect statistical data according to their manifestations. See Box 4–4 for definitions related to elder abuse.

The abuser may violate the rights of an older adult by eviction or placing the older adult in a long-term care facility against the individual's will, which deprives the older adult of autonomy. Of all the various kinds of abuses, the psychological abuse seems to be the most common type of abuse. Physical, sexual, and financial abuses are considered crimes in almost all states. Self-neglect is generally not addressed as a crime.

A typical profile of an abused older adult has been identified. Typically the victims of abuse are men and women older than the age of 75 years, although men are less often abused physically. Abused individuals are generally demented, physically disabled, or incontinent, or have chronic health problems and are dependent on their caretaker. The abused individual is usually too embarrassed to report abuse, is fearful of retaliation by caregivers, or may try to protect family member(s) by silence.

There is also a profile of the abuser. About two thirds of the abusers are family members of the victim. Adult children who take care of the parent(s) are the predominant abusers, followed by spouses, grandchildren, siblings, and even friends or neighbors. Adult abusers of elderly parents often suffer from emotional disorders, alcoholism, drug addiction, and financial problems.

Although physicians, nurses, or social workers are in ideal positions to detect abuse, especially when it results in physical trauma, they have not been very successful in identifying the problem. One of the main obstacles is that older adults have a tendency to fall and to bleed easily when traumatized. This can make it difficult for professionals to differentiate between abuse and natural trauma. The mal-

---

Box 4-4   DEFINITIONS RELATED TO ELDER ABUSE

Chemical restraints. Immobilization of the patient by sedating with psychoactive pharmacological agents such as sedatives and major tranquilizers.

Emotional or psychological abuse. Willful infliction of mental or emotional threats of violence, isolation and abandonment, humiliation, intimidation, or other verbal or nonverbal abusive conduct.

Financial or material exploitation. Unauthorized use of funds, property, or any resources of an older person by force or by misrepresentation.

Neglect. Willful or nonwillful failure by the caregiver to fulfill his or her caretaking obligations.

Physical abuse. Nonaccidental use of physical force that may result in body injury, pain, or impairment. It could involve slapping, beating, burning (by cigarette butts or hot water), or even murder.

Physical restraint. Material or equipment attached to or adjacent to the patient's body that prevents free bodily movement to a position of choice (turning, walking, sitting, lying, standing, and the use of the hands).

Self-inflicted abuse. When the elderly person may abuse or neglect himself or herself.

Sexual abuse. Nonconsensual sexual contact of any kind with an older person.

nourished or dehydrated older adult may be exhibiting self-neglect or caregiver neglect.

Nurses and physicians in the emergency department can be aware of cues that may suggest abuse or mistreatment, such as delay or neglect in seeking medical attention for the older person by the family, unexplained trauma, head injuries, failure to thrive, and injuries that do not fit with the explanations as to how they occurred (Jones, Dougherty, Schelble, and Cunningham, 1988).

The nurse is in a strategic position to perform a comprehensive assessment while looking for physical indicators of abuse, which may include bruises, burns, bites, abrasions, or marks in patterns reflecting use of instruments. The nurse should also look for an older adult's unusual gait, indicating sexual abuse (which is becoming a problem in long-term care facilities). The nurse may observe psychological indicators that include extreme withdrawal, agitation, infantile behavior, or expression of

ambivalent feeling toward caregivers (Jones et al., 1988). In the emergency department, the management of elder abuse is a team function.

To choose appropriate interventions, with specific emphasis on prevention, the nurse should first understand the dynamics of elder abuse, because each type of abuse requires a somewhat different strategy of intervention. Preventive interventions that the nurse can use to assist both the abused and the abuser include

- Educating the public about the natural aging process and its consequences
- Referring involved family members to stress management courses
- Providing counseling for families who are highly stressed
- Encouraging families to use respite care and other kinds of services
- Facilitating and encouraging caregivers to pursue other individual interests
- Offering information on resources for meals and help

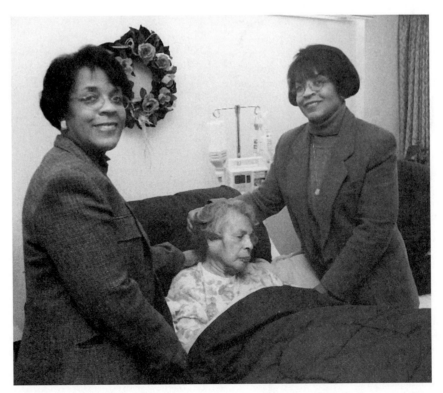

Problems may arise when family members disagree about the patient's treatment. This is when a guardian or surrogate is most important.

The nurse can also prevent or forestall physical and emotional conflicts for the older adult by early detection and long-term intervention to avoid prolonged, excessive stress on the caregiver (Patwell, 1988).

All 50 states have established some form of legislation to address domestic or institutional elder abuse and various mechanisms to report elder abuse offenders. However, statutes vary widely from one jurisdiction to another in both scope and types of abuse that are covered. Some states address both domestic and institutional abuse with one law, whereas others have separate legislation. States generally require that professionals such as employees of law-enforcement agencies, long-term care ombudsmen, physicians, and other health care professionals are mandated to report all suspected cases of elder abuse (they are similar to statutes for child abuse). In some states the public is also required to report suspected abuse. Agencies that receive such reports include the police department, district attorney's office, area agencies on aging, and other older adult organizations (Tatara, 1994).

Private and government protective agencies have taken a very active role to mitigate elder abuse and exploitation. The U.S. Department of Health and Human Services (USHHS) established an Elder Abuse Task Force in 1990 that directed several of its agencies to study the problem of elder abuse. The plan, which has been in operation since 1992, consisted of identifying and implementing various strategies to reduce elder abuse. The Administration on Aging (AOA) launched a National Eldercare Campaign to develop resources for elders who are abused, neglected, or exploited and at risk of losing their independence. The AOA also provided funds to operate the National Center on Elder Abuse (NCEA), which came into being through the 1992 amendment to the Older Americans Act.

The nurse and other health care professionals should be familiar with these agencies to make use of their resources when necessary. Although federal funds for these programs have not been adequate, it is encouraging that some strides have been taken. More important, elder abuse has been recognized as a national health problem that, according to some accounts, has reached epidemic proportions.

The older adult has a right to refuse protective services. He or she is assumed to be able to judge his or her own need. The court intervenes only if it finds the person to be incompetent. This differs from child abuse, in which the government assumes the right to intervene and protect the child even when the child has parents or adult caretakers (Jones et al., 1988).

RESTRAINTS

The use of any type of restraint can be classified as abuse under certain circumstances. Physical and chemical restraints are used in hospitals and long-term care facilities with the intent of preventing falls and incidents in certain categories of patients. These include patients with delirium, confusion, and wandering behaviors. It has been asserted that one impetus for restraints arises out of fear of litigation by the family.

Physical restraints consist of material or equipment attached to or adjacent to the patient's body designed to prevent free bodily movement; their overt purpose is to prevent falls or accidents, but they also prevent the patient from moving to a position of choice. Research clearly indicates that patients who are restrained continue to fall (in some instances, more often) and injure themselves, sometimes fatally. Besides acute physical discomfort, restrained patients have emotions of anger, fear, frustration, humiliation, and resignation (Stillwell, 1988; Stumpf and Evans, 1988; Tinetti et al., 1991). *Chemical restraints* are psychoactive pharmacologic agents that are used to sedate

C a r i n g

"*Advocacy for older adult patients includes becoming familiar with their advance directives and verbally expressed wishes and representing them to other members of the health care team.***"**

patients to immobilize them; they are frequently used in long-term care facilities. The pathological, physical, and psychological effects of the restraints are detrimental to the patient's well-being.

Because of the outcry from families of older adult patients and the public, the Omnibus Budget Reconciliation Act (1987) stipulated that restraints are to be used only as a last resort after other alternatives for patient safety have been tried and failed. Except in emergency situations, restraints may be used only on the written order of a physician, which specifies the type, duration, and circumstances under which restraints are to be used. If restraints have to be used to protect the patient or other patients, the least restrictive devices must be chosen. It is the responsibility of the nurse to assess, evaluate, and implement nonrestraint approaches to maintaining patients' safety. The nurse should focus on two main strategies: staff education and residents' environmental adaptation and modifications to prevent and reduce falls. Patients' dignity must be maintained regardless of what methods are used for safety. Further discussion of restraints can be found in Chapter 10.

Summary

In caring for older adults, it is important for nurses to include information on values, preferences, and advance directives in initial assessments. The patient's permanent medical record should be reviewed for inclusion of any documents. This information needs to be elicited while the person is still mentally competent and able to participate actively in decisions regarding care of self. Nurses should also individualize patient care according to the advance directives and the timing of these decisions.

The chances of litigation can be reduced by documenting the wishes of the patient on the medical record while the individual is still mentally competent. Written documentation about personal wishes may also reduce confusion and family conflicts and decrease the patient's anxiety about management of care, especially in situations of a terminal illness or condition. Advance directives and the appointment of a surrogate or proxy also make it easier for the health care professional to offer the kind of care the patient desires without going through legal proceedings. Regardless of the patient's written advance directives, nurses are obligated to give the best care possible to the dying person. Although caring may not always coincide with curing, it always demands that nurses provide care that offers dignity in dying.

REFERENCES

American Nurses' Association (1992). Position statement on nursing and the Patient Self-Determination Act. In Compendium of Position Statements on the Nurse's Role in End-of-Life Decisions. Washington, DC: American Nurses' Association.

Bates S. (March 7, 1993). Elderly abuse rises sharply. The Washington Post, pp A16, A18.

Coordinating Council on Life-Sustaining Medical Treatment Decision Making by the Courts. (1991). Guideline for State Court Decision Making in Authorizing or Withholding Life-Sustaining Medical Treatment: A Project of the National Center for State Courts. Williamsburg, VA.

Council on Scientific Affairs, American Medical Association. (1987). Elder abuse and neglect. JAMA 257: 966–971.

Drugay M, Gallagher C. (1993). Patient Self-Determination Act: Implementing an information program in a nursing facility. J Gerontol Nurs 12:29–34.

Ebersole P, Hess P. (1998). Toward Healthy Aging. 5th ed. St. Louis: CV Mosby.

Foster D. (November 15, 1991). Doctor warns against euthanasia. Rocky Mountain News, p 10.

Goldstein MK. (1992). Ethics. In Ham RJ, Sloane PD, eds. Primary Care Geriatrics, pp 213–214. St. Louis: CV Mosby.

Guido J. (1997). Legal Issues in Nursing. 2nd ed. Sanford, Connecticut: Appleton & Lange.

Janofsky JS. (1990). Assessing competency in the elderly. Geriatrics 45(10):45–48.

Jones J, Dougherty J, Schelble D, Cunningham W. (October 17, 1988). Emergency department protocol for the diagnosis and evaluation of geriatric abuse. Ann Emerg Med 17(10):1006–1015.

Matteson MA, McConnell ES, Linton AD. (1997). Gerontological Nursing: Concepts and Practice. 2nd ed. Philadelphia: WB Saunders.

Patwell T. (1988). Familial abuse of the elderly: A look at caregiver potential and prevention. Home Health Care Nurse 4(2):10.

Steinbrook R, Lo B. (1984). Decision making for incompetent patients by designated proxy: California's new law. N Engl J Med 310:1598–1601.

Stillwell E. (1988). Use of physical restraints in older adults. J Gerontol Nurs 14:42–44.

Stumpf N, Evans L. (1988). Physical restraints of the hospitalized elderly: Perceptions of patients and nurses. Nurs Res 37(3):132–134.

Swonger AK, Burbank PM. (1995). Drug Therapy and the Elderly, pp 77–78. Boston: Jones & Bartlett.

Taormina SF. (Winter 1996). Crimes against the elderly. Natl Conf Gerontol Nurse Practitioners Newsl, pp 1–2.

Tatara T. (1994). Elder Abuse: Questions and Answers. 4th ed. Washington, DC: National Center on Elder Abuse.

Tinetti ME, Speechley M, Ginter SF. (1991). Risk factors for falls among elderly persons living in the community. N Engl J Med 319:1701–1707.

Uniform Durable Power of Attorney Act (1983). Uniform Durable Power of Attorney Act 8A, U.L.A.

CRITICAL THINKING EXERCISES

Alicia Long is an 88-year-old woman who, with her 91-year-old husband William, moved to a continuing care retirement community. They relocated from out of town to be near their two adult sons and their families. Mr. Long has advanced Alzheimer's disease and needs assistance in both ADLs and IADLs. Mr. Long's primary physician wanted to perform tests, both for an enlarged prostate and to rule out any other causes that might be contributing to his dementia. However, the two sons informed the physician that further testing of their father is futile.

Because one of the sons has a durable power of attorney from his father, both for health and financial affairs, and his brother is in agreement, no treatment is being offered at present. Mr. Long is ambulatory and goes to the main dining room for meals; he has an aide for ADL care.

Mrs. Long has had situational depression, for which she is being treated. Earlier, she had one kidney removed because it was cancerous.

Now she has developed some problems with the other kidney, so her primary physician wants to refer Mrs. Long to a nephrologist for evaluation and treatment. However, the two sons are opposed to further investigations of their mother's health as well. Mrs. Long is able to take care of herself and interacts socially with the other residents, always winning at Scrabble.

1. As a nurse caregiver, what would be your responsibilities regarding cardiac resuscitation for Mr. Long? For Mrs. Long? How would you make the decisions?

2. As a member of the health care team, what specific observations can you make and document that will assist the physician to establish a plan of care for Mrs. Long?

3. In view of the actions of the sons vis à vis their father and their mother, do you suspect parental abuse? What actions of the sons would lead you to suspect it, and what actions would you take if you did suspect abuse?

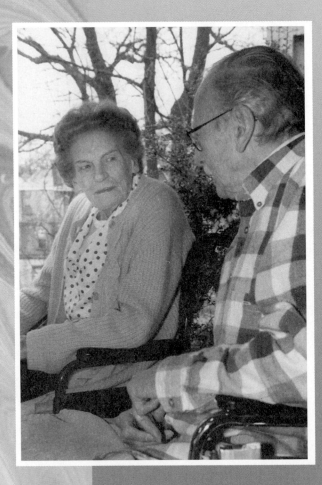

Psychosocial Health in Maturity

CHAPTER 5

Acknowledging the Whole Person:
Culture, Ethnicity, and Religion

Carol Sue Holtz, RN, BSN, MN, PhD

CHAPTER OUTLINE

Demographic Data
Cultural Sensitivity
Ethnic Groups
    Hispanic Older Adults
    African American Older Adults
    Native American Older Adults
    The Navajo Nation's Older Adults
    Jewish Older Adults
    Asian Older Adults

Spirituality and Religion
    Spirituality
    Religion
    Implications for Nursing Practice
Cultural Assessment Tool
Summary
References
Critical Thinking Exercises

OBJECTIVES

After completing this chapter, the reader should be able to:

1. Address the issues of increased ethnic diversity in the older adult population.
2. Write a teaching plan that addresses the special needs of the Hispanic older adult population.
3. Describe the history and special issues of African American older adults.
4. Formulate ways that nurses can better meet the health care needs of Native American older adults.
5. Apply your knowledge of the three Jewish subgroups to address the unique needs of their older adults.
6. Compare and contrast the Asian American and European American subcultures.
7. Distinguish between spirituality and religion and explain why they are important issues for the older adult.
8. Teach a classmate how nurses can integrate spiritual needs into nursing care for older adults.

KEY TERMS

culture
ethnic
ethnicity
ethnocentric
holistic
religion
spiritual distress
spiritual needs
spirituality

It is natural for humans to resist being categorized, yet each of us finds part of our identity through ties to family, friends, work, education, religious or spiritual expression, communities, nation, and lineage. The tremendous diversity that characterizes the **culture** of the United States has been both a strength and a source of confusion and mistrust. When **ethnicity** and cultural identities are obviously different, people sometimes tend to feel uneasy with each other until personal bridges are built. In the nurse/client relationship, the responsibility for building these bridges rests with the nurse. Nurses, thus, have an obligation to examine and understand their own ethnic and cultural ties as well as to be aware of the differing backgrounds of those for whom they provide care.

Sensitivity to the background of the older client can be placed in a still larger context. In an individual who has reached older adult status there has been an accumulation of life experience that, coupled with personal reflection, can change knowledge into wisdom. Our society, with its emphasis on consumerism and advertising, teaches us to value youthful beauty. There is an associated tendency to overlook qualities that are packaged in an aging wrapper. Nurses not only need to be aware of unconscious cultural bias but also of the widespread prejudice associated with the loss of youth. A truly holistic view of the older client takes these aspects into account and makes corrections for the biases of society.

Nursing as a profession is constantly striving to improve the delivery of nursing care to all clients. This includes addressing the cultural aspects of nursing care. Older clients from cultures other than that of the nurse may not benefit from nursing care because of misunder-standings, miscommunications, or conflicts of values and beliefs between themselves and the nurse. Only with knowledge of the client's culture can the nurse adequately assess, plan, implement, and evaluate care. Satisfaction with nursing care is significantly impacted by the nurse's cultural sensitivity.

■ DEMOGRAPHIC DATA

In recent years, the older segment of the U.S. population has become much more culturally diverse. African American, Hispanic, and Asian populations are increasing more rapidly than the non-Hispanic white population. Non-Hispanic whites made up about 80% of the population in 1980 but were 74% of the population in 1995; by the year 2050, the non-Hispanic white population in the United States will be 67% of the total (Treas, 1995).

W e l l n e s s

"In an individual who has reached older adult status there has been an accumulation of life experiences that, coupled with personal reflection, can change knowledge into wisdom."

Approximately 2 million American Indians and Alaskan natives share certain genetic traits and belong to groups with distinct social, political, and biomedical characteristics. This group, designated as *American Indian* by the U.S. government but referred to in this text as *Native Americans,* also exhibits great internal ethnic, cultural, and social diversity (Rhoades, 1996). A distinction exists between Native Americans living on reservations and those living in urban areas. Native Americans in recognized nations living on reservation land are eligible for a variety of government programs and benefits. Once they move to the city, these programs are usually not available. This is particularly crucial to the health care of older adults. Overall, 25% of Native Americans live on reservations, 36% live in rural areas, and 37% live in urban areas. Compared with the general population in the United States (as well as with other minority groups), Native

Americans have the lowest median age and the second smallest proportion of people older than 65 years of age (Gelfand, 1994).

By the year 2030, we can expect to have 7.3 million African American older adults in the United States. The median age of these African Americans is 6 years less than for whites and 4.8 years less than for all groups combined. African American men who live beyond age 75 have good life expectancies, and African American women older than 75 have even longer life expectancies (Sayles-Cross, 1995).

The Hispanic American older adult group will grow by the year 2000 to a population seven times what it was in 1990. This overall growth rate will be 4.5 times greater than for the entire aged population and 5 times greater than the growth rate among non-Hispanic white older adults. Thus, the Hispanic American older adults are the fastest growing segment of the American population older than age 65 (Gelfand, 1994).

According to the 1990 U.S. census, the Asian population has grown to 2.9% of the total American population. The Japanese and Chinese American groups have the largest number of older people (Gelfand, 1994).

Treas (1995) stated that the ethnic composition of the older "minority" population is also changing. African Americans and Native Americans are gaining proportionally; the largest growth will be among Hispanics, Asians, and Pacific Islanders. African Americans in 1995 were the largest ethnic group, with 8% of the 65-and-older population. In general, older adults of nondominant groups have fewer economic resources, are less educated, have fewer assets, and are less likely to own their own homes. Many older adult immigrants speak little English and continue to follow diets and health practices of their native cultures.

◼ CULTURAL SENSITIVITY

Many health care providers have limited knowledge, experience, or understanding of the health care needs of those different from themselves. To best serve the needs of clients from different cultures or subcultures, nurses must become more knowledgeable about differing values, experiences, social networks, communication styles, and perceptions of health and illness. Diversity is a reality of the 1990s, and the United States is becoming the most ethnically diverse society in the world. The needs and responses of many different racial and ethnic groups are competing for recognition, and nurses must learn how to meet the health care needs of this multicultural society (Spector, 1996). Culture defines who is old, establishes rituals for the elderly, sets acceptable roles and expectations for behavior, and influences the attitudes of others toward the aged. Nurses need to respect the older client and identify how kinship, psychological and cultural factors, and socioeconomic status affect their physical and psychological health as well as their functional status (Andrews and Boyle, 1995).

Future cohorts of minority older adults will have more diverse characteristics than those of today because of their life experiences, including historical events and trends, socialization, educational and cultural events, and a perception of the global village. The acculturation process, from immigration to old age, will determine the characteristics of the older adult who was born into another culture. Health care professionals who work with the elderly must be educated to work with a variety of individuals whose backgrounds may vary in socioeconomic status and education (Gelfand and Yee, 1991).

A sensitivity to and a knowledge of the similarities and differences between people of different cultural backgrounds are extremely effective in establishing relationships and communication with others (Leininger, 1970, 1997). Maintaining an open attitude and examining one's prejudices, attitudes, and stereotyped perceptions is an essential prerequisite that makes it possible to learn about people from other cultures. Because there is a natural tendency to be centered on self, many health care practices have been (unconsciously) devised to fit the nurse's own culture.

To administer culturally congruent care to clients of diverse backgrounds, a variety of cultural values that affect health care practices need to be more closely examined. Optimum health is considered to be a value and right for all people in U.S. society. No one should be denied optimal health, but even in the United States there are numerous factors that limit health services. In some other cultures, opti-

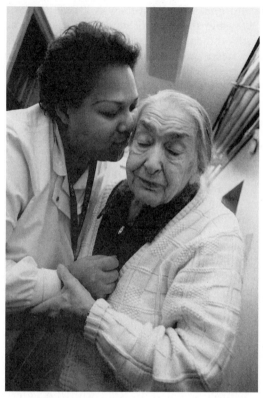

It is essential that this African American nurse be aware of the cultural background of her Greek American client.

mum health may not even be a primary concern or value.

In the United States, nurses run the risk of alienating people of other cultures by attempting to change their health practices so as to obtain their "optimum perceived level of health." It is a common practice among many cultural groups to show exterior signs of politeness but to feel anger, fear, or resentment. This becomes evident when cultural groups quietly refuse to follow suggestions of the health care providers. Individualism, another U.S. cultural value, characterizes the person as special and unique. Other cultural groups, such as Asians and Native Americans, value the group over the individual.

The cultural value of achieving is highly prized among some nurses. This U.S. middle-class value implies that those who work hard and keep busy can achieve success, which is often measured by material wealth. But such achievement is not a universal value. The cul-

tural value of time is of great importance for most nurses, but not always for their clients. In the professional world of the United States, time is to be used "well" and not "wasted." This perception has major implications for teaching about self-administration of medications, for treatment, and even for keeping health care appointments. One of the greatest injustices that health care providers can do is to label clients "noncompliant," "impossible," "difficult," or "uncooperative" when they are having trouble understanding a client's behavior. If culture-specific care is not given, clients will refuse to carry out the expectations of the health care providers, will withdraw, or will sign out against medical advice (Leininger, 1970, 1997).

Health beliefs of the various subcultures in the United States include a wide range of concepts regarding health and illness. Many Asian Americans (from China, Southeast Asia, Japan, and Korea) view health as a balance between *yin* and *yang* and illness as an imbalance. Elderly clients from Hispanic countries may see health as a balance between "hot" and "cold" and illness as an imbalance. Those of African, Haitian, or Jamaican origin may view health as "harmony with nature" and illness as "disharmony with nature." Spector (1996) states that many people who adhere to traditional practices base them on religious codes and view illness as a punishment for breaking them. For an elderly immigrant, cultural values often are deeply rooted in tradition. Culture affects how we perceive and define the meaning of illness and the expectations of caregivers and clients.

It is also important to emphasize that even well-intentioned, "culturally sensitive" nurses may naively err in stereotyping all members of a particular ethnic group. The goal of successful intercultural communication cannot be to discover a comprehensive set of communication tricks that when systematically applied to the correct culture, ethnicity, gender, or socioeconomic background will generate instant understanding (Nance, 1995). Nance (1995) states that she has some key concerns about transcultural nursing that takes a simplistic view of culture and fails to understand culture as dynamic and individually adaptive. Health care providers have a tendency to generalize and presume that what is true of the group is true of every individual in the group.

Culture influences how older adults determine illness and how they will seek care. Many older adults who are foreign-born use traditional sources of care. They may speak their native language, be suspicious of English-speaking health care providers, have limited incomes, and thus have transportation and financial barriers to accessing health care. Many desire having treatment by professionals who are culturally like themselves. Care of older adults in ethnically diverse cultures in the United States is often carried out by family members because (1) it is affordable, (2) it is consistent with cultural values and preferences, and (3) it avoids language problems. In addition, older family members may rely exclusively on younger family members for economic and social support because they have few financial resources (Andrews and Boyle, 1995).

> ### C a r i n g
>
> *"In the nurse/client relationship, the responsibility for building bridges rests with the nurse."*

Health care providers need to understand the impact of culture on their beliefs about health and illness; death and dying; health prevention, maintenance, and treatment; special foods; religious practices that relate to health and illnesses; family kinship ties; the cultural values of time and social distance to health; expressions of emotions (e.g., pain, joy); modesty customs; head of household and family decision-makers; and customs regarding care and respect for older adults. Nurses and other health care providers need to recognize that the older adult may be unable to cope with a complex health care system for ethnic or cultural reasons. Nurses may need to assist such clients to evaluate their support systems and to become comfortable with community services (Andrews and Boyle, 1995).

■ ETHNIC GROUPS

In attempting to describe any ethnic group, we inevitably identify characteristics that are present in some members and not in others. The word **ethnic** pertains to a religious, national, racial, or cultural group. In subcultures that are very traditional, sociocultural characteristics may be highly consistent, especially among older adults and recent immigrants. However, with younger members, or those who have assimilated into the majority culture, the identified characteristics may not be so consistent. As noted earlier, each individual is unique; therefore, when reviewing these cultural descriptions, nurses must remain aware of the risk of stereotyping.

Keeping this warning in mind, health care providers need to be cognizant of cultural identity when caring for older adults of diverse backgrounds. It is not possible to include within this chapter all ethnic groups in the United States. Yet, when caring for clients of backgrounds that differ from that of the nurse, the nurse needs to make the effort to become more familiar with the client's background. This caring behavior could be accomplished by talking to the client and family, utilizing a cultural assessment tool, and exploring the relevant literature at a library or on the Internet. When the client's language is unknown to the health care provider, every effort must be taken to communicate. The use of family members or an interpreter (many health care agencies now have a list of volunteers who are available when needed) is essential. The following are some brief overviews of ethnic groups (subcultures) represented among older adults in the United States.

Hispanic Older Adults

By the end of the 20th century, people whose origins are in countries once dominated by Spain will represent the largest minority group in the United States. There is significant disagreement among these people about how they wish to be called, and for convenience here we will respectfully refer to them as Hispanic Americans (*New York Times*, 1992). Sixty percent are Mexican Americans, 14% are Puerto Rican Americans, and the remainder originated in other countries of Central America and elsewhere (Miller, 1995). Hispanic Americans tend to share many common sociocultural characteristics, one of which is a focus on spirituality. Their spirituality provides a way to accept and cope with suffering and illness, often with the belief that suffering and illness are God's will (Miller, 1995).

The head of the household is traditionally the husband/father, who is also the breadwinner and family decision-maker. The husband/father thus makes all decisions regarding illness and treatment of family members. The wife/mother traditionally stays at home; the grandmother is usually consulted for child care advice. The family has strong kinship and extended family ties. Nurses may find that a patient's extended family members fill a waiting room to overflowing when a birth is imminent or surgery is in progress (Schiavenato, 1997).

The hierarchy of kinship relations is very strict. Authority runs from older to younger and from male to female. The relationships are for life, with parents in control of adult children, and older adults in control of their younger adult siblings. It is inappropriate to use a child as an interpreter for an older family member because it may be culturally unacceptable for a young child to tell the older family member all that he or she needs to know (Turner, 1995).

Beliefs about the causation of illness are important determinants regarding Hispanic American views about life support. Health is viewed as a gift from God, and illness (including accidents) may be due to punishment from God. People of this ethnic background often believe that we should not interfere with suffering—that there is always hope. To stop life support may cause the family great guilt (Turner, 1995).

Group members are very much oriented to the present; the sense of time is very relaxed, and patients may not adhere strictly to appointment times. The social distance preferred is very close, and there is a lot of physical touching among family and friends. Regarding expressions of emotion, Hispanic Americans are generally very demonstrative of happiness, pain, and discomfort (Dickason et al., 1994; Schiavenato, 1997; Spector, 1996).

Some Hispanics believe in the *mal ojo* (evil eye), which represents strength and power. Prolonged eye contact by strangers may be considered disrespectful and may be interpreted as harmful to health. In general, the belief is that as long as the person's strengths and weaknesses are in balance, that person will be healthy. The balance theory suggests that illness is treated by restoring the balance of "hot" and "cold." A *cold* condition, such as a respiratory illness, is treated with a *hot* environment, such as hot foods. Menstruation and giving birth are *hot* conditions that are treated with *cold* foods. There seems to be no general agreement as to which diseases or foods are considered hot or cold; the classification varies. If a Hispanic client refuses to eat meals offered, the nurse needs to ask what food is preferred. Among Hispanic Americans, illness is sometimes considered a punishment for wrongdoing, or the result of poor hygiene, poor air, poor food, poor water, or a hazardous lifestyle (Spector, 1996).

Traditional diet includes a variety of meat, poultry, and eggs. Dried beans and rice are staples. Starchy vegetables, chili peppers, and a variety of fruits are included. Milk is often excluded, but cheese is used in cooking. Sugar is used heavily in the diets of many traditional members (Williams, 1993).

Some Hispanic people believe in and utilize the healing power of the *curandera* (or *curandero*), a folk healer whose powers are considered a gift from God. The *curandera,* a powerful person in the community, uses prayer, rituals, and herbal treatments to heal. Practices that do no harm to clients should be respected and incorporated into the health care regimen. Some clients may wear amulets, medals, and other religious relics for protection against harm and promotion of healing. Health care providers should allow these to remain with the client, or if they must be removed, they should be replaced as soon as possible (Spector, 1996).

Traditionally, Hispanic Americans have been Roman Catholics, but now they include Protestants as well. As a group they are usually quite religious and believe that God awards people with health and punishes them with illness. Most Hispanic clients are extremely modest (especially women), and most prefer to be examined and treated by same-gender health care providers. They are usually very uncomfortable discussing sexual topics. Death, when it comes, is considered the will of God. There is a strong belief in the afterlife. After the death of a Catholic person, the body is prepared by a commercial mortuary and placed on display during a rosary ceremony. The funeral is held on the day after the rosary and subsequently *Novenarios,* or nine days of evening prayer services, begin on the Monday after death (Holmes and Holmes, 1995; Schiavenato, 1997).

Communication with the dominant culture may be one of the biggest problems for Hispanic Americans. Many, especially the older adults, lack knowledge of English, which can be a source of both stress and misunderstanding. Clients may simply smile or nod in agreement if they do not understand questions, directions, or explanations. The ideal situation would include a health care provider who speaks fluent Spanish. If this is not possible, improvisation and creativity are necessary (Holmes and Holmes, 1995; Schiavenato, 1997).

C a r i n g

66Satisfaction with nursing care is significantly impacted by the nurse's cultural sensitivity.99

The elderly have a strong sense of privacy and often feel they are able to handle their own problems within the family with the help of the church. Many believe that if they have enough faith in God, they will be helped. They value being respected and often prefer that health care providers call them by their last names with *Senor* or *Senora* preceding. Most older adults do not retire but continue to work as long as they are able. Old people, both men and women, serve as teachers of proper conduct, relating historical precedents. The decision-maker remains the most elderly man (Holmes and Holmes, 1995).

African American Older Adults

African American is a collective term used to describe people who identify themselves as black (Zack, 1993) and are from a variety of cultures, primarily (1) those born in Africa, usually relatively recent immigrants; (2) those born in Caribbean areas such as Puerto Rico, Haiti, and the Dominican Republic; (3) and those born in the United States, whose lineage may trace back to the time of slavery. Clearly, the African American community is composed of many subcultures.

Extended families have been an important part of African American culture since the days of slavery. During that time families were split up and sold, and the older adults on the plantations became the parents to all. An extended family could consist of parents, children, grandchildren, aunts, neighbors, and fellow church members. Today, extended families often provide financial as well as emotional support. Children and older adults are especially valued in the family.

Most African American older adults are highly respected, sometimes standing in as doctor, teacher, and disciplinarian. Although there are many households headed by singles, when there are dual-parent households the duties, responsibilities, and family decision-making are shared equally. All adults in the household are expected to contribute to the finances; this can include parents, grandparents, aunts, and uncles (Holmes and Holmes, 1995).

Family characteristics of some African American families may include the following: role flexibility, strong kinship bonds, strong work orientation, strong achievement orientation, and a strong religious orientation. Death may be viewed by some as a passage from one life to another. Funerals are often times for celebration, despite the grief of family members (Hassan, 1995).

Family decision-making, household chores, and childrearing are generally shared by husband and wife. The family unit usually has strong kinship ties with extended family members. Time orientation may differ from that of the dominant culture. For many African Americans time is very flexible; lateness up to 1 hour is socially acceptable. Orientation toward the present is common, and physical closeness is generally preferred. African Americans tend to be demonstrative about emotions and the expression of pain, are comfortable with touching and close social distance, and emphasize spontaneous self-expression. Religion is a very strong influence among families within the community (Holmes and Holmes, 1995).

For recent immigrants from Africa, English may be a second language. American-born clients may speak a nonstandard variant of English (Black English). Black English evolved during the period of slavery and combines English words with West African language patterns. These patterns are oral, rhythmic, and spontaneous, with many intonations and inflections (Ebersole and Hess, 1998). Traditional diets of African Americans from West Africa may include such foods as dumplings or gruel from millet, corn, yams, bananas, fresh fruits, okra, and hot peppers. Many exclude milk and milk products from their diets. Traditional diets of African Americans who live in the southern United States may include smoked meats, pork, poultry, stews, hominy grits, legumes, vegetables, and some fruits. There may be a high intake of sweets. Many are lactose intolerant, so that milk products can cause gas or diarrhea (Williams, 1993).

Many African Americans are reluctant to seek mainstream medical care when ill, often because of a basic mistrust of the health care system. When they are ill, other resources may be used. Religion is central to healing in this group. Chronic illnesses may be viewed as causing stress or additional financial burdens on other family members; this results in reluctance to seek treatment, especially because special diets and medications may not be affordable. African Americans do not often seek help outside their home, community, or church. Health care agencies may be viewed as the last resort, to be used when all else fails. This is because many view the health care system as an extension of institutional forces that negatively value the African American community (Hassan, 1995).

African American older adults as a group have generally not enjoyed the same social benefits as their peers in the dominant culture. Therefore, they are relatively less educated, less affluent, have less adequate housing, and have more difficulty in accessing health care; not surprisingly, they have more chronic health problems, including cancer, heart disease, stroke, hypertension, diabetes, accidents, and chemical dependency (Hassan, 1995).

Illness, death, and dying are considered to be a part of life. African Americans tend not to donate organs because of a general mistrust that another African American may not be accorded eligibility for the organ. In addition, a commonly held belief is that "you leave the world with all that God gave you." African Americans are less likely to be placed in nursing homes or rehabilitation facilities unless insurance is covering the stay. It is generally un-

derstood that the elderly or sick will be cared for at home (Hassan, 1995).

Nurses need to know about assessment of dark skin, special skin problems, and appropriate hair care when caring for elderly African Americans. Special skin problems may include

- Keloids—scars that form at the site of a wound that are sharply elevated and irregular
- Pigmentary disorders—postinflammation light or dark spots
- Pseudofolliculitis—razor bumps or ingrown hairs that may include papules, pustules, and even keloids

Nurses need to consult clients about special hair care needs. African American hair may become brittle and break if shampooed every day. Hair needs to be assessed as to amount of oil (dry, normal, oily), straight or curly texture, and hairstyle preference. After shampooing a client's hair, a pick or comb may be used before drying to prevent tangles.

Knowledge of physical assessment of a darker-skinned client is essential. *Pallor* can be assessed by observing for the absence of underlying red tones of the mucous membranes. Brown-skinned people may appear yellow, and black-skinned people may appear ashen (gray). *Erythema,* an inflammation, must be detected by palpation of the skin; the skin may feel warmer, tight, and/or edematous. *Cyanosis,* a condition of low oxygenation, may be observed by close inspection of lips, tongue, and mucous membranes for lack of rosy color. Conjunctiva, palms of hands, and soles of feet may appear ashen. *Jaundice,* the yellowish coloring, may be observed in buccal mucosa, palms of hands, and soles of feet (Berger, 1992; Dickason, 1994).

Holmes and Holmes (1995) state that it is possible to generalize the following statements regarding elderly African Americans' beliefs vis-à-vis those of the dominant culture. African Americans tend to

- See old age more as a reward than a disaster
- Have fewer anxieties about old age, and therefore higher morale
- Be less likely to deny their actual age
- Tend to remain part of their family structure to a greater degree, and consequently be respected and treated well

- Be strongly supported by bonds of mutual assistance (with friends, neighbors, and family)
- Be more likely to maintain useful and acceptable family functions
- Be more likely to be tolerated by their families in spite of behavioral peculiarities
- Be generally more religious but less involved in economic and political institutions
- Feel less integrated into society at large
- Have a life expectancy at birth of approximately 8 years less for men (64.8) and 5.5 years less for women (73.5)
- Live longer than other Americans once they reach the age of 75
- Be considerably less prone to suicide

Native American Older Adults

There are 307 officially recognized Native American political groups (nations, tribes, bands, and other designations) who speak approximately 149 different languages and reside in 26 mostly western states in the United States. Thus, it is not possible to make generalized descriptions about all Native Americans (Hanley, 1995; Holmes and Holmes, 1995). In addition, there is some disagreement about the designation of American Indian; some Native American organizations prefer that way of identifying themselves, others do not.

In the face of this diversity, there may still be some values and cultural characteristics that tend to be consistent among Native American groups. These characteristics include the following (Holmes and Holmes, 1995):

1. Respect for individual freedom and autonomy
2. A tendency to seek group consensus, not majority rule
3. Respect for the earth and all living things
4. A propensity to be hospitable
5. A dictum that one should avoid bringing shame on self, family, clan, or nation
6. A belief in a supreme being and life after death

Growing old in our society is generally associated with a loss of friends and family; this loss may lead to increased isolation and subsequent depression, especially if the aged lack a good support system. However, among Native Americans, social support need not decrease with age because it is possible to "make relations." Ceremonies are held as the number of older adults grows within the community, and more individuals are experiencing chronic illness, loss of friends through death, and a variety of transitions. In these ceremonies, one person forms a mutual contract with another and they become "related." This tie is equivalent to a kin relationship, so an older person may have accumulated many more family members than the original biological family. Not only does this custom serve to support the older adults, but young people may also benefit from mentoring relationships with the older adults of the community. For older adults, new ceremonies are needed both to strengthen the ties between relatives and for individual expression (Silverman, 1990).

The older Native American is seen as a family leader whose advice and social acceptance are sought by younger family members. Older adults are an integral resource and play a central role in family life by providing guidance to younger family members. Grandmothers often provide child care and perform household duties; in return, they are respected and cared for when they become too frail to care for themselves (Yee, 1990).

Native Americans generally prefer to speak in low tones and wish to have others be attentive to them in conversation. They frequently use nonverbal communication techniques. Asking a Native American to repeat a statement and taking written notes during a conversation are considered insulting behaviors. Instead of asking direct questions, the health care provider should make declarative statements. For example, instead of asking "Do you have headaches?" a statement such as "The pain in your head is interfering with your daily activities" would be a more culturally sensitive way of evoking a response (Yee, 1990).

Poverty is a familiar condition for many Native Americans. About 25% have incomes below poverty level, and for those who live on reservations the number increases to 40%. Social Security is a source of income for only 50%, less than 51% receive Medicare, and less than 40% receive Medicaid. Poverty in the older adults may be the result of a lifetime of deprivation of good housing, education, income, and health (Holmes and Holmes, 1995).

Many adults in the Native American population have shifted from having acute infectious diseases to chronic degenerative diseases. Tuberculosis and non–insulin-dependent diabetes mellitus are the two most common health problems. Deaths from pneumonia, influenza, tuberculosis, and gastrointestinal diseases have increased by 79% to 95% since the establishment of the Indian Health Service in 1955. In addition, deaths from chronic liver disease, cirrhosis, suicide, diabetes, hypertension, and malignant neoplasms have increased substantially. Of particular concern are the environmental stressors that increase the incidences of these diseases (Mercer, 1994).

Caring

"To administer culturally congruent care to clients of diverse backgrounds, a variety of cultural values that affect health care practices needs to be closely examined."

Many Native American groups live in the United States, each with their own special language, beliefs (especially health beliefs), customs, and practices. To include each group would be ideal but not realistic for this textbook chapter. The largest group, the Navajo Nation, is explored in greater detail in the next section. Nurses caring for other Native American subcultures need to obtain more specific data to provide culture-congruent care (as described by Leininger, 1997). Suggestions include talking with the client and family, use of the cultural assessment tool, exploring the literature in the library or Internet, and phoning the National Indian Health Service at (301) 443-1083 or writing them at 5600 Fisher's Lane, Parklawn Building, Room 6-05, Rockville, Maryland 20857-0001.

The Navaho Nation's Older Adults

The Navaho Nation is the largest Native American group, with a 1990 population of about 155,000, showing an increase of 3% since the 1980 census. The Navaho maintain a unique relationship to health and illness based on treating causal agents rather than the illness itself. Once the cause has been determined by the medicine person, a special ceremony is performed to negate its effects and to restore harmony (spiritual wellness) to the patient. A medicine man or woman may spend 4 or 5 days with the patient, using chants, holy objects, and herbal remedies. Members of the Native American Church employ peyote, a hallucinogen, as an important ingredient in healing ceremonies. It is common for the Navaho to seek western medical treatment for distinct conditions such as a broken bone, while at the same time consulting a medicine man or woman to determine what has brought on the problem. The medicine person's responsibility is not to cure the condition but to assist the person in integrating mind, body, and spirit, so as to live in harmony with that condition. Western health care providers need to include Navaho definitions and concepts or terms that describe health, illness, and cure. Other Navaho healers include *singers,* who perform direct healing ceremonies, and *herbalists,* who use herbs to diagnose and treat illnesses (Hanley, 1995).

Navaho people believe good health derives from being in harmony with nature. Health also includes congruency with family, livestock, and community. *Blessingway* is the main philosophy from which many health ceremonies are derived. Ceremonies include attempts to remove ill health by means of stories, songs, rituals, prayers, and sand paintings (Hanley, 1995; Spector, 1996).

The Navaho Nation is the only Native American nation to have two nursing homes on its reservation, Chinle nursing home and Toyei nursing home (an intermediate and custodial care facility) (Mercer, 1994). To grow old in harmony and to die naturally of old age are still mentioned in prayers; nevertheless, many older adults now feel they are a burden to their children. Some believe that reaching old age is no longer respected (Mercer, 1994). The Navajo Nation's Council on Aging is reportedly more supportive of the tribal group home program than of nursing homes. Nursing homes are less favored because of the council's position that it is the younger generation's responsibility to care for their own aging family members (Kunitz and Levy, 1991).

Instead of shaking hands when meeting another person, Navahos extend their hand and lightly touch the hand of the other person they are greeting. Direct eye contact with another person is considered a sign of disrespect. Many Navaho believe that shared space provides a spiritual security and a sense of trust. Hanley (1995) states that most are oriented in the present time (i.e., they value living in the present).

Jewish Older Adults

Most American Jews immigrated from Eastern Europe from the late 19th through the early 20th centuries, bringing with them a high value on education and experience with urban living. Their education and the skills brought with them from Europe were useful to a rapidly industrializing society. They have high expectations of health care, and many older Jews have sufficient income to afford good care. Jews highly value good relations between parents and children, and older Jews can usually count on their children for support if needed (Markides and Mindel, 1987; Schwartz, 1995).

European Jews were distinctive among immigrant populations in the United States because they were not landholders or peasants but artisans, merchants, and small businessmen. Family and communal obligations were based on scripture and the Talmud (commentaries on the scriptures). Family patterns and communal responsibilities for the needy and the aged were carried over to the United States and are still relevant today (Markides and Mindel, 1987; Schwartz, 1995).

The experiences of death and dying follow tradition. According to Jewish law, nothing may be done to quicken death, but if the use of mechanical systems would delay death rather than promote life, they should not be used. During the dying process, a constant vigil is kept by family members. Nurses need to be aware that, after death, members of the ritual burial society (from the synagogue congregation) may wish to wash the dead body. Funerals are usually held within 24 hours, with no embalming or cremation. Very traditional Jews choose a plain wooden casket and a burial shroud. Visitation takes place at the home of the family. Some Jews practice deep mourning for one week ("sitting *shiva*"), which is followed by a semi-mourning period for 1 year. No flowers are used at Jewish funerals, but food is taken to the mourning family and charity donations are made in memory of the deceased (Jakobovits, 1975). Judaism considers death to be the final stage of life. Repentance, confession, and getting family obligations in order are important in helping the Jewish older adult to experience death with dignity and meaning (Markides and Mindel, 1987).

Over the years, the practice of Judaism has developed three branches: Orthodox, Conservative, and Reform. Each has its own expression of religious practices and related cultural beliefs.

Orthodox Jews are very religious, with strict interpretation of scripture. They abide by ancient (kosher) rules for diet, observe religious holidays faithfully, and hold some traditional health beliefs and practices. Abortion (with exceptions for saving the mother's life) is forbidden, and birth control is not allowed unless giving birth would be harmful to the health of the woman. If during life a limb is amputated, the limb is buried and then later placed with the body of the deceased person for reburial.

If an organ transplant would save the life of another human, it is permissible to donate the organ. Removal of the heart for transplantation is allowed as long as the dying person has total brain stem death. Autopsy is usually not allowed unless (1) it is required by law, (2) the person has a hereditary disease and the information from an autopsy may help other family members, or (3) other people are known to be suffering from the same problem and knowledge from an autopsy may help them (Schwartz, 1995).

> # W e l l n e s s
>
> **❝**Only with knowledge of the client's culture can the nurse adequately assess, plan, implement, and evaluate care.**❞**

The traditional gender roles for a woman are those of homemaker and mother, and the men are expected to be the breadwinners. Modesty is extremely important. Women always cover their hair (typically, with a wig) except when in private with their husbands, and they cover their arms and legs at all times in public. Men wear beards, cover their heads with skull-caps (yarmulkes), and in some sects wear long earlocks, large black hats, and long black coats (Schwartz, 1995).

Conservative Jews are observant of religious practices but less fundamentalistic in interpretation of scripture. Some are strict in following rules for kosher diet and holiday observances, whereas others are more moderate. Most accept all birth control methods, abortion, autopsy, and organ donation and reception (Schwartz, 1995). *Reform Jews* are more liberal in religious observation of diet and in holiday observances.

Jews tend to be very expressive and verbal about their innermost thoughts. Many use their hands to express and emphasize what is stated. Social touching and close space between individuals is welcomed among most Jewish people, although among unmarried Orthodox Jews, male/female touching is not accepted. A nurse, when caring for an Orthodox Jewish client of the opposite sex, should use touch only for hands-on care. Casual touching of the Orthodox Jewish client at any other time would be considered offensive (Schwartz, 1995).

Visitation of the sick is considered an obligation and a good deed (*mitzvah*) and is done by family, close friends, and the rabbi. Much emphasis is put on health promotion through diet, and it is common to seek medical attention readily for unknown symptoms. Many are very demonstrative of pain and suffering and openly display emotions.

Time is oriented toward the past, present, and future. Jews are very much concerned about the past, especially in relation to the Holocaust. During the wedding ceremony, the breaking of a glass serves as a historic reminder of the destruction of the Temple and the dispersion of Jews all over the world. Jews are also present-minded and concern themselves with social causes and political issues. Their future orientation to time is exemplified by their interest in the education of children. During illness, adults may worry about the implications of their illness for the future of their jobs or their families. Most Jews tend to value punctuality and may be unhappy if they have to wait for their appointments; it is generally acceptable to be 10 to 15 minutes late (Schwartz, 1995).

Jewish people believe that prevention of illness and maintenance of health are very important. Family members warn each other about possible dangers and discuss the causes of illnesses or injuries. Proper exercise, adequate sleep, and good diet are stressed. When a family member gets sick, the whole family is concerned and each person makes an effort to help the person get well.

Demonstrativeness in complaining about pain and discomfort is socially acceptable. If the Jewish client is unable to verbalize about pain or problems, often other family members will do so. Jewish clients tend to want explicit information concerning their illnesses. They may seek many professional opinions, want to know their pathology, the prescribed treatment and how it works, and the names and action of drugs ordered (Schwartz, 1995).

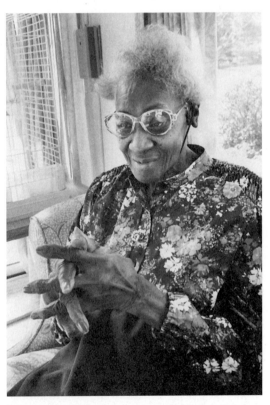

A lifetime habit of prayer signals deeply held beliefs that are of importance to the nurse/client relationship.

Orthodox (and many Conservative) Jews observe a kosher diet. The kosher diet allows meat only from animals with a cloven hoof that chew their cud. Meat and fowl are usually salted to drain the blood; this may present a problem for a client on a low-sodium diet. A special meat and fowl inspector (*shochet*) must observe all slaughtering, which is performed according to ritual. Meat and milk products are never served at the same meal. Separation of meat and dairy dishes, utensils, and cookware is necessary. Fish must have scales and fins, and no shellfish or scavenger sea animals are allowed. All food from a pig is forbidden. Fasting for 24 hours is required by all healthy adults on Yom Kippur (Day of Atonement). During Passover (*Pesach*) matzo and other special foods replace bread, leavened foods, and lentils (Williams, 1993). Nurses need to be aware that all Jewish clients are allowed to waive dietary restrictions if necessary for health treatment or if kosher food is unavailable. Furthermore, all commandments are suspended when a life is in danger, no matter how remote the possibility of death (Schwartz, 1995).

Asian Older Adults

The term *Asian American* includes people who are immigrants and people born here whose ancestors came from Asian countries, including Vietnam, Cambodia, Korea, the Philippines, China, or Japan. Asian Americans may be seen to have some similar physical, cultural, historical, and social characteristics, but it is important to understand that they view themselves as belonging to distinct ethnic subgroups and cultures.

The traditional head of the Asian American household is the husband/father. The authority is passed to the oldest son when the father is absent. The father is responsible for family decision-making, and the subordinate position of the wife/mother is firmly established. The family consists of the husband, his wife, and their children. Occasionally, there may be elderly people present in the household as well. Older adults are respected members and play an important role in the family. The traditional Asian American wife is devoted to the care of the home, children, and husband. Sons are considered a more valuable asset than daughters by some Asians (Yee, 1992).

Time orientation is toward the future. There is a great appreciation for the effective use of time. Appropriate social distance is important. Asian Americans tend to be restrained, formal, and polite. Spatial distance is appropriate in the health care setting. Emotions are not always outwardly expressed. Children learn the value of self-discipline and self-control. Avoiding conflict, confrontation, and disagreement is expected. Negative feelings of anger and pain are often suppressed. Close family members are not likely to be overt in expressing affection and warmth. Communication between health care providers and Asian Americans tend to be less verbal than with other groups. The health care provider should avoid prolonged eye contact and social physical contact. Language barriers may exist. A family spokesperson may accompany a client to the physician or the hospital to serve as an interpreter (Yee, 1992).

Caring

"*Health care providers need to be cognizant of cultural identity when caring for older adults of diverse backgrounds.***"**

Japanese Americans value self-control, and their response to pain is not verbalized. Children are not allowed to bring shame to themselves or to their family by unacceptable behavior. The Japanese value family piety, and children are expected to care for their parents when the parents reach old age. Good health is highly valued and is centered around *chi*, which is balance and harmony in relation to the environment. Harmony is represented by two opposing forces, *yin* and *yang*. Yin represents the female, which is the formless energy out of which creation emerges; it is sometimes interpreted as negative or empty, dark, and cold. Yang represents the male, which is manifested form; it is sometimes seen as positive or full, light, and warm. An imbalance in yin and yang is thought to cause illness. Application of heat to the skin (moxibustion), acupuncture, and careful mixtures of hot and cold foods are remedies for illnesses. There is a great reliance on herbs and the use of acupuncture for treating disease. The body is viewed as a gift from the ancestors that out of respect should be well maintained. Intrusive procedures are often believed to detract from harmony within the body (Yee, 1992).

Religions of Asian Americans are varied:

- Japanese Americans practice Shintoism and Buddhism.
- Southeast Asian Americans practice Buddhism, Confucianism, or Catholicism.
- Chinese Americans practice Buddhism, Confucianism, or Taoism.

The philosophy of holistic healing and care is present in most religions of Asia. The religions of Buddhism, Taoism, and Confucianism all emphasize the whole person, body and spirit. These religions each present a philosophy that permeates everyday life. Whereas western medical care is valued, many people of Asian lineage continue to keep their deeply rooted cultural philosophies, which include herbal remedies and acupuncture. Practices such as meditation and inner prayer are considered to be essential to good health and to healing of disease. Shintoism regards disease as the result of evil influences caused by contact with impure substances. Mental illness is considered a stigma, and clients who experience mental illness symptoms do not usually seek health care. Death and dying are considered to be a normal process of life, and life support technology is sometimes questioned (Yee, 1992).

Confucius instituted a cult of ancestors, in which one's actions are always measured in terms of how they will reflect on the family of origin. Confucianism is characterized by filial piety and respect for the family's older adults. The child is totally obedient to the father. Recent refugees from Asia find a yawning discrepancy between the roles of older adults in their homeland and those in the United States. Older adult refugees who lack the ability to speak English fluently find their credibility is decreased when advising younger family members, and they are gradually losing traditional family leadership roles. Although many older refugees provide child care assistance and perform household duties, they can no longer offer financial support and are no longer asked to offer their wisdom to the family (Yee, 1992).

Many older Southeast Asian refugees today find that they are not considered "elderly" by American society. In their traditional cultures they could be considered elderly by 35 years of age, coinciding with the time when they become grandparents. With grandparent status, in Asia they could have expected their children to support them financially (Yee, 1992). Korean older adults who are recent immigrants will have Confucian values, which emphasize family and authority, in contrast to the dominant society's emphasis on the individual. As children and grandchildren become more Americanized, the older adults perceive a loss of respect and authority (Andrews and Boyle, 1995).

Caring

❝ *Spirituality is highly personal and must be approached in a nonobtrusive and sensitive manner; all that may be needed is the nurse's silence and caring touch.* **❞**

In the United States, the majority of Asian Americans live on the Pacific coast. Most elderly Asian Americans live in urban neighborhoods, where they experience much insecurity and isolation. Because their children are able to acquire a better education and better employment skills, older adults expect help and support to come from them, as well as from friends and the community (Holmes and Holmes, 1995).

Diets of many traditional Asian Americans includes rice, tofu, eggs, chicken, pork, a variety of vegetables (often stir-fried), bean noodles, and fresh fruits. Most exclude milk and milk products because of lactose intolerance. They use rice milk and soy milk in many dishes (Williams, 1993).

■ SPIRITUALITY AND RELIGION

Spirituality

Spirituality may be defined as a basic or inherent quality in all humans that involves a belief in something greater than the self and a faith that positively affirms life (Miller, 1995), or a person's actual experience of or connection to God, or our capacity for self-transcendence, generativity, hope, inner meaning, mystical experience, and religious behaviors (Reed, 1992). Berggren-Thomas and Griggs (1995) state that **spiritual needs** may be defined as the need for connectedness to self, others, and a higher being; or the need for an ability to transcend the self, space, and time.

Although some people use spirituality synonymously with religion, they are not the same. Some people may be spiritual without any religious affiliation. Spirituality (or religion) often helps people make sense of the world and provides a healthful source for coping with life stresses. Spirituality may play a valuable role in eliciting health-promoting behavior. As a coping strategy, it may allow for greater emotional stability, which could protect against stress-related diseases.

Forbes (1994) conducted a descriptive study of 17 older adults and their primary caregivers and concluded that spirituality in older adults includes (but is not limited to) religious expression or experiences. Therefore, spirituality has meaning for those who are religious and also for those who are nonreligious. Spirituality is highly personal and must be approached in a nonobtrusive and sensitive manner; all that may be needed is the nurse's silence and caring touch. Forbes states that client needs may be assessed by thoughtful discussion of spiritual assumptions, beliefs, practices, experiences, and goals. Nurses should be aware of the changing spiritual needs of a client during different phases of illness and be responsive to these changes. Nursing interventions may include providing time for religious activities as well as for private expressions of spirituality.

Religion

Religion may be defined as a belief system with concepts that relate to something greater than the self. Common elements of religions include rituals that reflect feelings of awe, adoration, and reverence. Every religion includes such themes as a world view and the purpose of human existence; a belief in a supernatural being(s) or power(s); a moral system or code; and social organization (Miller, 1995). Many religions prescribe rituals associated with health promotion and treatment of illness, such as dietary directions or moral and social behaviors. In each culture, there is usually a set of beliefs about the meaning of health, about illness prevention, and about illness behavior. Medicine, prayer, and rituals often provide cultural solutions to anxiety, give one a sense of mastery over the unknown, and increase the sense of well-being (Miller, 1995).

Caring

"Nurses view the older client as a spiritual being who is on a journey through the life span; they see their own role as enhancing that journey."

Religion seems to help older adults cope with the changes in their lives. Older adults benefit from church attendance as a social interaction that also gives emotional support. Religious participation also seems to decrease depression rates in older adults and gives a sense of life purpose and an overall hardiness. Older adults need to find meaning in aging. Events such as illness, death of a spouse, or retirement may threaten the older person's sense of wholeness, value to society, and identity. Spirituality may help some older adults find the answers to why they are losing their previous roles, identities, and physical capacities. Some older adults believe in an afterlife, and their religion helps them cope with loss of a loved one, particularly if their belief includes a reunion in the afterlife with the person who has died (Berggren-Thomas and Griggs, 1995).

Religion or spirituality is a significant part of everyday life for most older adults. It is important not to miss this aspect of the whole person, because it is a strength for coping with adversity and loss as well as a support system that enhances the quality of life. The church or synagogue is in a unique position for older people because more of them belong to it than to any other organization. Today's older adults were reared in an era when religion was given more importance than it is now, and many have retained that emphasis in their lives. As people age, role transformation, deaths of loved ones, and physical changes cause them to reassess and restructure their own priorities. This reevaluation and reordering of priorities can occur because of the cognitive and emotional growth that enables older adults to think abstractly, tolerate ambiguity, and practice flexibility. The aging adult usually accepts mortality and views the world with objectivity (McFadden and Gerl, 1990).

The positive effect of religious attendance on the life satisfaction of older adults often persists even when health decreases. In some societies, old age is not a time of spiritual growth but of spiritual despair. Some believe that the world loses its luster and incentives, one's energy fails, and an indifference of the spirit takes over (Blazer, 1991).

The 1971 White House Conference on Aging addressed the spiritual well-being of older adults. Spiritual well-being was defined as the affirmation of life in a relationship with God, self, community, and environment that nurtures and celebrates wholeness. Areas of spiritual need include relief from anxieties and fears, preparation for death, personality integration, and a philosophy of life. Spirituality often provides the framework within which older adults evaluate the meaning of later years (Blazer, 1991). Donley (1991) defines *spiritual nursing care* as having the following:

- Compassion, or "suffering with"
- Helping the client to find a meaning for suffering
- Helping to remove the pain and suffering

Hope and emotional strength help many older adults to meet their own needs, especially when they lack health, wealth, or love from family members. Through a system of beliefs and rituals, religion provides a mechanism by which negative attitudes can be changed and life circumstances can be reevaluated. Religion can give an older person's life meaning and purpose and is immediately accessible and affordable regardless of the person's disability or circumstances. Religion contributes to the aged person's maintenance of hope; the regulation of depression, fear, and anxiety; and the protection of interaction with others. Many older adults use religion to find forgiveness. Ritual behavior contributes to a sense of personal community and emotional warmth (Nye, 1993).

Nye (1993), in his research with religion and identity among older African Americans, states that the black church serves several functions:

1. An expressive function or an outlet for deepest emotions
2. A status function whereby religious participation confers recognition that may be lacking or denied in the wider (white) world
3. A function of meaning, or source of order and understanding of one's life
4. A refuge function as a haven from an often hostile world
5. A cathartic function, or an avenue for the release of pent-up emotions and frustrations felt from oppression
6. A worldly orientation function, because it orients them toward an eventual fulfillment in the next life

Abromowitz (1993) states that it is generally accepted that religion grows in importance for older people, perhaps as a solace for increased isolation and dependency. "Even among the frail elderly and the demented there is an awareness of a higher being and a desire to establish contact" (Abromowitz, 1993). Familiar prayers are comfortable, and the activity is respectful and nonthreatening.

Implications for Nursing Practice

The North American Nursing Diagnosis Association lists a nursing diagnosis of **spiritual distress,** which can be defined as the state in which the individual or group experiences, or is at risk of experiencing, a disturbance in the belief or value system that provides strength, hope, and meaning to life (Carpenito, 1992). Berggren-Thomas and Griggs (1995) state that providing spiritual care for aging clients requires an understanding of where they are on their spiritual journey through life. Berggren-Thomas and Griggs believe that the components of spirituality help meet the unique challenges of older adults and provide a context for the aging process as an important step on life's journey.

When nurses do a spiritual needs assessment for an elderly client, they first make a nursing diagnosis of spiritual distress. This implies that the nurse knows what is the spiritual state of the client and what interventions are needed. Nurses may view the older client as a spiritual being who is on a journey through the life span; consequently, they will see their own role is to enhance that journey (Berggren-Thomas and Griggs, 1995).

Implications for assessment of spirituality or religion of the older adult may arise not only in the hospital environment but also within adult community programs. Program development for the older adult is an integral part of the activities that occur in senior centers, housing developments for older adults, and long-term facilities. Assessing the spiritual needs of those people for whom a program is intended will assist staff in better understanding the clients' needs and also provide clues as to why some behaviors may or may not be accepted. Concerns about separation of church and state have often affected the education received by many health care professionals, and thus they have not been taught how to implement plans to meet their clients' spiritual needs (Bracki et al., 1992).

W e l l n e s s

66 *Spirituality (or religion) often helps people make sense of the world and provides a healthful source for coping with life stresses. . . which could protect against stress-related diseases.*99

Nurses in existing jobs within the community, especially those who work with "minority" clients, may need to learn a foreign language (often Spanish) and pursue education that will help promote cultural sensitivity to their clients. In many cases, old ways of thinking and behaving will have to be deprogrammed; in their place, new lenses, or paradigms, will have to be supplied for health care to minority clients to be effective. This may be accomplished through several means: participating in in-service education, attending conferences that stress meeting the needs of the culturally diverse population, taking new courses or even obtaining new degrees from institutions of higher learning, or participating in focus group discussions. These activities, of course, are only examples of what can be helpful.

Increased interest in providing holistic care to clients has resulted in greater attention to religious and spiritual aspects of the client. Providers of **holistic** health care explore their clients' beliefs and practices as well as their spiritual support, supply spiritual or religious resources requested by their clients, and share beliefs without imposing values (Miller, 1995). Some clients may want to discuss their religious needs with the nurse, but they are not always given the opportunity. Health care providers may feel that it takes too much time or that they are uncomfortable in exploring something so personal. Delegating spiritual care to a religious member of the health team may be a solution. Older adults have an accumulation of life experiences, some positive and some negative, which give them an opportunity to look at their lives in different ways than younger people could. Physiological and psychological changes may have altered the person's functional capacities, yet changes in the person's roles, authority, and number and quantity of relationships have all impacted on the person's inner spiritual/religious life. Many have suffered physical and emotional experiences and often fear dependency on others as well as death as they continue to age (Fahey and Lewis, 1990).

■ CULTURAL ASSESSMENT TOOL

When caring for clients from backgrounds different from the self, it may be helpful for the nurse or other health care provider to use a structured instrument. The cultural assessment tool of Figure 5–1 is included as a guide (Holtz and Smith, 1994).

Summary

All individuals are unique, and at the same time they find a sense of self and identification with the values and practices of the subculture to which they belong. It is important that nurses be familiar with the values and practices of those for whom they care. Cultural diversity must be not only accepted but also understood and valued if nurses are to provide the highest level of professional care. The first step in this process is that nurses first examine their own cultural and religious values, noting any prejudices or **ethnocentric** practices, and resolving to increase sensitivity in relationships with clients.

This chapter defined ethnic, cultural, spiritual, and religious beliefs and values of a num-

CULTURAL CARE ASSESSMENT

I. DEMOGRAPHIC DATA

Name _____

Children _____ Ages _____

Grandchildren _____ Great-grandchildren _____

Siblings _____

Age _____ Date of birth _____ Place of birth _____ No. years living in U.S. _____

Marital status _____ Significant other _____

Gender _____

Education (highest grade or degree completed) _____

Job/profession _____

Present address _____ With whom do you live? _____

Socioeconomic status _____

II. ETHNIC BACKGROUND

Culture/ethnic background _____ Urban or rural _____

Place of birth _____ Length of time in present location _____

Number of generations within your family born in U.S. _____

Primary language spoken in home _____ Secondary language(s) _____

Religion. _____

Diet/special foods _____ Forbidden foods _____

Medications/treatments used _____

Alternative or non-western health practices used (acupuncture, healers) _____

What is good health and what do you do to stay healthy? _____

What is illness and what do you do to treat illnesses? _____

Who is family decision maker? _____

Who supplies your social support? _____

Who supplies your financial support? _____

Who do you take care of? _____

Who takes care of you? _____

What specific things do nurses need to know about your culture to better meet your health care needs? _____

_____

III. APPLICATION OF ASSESSMENT

A. List nursing diagnoses, rationale, and specific nursing interventions for client. _____

_____

B. Teaching needs _____ Goals _____ Time to be accomplished _____

_____

C. Interdisciplinary consults needed (dietitian, chaplain or rabbi, translator) _____

_____

IV. NURSING FACULTY COMMENTS _____

_____

Figure 5–1. Cultural care assessment tool.

ber of subcultures in U.S. society. Among these were the Hispanic, African American, Native American, Jewish, and Asian American older adult groups in the United States. Nurses may not have knowledge about various clients' religions or cultures, but they must be open-minded to learn and adapt nursing care plans to their clients' special needs.

REFERENCES

Abromowitz L. (1993). Prayer as therapy among the frail Jewish elderly. J Gerontol Soc Work 19(3/4):69–75.

Andrews M, Boyle J. (1995). Transcultural Concepts in Nursing Care. Philadelphia: JB Lippincott.

Berger K. (1992). Fundamentals of Nursing: Collaborating for Optimal Health. East Norwalk, CT: Appleton & Lange.

Berggren-Thomas P, Griggs M. (1995). Spirituality in aging: Spiritual need or spiritual journey? J Gerontol Nurs 21(3):5–10.

Blazer D. (Winter 1991). Spirituality and aging well. Generations 61–65.

Bracki M, Thibault J, Netting F, Ellor J. (Fall/Winter 1992). Principles of integrating spiritual assessment into counseling with older adults. Generations 55–58.

Carpenito L. (1992). Nursing Diagnosis: Application in Clinical Practice. Philadelphia: JB Lippincott.

Dickason E. (1994). Maternal-Infant Nursing Care. St. Louis: CV Mosby.

Donley R, Sr. (1991). Spiritual dimensions of health care: Nursing's misson. Nursing and Health Care 12(4):178–183.

Ebersole P, Hess P. (1998). Toward Healthy Aging. 5th ed. St. Louis: CV Mosby.

Fahey C, Lewis M. (Fall 1990). Principles of integrating spiritual concerns into programs for the aging. Generations 59–62.

Forbes E. (1994). Spirituality, aging, and the community-dwelling caregiver and care recipient. Geriatr Nurs 15(6):297–301.

Gelfand D. (1994). Aging and Ethnicity. New York: Springer.

Gelfand D, Yee B. (Fall/Winter 1991). Trends and forces: Influence of immigration, migration, and acculturation on the fabric of aging in America. Generations 7–10.

Hanley C. (1995). Navaho Indians. In Giger J, Davidhizar R, eds. Transcultural Nursing. 2nd ed. St. Louis: CV Mosby.

Hassan R. (1995). African-American concepts in health care. Nurse's Connection 13(1):6–7.

Holmes E, Holmes L. (1995). Other Cultures, Elder Years. Thousand Oaks, CA: Sage.

Holtz C, Smith K. (1994). Caring for culturally diverse families: A guide for health care professionals. Pamphlet (unpublished).

Jakobovits I. (1975). Jewish Medical Ethics. New York: Bloch.

Kunitz S, Levy J. (1991). Navajo Aging. Tuscon, AZ: University of Arizona Press.

Leininger M. (1970). Nursing and Anthropology: Two Worlds to Blend. New York: John Wiley & Sons.

Leininger M. (1997). Future directions in transcultural nursing in the 21st century. Int Nurs Rev 44(1):19–23.

Markides K, Mindel C. (1987). Aging and Ethnicity. Newbury Park, CA: Sage.

McFadden S, Gerl R. (Fall 1990). Approaches to understanding spirituality in the second half of life. Generations 35–38.

Mercer S. (1994). Navaho elders in a reservation nursing home: Health status profile. J Gerontol Soc Work 23(1/2):3–28.

Miller M. (1995). Culture, spirituality, and women's health. J Obstet Gynecol Neonatal Nurs 24(3):249–255.

Nance T. (1995). Intercultural communication: Finding common ground. J Obstet Gynecol Neonatal Nurs 24(3):249–255.

New York Times. (November 18, 1992). Latino? Hispanic? Quechua? No, American. Letters to the Editor.

Nye W. (1993). Amazing grace: Religion and identity among elderly black individuals. Int J Aging Hum Dev 36(2):103–114.

Reed P. (1992). An emerging paradigm for the investigation of spirituality in nursing. Res Nurs Health 15:349–357.

Rhoades E. (1996). American Indians and Alaska Natives—overview of the population. Public Health Rep 3(Suppl 2):49–50.

Sayles-Cross S. (1995). Aging, caregiving effects, and black family caregivers. In Johnson R, ed. African American Voices. New York: National League for Nursing Press.

Schiavenato M. (1997). The Hispanic elderly: Implications for nursing care. J Gerontol Nurs 23(6):10–15.

Schwartz E. (1995). Jewish Americans. In Giger J, Davidhizar R, eds. Transcultural Nursing. 2nd ed. St. Louis: CV Mosby.

Silverman H. (Fall 1990). Ceremonies and aging. Generations 51–54.

Spector R. (1996). Cultural concepts of women's health and health-promoting behaviors. J Obstet Gynecol Neonatal Nurs 24(3):241–45.

Treas J. (1995). Older Americans in the 1990s and beyond. Population Bull 50(2):2–43.

Turner T. (1995). Cultural diversity: Spanish-speaking Americans. Nurse's Connection 13(1):5.

Williams S. (1993). Nutrition and Diet Therapy. St. Louis: CV Mosby.

Yee B. (Summer 1990). Gender and family issues in minority groups. Generations 39–42.

Yee, B. (Summer 1992). Elders in Southeast Asian refugee families. Generations 24–27.

Zack N. (1993). Race and Mixed Race. Philadelphia: Temple University Press.

CRITICAL THINKING EXERCISES

Mrs. Min Chen, an 85-year-old Chinese American, is presently hospitalized for bilateral bacterial pneumonia. Mrs. Chen, who speaks only Chinese, lives with her married daughter, age 55, her son-in-law, age 57, and three grandsons, ages 19, 17, and 15. The daughter and son-in-law work full time and the grandsons are students. Mrs. Chen is presently taking oral antibiotics and is on nasal oxygen and a regular diet. She refuses to eat, does not want to take her medicine, smiles politely to the nurses and doctors, but is observed crying when in the room by herself.

The nurse, Mrs. Green, states in her nursing notes that Mrs. Chen is "noncompliant with the medical regimen and appears somewhat depressed. Because of a language barrier little more can be done to help her."

1. For the nurse to give more culturally congruent nursing care she could utilize the cultural assessment tool. Explain how additional data gathered from the tool could better meet Mrs. Chen's needs.

Mr. Sam Jackson, a 78-year-old African American man, is hospitalized for end-stage renal disease. He is currently alert and oriented, yet has a poor prognosis, of which he and the staff are aware. He had no family or friends visiting until one Sunday afternoon a group of six members of his church choir came to visit with him and conduct a mini church service at his bedside. The hospital staff at first were reluctant to have a large group of visitors come to Mr. Jackson's room at one time and perhaps disturb the other clients with the singing but eventually agreed.

2. Discuss Mr. Jackson's spiritual needs and how they could be met by the church choir group. Relate the strong emphasis of religion in African American older adults.

Sara Myerson, an 87-year-old Yiddish-speaking, Orthodox Jewish woman, is hospitalized for regulation of medication, diet, and activity for diabetes mellitus. Her primary nurse, Mr. James Thomas, wishes to learn more about his client's culture to better meet Mrs. Myerson's total health care needs.

3. Explain how each of the following potential problem areas could be solved.
   a. A male primary nurse
   b. Lack of kosher hospital food for an 1800-calorie adult diabetic diet
   c. Observance of Sabbath customs and practices
   d. Limited English, speaks mainly Yiddish

CHAPTER 6

Alterations in Lifelong Capabilities:
Social, Physical, Sexual

Suzanne S. Resner, RN, DNSc
Shirley Rose Tyson, RN, MA, EdD

CHAPTER OUTLINE

OBJECTIVES

After completing this chapter, the reader should be able to:

1. Teach a class in successful aging to a group of older adults in a community setting. Address social, physical, and sexual issues.
2. Analyze at least five stressors of later life and suggest ways to cope with them.
3. Teach a client four problem-solving skills for addressing unwanted changes in lifestyle.
4. Specify five ways to maintain healthy sexuality throughout life.
5. Compare and contrast health alterations that affect male and female sexuality and formulate options for continuing sexual expression.
6. Describe caregiver stress and formulate a plan for addressing it.

KEY TERMS

anxiety
caregiver stress
coping
crisis
fear
sexuality
stress/stressor

Capabilities are enabling factors that assist us in handling daily life in its mundane aspects as well as its challenges, problems, and changes. Among the enabling factors that lead to successful aging are mental and physical health, positive self-esteem, and adaptability, as well as heredity and personal endowment. Health problems, personal losses, or other life traumas are disruptions that assault the self and impact the equilibrium of an individual, which causes an alteration in the capacity to adjust or adapt.

The innumerable changes faced by one individual across the life span require myriad adjustments. People encounter life events that impact every aspect of their lives, including their behavior, attitudes, roles, status, and health. This chapter addresses some of the alterations that come with age in the social, physical, and sexual aspects of an individual's life and identifies ways of coping with them.

■ SUCCESSFUL AGING

Successful aging is a person's ability to adapt or adjust to the process of aging. Many factors contribute to successful aging, including the continuation of physical, mental, and social activity. Successful aging is accomplished by the maintenance of a person's capabilities throughout life (Seeman et al., 1996). Activity theory (see Chapter 1) proposes that individuals who continue their normal activities into old age probably age the most successfully. Older adults who continue to be physically and mentally active seem to be the healthiest and happiest. Figure 6–1 presents a model for incorporating wellness and successful aging.

Presently, there is an increasing trend toward focusing on the positive aspects of aging. Old age can be described as the period of clarifying and deepening what already has been attained from experience and from adaptation,

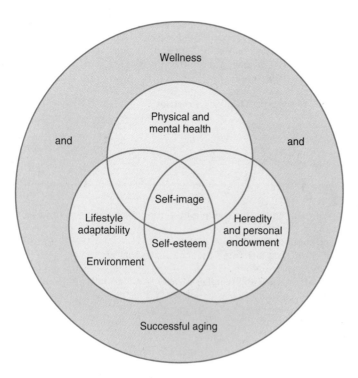

Figure 6–1. A model for incorporating wellness and successful aging: enabling factors.

across the life span. Table 6–1 presents an array of factors that contribute to successful aging and continuing life satisfaction. Successful aging is most readily achieved by older adults who have made every effort to incorporate the following into their lifestyles:

1. Financial resources to provide food, adequate housing, medical care, living expenses, and recreation
2. An environment that includes clean air, unpolluted water, sunlight, and fresh foods
3. Health maintenance through prevention and health promotion activities as well as periodic medical and dental examinations
4. Time spent with loved ones and others who give meaning to life, as well as a connection to the community

Many people actively enjoy life in later years and adjust well to changes that may occur as a result of the aging process. Successful aging and life satisfaction involve a positive self-image and the feeling that a person has made a difference (Fisher, 1995).

Self-Image

Positive self-perceptions and self-esteem enhance morale and mental health. Individuals who identify themselves as capable, active, valuable, and mentally healthy have achieved a positive sense of self. In later life, the older person's identification with family, culture, religious beliefs, and community are important contributors to maintaining a positive self-image. With a strong self-image, the older adult finds ways to move from a fully active life to one that may be more appropriate for age and capabilities. For instance, an activity such as part-time employment may be an excellent way to disengage—to slow down gradually while making the transition to older age (see Disengagement Theory, Chapter 1). Indeed, there are multiple adjustments that older adults make on a daily basis to deal with the transition from the middle to older years.

Changes in family dynamics or structure, retirement, widowhood, and declining function can have an effect on self-image with age; however, the personality and self-image achieved earlier in life remain relatively intact for most older adults. The older adults who adjust well and show adaptability are capable of increasing their life span and protecting their mental and physical health. When an older person's health is challenged and an alteration such as a disease process occurs, the nurse can assist the person to confront the stressor successfully through numerous **coping** (adaptive) mechanisms. The older adult can be empowered to take control of the situation to continue to live life in a productive manner (Strawbridge et al., 1996).

Personal interest in and maintenance of good physical and mental health, begun in early

TABLE 6–1. Factors Contributing to Successful Aging and Life Satisfaction

Physical Activity	Participation in moderate exercise several times a week increases health, vitality, strength, endurance, and flexibility.
Mental Activity	Participation in new careers, jobs, college courses, volunteer work, mentorship, and learning a new skill, new language, or how to play a musical instrument increases intellectual capacity.
Social Activity	Involvement in community and recreational activities enhances physical and mental health.
Heredity	Health and life span of parents have an impact on their children.
Attitude	People who are positive and creative usually live longer and adjust well to aging.
Rest and Relaxation	Adequate amounts of sleep (6 to 10 hours) and relaxation contribute to healthy life span.
Nutrition	Adequate nutrition with modest restriction of calories without malnutrition is said to increase life span.

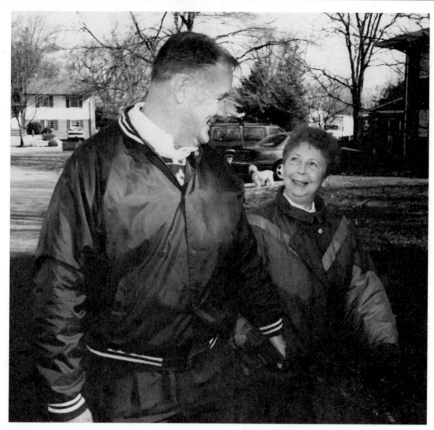

Active companionship is a source of strength in the later years.

life, promotes good physical and mental health in later life. Older adults need to participate in satisfying activities that stimulate their interests. The needs for intimacy, social interaction, acceptance, and belonging are innate in all humans, and they must be satisfied at all ages.

Intimacy and Social Interaction

Intimacy in a social relationship encompasses the concept of emotional bondedness. Emotional bondedness can be described as having three dimensions: (1) feelings of positive affect shared with another, (2) the sense that one receives emotional support from another, and (3) the sense of mutual sharing with another. The connections between mind, body, and social function are very important to the enhancement of mental health.

A person's social network is relatively stable over time until old age, when it may decrease rather abruptly. Those who are living alone for the first time or are under physical or mental stress may interact less with others than they did previously. Family and friends may become more important as buffers against the stress of life events or as support for health and personal care. When the older adult relocates to a congregate setting, continued social interaction with family and friends is a factor that influences a positive adjustment. Social interactions may often take place by telephone. The nurse in a long-term care setting needs to be aware that the most common result of loneliness is depression and identify resources that will assist the client to cope. Meaningful social interaction is crucial to maintaining a sense of well-being and self-worth.

Acceptance and Belonging

The need is universal for acceptance by an individual within a social network of family and others. In some cultures, respect for and recognition of older adults is paramount; the life experiences and accrued wisdom of older adults give them the highest status in intergenerational settings. In our own youth-oriented culture, often the opposite is true. Thus, perceived dignity, social status, and self-image are concerns for older adults. They are also concerned about the need for respect and recognition.

Interactional ties of non-kin relationships also relate to health. Friends and neighbors provide an important source of companionship and support. This social network provides a sense of belonging and is a source of positive self-image. Companionship and social interaction are important. While aging, it is healthy to be able to establish new relationships and live comfortably under new circumstances. Companionship is a basic human need; displaying affection is part of our sensual nature.

The Family

Today's families take on many nontraditional forms. We hear of the nuclear family and the extended family. Single parents also manage households. Because of the growth of the aging population, families of all varieties will be caring for their parents and their children at the same time.

The family unit is hoped to be a place of belonging and a source of joy and satisfaction. Older adults within a family can look back on their own achievements, applaud their children's successes, and enjoy those of their grandchildren and great-grandchildren. Family members are also a great source of support when older adults experience loss, death of a spouse, retirement, aging, and health alterations. Some older adults may feel a sense of loss as their childrearing years come to an end, but their grandchildren and great-grandchildren can bring new roles, new beginnings, and hope for the future. There are some older adults who have negotiated marriage, divorce, childrearing, remarriage, widowhood, and solitude very well.

As couples age and begin to lose physical or mental abilities, children assume the responsibility for parents and the power of handling the family structure. With role reversal can come abuse of power. The nurse can assess the power in the family by observing family interactions, taking a family history or review, and asking questions. A family history provides information on cultural values, religious preferences, feelings, obligations, and social class.

W e l l n e s s

66 *The spiritual dimension of a person's religion or philosophy of life enhances the person's ability to cope.* 99

Most adult children do not abandon or neglect their aging parents but care for them and maintain regular contacts. Today's older adults are independent, can usually provide for themselves in varying degrees, are less restricted in the roles of parenting and grandparenting, and are enjoying their later years.

Retirement

Retirement is a major change that affects all aspects of a person's life. Perceptions of retirement vary greatly, and this segment of life is handled differently by each individual. The time following years of work can be seen as an opportunity for happy and fulfilling activities or as a period when time drags and there is nothing to do. Many older adults enjoy retirement and the time they now have to devote to meaningful activities. After many years of employment in a career or job, and with preparation in advance for the free time, retirement can be a very welcome and rewarding time.

When the transition is easy and the older adult adapts and adjusts, successful aging and a positive self-image are inherent. Some older adults find retirement a threat to their financial and emotional security, having neither prepared for the eventuality nor adjusted to the change. If older adults no longer feel that they are useful, are no longer receiving compensation for their work, or perceive themselves as no longer having merit in the workplace or family structure, then their feelings of self-worth and their self-image are certain to be jeopardized. Table 6–2 presents factors that impact retirement and coping strategies for dealing with them.

Social Isolation

The opposite of social interaction is social isolation. Social isolation occurs when friends and relatives die or move away and when there is lack of a support system and possibly a lack of transportation; this can lead to depression and feelings of inadequacy. Interventions for social isolation include the following:

1. Support groups in which older adults can share similar problems and make new friends
2. Nursing actions that enhance the older adult's feelings of self-worth and self-esteem, especially those who may live alone in the community
3. Activities that promote health and wellness such as attendance at senior centers, exercise, nutrition counseling, recreational activities, and social interaction

With a positive self-image, older adults are better equipped to make life adjustments, to adapt, and to be aware of their own mortality. Older adults may experience some physical, mental, and emotional changes as they age. However, with the help and support of family and friends and nursing interventions, solutions can be found for most problems.

TABLE 6–2. Factors That Impact Retirement and Coping Strategies	
Factors	**Coping Strategies**
Psychological	Express emotions
	Verbalize feelings and fears
	Accept change in status and role
Social	Prepare for use of free time
	Participate in meaningful activities
	Develop social networks
Financial	Plan ahead for finances
	Investigate benefits and resources
	Apply for Social Security and other benefits
Spiritual	Explore the meaning of life
	Believe in a power greater than self
	Believe that coping is possible

Adjustments to Aging

Aging seems to come as a surprise to everyone. Those who wish to age gracefully and maintain health and vigor must come to terms with a plethora of new challenges. Among the many adjustments that older adults must make to survive are

- Adjusting to aging itself. This process includes changes in physical appearance, declining physical strength, and sometimes declining health.
- Adjusting to retirement. Issues include free time, reduced income, and loss of status that comes with a career or job.
- Adjusting to death of a spouse or significant other (widowhood).
- Adjusting to death of parents, friends, and long-term acquaintances (peers).
- Adjusting to change in residence. This happens when moving to a smaller house, retirement village, assisted living community, or nursing home.
- Adjusting to loneliness. This is a common problem for older adults with mobility problems and for those who are institutionalized.
- Adjusting to loss of independence. Physical or mental decline or impairment may necessitate dependence on others.

▩ MALADAPTIVE RESPONSES TO CHANGE

The experience of growing older brings changes that are not always welcome, yet they must be met and integrated if the individual is to continue to thrive. For many people, at one time or another the array of changes is overwhelming, and maladaptive responses can occur. Fear, anxiety, and stress are not peculiar to older adults; everyone is subject to them from time to time. However, the nurse who cares for older adults must be aware of their vulnerability to these negative states and be ready to help them move through them to a more positive stance.

Fear and Anxiety

Fear is an unpleasant emotional state that arises from a specific external threat or danger. **Anxiety** is also an unpleasant emotional state, but it arises from an unreal or imagined danger; it may arise spontaneously with no clear explanation as to its source. Fears may be more easily addressed because the specific cause may be removed, accepted, or transformed. Anxiety may be more complex to treat; regardless of its origin, severe and persistent anxiety can be disabling. Anxiety states may produce physical symptoms of palpitations, breathlessness, giddiness, abdominal discomfort, or even panic. Programs have been designed to reduce anxiety, and the caring nurse can be instrumental in assisting individuals to regain control.

Stress

Stress is the sum of the biological reactions to any adverse condition; it can develop from discrete events such as losing a job, loss of a loved one, an automobile accident, or a strained relationship with a family member. Chronic **stressors** (producers of stress) that may be disabling for some older adults include ongoing economic hardships, loneliness, and chronic or fatal illness.

Sources of stress arise from the challenges of everyday living—life events that are one-time occurrences and chronic conditions that are enduring stressors. Stress increases if physical problems are present. Older adults are especially likely to experience stress if the lack of resources leads them to feel vulnerable and powerless. Indicators of powerlessness are apathy, resignation, fatalism, and inability to make decisions. Decreased physical and intellectual capacity are causes of perceived powerlessness.

What is stressful for some individuals may not be perceived as stressful by others. Some life concerns producing stress are health, caring for others, maintaining independence, finances, household management, activity limitations, family and friends, health maintenance and illness management, time management, concerns about self-concept, care during periods of illness or disability, and a peaceful death. Stressors consist of pain or physical discomfort, alterations in social activities, physical activity, household activity, and activities of daily living (ADLs). Additional stressors are financial and psychological problems and loss of mobility about the community. The effects of stress can impact physical and psychological health. Although stress is a normal part of life that is encountered daily, some theorists believe that stress can lead to aging.

Abraham and Hansson (1995) describe successful aging as adaptation to developmental losses that produce stress. For example, hearing aids can provide compensation to a person who has a decrease in hearing acuity. Change nearly always produces stress at some level, but its acceptance is generally followed by a relief from stress. The caring nurse can have a major impact on, and influence a positive outcome of, the individual's functioning and adaptation to stressors.

Ineffective and maladaptive behaviors do not enhance individual growth; at times, such behaviors create the feeling of powerlessness. Maladjustment is characterized by immobility, dependency, anger and hostility, extended mourning, or self-destructive behavior. Loss of control and low self-esteem are experienced with responses such as drug and alcohol use, withdrawal from stressful situations, and distancing strategies that can consist of sleep, daydreaming, and other escape mechanisms. Coping mechanisms protect against stress, reduce anxiety, and facilitate the adjustment process, whereas overuse or maladaptive use of coping mechanisms can delay adjustment.

◼ STRESS MANAGEMENT AND THE CARING NURSE

By using a problem-solving approach, most older adults can reduce stress using stress management techniques. One method is to identify the stressor and systematically decrease or eliminate it. Another technique is to implement a time management plan. Other interventions used to manage stress are nutrition, rest and sleep, exercise, humor, assertiveness training, progressive muscle relaxation, and guided imagery. Stress management is also useful in treating chronic pain. Relaxation training is a widely used, nonpharmacological intervention with the chronically ill. Relaxation training decreases anxiety and nausea from chemotherapy and decreases pain. Various combinations of relaxation training and stress management, thermal biofeedback, and blood pressure monitoring have been beneficial in the treatment of essential hypertension. Stress management classes assist people to anticipate events, enhance perceived control or management abilities, and make available a greater variety of ways of handling future stresses.

An everyday method of reducing stress is through the use of touch. Touch is essential to well-being at every age. The nurse may be perceived as showing more caring through touch. Nurses' touching tends to be either *procedural* (instrumental or task-oriented) or *nonprocedural* (comforting or expressive). Using touch in the form of back massage (nonprocedural) decreases anxiety. To reduce stress, the slow-stroke back rub might be an effective noninvasive measure for promoting rest and relaxation.

Not all patients, however, are receptive to touch. It is important to develop a good nurse/patient relationship before using expressive touch during nursing interventions. The nurse should be sensitive to verbal and nonverbal cues when using either type of touch. Male and female nurses must use discretion in touching the leg, face, neck, and shoulder areas of an older adult.

During illness, physical contact may be perceived as an invasion because the patient is less able to defend personal space. Conversely, physical contact might be welcomed as a social contact and a caring response. The caring nurse needs to ascertain if the patient is able to tolerate touch or intrusion of personal territory (which can vary from 18 inches to 4 feet). The nurse may enhance the quality of the caring relationship by being aware of the effects that the act of touching may have on the patient.

Caregiver Stress

The manifestations of **caregiver stress** are varied and come from the physical demands on the caregiver's time and energy, as well as the mental distress of coping with the caregiving situation. The impact of caregiver stress may be reduced by the use of community-based care programs such as adult day care and respite services. Caregivers who participate in support groups staffed by community health nurses and social workers experience significant reductions in anxiety and depression.

A caregiver's checklist is included in the NIH publication No. 91-323 (March 1992, pp 58–59), from the U.S. Department of Health and Human Services, Public Health Service, National Institutes of Health, National Institute on Aging. People providing care, particularly for an older parent or a spouse, may find the following strategies helpful:

1. Give assurance to the person being cared for by expressing support and by showing that you can be depended on to help solve problems.
2. Become informed about areas relating to the older person's situation. This may include familiarity with legal matters (wills and property ownership), financial arrangements, health care resources, support services, housing and recreation resources, and knowledge about aging processes.
3. Obtain a professional assessment of the older person's problems. Seek out professionals trained in caring for older people by calling the local medical society, hospital, or medical school. A lawyer or a financial advisor may also be of assistance.
4. Help the person retain control of his or her affairs as much as possible. Limits often have to be placed on autonomy due to illness, finances, or for other reasons, but the older person's participation is still almost always possible.
5. Share caregiving responsibilities with family, friends, professionals, and paid helpers. Do not try to do everything alone.
6. Brainstorm with family and friends about ways to help an older family member remain active.
7. When making a change, start with the smallest step possible. This will help avoid becoming overwhelmed if many difficult decisions have to be made; they may not all have to be made at one time.
8. Seek professional counseling if a situation or relationship with an older person becomes too demanding.

9. Take time off. There is a need for recreation and time to pursue personal interests. Be honest with the older person about the limitations on time and energy.

As they age, husband and wife often assume the role of caregiver for one another. However, because both are older adults, the caregiver role may become burdensome and eventually lead to caregiver stress.

Women are often the caregivers: wives, adult daughters, daughters-in-law, or other females are called into the role. Many of these women also have full- or part-time jobs and younger family members to care for. Employers can reduce the stress of caregiving by offering programs at work such as alternative work schedules, caregiving fairs, lunch time seminars, weekly support groups, videotaped informational messages and programs, caregiving articles in company newspapers and newsletters, caregiving reference materials in the corporate library, and financial benefit plans that include dependent care allowance plans and unpaid personal leave.

The caring nurse should be alert to stress in family caregivers that could lead to deteriorating health and even possible burnout. The experience of caregiving full time has the potential to be emotionally draining, and the stress that arises from it can produce fear and inability to adequately address other aspects of life.

Respite Care

Respite care is a great help in the prevention of caregiver stress. It relieves the caregiver for a period of time so that the caregiver may have some time for relaxation, relief from stress, and recreation. Respite care provides a safe environment for older adults who need the service. Caregivers are also assisted by the knowledge that their family member is cared for by capable staff. Such institutions as Veterans Administration hospitals and nursing homes offer respite care programs. Beds are set aside for respite care, and families can make appointments and reservations for their use.

Nurses and Work-Related Stress

Nurses need to work closely with their employers to examine and monitor institutional and environmental variables that may contribute to work-related stress. When specific behaviors of their older adult patients produce stress in themselves, nurses should examine the underlying reasons why these factors produce stress. Relaxation techniques, leisure activities, support groups, nurses' groups, and mental health counseling for burnout and depression are of therapeutic value.

◼ COPING MECHANISMS, ABILITIES, AND RESOURCES

Coping mechanisms are learned behaviors used to manage, tolerate, or reduce stress. The behavior is effective and adaptive if it reduces stress and enhances the individual's ability to function. Family and friends often adapt routines and environments for older adults that act as coping mechanisms. These increase support and resources that can be utilized to overcome problems.

A repertoire of coping mechanisms, abilities, and resources is needed to survive. Three basic strategies can be used to approach the stresses of various losses: (1) anticipate the possibilities, (2) secure information related to the various issues, and (3) mobilize social support. To anticipate or prepare for events such as retirement or changing relationships, the patient might discuss and develop a plan of options for the possible event. Being prepared can assist the individual and speed adaptation. Securing information enables better patient understanding, facilitates decision-making, and gives the feeling of being in control. The social network of family and friends gives moral support and direct assistance during times of crisis.

It is important for the caring nurse to encourage the patient in adopting a repertoire that could include the following:

- Stay active.
- Pursue a healthy lifestyle (including diet, rest, and exercise).
- Cultivate lifelong interests.
- Socialize regularly.
- Keep working in activities that provide a sense of purpose.
- Have a positive, enthusiastic attitude.
- Seek consultation for health alterations when they occur.

These activities also stimulate older adults to maintain an interest in personal appearance, which can build self-esteem as they age. For example, if an older adult feels better after using cream for wrinkles or coloring the hair, the individual should be encouraged to pursue these activities. The goal of these activities is to build or enhance self-esteem.

Coping strategies to reduce stress include the use of diversional activities such as walking, reading, and gardening. Other stress reduction interventions include (1) discussing concerns and difficulties with support people, (2) using humor, and (3) respecting a value system and religious beliefs.

Health changes and forced retirement without adequate preparation create a sense of losing control and generate overwhelming feelings of dependency, fear, anxiety, or anger. Clients experiencing the uncertainties of a medical problem, pain, decreased resources, and possible impending dependence on others may be overwhelmed. Both formal and informal services are available to assist the client dealing with stress. Informal services are usually a combination of family, friends, and volunteer community support services. Formal services may include social work, respite care, day care, home-delivered meals, home maintenance services, and case management.

DEALING WITH CRISES

Loss of Body Part: Rehabilitation

Loss of a limb in the older adult patient is a crisis event. Rehabilitation is a challenge for this patient population. Coping strategies are needed to address this stressful experience, which can include grieving for the limb and phantom limb sensation. Nursing interventions should focus on understanding patient feelings, perceptions, fears, and stresses that relate to amputation. The caring nurse can provide support for both the patient and family through education and encouragement of participation in support groups.

> ## Caring
>
> **"** *The caring nurse acquires an understanding and respect for the sexuality of older adult patients and residents.* **"**

> ## Wellness
>
> **"** *A positive self-image helps the transition to retirement because it allows the older adult to adapt and adjust readily.* **"**

The caring nurse should be sensitive when discussing rehabilitation plans with older adults who are to undergo surgery for amputations. Patient education is a nursing strategy that can provide the older adult with a sense of control over the crisis of amputation and result in a better health care outcome. Education should focus on what can be expected and positive plans after surgery. A prosthesis can be vital to retaining function and independence. If hope can be offered for continued ambulation and independence, the procedure will be more favorably accepted.

Nurses' reactions strongly influence patient rehabilitation. The patient may be fearing social rejection or abandonment. Actual visits with other amputee patients or illustrated educational materials and audiovisuals may be used to allay such fears.

Patients who experience amputation of a limb are vulnerable to the phenomenon of phantom limb experiences. These include seeing, hearing, and feeling that the lost limb is still there. This is not imaginary but is thought to arise from continuing signals of nerves that formerly served the limb that was amputated. Phantom experiences may be treated by use of psychotropic medications, which can be a problem in older adults. The nurse assesses such patients by encouraging them to discuss their experiences to determine if these phenomena are present. If a caring nurse determines that patients are not bothered by these experiences, there may be no need for psychotropic medications.

CASE STUDY

Loss of Body Part, Phantom Limb Experience

Mrs. Brown, age 75, fractured her left hip at home. Her postoperative course progressed well and she looked forward to returning home to care for her husband of 42 years. However, on the third postoperative day she developed a deep-vein thrombosis that resulted in an amputation of the left leg. The loss was devastating to Mrs. Brown because she was a particularly independent person.

On transfer to a nursing home for rehabilitation, Mrs. Brown withdrew and did not participate in any self-care. She told her husband, who visited daily, that she might as well be dead. Mrs. Brown called the staff many times to complain of pain in the missing left leg. The phantom limb experiences caused her much anxiety as she grieved for the loss of her leg.

A caring nurse intervened. On her frequent visits to Mrs. Brown the nurse alllowed verbal expression of fears, anxieties, and stress related to the amputation. Specific patient education was initiated to prepare Mrs. Brown for adjustment to the loss and to a prosthesis. The nurse requested that Mr. Brown bring clothing and cosmetics for Mrs. Brown, which she had previously refused.

Over time, Mrs. Brown discussed the loss of her leg and other losses she had experienced. She maintained joint mobility through exercise. She began to participate in her care and appearance, requesting certain clothing from home. She discussed her plans for the future, which consisted of a left-leg prosthesis, discharge from the nursing home, and continuing with her life. Nursing intervention consisted of

- Emotional support
- Encouragement of verbalization and expression of feelings
- Coping strategies
- Improvement of functional capacity
- Patient education in preparation for prosthesis
- Involving family (patient's husband) in plan of care
- Preparation for return to community
- Referral to support group in the community

Treatment for breast cancer is often by mastectomy. Breast reconstruction procedures may restore a close-to-normal appearance, but there is still a need to become mentally prepared to begin adaptation for change. When loss of a breast is contemplated, the patient should receive advance preparation to maximize positive self-image. Peer counseling by other women who have undergone mastectomy is available. The nurse needs to be sensitive about sexual assessment and counseling, which are elements in the rehabilitation process for optimal functioning. Improving the functional capacity of older adults promotes a sense of independence, well-being, and a higher quality of life while enhancing self-image.

Chronic Illness: Adaptability

Understanding the meaning of chronic illness to the patient is a prerequisite for helping an older adult to cope with it for the first time. Caring for others requires both a knowledge of those cared for and a knowledge of self. To be effective, the nurse must be thoughtfully concerned with how others experience life. In addition, a professional understanding of the adaptation process will assist in designing effective interventions to promote realistic psychosocial adaptation to chronic illness. Authentic caring for those with a chronic illness is a part of life.

The nurse assists the patient to redefine the present by understanding the person's previous lifestyle and the adjustments required by the chronic illness as it relates to the past. Patients often define their experiences of health in terms of their abilities to perform functions independently. They want to care for themselves at approximately their previous levels of functioning. With a thorough knowledge of the health and personal history, the caring nurse is in a position to suggest ways patients can best manage and adjust to new, adaptive lifestyles.

The nurse can facilitate adaptive strategies by being sensitive to cues from the patient. Suggested adaptive strategies might be based on what has worked for the patient previously in times of stress. The caring nurse meets the needs of patients as sensitively as possible. The area of communication is important. When communicating with the elderly, the nurse might not understand the intent of the patient's statements. The thought from the patient's statement might differ from the literal meaning of actual words used. The nurse should gently clarify those statements that seem unclear to obtain a precise understanding of the patient's thoughts.

Coping with Health Alterations

Health alterations present a challenge for older adults. Nurses need to assess the older adult's coping strategies and encourage the patient to focus on the strengths developed through those earlier positive behaviors. As a full member of the treatment team, the patient must be given as much control as possible.

Caring

"Caring is shown through the act of reaching out and of touching in a way that is acceptable to the recipient."

Coping with physical or chemical treatment protocols may be difficult for older adults who are dependent on others for transportation or who have visual or hearing impairments. The nurse must take time to explain anticipated side effects, state realistic expectations from treatment, and correct any misconceptions. It is essential to maintain eye contact and speak clearly if the patient's hearing is impaired. Nurses can provide patient education by supplying written materials in large print, if needed. The patient who understands the treatment process has a higher tolerance for therapy.

Older adult patients with cancer may be treated primarily with radiation when medical problems preclude surgery. The nurse should be aware that these same problems may intensify the effects of radiation. Nursing care should focus on assisting the patient to manage the effects of therapy. Several areas might need special consideration. Nursing assessment to detect infections is critical because the immune system may be compromised due to illness or aging. Handwashing techniques and minimal contact with possible sources of infection are among the measures to prevent the spread of infection.

Many older adults live on fixed incomes. They are likely to cope by using the emergency department more frequently than those who are able to afford health maintenance and care for minor conditions. Common emergency department presentations by older adult patients include the conditions of myocardial infarction, acute abdomen, poisoning, hypothermia and hyperthermia, fractures, falls, and abuse.

Some elderly are survivors of incest, violence, and abuse. Once a patient has been identified as an incest survivor, goals for nursing care should include improving coping skills and increasing self-esteem by encouraging ventilation of emotions and communication.

If a particular stressor is determined, nurses can provide crisis intervention or assistance with active problem solving. The caring nurse should emphasize that the patient has survived the past and can successfully cope with the fu-

ture. Knowledge about coping strategies seems to make life more tolerable and to promote adaptability. Among the variety of coping strategies available to the patient to manage stress are being more assertive and using self-control.

Crisis Intervention

A turning point in life has been reached when patterns of interaction that worked in the past are no longer effective. To survive, the person must develop different coping strategies. The feeling of powerlessness involves a person's inability to cope with a situation. Conversely, successful coping involves overcoming powerlessness.

Several nursing interventions can be implemented to assist older adults to cope effectively when encountering a **crisis,** a transition or turning point in life or in health. The nurse should assess the individual's perceived meaning of the crisis, because the nurse's and older adult's perceptions may differ as to the meaning of the crisis and about strategies to be utilized in managing the crisis. Nursing interventions to assist older adults in coping effectively are implemented based on identified needs of the individual. Interventions should complement, supplement, or support the individual's effective coping skills to enable the achievement of positive outcomes that maintain or enhance quality of life.

One nursing role is to recognize and evaluate the stress level of the client in crisis. Nursing interventions consist of careful listening, providing explanations when and where appropriate, encouraging, and enabling a change in life patterns. Just providing an explanation about a medical or nursing procedure may reduce client stress.

Problem-Solving Methods and Skills

The nurse often assists older adults with adaptation to physical changes that occur with incontinence, mobility, altered sleep patterns, and altered appearance. Older people are faced with a myriad of changes, including altered nutrition and the psychosocial changes associated with retirement or relocation; some are at risk for depression, withdrawal, or isolation. The older adult who experiences stress may be a candidate for problem-solving methods. The nurse should encourage the individ-

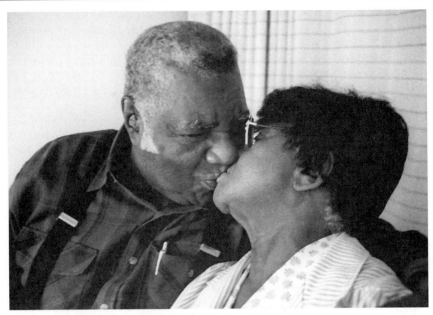

The need for expressing sexuality continues throughout life.

ual, who may be more cautious at this point in life, to use previous experiences and coping skills for possible solutions to new problems. A change in thinking or reframing skills might be useful. Problem-solving skills can also be developed by using a plan of action and approaching a problem with a solution in a systematic way. Nursing intervention can also be provided for other needs through phone-based case management.

Older adults succeed in reaching old age because of their strength, resilience, and ability to cope with stressors and changes throughout their lives (Jacelon, 1997). They have developed a repertoire of survival skills that include attentive listening, careful planning, strengthening relationships with helpers, and avoiding dependency by being able to lower aspirations to match their diminished abilities.

▰ HEALTHY SEXUALITY IN LATER LIFE

Sexuality does not change with aging. Sexual expression continues throughout life. Many older adults report feeling little difference between youth and old age. However, aging does relate to some changes in sexual physiology. The outcomes of these changes on sexuality vary. Some older adults find more barriers to sexuality and some older adults report greater sexual freedom.

Healthy sexuality is normally manifested by an attitude of enjoyment and a range of expression, interest, and ability. Sexuality in old age often includes tender affection and intimate sharing of companionship and life. Expressions of sexuality include eye contact, smiles, kissing on the cheek, and holding hands, in addition to sexual intercourse. While many older adults continue to engage in sexual intercourse, a concept of pleasuring has been described as any sexual experience that feels good.

Over the past two decades, a healthy attitudinal change of openness toward sexuality in later life has been occurring; included in this has been societal permission for older adults to choose alternate lifestyles. Health care professionals' efforts to improve sexuality emphasize the areas of nutrition, exercise, rest, and physical appearance.

Sexual interest may decline in older adults but for most it is never totally absent. All sexual activity—including kissing, petting, oral sex, partner masturbation, self-masturbation, and intercourse—is less prevalent among older adults. Vaginal intercourse remains the preferred sexual activity among older adults. Frequency of intercourse diminishes from about once per week for 30- to 39-year olds to once per year among 90- to 99-year-olds. Frequency, rigidity, and duration of erections are diminished in older males; most old-old males' erections are rarely adequate for vaginal intercourse, and other forms of sexual expression replace intercourse.

Alterations in Sexuality

Alterations in sexuality are experienced not because of changes arising from aging or from illness but also to disruptions in relationships. Alterations in health may lead to alterations in body image and self-esteem. A sexual relationship is intimately related to an individual's sense of self-worth. When that relationship changes significantly due to health alterations, the ability to communicate about the change is important. Maintaining sexual functioning in older adults is important because its premature loss can contribute to emotional and physical deterioration in later life.

ALTERATIONS THAT AFFECT MALES

Male sexuality peaks sharply around 17 years of age and then gradually declines. In contrast, female sexuality reaches full sexual potential around the late 30s or early 40s, with a slower decline than males. Many men in their 30s become concerned about sexual aging.

> ### *W e l l n e s s*
> "*Knowledge about coping strategies makes life more tolerable and promotes adaptability.*"

Male age-related biological changes relate primarily to diminished sexual desire, a lengthened time between ejaculations (which can be a few minutes at age 17 and up to 48 hours at age 70), softer penile erections, and a higher penile threshold for mental and physical stimulation. Male adaptations to these age-related biological changes might include less frequent intercourse, use of coital positions that facilitate intromission, and more reliance on partner-provided manual and oral stimulation. A de-emphasis on coitus with an exchange of

sensual pleasure in other ways can decrease male performance anxiety and increase female pleasure.

Males can maintain sexual functioning throughout life, especially if they have been sexually active in their earlier years. They need to be aware of the need to adapt to the age-related changes noted earlier and to utilize good communication skills with their partner.

The panel from the 1992 NIH Consensus Development Conference on Impotence found that (1) the term *erectile dysfunction* should replace the term *impotence;* (2) the likelihood of erectile dysfunction increases with age but is not an inevitable consequence of aging; (3) patients and health care providers do not discuss sexual matters candidly and thus contribute to underdiagnosis of erectile dysfunction; (4) many patients with erectile dysfunction can be successfully managed with therapy; and (5) education is essential.

Erectile dysfunction is diagnosed when there is an inability to obtain an erection adequate for sexual intercourse on at least 75% of attempts. Possible causes of erectile dysfunction are listed in Table 6–3. Medications associated with erectile dysfunction include antihypertensive agents and centrally active drugs; drugs of abuse include heroin, cocaine, alcohol, and tobacco. Obesity may be a factor in erectile dysfunction. Alterations in health often affect male sexuality. Nurses need to be familiar with the many therapeutic interventions that promote adaptation to these alterations.

ALTERATIONS THAT AFFECT FEMALES

Female age-related biological changes relate primarily to diminished sexual desire, vaginal dryness (generally occurring about 5 years after menopause), atrophy, and dyspareunia. Female adaptations to these age-related biological changes include use of nonsteroidal lubricants, estrogen replacement, and an assertive attitude.

Few alterations in health affect female sexuality. Menopause is accepted by most women as normal. Hormone replacement therapy for perimenopausal women and those older than 60 years of age should be considered on a case-by-case basis, because insufficient data are available for generalized recommendations. Conditions that do affect female sexuality in-

TABLE 6–3. Possible Causes and Drugs Associated with Erectile Dysfunction	
Possible Causes of Erectile Dysfunction	**Drugs Associated with Erectile Dysfunction**
Vascular changes	Antihypertensive agents
Hormonal changes including testosterone and bioavailable testosterone	Centrally active drugs
Endocrine alterations including diabetes mellitus	Drugs of abuse such as
Hypogonadism and thyroid disorders	Heroin
Neurological alterations including cerebrovascular accidents	Cocaine
Spinal injuries	Alcohol
Multiple sclerosis	Tobacco
Nutritional deficiencies including zinc and vitamin B_{12}	
Psychotropic illness including performance anxiety	
Widower's syndrome	
Depression	
Bereavement	
Anxiety	
Stress	
Medical illness including chronic illness	
Degenerative joint disease	
Obstructive pulmonary disease	
Parkinson's disease	
Chronic renal failure	
Sleep disturbances	
Prostate disease	
Cancer	

clude diseases related to the pelvic and genital organs, surgery that impairs body image, neurological and chronic illnesses, pain, anxiety, and depression.

Most women experience some vulvovaginal atrophy after menopause. Symptoms include burning, pruritus, insertion dyspareunia, discharge, and bleeding. Atrophy can cause vulvovaginitis, or the condition may be due to other causes, including sexually transmitted diseases (STDs), candidiasis, and vulvar dystrophies. Proper hygiene, pelvic muscle exercises, and continued sexual activity using adequate lubrication maintain healthy vulvovaginal tissue.

C a r i n g

“The caring nurse should be alert to stress in family caregivers that could lead to deteriorating health and even possible burnout.”

Urinary problems frequently occur because of reduced muscle tone of the bladder; stress incontinence is common. A hysterectomy or breast cancer may impair body image. The effect on sexuality of a hysterectomy with or without oophorectomy varies. Women whose self-esteem or body image is dependent on their breasts might be at risk after a mastectomy. Radiation therapy and chemotherapy can also impact sexuality. Specific health alterations that may affect female sexuality include

• Diabetes mellitus
• Arthritis
• Other painful conditions
• Medications
• Alcohol and drug abuse
• Hemodialysis
• Cerebrovascular accidents

Conditions associated with lack of pelvic support include vaginal-uterine relaxation, vaginal prolapse, urethrocele, rectocele, and enterocele. These conditions may affect female sexuality but are treatable through corrective surgery.

Gynecological malignancies resulting in genitourinary surgeries are associated with many sexual difficulties. These include vulvectomy, pelvic exenteration (en bloc excision of the uterus, cervix, and vagina and removal of bladder or rectosigmoid or both), radical cystectomy, or abdominoperineal resection (removal of the rectum). Nurses work with older women who have sustained these surgeries on a one-to-one basis, utilizing the patient's lifelong strengths and capabilities and using education to teach positive outcomes.

Sexual Health Care and Nursing

The caring nurse acquires an understanding and develops respect for the sexuality of older adult residents and patients. This involves recognizing the importance of assisting the patient to feel a positive sense of self-worth. Clothing, proper underwear, dentures, glasses, hearing aids, cosmetics, and attractive hairstyles are essential. They contribute to the feeling of well-being and enhance self-esteem. The nurse does not need to know all the answers but should function as a resource person to find help when necessary to increase the self-image of older adults. Continuing education is an effective means of influencing knowledge and attitudes that can help nurses become comfortable with discussing sexual health care, which is an important aspect of patient care. Nurses can teach older adults that sexual expression need not be restricted by age. This information presents sexuality in a positive light. An open atmosphere of trust and confidentiality that encourages discussion of the older adults' concern will promote a healthy attitude toward sexuality.

The management of sexual relationships among older adult residents of long-term care facilities should include the development of an individualized plan of care. A sexual history is part of nursing assessment and provides an opening for discussions. The plan should consider the resident's sexual needs and physical capabilities, provide for the resident's emotional comfort as well as that of family members, and ensure the resident's safety. All residents should be considered potentially infected with human immunodeficiency virus (HIV) and other blood-borne pathogens. Thus, precautions must be implemented to prevent the spread of infection and health teaching undertaken.

Wellness

"It is healthy to be able to establish new relationships as the person moves into old age."

When a sexual relationship appears probable, the resident's expectations need to be discussed with the nursing staff. During this discussion, questions and answers can be carefully considered. The resident's family may be involved, as deemed appropriate, with a nursing staff member present.

Nursing homes can promote a positive environment for sexuality among their residents. Nurses need to educate nursing home staff to understand that sexuality includes a range of sexual behaviors that express the residents' needs for closeness and tenderness. Three goals of the caring nurse to promote and increase sexuality in long-term care settings are

1. Teaching both licensed and nonlicensed staff accurate information about sexuality and the aging process
2. Facilitating the awareness of staff members about their own sexuality
3. Promoting an appropriately tolerant environment that fosters sexual freedom for residents

Sexually Transmitted Diseases

Older adults are not immune to STDs. The nurse should never assume that an older client is sexually inactive. STDs include

- Acquired immunodeficiency syndrome (AIDS)
- Gonorrhea
- Syphilis, primary and secondary
- Herpes simplex virus, genital
- Human papillomavirus infections, genital
- *Chlamydia trachomatis* infections
- Bacterial vaginosis
- Hepatitis B infection, sexually transmitted

At least 50 different organisms and syndromes have a role in STDs. Portal of entry or local sites of infection vary. Through education and counseling, older adults can learn to protect themselves from STDs by reducing risky behavior. Strategies for risk reduction of STDs are abstinence, monogamy, and safe sexual practices, including the use of a latex condom barrier.

In the United States, AIDS cases have been diagnosed in 10% of patients 50 years of age or older, and the number is growing. Older Americans are at risk of becoming infected with HIV because they are not protecting themselves. Many older Americans need counseling about HIV risk and condom use. Sexual and HIV risk assessments on older adult patients include questions on gender and number of partners, use of condoms, history of STDs, and history of blood transfusions or intravenous drug use. Nurses who understand the usual coping strategies of different cultures are able to assist individuals to seek the needed resources and facilitate acquisition of necessary knowledge and skills.

Summary

In this chapter capabilities were discussed that assist older adults in handling life's challenges, problems, and changes. Among these are positive self-image, capacity for intimacy, and social interaction. Nurses are particularly well positioned to assist older adults in managing and adjusting to the stressors that come with age. Health is the most significant of the variety of stressors that may concern aging individuals.

Nurses can teach or reemphasize coping mechanisms that allow patients to manage, tolerate, or reduce stress. New behaviors can be learned by most individuals at any age.

Individuals retain their sexuality throughout life. It is essential that nurses in all health care settings be sensitive to the sexual needs of older adult clients or residents and help them find healthy avenues of sexual expression.

REFERENCES

Abraham JD, Hansson RO. (1995). Successful aging at work: An applied study of selection, optimization, and compensation through impression management. J Gerontol B Psychol Sci Soc Sci 50B:94–103.

Fisher BJ. (1995). Successful aging, life satisfaction, and generativity in later life. Int J Aging Hum Dev 41(3):239–250.

Jacelon CS. (1997). The trait and process of resilience. J Adv Nurs 25(1):123–29.

Seeman T, McAvay G, Merrill S, et al. (1996). Self-efficacy beliefs and change in cognitive performance: MacArthur Studies of Successful Aging. Psychol Aging 11(3):538–551.

Strawbridge WJ, Cohen RD, Shema SJ, Kaplan GA. (1996). Successful aging: Predictors and associated activities. Am J Epidemiol 144(2):135–141.

U.S. Department of Health and Human Services, Public Health Service, National Institutes of Health, Consensus Development Conference on Impotence. December 7–9, 1992, 10(4):1–33.

U.S. Department of Health and Human Services, Public Health Service, National Institutes of Health, National Institute on Aging. Who? What? Where? Resources for Women's Health and Aging. NIH Publication No. 91-323, March 1992.

CRITICAL THINKING EXERCISES

1. Design a program for stress reduction for residents of a local nursing facility. Base your program on an actual visit where you do an informal assessment of the facility and interview at least three residents.

2. Interview a member of your community who is older than 75 years of age. What elements of satisfaction are present in this individual's life? What problems, if any, is the person facing? If health issues exist, what health care professionals are involved in helping to resolve them? Is the person being served adequately by your community? Summarize your findings and present them to the class.

3. Present a panel discussion in which class members express their feelings and ideas regarding sexuality and older adults. Create a series of questions to be addressed and then solicit additional questions from the class.

4. Visit three community facilities that serve older adults (e.g., senior center, retirement community, nursing home) and find out what their policies are regarding the expression of sexuality by their clients. Are the policies written? Are they the result of consensus? Are they missing? Conduct a class discussion about your community's readiness to acknowledge sexuality throughout the life span.

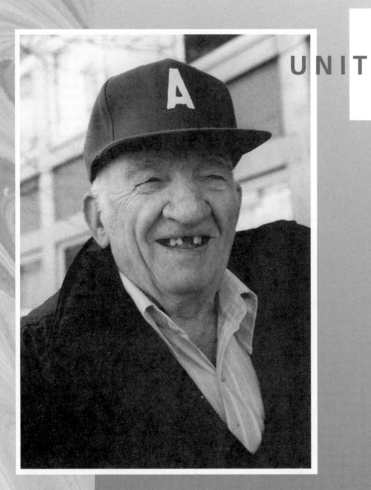

UNIT III

Physiological Health in Aging

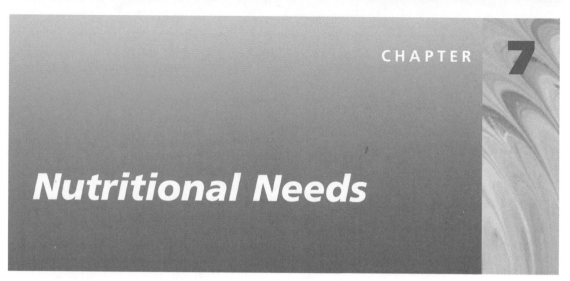

CHAPTER 7

Nutritional Needs

Paula Fishman, RD, EdD

CHAPTER OUTLINE

OBJECTIVES

After completing this chapter, the reader should be able to:

1. Apply the Food Guide Pyramid to teach normal nutrition to older adults in a community setting.
2. Analyze the nutritional status and identify any nutritional problems of an older adult client.
3. Describe the elements of interdisciplinary nutritional assessment and be able to obtain and use the appropriate tools.
4. Demonstrate how to gain access to current nutritional support programs available to older adults in your community. Include Internet sources.
5. Analyze the role of culture and ethnicity in the food habits of an older adult client.
6. Apply common dietary modifications in long-term care settings.

dysphagia
osteopenia
osteoporosis, menopausal
pica
recommended dietary allowances (RDAs)
xerostomia

Achieving and maintaining a healthy nutritional status is possible for a person of any age, and today there are many resources for older adults interested in maintaining wellness throughout their life span. For those older adults who are not attuned to the current emphasis on healthful living, however, the changes brought about by aging provide physical, environmental, and social challenges that may lead to malnutrition. Untreated malnutrition, which includes both deficiencies and excesses, can shorten the life span, decrease the functional capacity, and lower the quality of life of older adults. Unfortunately, the signs of malnutrition are easily overlooked or mistaken for "normal aging," even by health care professionals. Nurses can work with professionals of all disciplines to prevent, assess, and control malnutrition among older adults.

This chapter describes the common risk factors for malnutrition in older adults and how nutritional risk can be assessed by interdisciplinary teamwork. It outlines the prevalent nutritional problems that older adults encounter in community and institutional settings. Teaching tools and general dietary guidelines for nutrition education, as well as the various forms of nutritional support available across the United States, are included.

Although some brief discussion of dietary management is integrated throughout, this chapter was not meant to substitute for a diet manual or a diet therapy textbook. This chapter is designed to stimulate your interest in assessing the nutritional status of geriatric clients, because nurses play a vital and expanding role in team-based nutrition care, and a thirst for learning can go a long way toward maximizing the nutritional health of all older adults.

NUTRITION AND OLDER ADULTS

Effects of Aging on Nutritional Status

As in so many areas of geriatric health, there is wide variability in the older population's nutritional status and nutrition care needs. Malnutrition encompasses both undernutrition and overnutrition, and elderly people can manifest either or both of these types of problems, from iron-deficiency anemia to obesity.

Multitudes of healthy, vibrant, well-nourished older adults provide evidence that malnutrition is by no means an inevitable consequence of the aging process. On the other hand, the normal processes of physical degeneration, the lifestyle and environmental alterations common in this age group, and the increasing incidence of multiple disease conditions over the life span can put a strain on the body's ability to maintain optimal nutritional health. Collectively, older adults are classified nutritionally as a high-risk group, and some studies have found malnutrition in as many as 59% to 65% of institutionalized older adults (Phaneuf, 1996; Silver et al., 1988).

The prevention, assessment, and treatment of malnutrition in older adults takes place both in community and institutional settings. It includes identifying the existing and potential problems and their causes and providing services such as individual nutrition counseling, group nutrition education, congregate and home-delivered meal programs, dietary supplements, and food shopping assistance. These functions are often shared among nurses, physicians, dietitians, social workers, and other members of the health care team, because they require skills and include tasks that can be performed by a variety of health care providers and are best accomplished through interdisciplinary teamwork.

If undetected and untreated, undernutrition can abort or delay the healing process, shorten the life span, diminish functional capacity, and lower the quality of life of the aged person. Overnutrition can increase the risk or hasten the onset of chronic diseases and limit functional capacity. It is therefore in the interests of all health care professionals and their clients to ensure that the prevention, detection, and treatment of malnutrition is a routine part of geriatric health care.

Factors Associated with Nutritional Risk

Many physical, psychological, and environmental factors contribute to poor nutritional status within individuals and among subgroups of older adults. It is impossible to generate an exhaustive list of malnutrition antecedents or rank them in the order of their importance or areas most densely populated by people at highest risk.

The most common risk factors for malnutrition (undernutrition) among the elderly are as follows (Morley, 1988; White, 1994; White et al., 1991):

- Advanced age—especially 80 years of age and older

- Inappropriate food intake
- Frailty
- Limited ambulation
- Institutionalization or homebound status
- Having one or more chronic or acute nutrition-related health conditions, including alcohol abuse
- Taking multiple prescription and over-the-counter drugs
- Insufficient income
- Diminished mental capacity brought about by depression, dementia, or nutrient deficiencies
- Social isolation
- Low literacy, resulting in inadequate nutrition knowledge and food-preparation ability
- Being a member of a minority group
- Being edentulous

Refer to Box 7–1 for more detail on the risk factors for malnutrition.

Box 7-1   RISK FACTORS FOR MALNUTRITION, DIVIDED BY ETIOLOGY

Factors Likely to Impede the Ability to Consume an Adequate Diet
- *Loss of dentition and oral cavity problems.* Fifty percent of Americans age 65 and older have lost their teeth. Oral abscesses can distort taste or make chewing painful. Weight loss can produce ill-fitting dentures. Dry mouth can make chewing painful; this is a side effect of many psychotropic and antihistamine drugs, and may occur in normal aging in some people.
- *Swallowing problems* (see section on dysphagia).
- *Reduced ability to obtain food and/or to feed self.* This can be due to economic circumstances or to conditions that impede mobility, such as arthritis, vision problems, strokes.
- *Cognitive impairments and psychological problems,* such as dementia, anxiety disorders, depression, and paranoia about poisoned food.
- *Behavior problems in institutional settings,* such as wandering, social withdrawal, throwing food, and pacing.
- *Inability to communicate,* such as aphasia, difficulty in hearing, and difficulty in understanding others.
- *Taste alterations,* such as those that result from chemotherapy or zinc deficiency. There is some normal decline in taste acuity with aging, which may produce disinterest in food.
- *Overly restricted therapeutic diet, mechanically altered diet, and syringe oral feeding.* Weight loss should be carefully monitored, and food consumption measured. The efficacy of the diet should be reviewed regularly.
- *Enteral feedings.* Although necessary when oral intake is not possible, tube feeding for long periods increases the risk of side effects. Complications of tube feeding can include anxiety, depression, lung aspiration, self-extubation (patient pulls tube out), infections in lung/trachea or at the site of the stoma, pneumonia, constipation, diarrhea, fecal impaction, dehydration, abdominal distention, respiratory problems (airway obstruction, respiratory distress), and cardiac distress/arrest.

Continued

Box 7-1   RISK FACTORS FOR MALNUTRITION, DIVIDED BY ETIOLOGY
(*Continued*)

- *Constipation.* When chronic, it produces anorexia. Causes include laxative abuse, low food and fluid intake, low-fiber diets, inadequate exercise, and decreased intestinal muscle tone.
- *Inadequate knowledge about nutrition.*
- *Anorexia from medications.* Drugs that cause dry mouth can make chewing and swallowing painful. Oversedation can cause loss of appetite. Digoxin may suppress appetite or cause nausea.

Factors That Impede the Ability to Absorb and/or Utilize Nutrients Adequately

- *Reduced secretion of digestive juices.* Achlorhydria is a common problem of the aged that decreases body pools of vitamin B_{12}, iron, and calcium.
- *Drug–nutrient interactions.* Histamine-2–receptor antagonists cause fluid, vitamin B_{12}, calcium, and iron malabsorption. Cholesterol-lowering drugs bind bile acids and nutrients, causing malabsorption of vitamins B_{12}, folacin, A, D, E, and K and iron. Furosemide decreases calcium absorption. Sulfasalazine decreases folic acid absorption. Diuretics can cause hyponatremia, hypokalemia, and magnesium deficiency. Laxatives can cause malabsorption of calcium and vitamin D and can increase excretion of potassium. Aspirin and other nonsteroidal anti-inflammatory drugs can cause iron and vitamin C deficiency. Alcohol intake at 15% or more of calorie intake may result in deficiencies of vitamins B_1, B_6, and B_{12}, folacin and zinc, calcium, and magnesium.
- *Overdoses of nutrients.* Excess supplemental iron can cause zinc and calcium malabsorption. Megadoses of vitamin A can cause hypercalcemia, as well as anorexia, headaches, fatigue, necroses, and increased intracranial pressure. Megadoses of vitamin D can cause symptoms similar to those associated with megadoses of vitamin A, plus deficiency of vitamin K. Pharmacological doses of vitamin C can cause false-negative Hemoccult results, decrease vitamin B12 absorption, and dangerously increase iron absorption in individuals who are sensitive to iron toxicity.
- *Gastrointestinal diseases* such as esophageal stricture, gastritis, peptic ulcer, colitis, and diverticular disease interfere with intake, absorption, and utilization of nutrients. They are associated with malnutrition.

Factors That Increase Protein Needs and/or Overall Nutritional Requirements

Fever and inflammatory diseases
Surgery
Burns
Injuries
Pressure ulcers
Immobility

Note: The NSI screening tools can be ordered from: Nutrition Screening Initiative, 1010 Wisconsin Avenue NW, Suite 800, Washington, DC 20007; (202) 625-1662.

Nutritional Risk Factors by Group

Older adults constitute a heterogeneous group, so it is better to discuss common nutrition problems by subgroups. It is known that there are differences according to variables of age range, health status, income, geography, living arrangement, and gender. Unfortunately, there is also variability in the type and extent of data available for these diverse groups. Much less is known about the nutrition status of isolated and hard-to-reach groups such as homebound older adults than about ambulatory older adults younger than the age of 75, for instance. This limits comparisons among these groups. The nutrition problems of 60-year-olds who are concerned with lowering health risks such as hypertension and obesity tend to be quite different from those of 90-year-olds, who are more likely to manifest unintentional weight loss, protein–calorie malnutrition (PCM), or vitamin B_{12} deficiency. Noninstitutionalized, ambulatory older adults generally present quite a different set of problems and needs from those who are homebound or in acute or long-term care facilities. Even within the free-living ambulatory group, males and females tend to vary in the types and extent of osteoporosis and other nutrition problems encountered.

In 1990, The Nutrition Screening Initiative (NSI) was formed to address the limitations of the database on the nutritional status of older Americans and to promote better nutritional care for the older adult population in the United States. It is a joint project of the American Dietetic Association, the American Academy of Family Physicians, and the National Council on Aging, Inc. The NSI distributes a set of nutrition screening tools that can be used by older adults themselves and by a variety of health care and service providers. In this chapter, the section on nutrition assessments contains a discussion of these tools and their use.

Although the screening tools focus on undernutrition and are not diagnostic, the data generated from these screening surveys are beginning to provide information on the nutritional risk status of subgroups of older adults who have thus far not been represented in the ongoing nationwide nutrition surveys (largely those who are younger than age 75, ambulatory, relatively healthy, and willing to participate in extensive interviews and medical examinations—this group showing relatively few signs of undernutrition) or in independent, small-scale nutrition assessment research studies (which have tended to focus on frail or

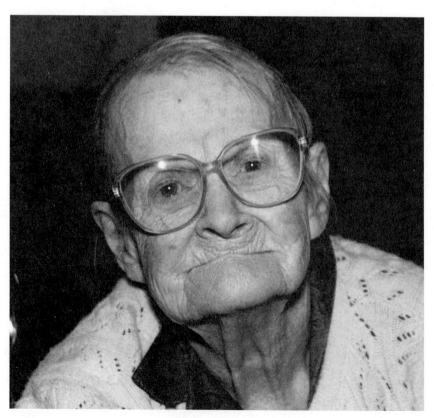

It is difficult to maintain adequate nutrition when the patient is edentulous.

acutely ill institutionalized populations—this group showing widespread undernutrition).

The 1990 national NSI survey revealed that 30% of the respondents skipped meals almost daily, one third of noninstitutionalized people older than the age of 65 lived alone, 45% engaged in polypharmacy with drug–nutrient interaction potential, and 25% had incomes below $10,000 (Netterville, 1991). All of these factors are included in the list of risks for undernutrition, suggesting that malnutrition is more widespread in older adults than previous nationwide cross-sectional nutrition surveys have documented.

Variability in Interpreting the Data

Even when objective assessment data are available, perceiving, prioritizing, and treating nutrition problems in the elderly can be subjective and variable, depending on the age and total health picture of the individual, the attitudes and knowledge of the person who is being assessed, and those of the health care providers and program planners who are providing the services.

There is no consensus on the maximum age at which to recommend lowering elevated blood cholesterol to reduce the risk of heart disease, for instance (Dwyer et al., 1993). Therefore, a total blood cholesterol of 320 mg/dL in an otherwise healthy 70-year-old man might be perceived as a treatable nutrition problem by some health care providers but not by others.

Should that 70-year-old also manifest an unbalanced diet and a recent decrease in dietary intake of minerals such as zinc and iron (due perhaps to loss of a spouse and subsequent depression), the desire to recommend reducing total fat and saturated fat intake would have to be balanced against this individual's food preferences, the substantial mineral contributions made by red meats, and his need to maximize mealtime pleasure and resume eating. In this case, preventing nutritional anemias and protein deficiency, which could lead to a downward spiral of anorexia, infection, and death, would be considered the major nutrition problem and take priority over dietary means of lowering heart disease risk.

The definition of obesity as a problem and the efficacy of recommending weight loss in older adults are other areas lacking in consensus (Andres, 1985). An otherwise healthy, nor-motensive 65-year-old woman who is 135% of ideal body weight but who has been obese all her life and carries her weight in the "pear-shaped" pattern (relatively small waist in proportion to her hips, thighs, and buttocks) may not have a nutrition problem requiring intervention. A hypertensive, diabetic person with the fat primarily distributed over the abdomen, however, definitely merits intervention at 120% of ideal body weight (Johnson et al., 1992).

In addition to the variability of nutrition problem definition and prioritization owing to the unique circumstances of aging, there are inequalities in nutrition problem identification and distribution of care services arising from factors of income and geography alone. Unless and until health care reform provides comprehensive health promotion services for all Americans, upper- and middle-income healthy older adults in the large urban centers will continue to have greater access to private, outpatient dietary counseling and support groups such as Weight Watchers and are therefore more likely to be perceived by nurses and other health care providers as people who are willing and able to make health-promoting lifestyle changes. These risk factors are also more likely to be identified as treatable problems in such urban settings.

Overnutrition problems, such as obesity, hypertension, elevated blood cholesterol, diabetes, and cardiovascular disease, obviously also occur in low-income older adults, who are disproportionately minority group members (Miller, 1996). Because free and low-cost disease prevention oriented nutrition care services such as counseling and group nutrition education can be very difficult to obtain, these elderly individuals are less likely than their more affluent counterparts to be recognized as needing help for overnutrition risk factors.

Box 7–2 lists nutrition support programs and services provided to the elderly population in the United States.

■ COMMON NUTRITIONAL PROBLEMS

As mentioned earlier, both undernutrition and overnutrition are found in older adults. Undernutrition is a more immediate and readily treatable problem, and it becomes increasingly

Box 7-2   NUTRITION SUPPORT PROGRAMS AND SERVICES

- *Food stamps* (for low-income people only). Administered by the U.S. Department of Agriculture, these coupons can be used to purchase grocery items and pay for meals at some participating restaurants. Several special considerations are made for elderly participants, including the designation of a representative to go to the Food Stamp Office and a larger admissible savings account.
- *Congregate meals at senior centers* (no income ceiling). Funded under Title IIIc of the Older Americans Act, this program provides a nutritious cooked lunch to anyone older than 60 and their spouse. Payment is voluntary. It also provides socialization, recreation, social services, and sometimes health and nutrition lectures.
- *Meals-On-Wheels,* both federally funded and private. A home-delivered lunch (sometimes supper also) is delivered to isolated homebound people older than 60 years of age. Eligibility and payment requirements vary.
- *Soup kitchens, food banks, and emergency food pantries.* Privately run, these programs provide a cooked meal (soup kitchen) or take-home groceries to people without food and money.
- *Homemaker, Home Health Aide* (low-income people). Provided through the Welfare Office, these workers will shop, cook, and provide light homemaking services for frail or ill adults.
- *Food shopping assistance.* A variety of federal and privately run programs provide help with food shopping. Local agencies on aging maintain lists.
- *Adult day care.* Meals and care are provided for frail, ill older adults who live alone or with people who work or need daytime respite from care provision.
- *Nutrition Education and Counseling.* The American Dietetic Association hotline (800-366-1655) can provide names of registered dietitians in private practice and referrals to agencies that may provide group education to consumers, such as the American Cancer Society and the American Heart Association. One can also contact the NSI for resource lists.

prevalent with acute disease, institutionalization, poverty, and advancing age.

Protein–Calorie Malnutrition

Protein–calorie malnutrition is the most severe nutrition problem, follows an unintentional significant weight loss (5% or more in a month or 10% over 6 months), and is usually secondary to a primary disease, such as a cerebrovascular accident or Alzheimer's disease.

Some other factors that impede the ability to consume food and/or cause abnormally high metabolic losses of calories and protein—and therefore lead to PCM—include chewing and swallowing problems, reduced ability to self-feed, and medical causes such as cancer and its therapies, anorexia from medications, septicemia, pneumonia, fever, diarrhea, ostomy losses, chronic obstructive pulmonary disease, and shortness of breath. The last two conditions interfere with food intake through the patient's fear of choking when eating or drinking. Parkinson's disease, with tremors, vomiting, burns, and pressure ulcers, can also cause increased metabolic losses of calories and protein. Depression and social isolation can lead to poor appetite and decreased motivation to eat.

When it is correctable, PCM requires immediate and aggressive intervention, because patients with hypoalbuminemia are at greater-than-normal risk for complications from medical and surgical interventions, and wound healing is delayed. There is decreased cardiac output and lower immune function with increased infection rate—and malnutrition worsens because of decreased absorption capacity caused by gastrointestinal tract atrophy and bacterial overgrowth.

PCM is most prevalent in institutionalized geriatric patients but is found in smaller numbers in old-old free-living people with extremely poor food intake and/or with diets high in starches and simple sugars, which can lead to gastric distention and early satiety. Prolonged mental confusion will eventually lead to improper diet and to PCM in the noninstitutionalized person living alone. Clients with PCM often present with altered mental status, but confusion can be caused by a variety of nutritional and nonnutritional problems, so definitive diagnosis must be made biochemically. If the PCM is severe and of long standing, other clinical signs of malnutrition may be present, such as flaky-paint dermatitis, glossitis, brittle hair, edema, muscle wasting, loss of subcutaneous fat, and diarrhea.

Serum albumin is a readily available and useful indicator; levels less than 3.5 g/dL (35 g/L) in the absence of dehydration are considered too low. Because of the long half-life of protein, depression in serum albumin shows up several weeks after the initial protein depletion.

If the patient is able to eat by mouth and has no renal problems, treatment consists of vitamin and mineral supplements and a high-protein, nutrient-dense diet, with protein-rich between-meal snacks and supplements. Commercially prepared high-protein beverages and solid food snacks are available, but the intense sweetness of many of these products might cause diminished appetite for meals. The patient's total food, nutrient, and calorie consumption should be carefully monitored by the nursing and dietetics staff and constantly adjusted. Depending on the nature of the food intake problem, adjustments might be in the form of finger foods, encouragement to take small bites, or the use of adaptive eating instruments to enhance self-feeding and further self-esteem and the desire to eat. Patients who are unable to eat, or eat sufficiently by mouth, require enteral (tube) feeding, often for prolonged periods. Oral feeding is clearly preferred in terms of functional status, quality of life, and safety.

Pressure Ulcers

One common sequel to PCM and other forms of undernutrition is pressure ulcers. They are caused by a lack of oxygen and nutrition to a body area—predominantly areas over bone or cartilaginous prominences, such as hips,

sacrum, and elbows. Nutritional therapy consists of correcting the underlying malnutrition. The diet is generally supplemented with multivitamins—especially vitamins A, C, and thiamine—and the mineral zinc. The best therapy, however, is prevention; pressure ulcers are not likely to form in well-nourished patients, even those who are immobilized.

Iron-Deficiency Anemia

Iron-deficiency anemia is a relatively common problem in the elderly, both institutionalized and free living. It is infrequently due to inadequate dietary intake (especially because postmenopausal women require modest quantities of dietary iron, and national nutrition surveys suggest that the majority of healthy, mobile older men and women tend to meet the daily iron intake recommendations) (Reuben et al., 1995).

The major causes of iron-deficiency anemia are (1) blood loss from chronic diseases such as malignancies and medications such as aspirin, histamine-2 blocking agents, antacids, and corticosteroids; (2) fevers (sweat loss); and/or (3) reduced iron absorption secondary to absent or diminished stomach acidity (achlorhydria). Acid is needed to reduce ferric ions to the more absorbable ferrous form. Tannic acid in tea interferes with iron absorption, however, so tea intake should be investigated in patients with iron deficiency of unknown etiology. Dietary insufficiency should be suspected in patients displaying one or more of the risk factors for malnutrition.

When iron deficiency is caused by inadequate diet, it may take years to produce symptoms, because the body maintains iron stores. Symptoms and signs include fatigue, anorexia, glossitis, pale skin, ankle edema, palpitations, and tingling extremities; a definitive diagnosis must be made biochemically. Iron-deficiency anemia is easily overlooked in older adults, because it develops slowly and patients rarely complain of the symptoms, which they mistake for normal aging.

None of the routine biochemical tests measure dietary intake levels but rather reflect body stores. The prevalence of iron-deficiency anemia depends on the criteria used for diagnosis. A normal decrease in hemoglobin values has been demonstrated in men older than 60 years of age, whereas women's values did not decrease into their mid 80s. Iron-deficiency anemia in older adults should be determined by a combination of low hemoglobin, low hematocrit, low serum iron, low transferrin saturation, and elevated iron-binding capacity. The early stages of iron depletion can usually be determined through depressed serum ferritin levels. In the elderly, however, inflammatory conditions can elevate serum ferritin levels, even in the presence of iron deficiency (Lynch et al., 1982).

Treatment of iron-deficiency anemia includes iron supplementation. Achlorhydric patients should have an ascorbic acid supplement combined with the oral iron. Oral iron needs to be ingested after meals to avoid epigastric symptoms such as nausea, indigestion, diarrhea, and abdominal cramping. When oral iron cannot be tolerated or malabsorption is the cause of the deficiency, parenteral iron may be needed.

Dietary treatment is important to prevent recurrence; it includes a diet high in total iron, especially heme iron, which is abundant in red meats and organ meats. This is because the elderly have a normal capacity to absorb heme iron but their ability to absorb nonheme iron is diminished. Nonheme iron sources (legumes, dark leafy greens, whole grains, dried fruits, and molasses) should also be included. Hemoglobin is made from protein, iron, and copper, and a well-balanced diet plentiful in the foods listed here and not dominated by milk will contain adequate quantities of protein and copper as well. A source of vitamin C (citrus fruits, strawberries, cabbage, broccoli, potatoes) taken with meals will enhance iron absorption. Coffee and tea consumption with meals is discouraged because they may reduce iron absorption. If **pica** (bizarre eating compulsions) is also present, it should be monitored and an attempt made to correct it. Excessive consumption of ice, Life Savers, snack chips, and chocolate is a common form of pica seen in iron-deficient patients. The etiology of pica is unknown.

Alzheimer's Disease

Malnutrition due to Alzheimer's disease and other forms of chronic organic brain syndrome is another common nutrition problem in the very old geriatric population, because the incidence of dementias increases with advancing age. Demented patients are at a significant risk for malnutrition, especially significant unintentional weight loss (Silver, 1993). This may be because the confusion and distractibility characteristic of the later stages of the disease can diminish food recognition and food intake, while wandering behaviors cause elevated losses of calories. Patients with cerebrovascular accidents, Parkinson's disease, Alzheimer's disease, and other dementias may show tremors, aspiration, decreased ability to self-feed, eating confusion, and swallowing impediments. With Alzheimer's disease there are also decreased function levels of the neurotransmitters that stimulate appetite.

To improve the nutritional status of demented individuals in any setting, it is suggested that the body weight be monitored at weekly intervals. Weight loss should signal the need for nutrient-dense supplements; otherwise a normal geriatric diet geared to meeting the food pyramid guidelines (discussed later in this chapter) should be sufficient. Meals should be small, simple, and regularly timed, with frequent snacks of favorite foods (including desserts, because sweets are well liked) supplemented throughout the day. Rather than forcing the person to sit for a meal, finger foods can be offered that can be consumed while wandering. Finger foods are also useful when the person forgets how to use eating utensils, and they avoid the risk of accidents by eliminating the need for sharp instruments. The nurse should try to be patient and allow extra time for meals when the patient's coordination is deteriorating.

A routine reminder of mealtime, such as a regularly scheduled before-lunch walk, may help to increase receptivity to the meal. Offering one food or course at a time will also help to alleviate confusion, and limited choices keep anxiety down. Foods should be cut into small pieces and the risk of choking avoided by eliminating tough skins, seeds, and dry, sticky foods.

> **Wellness**
>
> **"Multitudes of healthy, vibrant, well-nourished older adults provide evidence that malnutrition is by no means an inevitable consequence of the aging process."**

The diet should be adequate in calories and provide enough fiber and fluids to prevent constipation and dehydration. Adequate vitamin E in the form of polyunsaturated oils and choline from eggs and soybeans may also be useful in depressing symptomatology. When swallowing is impeded, the texture of the foods should be adjusted to prolong oral feeding as much as possible. (See later section on dysphagia.)

Cognitive Impairment Due to Malnutrition

Although it is clear that dementia can cause malnutrition, there are also indications that malnutrition can impede cognition. Subclinical malnutrition of certain water-soluble vitamins can cause cognitive impairments and dementia-like behaviors in the elderly. Some research has suggested that there may be significant links between moderate, long-standing nutrient deficiencies and the loss of cognitive function in aging. One study on 200 normal older subjects found that those with low blood levels of vitamin C or B_{12} scored worse in tests of short-term memory and problem solving than better-nourished subjects (although scores were still within acceptable range). Low blood levels of riboflavin and folacin were also related to diminished problem-solving ability in this study (Rosenberg and Miller, 1993).

Although of limited current clinical application, repletion of subclinical deficiencies of one or more nutrients in some documented cases of geriatric dementia have restored all or part of cognitive functioning (Goodwin et al., 1983). When a geriatric patient presents with cognitive impairments of unknown etiology, it is advisable to include a complete nutritional assessment, including functional levels of vitamin C, folate, vitamin B_{12}, and riboflavin. Serum folate levels are sensitive to dietary fluctuations; therefore, the red blood cell folate level is more specific evidence of a folate deficiency.

Dysphagia

Malnutrition due to **dysphagia** (swallowing disorders) occurs in people with oral, pharyngeal, and/or esophageal dysfunction. This could be caused by problems as diverse as stroke, multiple sclerosis, Alzheimer's disease, chronic obstructive pulmonary disease, carcinoma, systemic lupus erythematosus, or dry mouth (**xerostomia**). Dysphagia is a prevalent problem in the nursing home population, where as many as 59% of the patients may display swallowing impediments (Martin, 1991).

Undetected, dysphagia can lead to dehydration, aspiration pneumonia, or respiratory problems, as well as malnutrition. Dysphagia may also lead to emotional fear of eating, which can progress into a behavioral aversion to oral intake. Nurses need not wait for severe symptoms to develop in geriatric patients; assessment of swallowing function is recommended as a routine part of the nursing assessment and monitoring protocols for geriatric patients.

The goal of feeding the dysphagic patient depends on the etiology of the problem, but in general it is to maintain or restore as much oral intake as possible and to progress as far as possible back to a normal diet, while avoiding complications. Patients who have been on prolonged tube feedings should be monitored and evaluated for the reintroduction of solid foods whenever possible. This requires interdisciplinary assessment and implementation, with essential roles for the nurse, physician, dietitian, and speech-language pathologist.

The proper food texture for safe and comfortable swallowing is essential. Patients with delayed triggering of the pharyngeal swallow can be helped with cold foods that are mashed and pureed, are sufficiently thick, and are neither too dry nor too sticky. Patients with reduced lingual control do well with chopped, ground, or pureed foods, with gravies or sauces added to keep them cohesive. Patients with reduced oral sensitivity do best with bites of cold foods alternated with foods of other temperatures.

The diet should be tailored to the individual and the nature and stage of the swallowing disorder. To avoid malnutrition, oral feeding may be gradually introduced while enteral feeding is continued. Initially, a soft mechanical diet with thickened liquids (about the consistency of honey) may prevent aspiration better than a traditional pureed diet with water. Foods such as mashed carrots, pureed meats, mashed potatoes moistened with meat broth, oatmeal, and thick fruit purees hold their shape and have adequate texture to stimulate swallowing; watery liquids can leak down the throat and cause choking. Commercial thickeners offer the opportunity to turn thin vegetable and fruit purees into acceptably thick foods. Progress back to solids and liquids should be a goal when medically indicated. Milk products may be contraindicated when they stimulate mucus secretion. Fiber intake should be adequate to prevent constipation. Crushed bran stirred into foods is helpful for this, as are high-fiber commercial supplemental beverages.

In 1990, the journal *Dysphagia* (vol. 4, no. 4) devoted an entire issue to the nutritional aspects of swallowing disorders. It is an excellent review of the subject.

Osteoporosis/Osteomalacia

Osteoporosis, and to a lesser extent osteomalacia, are problems that are partly nutritional in origin and affect millions (over 50%) of older women, especially thin Caucasians and Asians, and about a fourth of older men (Mobarhan and Trumbore, 1991).

There are two main types of osteoporosis in older individuals. Type I, or *menopausal osteoporosis,* is characterized by significant loss of trabecular bone and is due to estrogen deficiency. Symptoms include pain in the vertebrae, rounded shoulders, height loss, and susceptibility to fractures. This type of osteoporosis is responsive to estrogen replacement therapy.

Type II (senile type) affects men as well as women. It has elements of both osteoporosis and osteomalacia (adult rickets, caused by a deficiency of vitamin D, calcium, or phosphorus), hence the name **osteopenia** is probably more appropriate for it. It involves loss of both trabecular and cortical bone. Aging itself is thought to be the primary etiology, but risk factors include family history, lactase deficiency, cigarette smoking, alcohol, caffeine (equivalent of 4 or more cups of coffee per day), lack of weight-bearing exercise, long-term inadequate calcium intake, dietary protein excess, vitamin D deficiency or excess, unbalanced calcium:phosphorus ratio (1:1 is ideal; red meats, carbonated beverages, and processed foods are rich in phosphorus), and renal disease.

Because bone density reaches its maximum levels before the age of 30, dietary prevention of osteoporosis should begin long before the onset of geriatric care. Incredibly, most adult women consume about half of the recommended 800 mg of calcium daily. Some studies do suggest, however, that bone loss can be slowed in the older population, particularly with a multipronged approach that works on the reversible risk factors and provides estrogen replacement therapy when appropriate.

Type II osteoporosis has been responsive to calcium and fluoride supplementation (although some studies suggest that fluoride may actually increase fractures), along with a recommended level of vitamin D when possible from diet and sunlight. Some elderly individuals have diminished production of the active form of 1,25 vitamin D by the kidney and may require a vitamin D supplement in the form of 1,25(OH) vitamin D_2.

Calcium intake in optimal quantities is believed to help build strong, dense bones in early life and to decrease the rate of bone loss in late life. In June 1994, the National Institutes of Health sponsored a consensus development conference on optimal calcium intake. The results of this conference, which recommended 1500 mg/day of calcium for postmenopausal women, should help to shape calcium intake recommendations for the U.S. population in the next revision of the recommended dietary allowances (RDAs).

If a 1500-mg calcium intake is desired, this is hard but not impossible to achieve with a low-fat, calorie-controlled diet (which most menopausal women should be following) and without supplementation; it can be accomplished, for instance, by drinking 24 ounces of skim milk daily with an additional tablespoon of dry skim milk powder in each glass, plus 8 ounces of fat-free plain yogurt.

> ## C a r i n g
>
> **❝***The most successful approach to the challenge of obesity in older adults emphasizes dietary fat reduction, group support and follow-up care, exercise, and behavior modification.***❞**

Lactase replacement products such as treated milk, tablets, and liquids can be helpful for lactose-intolerant people who are motivated to obtain a high calcium intake from dietary sources only. Calcium supplements are a way to boost intake, but it is generally agreed that food sources of calcium are superior. Calcium carbonate, for instance, temporarily decreases gastric acidity, which is needed for calcium absorption. Calcium citrate is the most easily absorbed form, but it is also more expensive. Added vitamin D can cause bone loss if the total amount of daily vitamin D intake exceeds twice the RDA. In the absence of sufficient fluids, supplements can cause hypercalcemia or calcium stones.

Diabetes/Glucose Intolerance

Type II diabetes and glucose intolerance are prominent overnutrition problems in the geriatric population. Defining the onset of diabetes (as opposed to glucose intolerance) in the aged population is subject to debate, because use of the standard ranges for younger people would label as diabetic about half of the older adults in the United States. Some physicians accept a fasting blood sugar of greater than 140 mg/dL as the definition of geriatric diabetes; others use a nanogram developed by Andres and colleagues (Reed and Morradian, 1990). Using age-adjusted standards, about 18% of the geriatric population are diabetic or glucose intolerant (Reed et al., 1990). Type I insulin-dependent diabetes is less common in older adults; the majority are treated with diet (and, ideally, weight control and exercise), with or without the addition of oral medications.

There are limited data on the nutritional status of the older diabetic and on the role of diet in correcting hyperglycemia, normalizing blood lipids, and preventing the complications associated with this disease (Schaefer et al., 1995). Common sense would suggest that dietary adherence to prevent complications would be most useful in the young-old population and that correcting undernutrition in the frail elderly would take precedence over tightly controlling elevated blood sugar levels.

We do know that diabetes induces a catabolic state, causing increased demand for vitamins and minerals. Additional minerals are lost through polyuria, placing the older diabetic, particularly one who is in poor control, at high risk for nutrient deficiencies.

No matter what the age, the optimal diet for every relatively healthy and mobile diabetic patient is one that is adhered to and results in good metabolic control. Because older adults can easily slip into hypoglycemic states, tight control has to be balanced with sufficient blood glucose levels to meet energy needs. Health care providers often err on the liberal side, believing that older patients cannot understand the diet or make food and lifestyle changes, or they may think that an old person's enjoyment of food is more important than the long-term prevention of medical complications such as blindness, visual impairment, renal failure, and amputation. Such providers do not allow the patient the full benefit of informed consent in the matter of choosing to adhere to a diabetic diet, however; complete nutrition education on diabetes should include information on the risks associated with prolonged hyperglycemia and the potential benefits of dietary changes. The diet instruction should be tailored to the literacy level and food acquisition and preparation skills of the patient, with instructions simplified and exchange lists eliminated when needed. In 1995, the American Dietetic Association liberalized the dietary guidelines for diabetic diets, allowing moderate amounts of sucrose.

If the patient is obese (which nearly 80% of type II adult diabetics are, although long-term care patients with diabetes can frequently be of normal weight or thin), the normalization of body weight should be the primary goal, because a weight loss of as few as 10 pounds can greatly improve glucose tolerance and reverse diabetic symptoms in some people (Johnson and Klignan, 1992). Calorie levels should be set to allow a reduction of 1 to 2 pounds/wk, and for most people should not be below 1000 calories/day.

Because regular exercise burns calories and improves blood glucose and lipid profiles in individuals of any age, an appropriate exercise regimen should be prescribed and exercise routines facilitated, especially in institutional settings. Swimming pools and exercise equipment rooms with appropriate "trainers" would greatly increase the amount of regularly scheduled aerobic exercise accomplished by long-term care patients who have good mobility; daily chair-bound exercise routines can be scheduled for less mobile residents. A few studies on well-conditioned elderly people show glucose tolerance, insulin sensitivity, and lipid profiles that are comparable to those of active younger people (Astrand, 1992; Elward and Larsen, 1992).

The optimal proportion of carbohydrate, protein, and fat in the geriatric diabetic diet is unknown. Increasing the carbohydrate calories to 60% of the total intake (which has been recommended for young and middle-aged adults) could push blood glucose levels too high and might elevate triglycerides (Reed and Morradian, 1990). Permitting too much simple sugar might also elevate blood glucose levels too high, although studies have suggested that sweets need not be eliminated completely (Reed and Morradian, 1990). A modest increase in complex carbohydrates from legumes, whole grains, and fruits—amounting to about 50% of total calories as carbohydrates—is probably a safe recommendation for most diabetic older patients.

Cutting fat calories down to 25% to 30% of the total intake (as recommended for younger diabetics) might help to lower heart disease risk in the young-old population but would be contraindicated in a malnourished octogenarian, because it is very difficult to obtain adequate calories and protein from primarily complex carbohydrate sources.

Excessive protein intakes might tax the diabetic kidney, but cutting protein below 0.8 g/kg of ideal body weight (about 12% to 15% of total calories for most people) in the frail population could increase their risk of PCM.

The optimal amount of soluble fiber (psyllium, oats, pectin) to improve lipid profiles and lower blood sugar levels in the diabetic also depends on the age and physical state of the patient. Immobile patients are at high risk of bowel impaction from excessive fiber intake, even from food sources such as bran cereals. Ambulatory individuals might benefit from 25 g/day of total dietary fiber, preferably using food sources (citrus fruits, apples, oat products) rather than purified commercial supplements.

The proper use of insulin depends on a sufficient supply of chromium. Dietary chromium is low in highly processed diets. Good food sources include legumes and grains, which are recommended for their fiber and complex carbohydrates as well.

Hypertension, Elevated Blood Lipids, Obesity

Other nutritional problems encountered frequently in older adults include hypertension, elevated blood lipids, and obesity. These problems are often but not always intertwined. The more of them that are present as co-risk factors in an individual, the greater that person's risk of cardiovascular disease. For each condition, there are nutritional aspects unique to aging.

Hypertension in the older adult is frequently treated with diuretics and sodium restriction. This can be problematic because both treatments increase water excretion, and older adults are prone to dehydration. Hyponatremia is another danger of severe sodium restriction that has been encountered in institutionalized individuals. If diuretics are used, 2 g sodium should be an adequate restriction. Sodium restriction is beneficial only in salt-sensitive individuals, so the use of low-sodium diets should be monitored for efficacy and discontinued when they do not work. Alternative nutritional manipulations (which may take 6 to 8 weeks to show an effect) include weight normalization and increasing calcium, magnesium, and potassium intake, which are postulated to have a protective effect in reducing the hypertensive effect of sodium (Dreosti, 1995).

If caffeine and alcohol intake are excessive, they should be reduced. If total fat intake is not restricted, it may also be beneficial to include sources of omega-3 fatty acids (e.g., mackerel, salmon, haddock) several times a week. Uncontrolled hypertension can lead to stroke, coronary events, and cognitive losses arising from multiple cerebral infarcts; dietary intervention can be effective and may eliminate or reduce the need for pharmacological treatments, even in the old-old population.

It is well established that normalizing blood lipid profiles in young and middle-aged people will lower their risk for coronary heart disease. Hypercholesterolemia in older adults is also a risk factor for heart disease, but the magnitude of its importance is less clear. In this age group, coronary events are likely to be caused by competing risk factors such as diabetes and hypertension. The current consensus is that lowering low-density lipoprotein (LDL) and raising high-density lipoprotein (HDL) blood cholesterol, even in the old old, may be a useful health promotion step, although the risks versus the benefits in the context of the individual's overall health and nutrition status are paramount.

If a person older than 70 years of age with hypercholesterolemia has a concomitant illness such as congestive heart failure, chronic obstructive pulmonary disease, cancer, or dementia, a cholesterol-lowering diet would probably be of little value, because it would not increase overall longevity or significantly improve quality of life. On the other hand, a motivated and relatively healthy 70-year-old with two or more congestive heart disease risk factors could undergo a regimen of diet, exercise, and other risk reduction steps with more positive expectations, particularly if LDL cholesterol levels of less than 130 mg/dL can be achieved.

To prevent malnutrition, the diet should not be extreme and should meet overall health requirements. The National Cholesterol Education Program (Dwyer et al., 1993) recommends 30% of calories from fat and no more than 300 mg of cholesterol a day. Because of the benefits of its mineral and vitamin B contributions, meat need not be eliminated, but use of lean cuts of beef, skinless chicken, and low-fat fish should be emphasized. Adding soluble fiber in the form of food sources, pectins, oat bran, or psyllium may have a slight additional cholesterol-lowering effect.

Low blood cholesterol levels are not always a positive sign in the elderly. An unplanned drop in total blood cholesterol to less than 160 mg/dL could indicate that the patient is severely malnourished and close to death.

Intervention in geriatric obesity is a matter of much debate. Dr. Reuben Andres, of the Gerontology Research Center, National Institute of Aging, examined data from the Baltimore Longitudinal Health Study and the Rancho Bernardo Study (Andres, 1980) and found that risk of mortality actually decreases with a modest weight gain over time. The highest incidences of mortality occur at the leanest and heaviest ends of the quadratic curve. For women, he found that the optimal body mass index (weight divided by [height squared]) is 22 for a young adult but increases to 27 by the age of 70 (Figure 7–1). These data may be somewhat misleading, however, because people tend to lose a lot of weight during terminal diseases, and that would make it appear that thin people experience greater mortality.

We know that obesity (20% or more over desirable body weight) can be a significant health risk and that it is associated in all age groups with increased hypertension, hyperlipidemia, and heart disease, liver and gallbladder disease, diabetes mellitus, accidents, respiratory problems, gout, and cancer of the colon and breast. We also know that losing as few as 10 pounds has been associated with improvements in blood pressure, blood glucose levels, and blood lipid profiles in many individuals. In terms of 5-year success rates, however, intervention in body weight has not proven highly successful in any age group. The minority who do manage to maintain significant weight loss have done so by constantly monitoring dietary fat and total calories, performing regularly scheduled aerobic exercises, and changing eating behaviors. To complicate the matter, regaining lost weight is probably more of a health risk than remaining obese.

What treatment should be offered a patient with geriatric obesity? It must be carefully individualized. First, the number of concurrent risk factors should be determined, as well as the history of body weight, the motivation of the patient, and the overall nutritional status. If the obesity is lifelong and hypertension, impaired glucose tolerance, and elevated blood lipids are absent, for instance, nonintervention may be the wisest policy. If the obesity is centered in the upper body and over the abdomen, and one or more additional risk factors are present, or mobility is compromised by arthritis or hip fracture, then multifactorial intervention in body weight is advisable. The most successful approach in older adults emphasizes dietary fat reduction, group support and follow-up care, exercise, and behavior modification (Wylie-Rosett et al., 1993).

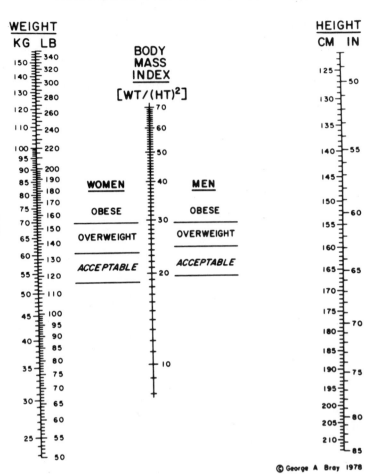

Figure 7–1. Nomogram for estimating body mass index. (Copyright George A. Bray, M.D., 1978.)

DETECTING MALNUTRITION

Assessment of Nutritional Status

Even in the clinical setting, geriatric malnutrition is often unrecognized and untreated, yet anyone who comes in contact with older adults can and should participate on some level in identifying and obtaining treatment for nutrition problems. Inherent in the nature of nursing assessments and nursing care plans is a significant role in nutritional assessment and intervention. This role can be expanded even further with a systematized approach and standardized assessment and follow-up tools such as those offered by the Nutrition Screening Initiative (White et al., 1991).

A thorough nutrition assessment includes diet, medical, drug, and social history data, anthropometric measurements, physical examination, and laboratory data. The nurse is often the first contact in the assessment process and the one best able to work with a dietitian to monitor patient motivation and compliance, food intake, and the overall success of nutrition education and nutritional therapies.

In many settings, it is the nurse who teaches family members and other health care providers to recognize and combat malnutrition and who coordinates team-based nutritional interventions in hospitals and long-term care settings. Other team providers can be any combination of physicians, dietitians, pharmacists, dentists, social workers, psychologists, physical and occupational therapists, and speech therapists.

Caring

66*In many settings, it is the nurse who teaches family members and other health care providers to recognize and combat malnutrition and who coordinates team-based nutritional interventions in hospitals and long-term care settings.***99**

To systematize and increase the practice of nutritional assessment and referral for care, the Nutrition Screening Initiative developed a self-assessment checklist (DETERMINE Your Nutritional Health Checklist), as well as a level I screen that can be administered in community settings by a variety of health or social service professionals, and a level II screen, which includes biochemical data and can be administered by nurses, physicians, and dietitians in a clinical setting. Copies of these tools can be obtained by writing to the NSI (White et al., 1991). The DETERMINE self-checklist assigns a score to a variety of physical and environmental warning signs of malnutrition. DETERMINE is an acronym for these signs: (D)isease, (E)ating poorly, (T)ooth loss/ mouth pain, (E)conomic hardship, (R)educed social contact, (M)ultiple medicines, (I)nvoluntary weight loss or gain, (N)eeds assistance in self-care, and (E)lder years above age 80. The reader can refer to the list of malnutrition antecedents earlier in this chapter to review the significance of these warning signs. Individuals who obtain a score that places them at moderate or high nutritional risk are directed to seek information and help. Nurses can play a role in ensuring that the DETERMINE checklist is distributed and collected in community settings where older adults gather, such as places of worship, health fairs, and senior centers, and that lists of local referral sources are available at the site that distributed the form.

The level I screen contains a nanogram for the body mass index (see Figure 7–1), with directions to refer the individual to a doctor for significant involuntary weight loss and when the index is above 27 or below 22. Via a checklist, it elicits more detailed information on eating habits, living environment, and functional status. Referral to a dietitian is recommended for people who have significant problems in selecting, preparing, or eating a healthy diet. Referral to a dentist is recommended when there are problems with chewing or swallowing. Referral to nutrition support programs such as congregate meals and food stamps is recommended when income, lifestyle, and/or functional status are compromised. Nurses can see that these forms are administered by the appropriate professional in community settings where older adults see social workers, senior center managers, dental hygienists, and others. The nurse can also provide the list of local referral sources.

The level II screen should be administered by a nurse, dietitian, or physician; it should be implemented in all clinical settings that do not already perform routine nutritional assessments. In addition to the measurements in the level I screen, this tool includes measurement of mid-arm circumference and triceps skinfold, serum albumin and serum cholesterol, clinical signs of malnutrition, and cognitive/mental status test results.

In this chapter, we have reviewed the major risk factors for malnutrition in the elderly. Nurses who work with this population in any capacity should be aware of conditions and situations that predispose an individual to correctable overnutrition or undernutrition; they should be able to recognize clinical signs of malnutrition; they should be familiar with how to network for the appropriate referrals and services when malnutrition is present or imminent. The reader is referred to Box 7–1, which presents common risk factors for malnutrition divided into categories by etiology and provides in-depth information to aid in their detection.

NUTRITION EDUCATION AND SUPPORT SERVICES

General Dietary Guidelines

Although there is a set of **recommended dietary allowances (RDAs)** for healthy older people (everyone older than 51 years of age is included in a single category), we do not yet have complete knowledge of the nutrient requirements of older adults. This is because the term *elderly* encompasses an age span of 40 years or more, because recommendations for "healthy" individuals (on whom the RDAs are based) are not as widely useful in this age group, and because too few nutrient requirement studies have been performed on people older than 65 years of age. In the past decade, research on the nutrition needs of older adults has been increasing. Many experts agree that the vitamin and mineral requirements of people over 75 years of age appear to be significantly different from those aged 51 to 74 (for some nutrients, such as vitamin B_{12} and vitamin D, perhaps higher; for some nutrients, such as vitamin A, perhaps lower). The RDAs may eventually add an additional age category of nutrient intake recommendations, as more age-specific data become available.

In the 1989 edition of the RDAs, the recommendations for older adults are almost identical to those for young adults. None of the nutrient level recommendations are significantly higher for older adults. In women, one recommendation drops substantially; the need for iron goes from 15 to 10 mg/day, owing to cessation of menstruation. In terms of preventing nutritional deficiencies, the general dietary recommendations for older adults are approximately the same as the recommendations for younger adults, and the same teaching tools—the Basic Four Plan and the Food Guide Pyramid (Figure 7–2)—can be used.

As the body ages, weight and appetite change, and food intolerances and gastrointestinal disturbances may occur. There can be problems with constipation, diarrhea, and chronic indigestion, and newly acquired food intolerances can develop. The existence of these issues should be assessed and brought into consideration when offering general dietary advice to an older person.

While recognizing the limitations of the RDAs and the controversies about disease-prevention diets discussed earlier in this chapter, older clients who are not on a therapeutic diet do need some general dietary guidelines on how to avoid both nutrient deficiencies and the excesses that can predispose them to cancer, heart and circulatory problems, and diabetes mellitus.

The Food Guide Pyramid (see Figure 7–2), developed and distributed by the U.S. Department of Agriculture, is an updated general eating guide. Its predecessor, the Basic Four Food Guide, was focused on the prevention of vitamin and mineral deficiencies but did not adequately emphasize fiber or teach dietary "prudence" for fat, cholesterol, added sugar, and calories. The Pyramid added a fifth (fruit) group and a "cautionary" category for fats, oils, and sweets. This caution is especially useful for older individuals who must obtain nutrient-dense diets (maximum nutrients per calorie consumed) because their calorie expenditures decline with a more sedentary lifestyle and a loss of lean body mass.

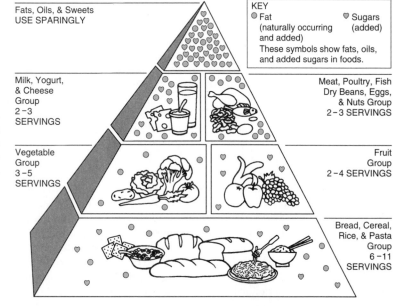

Figure 7–2. Food guide pyramid. (From U.S. Department of Agriculture and U.S. Department of Health and Human Services, Washington, DC.)

Fats, Oils, & Sweets
USE SPARINGLY

KEY
◦ Fat (naturally occurring and added)
♡ Sugars (added)
These symbols show fats, oils, and added sugars in foods.

Milk, Yogurt, & Cheese Group
2–3 SERVINGS

Meat, Poultry, Fish Dry Beans, Eggs, & Nuts Group
2–3 SERVINGS

Vegetable Group
3–5 SERVINGS

Fruit Group
2–4 SERVINGS

Bread, Cereal, Rice, & Pasta Group
6–11 SERVINGS

Looking at the Food Guide Pyramid (see Figure 7–2) from the bottom to the top, the shape of the five food groups visually reinforces the concept that the diet should be largely based on grain products, fruits, and vegetables; dietary balance is completed with servings of foods from the meat and milk groups. A handy way to remember this is that the plate should be about three-fourths full of carbohydrates, including grains, fruits, and vegetables. The remaining fourth is reserved for lean protein sources. The tip of the pyramid reinforces the

---

W e l l n e s s

"*A few studies on well-conditioned elderly people show glucose tolerance, insulin sensitivity, and lipid profiles that are comparable to those of active younger people.*"

---

fact that foods high in fats, oils, and added sugars are to be used sparingly.

The Food Guide Pyramid gives a range of servings in each of the five food groups. The number of servings that are right for each person depends on their calorie needs—as determined by age, lean body mass, gender, and activity level. The majority of older people consume no more than 1800 calories/day, and many women consume as few as 1200 to 1500 calories/day. As a quick rule of thumb, sedentary people can maintain current weight by consuming their weight in pounds times 10 calories (times 15 for moderate activity). In other words, 1600 calories would be appropriate for a 160-pound person. This would be achieved with the lowest number of servings in each of the groups.

In a 1600-calorie diet with 30% of the calories as fat, about 53 g of fat would be the daily allowance (1600 × 0.3 divided by 9 calories per gram of fat = 53 g). The amount of fat per serving of most packaged foods is available on the nutrition label, which has been revised to make it easier to understand. Foods with 8 g or more per serving should be used especially carefully, keeping the daily fat total in mind. Cholesterol should be limited to 300 mg/day or less. This can be achieved by using no more than three eggs per week and keeping meat servings lean (turkey breast, fish, beef sirloin, top loin, pork

tenderloin, skinless chicken) and modest (2 to 3 ounces per serving).

Sodium should be limited to 2400 mg/day or less. One teaspoon of salt has almost that amount (2000 mg). Again, nutrition label information on sodium content is helpful when making food choices.

Older adults often have blunted thirst and loss of kidney function. It is therefore important to remind older adults to drink plenty of fluids and to aim for eight glasses or more of liquid a day. Because overhydration also occurs, owing to retention of sodium and decreased ability to excrete water, fluid intake and output should be monitored whenever older adults undergo medical therapy.

Older adults should introduce high-fiber foods (e.g., legumes, oats, wheat germ, bran cereals, raw vegetables) gradually, especially when they are frequently constipated, diabetic, obese, or have an elevated blood cholesterol level and are unaccustomed to high-fiber foods. If they are well tolerated, legumes are a good choice several times a week. Dark, leafy green vegetables are also excellent choices for their vitamin and mineral contributions.

The Food Guide Pyramid is a simple, concise guide to healthful eating. In the final analysis, it is the moral and legal right of every competent older adult to make informed choices about food and diet—whether in the community setting or in an institution.

Cultural Influences

Older adults, whether living in the community or institutionalized, have food habits that have been shaped by past and present circumstances. Food patterns are an important part of an individual's identity, and maintaining autonomy and cultural identity at mealtime can enhance self-esteem and promote well-being. Food symbolism and preferences are developed through external and internal influences. These influences include ethnicity and culture, family interactions, and personality.

All nutrition services for older adults should consider culture and recognize the specific needs of people from diverse backgrounds. A 1991 study done by Lopez and colleagues in Indiana found that only 13% of the eligible Mexican American population were utilizing the congregate meal program. This underrepresentation could have been due at least in part to senior centers that were not accommodating to the language, food, and recreation preferences of the Mexican American older adults. To address these deficits, many communities across the country have since adopted culturally specific congregate meal programs.

To target support programs to those most in need, and to plan services that are culturally sensitive and address the most common nutrition problems in specific groups, more data are needed on the food habits by culture of the elderly population in the United States. Research in the area of aging and cultural foods has been sparse, but ethnic differences in nutrient intakes of older adults living in the United States have been described in some studies. Lam (1981) described lower intakes of riboflavin, calories, and vitamins A and C in Chinese Americans compared with "Anglo-Americans." In another study, "Anglo-American" males had higher intakes of riboflavin, vitamin A, and thiamine than did Hispanic Americans of the same age group (Hart and Little, 1986). Although individuals vary, these and other studies confirm that membership in a minority group places one in a high nutritional risk category (Miller, 1996). (Refer to the risk factors for malnutrition at the beginning of this chapter.)

Providing successful nutrition counseling and feeding services requires cultural sensitivity and sometimes cultural specificity. Culture and ethnicity help to shape food preferences and determine the symbolic meanings of foods, whether for religion, comfort, self-identity, or celebration. Older adults cope with physical, medical, environmental, social, and financial obstacles; some of these factors, along with culture and family background, shape dietary realities. Sometimes the stress of institutionalization actually increases a person's need for the cultural food patterns of more youthful times; providing these foods can promote a sense of belonging and reduce anxiety.

Nutrition Education and Counseling

There is no single menu or food pattern that is "healthy" for every older person, nor do our nutrition needs remain static as we age. The "right" food choices for each individual depend on a myriad of variables in the areas of health status, personal attributes, and social conditions. One man's meat may literally be another man's poison!

Given the depth and complexity of decisions that go into choosing food wisely, it is imperative that effective nutrition education and counseling be available to all older adults and that it be offered by a variety of care providers in the settings where older adults congregate. At present, the availability and level of professionalism of such services is limited and unevenly distributed. Registered, certified and licensed dietitians (who may be called "nutritionists" in nonhospital settings) have been trained and supervised in the art and skill of providing nutrition education. They keep abreast of current research findings, are able to sort out preliminary findings from established facts, and are able to translate complex information into "consumer friendly" terminology. They offer education and counseling services in hospitals, long-term care facilities, older adult day care agencies, outpatient and community health settings, and private practice. The American Dietetic Association (its hotline number is listed in the Resources section at the end of the chapter) maintains lists of qualified nutrition educators, as well as a resource list of nutrition education materials. Anyone may call the hotline number to have specific nutrition questions answered.

Caring

"All nutrition services for older adults should consider and recognize the specific needs of people from diverse backgrounds."

Nurses, physicians, health educators, pharmacists, and other professional and paraprofessional health care providers also deliver nutrition education services, often in settings where they function in the absence of a nutrition specialist. This section briefly describes the process of effective nutrition communications with the understanding that good nutrition advice must be based on accurate, current information. When the counseling goes beyond coursework completed by the person offering the education, it is wise to refer the client to a nutrition specialist or to seek a consultation with a specialist.

Effective education in any setting mandates a preassessment to tailor the content, methods, and materials to the individual or group being taught. The depth and scope of a preassessment depend on the purpose and structure of the education to be offered. Obviously, less information is needed for a one-time lecture than for a multi-session curriculum. This can be done by a written or oral survey of the clients or by gathering information from medical records and through interviews with people who know the target audience.

Examples of the types of preassessment data needed include physical status and demographics such as gender, age, ethnicity/culture, religion, and socioeconomic level. These data help to tailor the instruction to the context of the client. Because of vision changes, people of very advanced age may require specialized printed materials in large type on nonglossy paper and illustrations in vivid and contrasting colors (sometimes only black on white is perceptible readily). A preassessment of age range in the target audience may indicate the need for such specialized teaching tools.

It is also important to determine the education level attained, the primary language spoken at home, and any existing knowledge of nutrition. Written materials can then be designed at the appropriate reading level and translated into the required language. A small proportion of the older adult population is illiterate, but nonreaders can learn from well-designed pictorial materials. The diabetic exchange list is an example of a teaching tool that has been produced in picture format.

If the topic area for the education is open ended, it is a good idea to find out what interests the target audience, because people always learn best what they are motivated to learn. This is particularly true of the geriatric population. Studies have repeatedly found that, unlike children, older adults in general are not readily motivated to learn anything you wish to teach them, simply for the sake of learning. They want the information to be personally relevant and immediately practical. Even when there is no possible flexibility in the topic area, it is wise to preassess the aspects of the topic that are most familiar and useful to the audience and begin the session with these.

It is important to know the prevalent and potential nutrition problems of the target group and something about their eating habits and preferences. The level II screening tool mentioned earlier in this chapter can be used to survey this information. A sample survey for demographic and motivational information is included at the end of this section (Box 7–3).

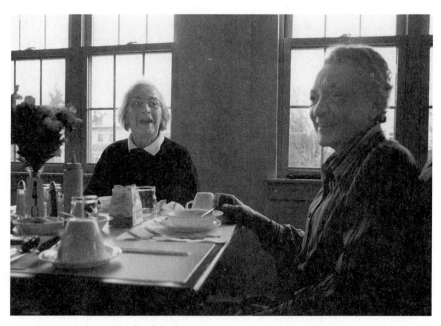

Appetite is stimulated by the social interactions around the dining table.

Box 7-3 NUTRITION SURVEY

This is a sample survey for the purposes of nutrition education preassessment in a site such as congregate meals. Actual knowledge and interest questions should be tailored to the target population and the potential topic areas. Be sure to use large type and leave adequate space for responses. Surveys such as this can be done in small groups, with participants helping each other to fill in the responses. Questions can be read aloud by a group leader. Combine this with the information from NSI level II screen.

This information is confidential and for the purposes of planning classes only. Your name is not required. Thanks for your help.

Check and fill in where requested:

Male _____ Female _____ Age _____ Race/ethnicity_____
Languages spoken _____ Current or former occupation _____
Following a special diet? Yes _____ No _____ If yes, check all types of diet modifications that you are following:
Diabetes _____ High blood pressure _____ Allergies _____ Cholesterol lowering _____
Liver or kidney diet_____ Weight loss_____ Ulcers or other digestive problems _____
Anemia_____ Osteoporosis _____ Other(s) Fill in _____
Where did you get the information about your diet?_____
Are you eating healthfully? Yes _____ No_____
If you could be eating more healthfully, what do you think you should be doing better?_____

Choose the five topics that interest you the most. Rank them from #1 (the best choice) to #5.

_____Saving money on food
_____Getting enough fiber
_____Preventing food poisoning and kitchen safety
_____Lowering blood cholesterol
_____Lowering blood pressure
_____Losing weight
_____Getting enough calcium
_____Cooking for one
_____Other(s) Fill in _____
Answer the following questions with T for true, F for false.

1. Egg white is free of cholesterol. T_____ F_____
2. Cooked meat must be refrigerated within 2 hours. T_____ F_____
3. Raw apples are high in sodium. T_____ F_____
4. Eight ounces of yogurt daily meets the calcium recommendation for an elderly man. T_____ F_____
5. A teaspoon of regular stick margarine is equal in calories to butter. T_____ F_____

Planning Group Lessons

Effective education begins with well-written goals and objectives. It is ideal to include the target audience in the planning stages of the educational process. Even when this is not possible, the goals and objectives are best directed at the potential achievements of the clients, rather than what the teacher hopes to accomplish. It is imperative that the nurse be sensitive to the knowledge levels of the audience, many of whom—especially if they are obese—may have been exposed to repeated nutritional lectures over their life span. A client-centered lesson on weight control could have several goals:

1. The clients will be motivated to reach and maintain an appropriate body weight.
2. The clients will incorporate an appropriate level of exercise daily.
3. The clients will read food labels when shopping and choose items that are low in total calories and fat (see an objective for this goal illustrated below).

Goals are broad expectations about long-term results. They do not have to be measurable or immediately achieved. Goals define the purpose of the education and suggest methodologies and materials that would suit these expectations. Objectives are concrete and measurable. They form a framework for the evaluation component of the lesson. To achieve goal 3 in an obesity class, an objective might read: *By the end of the lesson, all of the clients will correctly determine the fat and calorie information on a sample food label and choose the lowest fat per serving of frozen yogurt from samples of three labels.*

Concepts are sets of related ideas. Examples of concepts that clients will need to read and utilize the information on food labels include the following:

1. What information is available on a food label and in what format is it presented?
2. Which food items are required to carry the nutrition labels?
3. How does one use a food label to determine the calories and fat in a serving of food?

As a quick rule of thumb, three concepts are sufficient for a 30-minute lesson. To draw the audience into the lesson, the first concept can be a personalized one: *Why are food labels important to me?*

For each concept presented, the nurse must select a teaching method and materials. Examples of teaching methods include lecture, audiovisual presentations, and computerized learning. Any method can be used with geriatric audiences, but lecture is the least effective because it allows no interaction or student practice of skills. Older adults generally work well in small, structured problem-solving or hands-on teams. They do best when they build on earlier knowledge and skills and proceed from the familiar to the new. The assigned task must be clear, uncomplicated, and structured for the audience. Peer learners can help each

other to overcome physical or academic deficits, and no single individual is put in the "hot seat" with the team approach.

Materials could be posters, transparencies, films or videos, actual objects or models, computer programs, or printed matter. The American Dietetic Association produces excellent nutrition materials for geriatric audiences, as do the National Dairy Council and groups such as the American Heart and Diabetes Associations. It is wise to include some take-home materials for an older audience, because they need reinforcement and cues to carry out new behaviors. Choose commercial audiovisual software carefully, because many films and videos present too many concepts in a short period of time. A well-planned introduction, follow-up activities, and handouts can help to compensate for some "overkill" in a film or video. As a general rule, these complementary activities are used to stress the vital information and provide practical applications and skill development.

Effective education includes evaluation during the learning process as well as on its completion. Evaluation provides feedback to the student and the teacher, ensuring that new concepts are introduced only after previous concepts have been mastered. Paper-and-pencil tests are possible, but in general they are unattractive to older adults. Games, such as one built on reading a nutrition label, are a less threatening but equally effective approach. The level of teaching should be aimed at the sophistication of the audience.

One-to-One Counseling

Many of the same principles of group education apply to individual counseling sessions. Preassessment consists of a diet and social history that elicits information on the environment, skills, and habits of the client. The counselor can use this preassessment time to establish rapport with the client and to determine the client's amount of knowledge about nutrition.

Learning a diet or a set of new food-related behaviors necessitates motivation and comprehension. Making the appropriate behavior changes requires daily implementation of a new set of food-related skills. These are often enormous changes, with positive results difficult or impossible to detect for many weeks.

Clients do not undertake major food behavior changes easily or lightly.

Goal setting in individual counseling should be a mutual agreement between the counselor and the client. The setting of personal goals is a commonly used behavior modification technique. Modest goals can be achieved in the time between revisits. In weight management counseling, a goal for 1 week might read: *I will substitute diet jelly for butter and eat egg whites instead of whole eggs.* As in the process of "informed consent," the client needs to understand why and how changes would be of benefit and what risks accompany noncompliance.

Active learning methods and evaluative feedback are required for effective learning. For instance, a client can demonstrate to the counselor how to plan an actual menu using the diabetic exchange list. Models or pictures of foods to illustrate portion size are a great help, as are measuring utensils. Take-home materials are essential, because they are memory cues and provide needed repetition of the essential information. Computer-literate clients can use nutritional-analysis software to tailor their own menus. A Chinese client on a low-sodium diet can thereby include soy sauce yet remain within the diet prescription.

The purpose of nutrition counseling and nutrition education is to empower the client to make rational choices and positive behavioral changes. The role of the counselor is to motivate, instruct, and provide support. It is the client or the caregivers who must make the decisions and take the appropriate actions, because dietary changes are self-care behaviors. It is therefore important that the nutrition educator assume the role of a supportive helper, rather than a punitive authority figure.

Follow-up phone calls and revisit appointments create a supportive environment and provide information as questions arise. Self-help groups can be a useful adjunct to counseling, because they build in peer support and offer practical solutions to problems. In summary, nutrition education and counseling should be viewed as a means to support and empower self-care. The educator should tailor the content and methods to the students, build in participation and feedback mechanisms, keep the contents practical, provide written take-home materials, and maintain postcounseling contact through revisits or telephone calls.

Feeding Frail and Physically Challenged Older Clients

A common fear of the aged is the loss of self-mastery. Being able to perform the essential activities of daily living boosts morale and enhances self-esteem, particularly in an institutional environment. When physical or cognitive challenges diminish or eliminate the ability to feed oneself, it is essential that feeding assistance be tailored to maximize the efficacy and self-esteem of the person being assisted. Assistive eating utensils and rehabilitation with an occupational therapist can restore all or part of self-feeding functions in many cases, thereby minimizing the risk of nutrition status decline. Some patients cannot be rehabilitated and require total feeding assistance to maintain oral intake. Because choking is a potential risk when being fed, safe feeding techniques are imperative.

When the patient is sitting in a chair or in bed, proper feeding positioning is imperative. The person's head and back must be aligned at a 90-degree angle, and there should be no leaning to either side. Pillow supports at the hips and behind the head can help in some cases. An occupational therapist should be consulted when positioning is a problem.

If the patient requires feeding assistance, the experience should be aesthetically and emotionally positive for both parties, and delays (or rushing) should be minimized. It can be extremely distressing to wait for assistance in front of a tray of food for 15 to 20 minutes, watching the hot foods go cold and the cold foods grow warm! Adequate staffing at mealtimes can prevent undue delays and rushing, as can the use of trained volunteer feeders, regulations permitting.

W e l l n e s s

"Studies have repeatedly found that older adults in general are not readily motivated to learn simply for the sake of learning. In their world they want information to be personally relevant and immediately practical.**"**

Each mouthful of food should be swallowed before the next spoonful is introduced. Patients with cognitive impairments and some forms of dysphasia can benefit from gentle verbal reminders to swallow. Moistening the foods with gravy or sauce and offering intermittent swallows of a beverage can help adults with severe dry mouth. The use of a bulb syringe to "force feed" is illegal in some states and is to be discouraged. The practice of feeding several patients at once (seated in a semi-circle, for instance) increases the risk of choking accidents.

When the patient can self-feed with some assistance, the nurse should be sure that the entire meal is in view (patients with limited peripheral vision may have to be directed to turn their heads to view the foods) and that wrapped and sealed portions are opened, with bread buttered and seasonings applied. The atmosphere in a group dining room, especially one that is segregated to frail and severely impaired diners, can make a crucial difference. Background music, peach-toned walls, aquar-

ium tanks, pleasant talk, the smell of brewed coffee and freshly toasted bread—these and other aesthetic touches are appetite and mood stimulants. A scheduled pre-meal grooming can also raise the spirits of the diners and help them to anticipate the meal to come.

In general, remember that a positive atmosphere must be created in any eating environment; it does not develop spontaneously. To encourage proper nutritional intake, it is crucial to create an aesthetically pleasing atmosphere and to project a positive attitude toward the diners. Just as a meal would taste much better in a fine restaurant than in a "greasy-spoon" diner, the attitudes and procedures used to feed impaired elderly clients can make all the difference in their health and well being. Table 7–1 outlines some common dietary modifications in long-term care settings. The reader is referred to Box 7–2 for nutrition education materials.

TABLE 7–1. Some Common Dietary Modifications in Long-Term Care

This is a summary with common examples, not a diet manual. Hospitals and Long Term Care facilities maintain individual diet and nutrition care procedure manuals, with regulations specific to that facility.

Diet Name	Why Prescribed	Not Permitted	Allowed
Mechanical soft	Chewing or swallowing limitation		Whole, cut up, ground, chopped foods, as tolerated. Fried and gassy foods as tolerated.
Blenderized or pureed	Tendency to choke, dysphagia	Solids, unless puree consistency	Blenderized or pureed foods such as cooked cereals, mashed potatoes, blenderized soups and vegetables, puddings, ice cream milk shakes. Fiber can be added with blenderized salads and with oat bran. Visual appeal can be enhanced with garnishes such as cranberry sauce.
Full liquid	Dysphagia and transition from clear liquid after surgery	Solids at room temperature or that are hard to digest	Liquids at body temperature such as gelatin, milk, ice cream, diluted blenderized cream soups, yogurt, butter, and strained farina; can be used long term if fiber and protein boosters are added to the foods.
Clear liquid	Temporary use before and after surgery for vomiting, nausea, diarrhea	Solids at room temperature. All foods with fiber or residue	Bouillon, carbonated beverages, coffee and tea (no milk), fruit ices, popsicles, strained fruit juices, gelatin, and hard candy.

Table continues on facing page

TABLE 7–1. Some Common Dietary Modifications in Long-Term Care (*Continued*)

Diet Name	Why Prescribed	Permitted	Allowed
Bland	Gastritis, peptic ulcer, reflux esophagitis, and post-congestive heart failure (to avoid gas)	Traditional diet prohibits spices and fibers.	Liberal diet tailors to the resident and allows everything that does not cause distress except caffeine and alcohol. Milk is limited when it causes rebound acidity.
Low fat	Heart disease, gallbladder disease, AIDS, inflammatory bowel disease, liver disease, reflux esophagitis, and obesity	Whole or 2% fat dairy products no more than 3 to 6 daily servings of fats: avocado, butter, mayonnaise, bacon, nuts, olives, oil, cream, chocolate, fatty meats and poultry, and poultry skin	Skim milk, 1% fat dairy products, 3 to 6 oz. from meats group (lean), 1 to 3 egg yolks/wk, and all vegetables and fruits and grains
Low fiber/ residue	Obstruction, inflammation, and slow motility of the gastrointestinal tract; prolonged use can lead to diverticulitis and nutritional deficiencies.	Foods with moderate to high fiber or residue. Milk is low in fiber but leaves a residue.	Well-cooked, skinless and seedless fruits, and ripe banana. Potatoes, green beans, beets, carrots, winter squash, strained peas, and strained spinach. Refined grain products.
High fiber	Constipation, hemorrhoids, asymptomatic diverticulosis, and weight loss.	Anything that causes excess gas or digestive distress	Four or more servings each of raw fruits and vegetables and whole grain products daily. Prune juice and oat bran in gradual increments.
Low sodium	Hypertension, congestive heart failure, kidney disease, cirrhosis, coronary heart disease, and corticosteroids	Dependent on level prescribed. High-sodium foods include milk, bakery products, meats, celery, spinach, sauerkraut, canned and other processed foods and snacks, cold cuts, bottled sauces kosher meats, pickled foods, and condiments.	Permitted quantities of foods from the Food Pyramid Guide
Type II diabetes	Normal or underweight non–insulin-dependent diabetes	Nothing is completely prohibited. Examples of foods to restrict include cakes, candy, honey, chocolate, jelly and jam, regular canned fruits and frozen desserts, and sweetened yogurts.	All foods in reasonable quantities; depends on blood sugar and blood lipid profiles

Summary

Nutritional status is an essential concern of nurses when assessing older adults. The changes brought about by aging can present an array of challenges that lead to malnutrition. Malnutrition is never a sign of "normal aging," and health care professionals need to make every effort to address the risk factors that have brought it about. Untreated malnutrition, which includes both deficiencies and excesses, can shorten the life span, decrease the functional capacity, and lower the quality of life of older adults.

This chapter described the common risk factors for malnutrition in older adults and how nutritional risk can be assessed by interdisciplinary teamwork. It outlined the prevalent nutritional problems that older adults encounter in community and institutional settings. After setting forth guidelines for good nutrition it presented practical suggestions for implementing dietary goals for older adults ranging from free-living individuals to those who may be physically or mentally challenged. Teaching tools and general dietary guidelines for nutrition education, as well as the various forms of nutrition support available across the United States, are also included here.

RESOURCES

The following resources provide catalogs of commercial-free nutrition information and materials for counselors and clients. Printed and audiovisual materials generally carry fees.

The American Dietetic Association
216 West Jackson Boulevard
Chicago, IL 60606-6995
(312) 899-0040

The American Diabetes Association
Diabetes Information Service Center
1660 Duke Street
Alexandria, VA 22314
(800) 232-3472

Center for Science in the Public Interest
1779 Church Street NW
Washington, DC 20036
(202) 322-9110

Food and Drug Administration, United States Public Health Service Division of Health and Human Services

5600 Fishers Lane
Rockville, MD 20857

The High Blood Pressure Information Center
National Institutes of Health
Bethesda, MD 20205

National Cholesterol Education Program
NECP Information Center
NHLBI, c-200
Bethesda, MD 20892

The National Dairy Council
6300 N. River Road
Rosemont, IL 60018

National Institute on Aging
Public Affairs Officer
USDHHS Building 31, Room 5c-35
9000 Rockville Pike
Bethesda, MD 20892

Nutrition and the Elderly
Selected Annotated Bibliography
U.S. Government Printing Office
Washington, DC 20502
Stock# 001-024-0028-6

REFERENCES

Andres R. (1980). Effect of obesity on total mortality. Int J Obesity 4:381.

Andres R. (1985). Impact of old age on weight goals. Ann Intern Med 103(2):1030.

Astrand P. (1992). Physical activity and fitness. Am J Clin Nutr 55:12–15.

Dreosti I. (1995). Magnesium status and health. Nutr Rev 53(9):S23–S27.

Dwyer J, Gallo J, Reichel W. (1993). Assessing nutritional status in elderly patients. Am Fam Physician 47(3):613.

Elward K, Larsen E. (1992). Benefits of exercise for older adults: A review of existing evidence and current recommendations for the general population. Clin Geriatr Med 5:35.

Goodwin JS, Goodwin JM, Garry P. (1983). Association between nutritional status and cognitive functioning in a healthy elderly population. JAMA 249:2917.

Hart W, Little S. (1986). Comparison of diets of elderly Hispanics and Caucasians in the urban Southwest. J Nutr Elderly 5(3):47.

Johnson K, Klignan W. (1992). Preventive nutrition: Disease-specific dietary interventions for older adults. Geriatrics 47(11):39–40, 45–49.

Lam F. (1981). A comparison of the nutritional adequacy of elderly Anglo-American and Chinese living in Houston, Texas. Unpublished professional paper, Texas Women's University.

Lopez C, Aquilera ES. (1991). On the Sidelines: Hispanic Elderly and the Continuum of Care. Washington, DC: National Council of La Raza.

Lynch S, Finch C, et al. (1982). Iron status of Americans. Am J Clin Nutr 36:1032.

Martin A. (1991). Dietary management of swallowing disorders. Dysphagia 6:129.

Miller D. (1996). Nutritional risk in inner-city-dwelling of older black Americans. J Am Geriatr Soc 44:959–962.

Mobarhan S, Trumbore L. (1991). Nutritional problems of the elderly. Clin Geriatr Med 7:191.

Morley J. (1988). Nutrition in the elderly. Ann Intern Med 109:890.

Netterville J, ed. (Spring 1991). Gerontological Nutritionists Newsletter. American Dietetic Association Practice Group (available only through the American Dietetic Association).

Phaneuf C. (1996). Screening elders for nutritional deficits. Am J Nurs 96(3):58–60.

Reed R, Morradian A. (1990). Nutritional status and dietary management of elderly diabetic patients. Clin Geriatr Med 6:883.

Reuben D, Greendale G, Harrison G. (1995). Nutrition screening in older persons. J Am Geriatr Soc 43:415–425.

Rosenberg I, Miller J. (1993). Nutritional factors in physical and cognitive functions of elderly people. Am J Clin Nutr 55:12–75.

Schaefer EJ, Lichenstein AH, Lanion SS, et al. (1995). Lipoproteins, Nutrition, Aging, and Atherosclerosis. AM J Clin Nutr 61:726S–704S.

Silver A, 1993. The malnourished older patient: When and how to intervene. Geriatrics 48(7):70–74.

Silver A, Morley J. (1988). Nutritional status in an academic nursing home. J Am Geriatr Soc 36:487.

White J. (1994). Risk factors for poor nutritional status. Primary Care 21(1):19.

White J, Lipshitz D, Brown D. (1991). Consensus of the Nutrition Screening Initiative: Risk factors and indicators of poor nutritional status in older Americans. J Am Diet Assoc 91:783.

Wylie-Rosett J, Wassertheil-Smoler S, et al. (1993). Trial of antihypertensive intervention and management: Greater efficiency with weight reduction than with sodium-potassium intervention. J Am Diet Assoc 93:408.

CRITICAL THINKING EXERCISES

1. Describe three common physiological changes of aging and thoroughly analyze the way each can affect the nutrition status of an older adult. Formulate a care plan to combat the problems you described.

2. Describe three common social/environmental changes of aging and how each can affect the nutrition status of an older adult. In your community, find and evaluate existing nutrition support programs that could address the nutritional lacks you described.

3. Develop three potential research questions in geriatric nutrition, based on areas in which there are deficits of data.

4. Develop a case study for the nutritional assessment of a homebound older client with osteoporosis and cognitive impairment. What would you measure and with what tools? What laboratory data would be needed?

5. Construct a lesson plan about osteoporosis for a group of English-speaking Chinese participants in a congregate meal program. What are the goals and objectives? What methods and materials will be used? What data had to be gathered through pre-assessment? How will the lesson be evaluated?

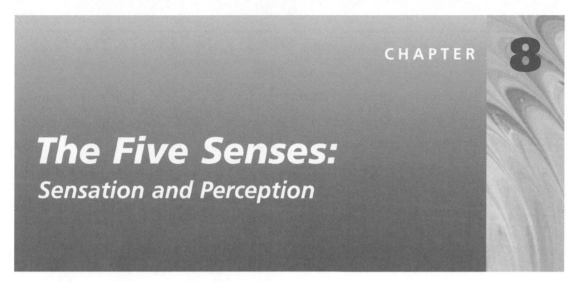

CHAPTER 8

The Five Senses:
Sensation and Perception

Shirley Rose Tyson, RN, MA, EdD
Sydney L. Tyson, MD, MPH

CHAPTER OUTLINE

OBJECTIVES

After completing this chapter, the reader should be able to:

1. Assess sensory-perceptual changes in an older adult client and apply the knowledge in planning an appropriate care environment.
2. Research the assistive devices available for visually impaired individuals and apply this knowledge to a specific older adult patient.
3. Formulate specific communication techniques to be used by the nurse in the care of a hearing-impaired older adult.
4. Design a teaching plan that encompasses the role of oral health in meeting nutritional needs of older adults.
5. Teach a classmate how to assess for pain sensitivity in an older adult client with rheumatoid arthritis who comes to a community facility for care.

We live in a beautiful world that we perceive largely through the five senses. A bouquet of colorful flowers, a glowing sunset, a vanilla ice cream cone, a baby's smile of recognition, a concert in the park, the fragrance worn by a special person, freshly baked cookies, wind chimes in the breeze, a cuddly kitten, freshly cut grass, a kiss—all make us aware of ourselves and our relationship to everything around us. Our sensory perceptions are the pathways through which we interact with the physical world and with one another. The senses, especially sight, smell, and hearing, affect personal interactions and influence mood and behavior. They also help us to maneuver safely in our environments. Because of this, the five senses could be considered our most valuable assets.

Sight, hearing, taste, smell, and touch are essential to living. Across the life span, the senses may often be taken for granted; however, they are much more appreciated when age-related changes begin to emerge. Many older adults have intact senses that enable them to enjoy their lives and the world around them, but some experience losses and alterations as they age.

A *sense* is a faculty or capacity by which objects are perceived. **Sensation** is an awareness made possible by one of the five senses. The interaction between the sense organs, nervous system, neurotransmitters, and hormones leads to perception. **Perception** is the evaluation of information gathered by the senses and the interpretation or meaning attached to it.

Wellness

"Many older adults retain intact senses throughout their lives, with healthy sensation and perception."

■ SENSATION AND PERCEPTION IN THE OLDER ADULT

Aging is often accompanied by sensory loss. Although many older adults have healthy sense organs and intact senses, there can be loss in varying degrees of some components of the five senses. Taste, smell, and touch remain responsive and emotionally potent long after sight and hearing may begin to show some age-related changes (Beauchamp, 1992). Changes in sight and hearing can have a deleterious effect on individuals experiencing such a change, whether it is decline or loss. For many, dependence on others for assistance at this time may affect self-esteem and other mental health issues such as helplessness and social isolation.

Because the senses provide the first line of protection for the body, if they do not function properly there is risk of suffering from hazards in the environment. Everyday experiences such as driving a car may have to be eliminated. Reading a book or listening to the radio may require special interventions for eyesight and hearing adjustments. The senses of smell and taste, when curtailed, diminish pleasures taken for granted throughout a lifetime and can lead to failure to identify spoilage and contamination of food. When senses deteriorate, not hearing doorbells, smoke alarms, or telephones, smelling gas odors, or perceiving temperature changes can become hazardous to the safety of older adults.

Much of the environmental information that individuals receive and respond to comes through the senses of sight and hearing. Reduced ability to protect oneself from the environment because of sensory deficits may present challenges as the older adult lives longer. Decreased sensation and perception contribute to the vulnerability of older adults to accidents. Sensory deficits can exacerbate physical and mental health (Kelly, 1995). However, many older adults retain intact senses throughout their lives with healthy sensation and perception.

Although millions of people experience alterations or decline in *taste*, significant changes related to aging are unlikely before the age of 70. As individuals age, most are unaware of a decline in their sense of *smell;* but by the sixth or seventh decade of life many begin to notice differences in the taste of food (The Monell Connection, 1992).

Touch is a body sensation produced by contact with another person that has social ramifications, especially for older adults who are often isolated from human touch. When some senses decline, nursing interventions should be directed toward stimulation of the older adult's other senses. The individual's level of sensory function should be maintained at its optimal level throughout the life span.

Vision impairment is one of the three most common medical problems among older people. Twenty-five percent or more of people older than the age of 85 have sufficient visual difficulty that they have trouble reading or independently conducting activities of daily living. As the population older than the age of 85 continues its rapid growth, it will become increasingly important to understand the causes and treatment of these visual disabilities; it is a truism that everyone who lives long enough will experience some visual changes. Yet, central visual acuity remains good for up to 85% of those younger than 90 years of age (Jarvis, 1992).

Twenty million people in the United States suffer from some type of hearing impairment. There are, however, many older adults who never experience a hearing loss. Hearing impairment is the second most common health problem affecting the gerontological population (Mhoon, 1992).

Sensory changes begin to occur at about age 65; some occur gradually and vary with each individual and each sense organ. Other changes or decline in sensory abilities may be the result of some disease manifestation. The way in which an individual perceives a stimulus or reacts through sensation is dependent on life experience, health status, intensity of the stimulus, and the context of the situation.

Because age-related sensory loss is not necessarily a normal part of the aging process, any change, loss, or decline should be monitored for appropriate intervention and treatment to be implemented as soon as possible. The older adult's sensory-perceptual function is extremely important to mental competency and

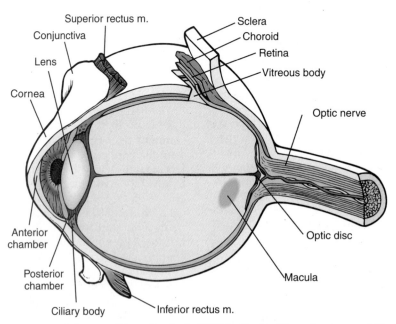

Figure 8–1. The structure of the eye. (From Jarvis C. [1992]. *Physical Examination and Health Assessment.* Philadelphia: WB Saunders.)

mental status. Decline in sensory function can greatly curtail the ability to respond appropriately and can produce reversible confusional states with consequent misdiagnoses.

THE EYE AND VISION

Assessment of Sight

Examination of the eye is an essential component of the physical examination (Figure 8–1). Older adults should have annual, or more frequent, examinations as recommended by their primary care physician or ophthalmologist. History taking is an important part of the assessment and should include questions about glaucoma, cataracts, diabetic and hypertensive disease, eye trauma, and other disorders that curtail vision.

Vision screening for acuity is tested by using a Snellen chart. Most adults are familiar with this test. The test should be performed without and with glasses (for those who wear them). Individuals are instructed to read the words on the chart, located approximately 20 feet away, until they are no longer able to do so. For those individuals who cannot read, alternative charts are available. The examination also includes evaluating visual fields and extraocular motility.

Diagnostic procedures should include measurement of intraocular pressure every 1 to 2 years as a test for the presence of glaucoma. When pressure builds up, it is caused by inadequate drainage of aqueous fluid in the anterior portion of the eye. This fluid is secreted continuously to provide nutrients. When, because of anatomical changes, the fluid cannot leave the eye at the rate it is produced, pressure within the eye increases, causing damage to the optic nerve and other parts of the eye.

Preventive Eye Care

Aging causes many expected changes in the eye. Even though the changes are well defined, the distinction between natural changes and disease is not always well understood. For this reason it is important that all older adults have regular examinations. It is often reassuring to know that a problem such as a cataract is part of a "normal" process rather than a specific ill-ness. With diseases that cause visual disability, it is important for the older adult to receive adequate advice from an ophthalmologist or other qualified health care professional. A thorough examination and explanation of the disease or problem will not only reduce the older adult's anxiety but also improve understanding of and compliance with treatment.

Eye Disorders

There are many eye disorders that are common to all ages but that affect older adults more adversely, particularly those eye disorders associated with systemic diseases such as diabetes. However, there are four disorders that are most common among older people and are responsible for the majority of their visual disability. These are glaucoma, cataracts, macular degeneration, and diabetic retinopathy.

GLAUCOMA

Glaucoma is the second leading cause of blindness in the United States and the first cause of blindness among African Americans. Some 3 million people have glaucoma (Eastman, 1993) and currently 50,000 Americans are blind from it. Although glaucoma can occur at any age, the proportion of people with glaucoma increases rapidly after age 40. There is no known cause for glaucoma, but several risk factors for the disease include a positive family history for the disease, diabetes, and being African American. Fortunately, much of the blindness this disease produces is preventable if the disease is detected early and treated promptly.

The most common form of glaucoma—chronic open-angle glaucoma—is painless. Individuals have no idea that they have the disease until it is advanced to the point where it is too late to restore lost vision. The loss of vision occurs gradually over time owing to an abnormally high fluid pressure in the eye. The fluid pressure becomes high as a result of a disruption of the normal drainage systems in the eye. This high pressure causes damage to the optic nerve at the back of the eye, which is responsible for the transmission of all vision, both central and peripheral, to the brain. When glaucoma damages the nerve, it does so in a piecemeal manner.

First the peripheral or side vision, then, over time, the crucial central vision is affected.

There is no change in the appearance or sensation of the eye. Only an ophthalmologist or optometrist can measure and detect this elevation in eye pressure and any abnormal appearance of the optic nerve or visual field.

Once a patient is diagnosed with glaucoma, the goal is to control the eye pressure and to keep it at a level safe enough to prevent visual field loss. The treatment of glaucoma should be undertaken by an ophthalmologist. It consists of three modalities—drops and/or pills, laser therapy, and surgery. (A new surgical procedure is called argon laser surgery.) The treatment modality chosen depends on several factors, most important being the severity of the disease. Treatment must start before serious damage to the optic nerve has occurred. The best treatment for glaucoma is prevention by early detection through regular eye examinations for all people older than age 60 and all African Americans over the age of 40. Acute (angle-closure) glaucoma occurs suddenly as a result of complete blockage and requires medical attention to avoid severe vision loss. Symptoms include severe eye pain, blurred vision, nausea and vomiting, rainbow halos surrounding lights, and pupil dilation. Treatment consists of normalizing intraocular pressure and application of eyedrops.

In chronic open-angle glaucoma, pharmacological treatments are based on the patient's history and current condition. Treatments include

- Miotic drugs (e.g., pilocarpine), which contract the pupil and the iris to draw away from the cornea, allowing fluid to drain

- Carbonic anhydrase inhibitors (e.g., acetazolamide [Diamox] and timolol [Timoptic]), which decrease the production of aqueous humor

In angle-closure (acute) glaucoma, medications are given for emergency treatment; if they are ineffective in lowering the intraocular pressure, laser iridotomy or iridectomy becomes necessary.

For patients having glaucoma, medical follow-up and eye medication will be prescribed for daily use for the remainder of the life span. Eye drops must be continued as long as prescribed, even in the absence of symptoms (Box 8–1). If the older adult is being treated for another medical problem, attention must be paid to other medications prescribed and possible side effects or interactions.

CATARACTS

Cataracts are the primary cause of poor vision among adults and the leading cause of preventable blindness in the world. More than two thirds of the population older than the age of 60 have cataracts to some degree, and about 90% of the population older than age 70 are affected. **Cataracts** are a natural, painless, age-related clouding of the transparent human lens. With time, the lens becomes progressively more cloudy, with concomitant worsening of vision.

The lens of the eye can be compared with the lens of a camera. In each case, if the lens is dirty or smudged, light rays passing through the

Box 8-1   INSTILLATION OF EYE DROPS BY NURSE OR OLDER ADULT

1. Wash hands before having any contact with the eye.
2. Ensure adequate lighting.
3. Clean the eye if there is any crust or discharge present.
4. Place the head backward.
5. Lift the lower lid up and outward.
6. Place the number of drops prescribed into space on lower lid.
7. Remove the hand from the lower lid and gently close the eye for drops to absorb.
8. Avoid touching the eye with the dropper.
9. Advise older adults to take their drops with them on their person when traveling, not in their luggage.
10. Stress that any symptom reappearance should be reported promptly.

1. Extracapsular surgery, in which the lens is removed and the posterior capsule is left in place
2. Extracapsular surgery, with phacoemulsification, in which the lens is softened by ultrasound and removed through a needle
3. Intracapsular surgery (not as frequently used), which can be an option if there has been trauma or if there is poor support for the lens. A cryoprobe is used in this procedure.

MACULAR DEGENERATION

The macula is the region of the retina that is responsible for detailed central vision. Age-related **macular degeneration** is the leading cause of visual deficiency and permanent reading impairment in patients older than 65 years of age. The condition is characterized by progressive deterioration of the retinal cells in the macula due to aging. The remainder of the retina, outside the macula, remains remarkably unaffected. Apart from aging, no other causes of macular degeneration have been proven. There are two types of macular degeneration, a wet form and a dry form. The dry form is a very slow and gradual deterioration of the function of the macula. The effect on vision is often very subtle and may go unnoticed by the patient for many years. Typically, patients note distortion or blind spots in their vision.

In spite of the fact that there is no known effective treatment for the "dry" form of macular degeneration, most patients with dry macular degeneration retain useful levels of vision indefinitely. The wet form of macular degeneration is more serious and is responsible for the majority of cases of severe visual loss with this condition. The term *wet form* derives from the leakage of fluid from abnormal vessels under the retina. The leakage of this fluid, which the ophthalmologist detects with a special test called a fluorescein angiogram, causes damage and degeneration of the overlying retinal cells. Although occasionally lasers can be used to "seal off" these leaking vessels before they reach the center of the macula, they often originate in the center. Because the laser destroys the area treated, it is usually not used in the center of the macula if it is already occupied by abnormal vessels. At this stage, the outlook for recovery of useful vision is poor.

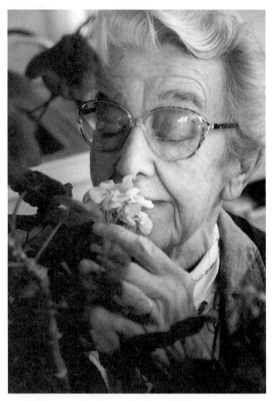

Although the senses may diminish, it remains important to stimulate them in a variety of pleasurable ways.

lens become blocked or scattered, resulting in a blurred picture. Changing the prescription of eyeglasses (i.e., the focus) will not correct the blurring that is caused by a cataract. In addition to blurry, hazy vision, other common early symptoms of cataract are distorted or double images, disturbing glare or haloes with bright lights, or the feeling that there is a film over the eye. Although there is no medicine or diet to cure cataracts, for most patients, surgical removal of the cataract and replacement with an artificial lens implant can restore vision and allow continuing active function. In fact, more than 1 million people in the United States undergo safe, successful cataract surgery each year. The intraocular implant of an artificial lens made of acrylic, plastic, or silicone is very beneficial in restoring vision. Performed as ambulatory surgery, the older adult is premeasured for the lens before the day of surgery. Postoperative care requires follow-up visits to the ophthalmologist and instillation of eye drops. There are three types of cataract surgery:

It is important to inform patients that even in the most severe cases of macular degeneration they will never go completely blind. Because only the macula is affected, these patients retain their peripheral vision and can walk without assistance. They can also learn to perform many activities by using this "side" vision and continue to lead productive lives. In this regard, low-vision clinics provide an important service to those afflicted by this condition. They can provide specialists who assess the individual needs of patients with limited vision. Patients are taught how to use low-vision aids such as magnifiers, high-power lenses, and telescopes to compensate for central vision

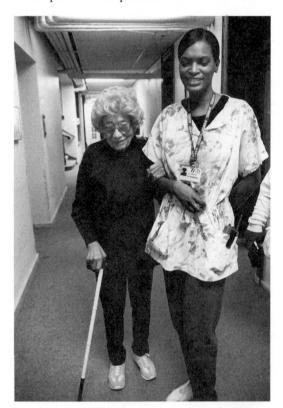

To preserve autonomy, the client with a visual impairment must always be allowed actively to take the arm of the helper.

loss. These items help improve the functional status of the visually impaired patient with macular degeneration.

DIABETIC RETINOPATHY

Only older adults with diabetes are at risk of developing a complication called diabetic retinopathy, which damages tiny vessels in the eye's retina and causes leaky, fragile, vision-interfering new blood vessels to form. Because there are often no early warning signs of diabetic retinopathy, the National Eye Institute urges all diabetics to have an eye examination at least annually.

When therapeutic intervention is indicated, ophthalmologists can often perform a type of laser surgery called photocoagulation to make tiny burns on the retina that cause regression of the leaky blood vessels. The procedure of photocoagulation, though very successful, does not become available to half of those who would benefit from it. Left unattended, diabetic retinopathy can cause blindness, as it does every year in approximately 8000 Americans (Eastman, 1993).

DETACHED RETINA

Detached retina, experienced in older adults, is a forward displacement of the retina from its normal position against the choroid. Symptoms include the perception of spots moving across the eye, flashes of light, and a coating over the eyes. Blank areas can progress to loss of vision. Prompt intervention and treatment are required to prevent further damage or loss of vision. After bed rest, surgery may be performed. Periodic examination is of great importance because the condition could occur in the other eye.

FLOATERS

Floaters can appear as dots, wiggly lines, or clouds that a person may see moving in the field of vision. They are more pronounced against a plain background and occur more often after the age of 50 as small clumps of gel or cellular debris floating in the vitreous humor in front of the retina. Floaters are caused by degeneration of the vitreous gel. They are normal and harmless but could be a warning sign and require a complete examination by an ophthalmologist.

FLASHERS

Flashers occur when the vitreous fluid inside the eye tugs or pulls on the retina. This produces the illusion of flashing lights or lightning streaks. Flashers commonly occur with advancing age, but the older adult should be examined by an ophthalmologist if a large number, or new ones, appear.

PRESBYOPIA

Presbyopia is the most common complaint of adults older than the age of 40 years. It is the diminished ability to focus clearly on close objects and fine print. This is not an eye disease from an age-related degeneration. Accommodation is impaired; the lens loses its elasticity and is not able to focus on close objects. These changes cause farsightedness, necessitating that individuals hold objects at a distance for reading. For most adults, magnifier reading glasses can correct presbyopia.

DRY EYES

Dry eyes are common in older adults. Stinging, burning, scratchiness, and even increased tearing are some of the symptoms. Dry eyes occur when tears are diminished as part of the aging process. This occurrence can also be the result of some medications. Intervention by an ophthalmologist can close off drainage of tears via the lacrimal ducts. Artificial tears, which can be purchased over the counter, help to relieve the symptoms and can be used as often as needed to replace the fluid that lubricates the eye.

Box 8–2 presents ways to adapt to age-related changes in visual acuity.

Interventions for Alterations in Vision

Interventions by the nurse on behalf of older adults who are experiencing alterations in vision include the following:

- Encourage regular eye examinations by an ophthalmologist.
- Inform the older adult simply and calmly of the activities to be done.
- Do not rush the older adult—this causes anxiety.
- Provide the individual with assistive items such as a transistor radio, books and cards with large print, or clocks and telephones that glow in the dark. Provide hand-held magnifiers, needle threaders, and better lighting.

To maximize the individual's vision, the nurse should keep the person's eyeglasses clean and handy for use and encourage the person to use any remaining vision. The nurse should talk directly to the older adult, speaking slowly, clearly, and distinctly. When entering the room, introductions should be made as to who the nurse is, the purpose of the visit, and the type of assistance to be offered.

The nurse can be creative in initiating activities and conversation. The individual's other senses of hearing, smell, taste, and touch can be stimulated. The nurse can play the individual's favorite music and enhance smell through flowers and pleasant odors, taste through preferred foods, and touch through different objects, fabrics, or small animals.

The individual's uniqueness in terms of culture, personality, and positive and negative attitudes should be considered. The level of function is maintained at its optimum. The older adult is asked for suggestions about his or her

---

Box 8-2   WAYS OF ADAPTING TO NORMAL AGE-RELATED CHANGES OF THE EYE

- Wear eyeglasses; keep them clean.
- Increase the amount of light when reading.
- Allow extra time for eyes to accommodate to the darkness.
- Avoid nighttime driving.
- Wear dark glasses to reduce the sun's rays or glare.
- Have regular examinations by an ophthalmologist.

Box 8-3   INTERVENTIONS FOR ALTERATION IN VISION

1. Allow the older adult to verbalize feelings concerning loss of vision or vision impairment.
2. Be a good listener, be supportive, and develop strategies that will allow the older adults to function at optimal level.
3. Teach and reinforce safety at all times. The bathroom should be equipped with grab bars, suction mats in the bathtub, and shower stool with hand rail in the shower. Doorways and hallways should be free of objects that could cause injury.
4. Be aware of environmental hazards. Do not move furniture around. This could be disruptive to routines. The older adult's home or room in the institutionalized setting should be hazard free.
5. If severely visually impaired older adults are to be left alone, leave something familiar with them that they can touch to maintain contact with the environment.
6. If the older adult has a guide dog, do not pet or distract the dog. The dog has a job to do.

---

care to maintain this level. Low-vision clinics where specially trained personnel can assist with the right type of optical aids are available.

Visually impaired individuals who are diabetic can be helped in monitoring their blood glucose level and insulin administration by a number of devices. A marking system of tactile markers can be used to identify medications. Daily or weekly pill dispensers and "talking" or alarm watches or clocks can help patients to take medications on schedule.

Good health practices and early detection of eye disease can retain adequate vision for most older adults. Any person with vision problems, eye diseases, or eye disorders should receive prompt attention by health care professionals (Box 8–3).

THE EAR AND HEARING

Assessment of Hearing

The ear is a sensory organ with complex functions related to hearing and the maintenance of equilibrium (Figure 8–2). Examination of the ears and tests for hearing should be a routine part of any physical assessment, and special attention must be paid when assessing an older adult. As people age, the ability to hear high-pitched sounds decreases. Hearing loss can be a chronic disability among older adults, but it should not be accepted as part of normal aging and left untreated or ignored.

Very often nursing assessment is the first step in identifying a hearing problem and directing an individual to the correct type of intervention. History taking is an extremely important part of the assessment. Instead of asking "Do you hear well?" the interviewer should ask "Does anyone complain that your television set is playing too loudly?" Because some older adults may deny that there is a hearing problem, the nurse needs to be alert when the individual asks for questions to be repeated. Other questions that could be asked as part of assessment are listed below:

1. Do you have any problems with your ears, hearing, or balance? If so, describe them. Have you ever had surgery on your ears to improve hearing? If so, when and for what? Did it help?
2. Have you ever had your hearing tested? If so, when was it done and for what reason?
3. Do you clean your ears often? How do you clean them?

These questions can elicit information necessary to make a plan of care. Information on cleaning the ears can lead to whether there is cerumen impaction, which is a common cause of hearing loss.

Individuals should be assessed for pain, vertigo, infection, excessive cerumen, hygiene practices, and tinnitus. The ear is examined by inspection and palpation of the external and middle ear. Assessment of auditory acuity should be included in every physical examina-

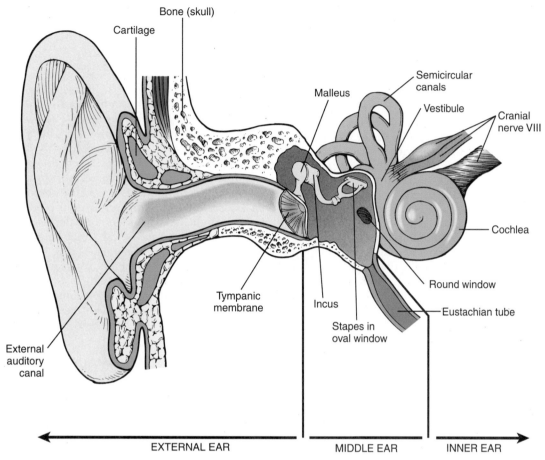

Figure 8–2. The external ear, middle ear and inner ear. (From Jarvis C. [1992]. Physical Examination and Health Assessment. Philadelphia: WB Saunders.)

tion. If problems seem to be present, an ear examination should be performed by an otologist or otolaryngologist to determine the exact type and degree of hearing loss. Auditory acuity is evaluated by voice, watch tick, tuning fork, and/or audiometer.

Medications, illness, fatigue, and anxiety can exacerbate hearing impairment. Age-related sensorineural hearing loss cannot as yet be cured. Some hearing loss can be corrected by medication, surgery, or a hearing device.

Hearing Disorders

There are many hearing disorders that are common to all ages but that affect the older adult more adversely. Disorders that occur in older adults and are responsible for the majority of their hearing impairment include oto-sclerosis, presbycusis, and sensorineural and conductive hearing loss.

OTOSCLEROSIS

Otosclerosis is the most common cause of progressive deafness in adults; it is caused by the formation of new, abnormal spongy bone. Immobilization of the stapes then occurs, preventing it from carrying the stimulus of the vibrating malleus and incus to inner ear fluids. The result is a conductive hearing loss that is usually bilateral, believed to be inherited, and more common in females. This loss is due to degenerative changes in the auditory nerve neurons, ossicles, and cochlea and leads to decreased ability to hear consonants. Surgical intervention by a stapedectomy is a treatment option.

PRESBYCUSIS

Presbycusis is a progressive hearing loss that may progress rapidly over a short time or slowly over a period of 5 to 10 years. It usually progresses gradually, and the older adult learns to adjust over time to decreased hearing. The condition affects both ears and is more common and more severe in males. The severity is dependent on several factors, including heredity, the status of the individual's circulatory system, and exposure to loud noises over time. Hearing loss is predominantly in the higher frequencies. *Tinnitus* usually accompanies presbycusis. Presbycusis affects many older adults during the aging process. Because there is as yet no medical or surgical treatment, over time the amount of hearing loss may necessitate a hearing aid. Presbycusis is the most common form of sensorineural hearing loss and is especially common in older adults (Thompson and Wilson, 1996).

SENSORINEURAL HEARING LOSS

Sensorineural hearing loss is the most common inner ear disorder. It results from disease or trauma to the sensorineural structures or nerve pathways in the inner ear that lead to the brain stem. The hearing loss may fluctuate, but a progressive loss usually results. This loss is usually permanent and precludes any medical or surgical intervention.

CONDUCTIVE HEARING LOSS

Conductive hearing loss is any interference with sound impulses through the external auditory canal, the eardrum, or middle ear when sound does not reach the inner ear. The inner ear is usually not involved in a conductive loss, and sound amplification can reach the inner ear. Most conductive loss is correctable by medical or surgical intervention because the original interference is often caused by a blockage such as impacted cerumen, otosclerosis, foreign bodies lodged in the ear canal, tumors of the middle ear, or otitis media.

Other contributing factors to hearing loss are certain disease processes such as heart or kidney disease, diabetes, and emphysema. Medications with ototoxic side effects can contribute to a hearing loss (Box 8–4).

HEARING LOSS AND SELF-IMAGE

The function of hearing meets basic human needs in the following ways:

1. Safety and survival, by detecting warning signals such as a smoke or a fire alarm

---

Box 8-4	MEDICATIONS WITH OTOTOXIC SIDE EFFECTS

Older adults should be taught to read literature accompanying the prescription, make inquiries of their doctor and pharmacist and to be aware of any changes in hearing impairment. They should also be taught side effects of medications they are taking. Medications that may cause side effects include

- Aspirin
- Cisplatin
- Erythromycin
- Furosemide
- Gentamycin
- Indomethacin
- Kanamycin
- Neomycin
- Quinidine
- Quinine
- Streptomycin
- Tobramycin
- Vancomycin

Data from Hall D. (1993). Do Not Neglect Your Hearing. Health News 10(3):4–5.

2. Enabling communication with others through the use of language and speech
3. Self-esteem and self-actualization through hearing environmental noises such as a laugh, music, conversation, or a baby's cry

Hearing loss is the sensory problem most closely related to mental health problems in the older adult; it can create anxiety, depression, and even paranoid states. Hearing impairment may lead to personality changes because it interferes with the communication process, causing loneliness and isolation. Hearing loss may exclude an individual from certain parts of a conversation, and the person may begin to think that others are talking about him, thus causing withdrawal from the environment and related depression.

A major hearing loss often leads to decreased feelings of self-worth and self-esteem. Insecurity and a lack of self-confidence may develop because of the person's inability to communicate with others and the environment and to protect the self as awareness of the deficiencies dawns. A person with a hearing loss may use denial or try to compensate in some other way for the loss. Also, an older adult may refuse to seek medical attention, equating hearing loss with signs of advancing age.

Hearing impairment changes the way people feel about themselves and influences how satisfied they are with their lives. Hearing-impaired individuals experience emotions of grief, loss, anger, and fatigue from trying so hard to understand what others are saying.

■ INTERVENTIONS FOR ALTERATIONS IN HEARING

Assistive Listening Devices

It has been estimated that approximately 30% of adults age 65 through 74, about 33% of those age 75 through 84, and about 48% of individuals older than age 85 suffer some degree of hearing loss (Thompson and Wilson, 1996). If there is no cause for hearing loss that can be treated by either medication or surgery, a hearing device is usually recommended. A hearing device should not be purchased until the person knows whether it will help his or her type of hearing loss.

Hearing aids have undergone significant engineering improvements in recent years. A hearing aid is an instrument worn behind the ear, within the ear, concealed on the frame of eyeglasses, or on the body. Age-related hearing impairments can be treated with properly fitted hearing aids or assistive listening devices designed for specific listening and hearing needs.

An ear specialist (otologist, otolaryngologist) should be consulted for an accurate medical diagnosis and management and an audiologist (specialist in nonmedical evaluation and rehabilitation of hearing disorders) for an accurate hearing assessment. This team of hearing specialists diagnoses sensory impairments and recommends therapeutic interventions. **Audiometry** (testing of the acuity of the sense of hearing) is the best assessment test for hearing.

Many hearing devices are available to assist older adults with mild to moderate hearing loss. These include telephone, television, and radio amplifiers; captioned television; teletypewriters; doorbells and telephones that light up as well as ring; flashing smoke detectors and alarm clocks; and other alerting devices. Hearing aids allow sound to be magnified, converting it into electrical signals and then into acoustic signals. A variety are available. The most expensive does not necessarily ensure the most benefit for the person.

Other assistive devices include those that can be carried from place to place. The Food and Drug Administration (FDA) has established regulations on hearing aids to protect the health and safety of people with hearing impairments. International Hearing Dog Incorporated trains dogs for hearing-impaired individuals who live alone. These hearing guide dogs alert the person by physical contact and then run to the source of the noise.

Another device approved by the FDA for individuals with severe hearing loss that affects their quality of life is the **cochlear implant.** A multichannel device is implanted into the cochlea, located in the inner ear. It has been greatly beneficial for adults older than age 65. The average rehabilitation period for a cochlear implant is 10 months to 1 year. Individuals must be evaluated by the otologist and audiologist. Use and care of the implant, auditory education, and training sessions are an important part of rehabilitation. Many local chapters of hearing and speech associations and organizations serving the hearing-impaired can provide assistance.

CARE OF HEARING AID

If a hearing aid is recommended, a number of adaptations should be made by the audiologist to maximize acceptance. In-the-ear or behind-the-ear aids are models appropriate for the older adult population.

Hearing-impaired individuals need to be taught how to care for their hearing aid. This involves cleaning the device and checking batteries. If servicing is needed, a reputable agency should be contacted. It is essential that the hearing-impaired person have a functioning hearing aid. The nurse should emphasize the importance of periodic testing or adjustments, because hearing loss that declines over time may necessitate changes in the hearing aid for optimal function. Box 8–5 presents interventions that can be used in communicating with hearing-impaired older adults.

HEARING REHABILITATION

Aural (hearing) rehabilitation is a comprehensive program of teaching and follow-up that helps an individual to maintain contact with the environment through enhanced communication skills. These services should be provided as soon as a hearing loss is identified. Family members should be included in the health teaching and plan of care incorporating speech reading, auditory training, education in the hearing process, amplification assessment, and counseling.

Because most hearing loss is permanent, the use of assistive devices should always be considered (see Assistive Listening Devices). Hearing education and auditory training are approaches used to enhance listening skills.

Still important today for hearing-impaired individuals is sign language. Various hand signals represent different letters of the alphabet, words, and phrases. Sign language is used globally with many recent advances such as in the entertainment field—theaters, plays, television, in other public places, and in colleges. Learning sign language is an important aspect of rehabilitation.

■ THE ORAL CAVITY AND TASTE

At birth, humans have several thousand taste buds often distributed among the 200 to 500 fungiform **papillae** on the surface of the tongue (Figure 8–3). The taste buds have the ability to distinguish four taste sensations: sweet, sour, salty, and bitter. In general, these

---

Box 8-5   INTERVENTIONS FOR ALTERATION IN HEARING

1. When speaking to the older adult, face directly. Speak slowly and clearly to be better understood.
2. Do not shout. Older adults often lose the ability to hear higher pitches. Adjust or lower the pitch of your voice.
3. If hearing loss is greater in one ear, direct speech to the *less* affected ear.
4. Speak at a moderate rate. Do not speak rapidly.
5. Keep voice at the same volume throughout the conversation.
6. If the listener does not understand what was said, rephrase.
7. To get the listener's attention, touch the listener's hand or lower arm lightly.
8. Be alert to nonverbal communication such as body language and facial expression. These can be helpful in interpreting what is being understood and communicated.

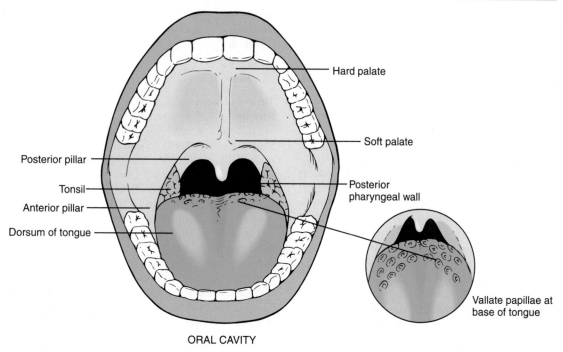

ORAL CAVITY

Figure 8–3. The structure of the oral cavity. (From Jarvis C. [1992]. Physical Examination and Health Assessment. Philadelphia: WB Saunders.)

sensations are perceived in separate areas of the tongue. Assessing the ability to taste and to identify taste sensations is facilitated by the use of sugar, lemon juice, salt, and quinine.

The acuity of the taste buds decreases with age. This can cause decreased appetite in older adults. Extra seasonings contribute to taste enhancement, increasing food intake.

Assessment of Taste

Because taste takes place in the oral cavity, older adults need to participate in regular dental examinations as part of good oral health care. Oral hygiene (including care of dentures, when present) after each meal contributes to oral health and improved taste. During the assessment process, the nurse should elicit information concerning an older adult's oral health. Pertinent questions include the following:

- Are there any physical conditions that interfere with performing oral hygiene tasks?
- How good is the appetite?
- Are there signs of irritation in the mouth?
- What is the condition of the teeth? Of the gums?
- Are the original teeth present?
- Are any teeth loose or decayed? Is there halitosis?
- Are dentures worn?
- How do the dentures fit? Are they worn during meals or removed?
- Is tobacco used?

Oral Disorders

DYSGEUSIA

Dysgeusia is a condition in which a person experiences strange taste sensations. These individuals are usually first seen in a dentist's office. Some reasons for the strange taste are

- Cigarette smoking
- Poor oral hygiene
- Mouth infections, which can be easily treated with appropriate medications
- Vitamin deficiency, particularly of riboflavin, niacin, and vitamin C
- Use of certain antibiotics, anticholinergics, and chemotherapeutic agents. Depapillation

of the tongue may occur but can be reversed with discontinuation of the medication.

The taste and smell of food influence nutritional intake profoundly. Healthy senses encourage a person to eat and thus enhance health, nutrition, and quality of life.

DECREASED SALIVARY FLOW

Saliva plays many roles in the oral cavity. It lubricates, digests, destroys microbes, and acts as a buffer. Saliva washes the hard and soft tissues of the oral cavity and moves food into the digestive tract. In an older adult, the process may be disrupted when salivary flow is reduced by illness and/or medication. As saliva decreases, a "burning mouth" syndrome develops, associated with avitaminosis, candidiasis, or drug toxicities.

Dry mouth, or xerostomia, is often a side effect of some medications, and it can cause discomfort and an increase in tooth decay. Because of the discomfort, artificial saliva is used to lubricate the mouth. Lemon juice and sugar-free candy have been beneficial in increasing the flow of saliva in preparation for mealtime.

Mandated oral care after meals is imperative to remove food particles that, if left in the mouth, can cause mouth infections. Some individuals do not feel ulcers in the mouth. Assessment by a dentist should lead to appropriate intervention and treatment.

Wellness

"*Older adults need to participate in regular dental examinations as part of good oral health care.***"**

SJÖGREN'S SYNDROME

Postmenopausal women sometimes exhibit a painful, reddened tongue, which is thought to be associated with an endocrine malfunction. This chronic inflammatory autoimmune disease called Sjögren's syndrome affects the salivary glands (McDonald and Marino, 1991). Approximately 1 million older adult women in the United States are affected. These women should be treated by an endocrinologist. Nursing care would be to treat the symptoms with

oral hygiene, with medications for pain and inflammation, and by keeping the patient comfortable.

DECREASED TASTE SENSATION

Taste can be temporarily affected by several factors including smoking (especially pipe smoking), new dentures, dentition status, radiation therapy, and mouth ulcers. Any of these can adversely affect an older adult's nutritional status. Because taste and smell guide food choices and influence nutrition and health, decline in taste buds can lead to loss in taste perception, loss of appetite, and poor nutritional status.

Decline in the number of taste buds is an age-related sensory change. Complaints about the taste of food often are a socially acceptable way for residents of a nursing home to express feelings. A disorder in the sense of taste can be a result of conditions such as nasal polyps, head injury, sinusitis, exposure to chemicals, and side effects of medications.

Interventions for Alterations in Taste

The use of multiple medications by older adults makes them more susceptible to xerostomia (absence of saliva). In assessment, the number of drugs taken is correlated with the prevalence of xerostomia. A careful assessment by the nurse of medications being taken and monitoring of their effects are of great importance. If symptoms are severe, medications can be substituted or eliminated. Because a dry mouth is more prone to fungal infections and ulcerations, oral hygiene should be administered both before and after each meal and at other times as indicated.

Older adults receiving liquid or soft food diets that do not require chewing will have a reduction in the flow of saliva, and masticatory stimulants such as sugarless gum are recommended to stimulate the flow (McDonald and Marino, 1991). Fluids with and between meals must be given to maintain fluid intake and decrease xerostomia. Older adults with xerostomia may experience taste alterations and report that food tastes salty, bland, or bitter. Difficulty with mastication may cause selection of less nourishing soft foods and result in compromised nutrition.

Caring nurses and nutritionists should work together to present food in as attractive a manner as possible. Flavor enhancers of condiments, herbs, and seasonings help. Effective dietary intervention strategies are as important as the nutritional value of the food. Interventions for meeting the needs of older adults with taste sensation alterations are found in Box 8–6. For more on nutritional status, see Chapter 7.

Poor dentition is a factor in older adults and could lead to altered food choices with decreased nutritive value. Older adults may compensate for the loss in taste acuity by excessive use of salt and sugar. This is undesirable, because additional health problems may result from this usage.

Nurses are in a position to promote better nutrition. Older adults should be involved in the selection, preparation, and serving of foods because this involvement can contribute to increased interest in taste and food.

THE NOSE AND SMELL

The nose is the sensory organ associated with smell (Figure 8–4). Decline in the sense of smell is caused by atrophy of olfactory organs and increased hair growth in the nostrils. Humans have 10 million olfactory nerve cells with six cilia attached to each cell. Damaged cells can reconstitute by regenerating.

Caring

"Caring nurses and nutritionists should work together to present food in as attractive a manner as possible."

Assessment of Smell

Examination of the nasal cavity is performed by the use of an instrument called the conchoscope. Assessment of olfactory function is implemented by a standardized test called UPSIT (University of Pennsylvania Smell Identification Test) (Aging and Research Training News, 1993). Subjects are requested to answer a multiple-choice questionnaire even if no smell is perceived. The test is sensitive to olfactory deficits, including those associated with aging, smoking, and some disease conditions. Results show that odor identification declines after 70 years of age, that women have a stronger sense of smell, and that nonsmokers have a greater ability to detect odors.

Alterations in olfactory sensitivity may be caused by cognitive deficits, respiratory problems, epistaxis, nasal polyps, or smoking. Olfactory dysfunction is observed in a number of age-related diseases, including Alzheimer's disease and Parkinson's disease. Decreased estrogen levels in postmenopausal women may affect odor perception. If a person cannot identify an odor, it should be clarified whether

---

Box 8-6   INTERVENTIONS FOR ALTERATION IN TASTE

1. If the older patient needs assistance with eating, foods should not be mixed together but served separately.
2. Food seasonings can be added if dietary compliance is adhered to (e.g., low-sodium diets should have no addition of salt).
3. Small amounts should be served attractively on bright colored dinnerware. Foods of the same color should not be served together (e.g., cauliflower and mashed potatoes).
4. Provide comfortable, colorful surroundings that are quiet and pleasant. If preferred, soft music could be an appropriate addition.
5. Ask about food likes and dislikes and provide accordingly if within dietary plan.
6. Hot foods should be served hot and cold foods served cold.
7. Stimulate the other senses of sight, hearing, and touch.

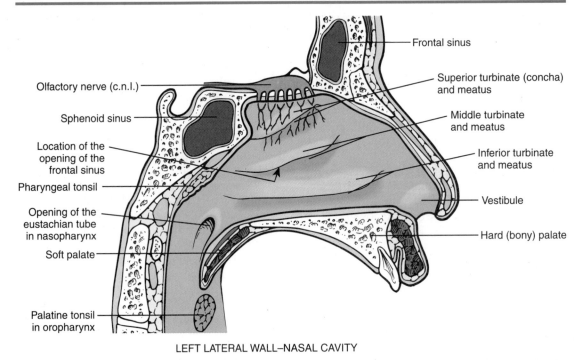

Olfactory nerve (c.n.l.)

Sphenoid sinus

Location of the opening of the frontal sinus

Pharyngeal tonsil

Opening of the eustachian tube in nasopharynx

Soft palate

Palatine tonsil in oropharynx

Frontal sinus

Superior turbinate (concha) and meatus

Middle turbinate and meatus

Inferior turbinate and meatus

Vestibule

Hard (bony) palate

LEFT LATERAL WALL–NASAL CAVITY

Figure 8–4. The structure of the nasal cavity. (From Jarvis C. [1992]. Physical Examination and Health Assessment. Philadelphia: WB Saunders.)

it is the detection of the odor or its identification. Most people with limited olfactory sensation enjoy food less, have diminished appetites, and alter their eating patterns.

Individuals who report deficits in smell and/or taste should receive sensory evaluation and medical, dental, nursing, and nutritional assessments. Research (Cowart, 1993) has revealed that 23% of individuals with nasal allergies suffer loss of the sense of smell. In the United States there are 20 to 30 million sufferers of allergic rhinitis. These findings suggest there may be as many as 4.5 million Americans experiencing smell loss from allergies alone, and the prevalence of smell disorders has been underestimated.

A decline in the ability to smell is not considered a disorder, but smell has many functions. The loss of the sense of smell may present life-threatening situations for vulnerable older adults. The odors of contaminated food, smoke, fire, noxious fumes, and leaking gas may not be detected by people with a loss in the sense of smell. Altered olfactory (smell) and gustatory (taste) senses can contribute to decreased appetite. Odor and taste of food

have direct impact on the older adult's nutritional health status.

Interventions for Alterations in Smell

The caring nurse acknowledges individual differences in sensory experiences, attitudes, and preferences for smells and tastes that are a function of culture. Box 8–7 presents interventions for alterations in the sense of smell. Tastes of food are often interpreted through the sense of smell, and modifications in nutrition can be made according to the individual's cultural food patterns. Often an early indication of lessening in the ability to smell is the loss of appreciation for or awareness of food flavor (Gold, 1993).

Health teaching needs to include the information that smoking affects the function of smell. If smoking is stopped, the sense of smell tends to return. Older adults should be informed that diminished smell may place them at risk for food poisoning through eating contaminated food. Health and nutritional teach-

Box 8-7 INTERVENTIONS FOR ALTERATION IN SMELL

1. There should be frequent checks for gas leaks at the older adult's residence.
2. If there are family members in the household, they can smell food before it is to be eaten. If the older adult lives alone, food that has been prepared should be dated and discarded by a designated deadline.
3. Personal hygiene should be a priority.
4. Meals should be attractively prepared and served.
5. Texture, color, variety, and size of portions are important.
6. An attractive, comfortable, pleasant environment at mealtime will contribute to the success of the activity.
7. The other senses of sight, hearing, and touch should be stimulated during mealtime activity.

ing should be directed to the use of fresh and freshly cooked foods.

TOUCH

The need for touch extends across the life span. Touch reinforces trust, portrays care, and conveys that a person is worthy of care. Touch is a means of communication between the person giving and the person receiving the tactile stimulation. Touch, as tactile stimulation, conveys nonverbal messages. Tweaking the cheek of an older adult can elicit anger. Patting an older adult on the back can be interpreted as demeaning. The back of the hand and lower arm are the best places to touch an older adult; this may be done during feeding, conversation, and caregiving.

Tactile deficits, or the inability to identify tactile sensation through the fingertips, is assessed by neurological examination. Sensory impairments are the result of a decrease in the number of areas of the body responding to all stimuli and the number and sensitivity of all receptors. Degenerative changes in receptors and the peripheral nervous system lead to difficulty in identifying objects by touch.

Assessment of Touch and Pain Sensitivity

Thorough physical assessment is necessary to identify conditions underlying complaints of pain and discomfort. Pain sensitivity is assessed

through the ability to distinguish between sharp and dull sensations. Older adults tend to experience decreased sensitivity to pain.

The sense of touch influences skin areas of temperature. Temperature regulation and **thermal sensitivity** alterations occur with aging and are assessed through a test identifying heat from cold. Extremes of heat and cold should be carefully monitored in older adults. The greatest changes in touch sensitivity of the skin occur on the palms of the hand and soles of the feet, requiring appropriate clothing and covering for temperatures being experienced. The identification of bruises, discolorations, burns, and pressure areas on the body may go unnoticed by the older adult and is therefore a crucial part of observation during the nursing assessment.

Interventions for Alterations in Touch and Pain Sensitivity

In older adults with circulatory problems or diabetes, nursing assessment and intervention lead to prevention of more serious health problems. Interventions for alterations in touch are found in Box 8–8.

Caring

The caring nurse acknowledges individual differences in sensory experiences, attitudes, and preferences for smells and tastes that are a function of culture.

Box 8-8   INTERVENTIONS FOR ALTERATION IN TOUCH

1. Provide additional touching if well received by the older adult. In an institutionalized setting a "hug therapy" program could be initiated, where nursing staff could reach out physically and emotionally, on a regular basis, to older adults in their care.
2. Involve family in the importance of touch to their older adult family members. If necessary, teach about the styles of touch.
3. Use a firmer, more positive touch where necessary; it sends a message of feeling, warmth, and caring.
4. Alert older adults to the temperature (warm or cold) of baths, liquids, and food when administering nursing care. Prepare them by telling them what to expect.

Hot and cold water used for bathing or washing should be carefully checked because of the temperature sensitivity of older adults. Nursing safety in the application of heat and cold is most important. A higher room temperature may be required at home or in an institutionalized setting. Cold temperatures are felt more easily than hot temperatures, requiring extra clothing during seasonal changes or extra covering while in bed. Neurological changes occurring with age may delay the time needed to alert the older adult about a burn or frostbite. Often the discomfort is experienced after some damage has already taken place.

Touch as tactile stimulation for older adults is experienced through visitation by family, friends, volunteers, and pet therapy. These interventions provide a sense of caring and reach out to those who may be isolated from human touch. Pets can be companions giving a feeling of someone to care for as well as a pet that cares; pet therapy is an established therapy.

Interventions for pain sensitivity are found in Box 8–9. Interventions for pain management include lessening anxiety, relaxation techniques, medication, and the addition of foods that contain tryptophan (a precursor to serotonin) to the individual's diet. Some such foods are yogurt, milk, bananas, pineapple, poultry, and beef. These foods are important to the descending inhibition of pain, contribute to a person's sense of well-being, and are nonpharmacological interventions.

Older adults tend to experience decreased sensitivity to pain. In assessing pain, the cause, onset, and duration should be determined. Effective ways of pain management that were used by patients over a lifetime should be encouraged. Culture and past experience form the basis for how a person copes with pain.

Box 8-9   INTERVENTIONS FOR ALTERATION IN PAIN SENSITIVITY

1. Pain and temperature sensitivity are often manifested by irritability, restlessness, and confusion. Such changes in the older adult should be reported immediately.
2. Be alert when giving skin care, baths, and other care. Soap products and towels could be harsh to the skin.
3. Be careful in turning older adults in bed because sheets may cause abrasions on the skin. Any evidence of bruises, burns, or pressure ulcers on the body must receive prompt attention. They could go unnoticed; because of the alterations in pain sensitivity, the older adult may not have any pain.

Summary

Sensation and perception are dependent on the quality of the five senses—sight, hearing, taste, smell, and touch. Aging is often accompanied by some degree of sensory loss. Nurses can assist the visually and hearing impaired client to communicate with others and the environment. Nurses are becoming more aware of and knowledgeable about alterations in the senses of taste and smell and their relationship to the health and nutrition of older adults. The sense of touch relating to tactile stimulation, pain, and thermal sensitivity provides areas for health teaching and client safety.

The emphasis of this chapter has been on what the nurse, the older adult, staff, and family can do to make sensory alterations less stressful. Human-environmental interactions and the quality of life can be greatly enhanced when older adults are taught how to respond to alterations with promptness and how to work with health care professionals who are able to assist with interventions that prevent further decline.

REFERENCES

Aging Research and Training News. (1993). Research findings: University of Pennsylvania Smell Identification Test (UPSIT). Aging Res Train News 16(3):21.

Beauchamp G. (1992). Multidisciplinary Approach at Monell: A Perspective. Philadelphia: Monell Publications.

Cowart B. (1993). Clinical Research in Smell and Taste. Philadelphia: Monell Publications.

Eastman P. (1993). The newest look: High tech medicine for the eyes . . . experts debate its usefulness. AARP Bull 34(4):6–7.

Gold G. (1993). Receptor Mechanisms for Olfaction. Philadelphia: Monell Publications.

Hall D. (1993). Do not neglect your hearing. Health News 10(3):4–5.

Jarvis C. (1992). Physical Examination and Health Assessment. Philadelphia: WB Saunders.

Kelly M. (1995). Consequences of visual impairment on leisure activities of the elderly. Geriatr Nurs 16(6):273–275.

McDonald E, Marino C. (1991). Dry mouth: Diagnosing and treating its multiple causes. Geriatrics 46(3):61–63.

Mhoon E. (1992). Otology. In Cassel C, et al., eds. Geriatric Medicine. 2nd ed. New York: Springer Verlag.

The Monell Connection. (1992). Does the World Become Less Fragrant As We Age? Philadelphia: Monell Publications.

Thompson J, Wilson S. (1996). Health Assessment for Nursing Practice. St. Louis: CV Mosby.

SUGGESTED READING

Absher K. (1996). Stop age-related cataracts. J Longevity Res 3(9):36–39.

Duarte A. (1994). Cataract Breakthrough. Eau Claire, WI: Doyle Maloney.

Margolis S, Schachat A. (1995). Vision Disorders: Johns Hopkins White Papers. New York: Medletter Association.

Marko R. (1990). Eye disease of people with diabetes. Aging Vision News 3(1):1–8.

CRITICAL THINKING EXERCISES

Miss Torres, age 76, a retired librarian, comes to the senior center/clinic for lunch every day. She lives alone and chooses to walk the half mile in each direction. Miss Torres says that she is afraid if she stops walking to the center each day she will lose the ability to do so. "Use it or lose it," she chuckles. Miss Torres has had cataract surgery and wears eyeglasses with very heavy lenses. In addition, the staff has become aware that she often has difficulty hearing peers and others in the dining room. Yesterday Miss Torres walked into a swinging door and sustained ecchymoses and swelling above her right eye. The staff is concerned that Miss Torres may sustain other injuries if she continues to walk alone to the center each day. As the nurse on staff at the center, you are asked to intervene with Miss Torres.

1. In two to four paragraphs, explain how you would approach Miss Torres about the potential dangers of her walking to the center each day. Include your desired outcome and any options that may be available to her.

2. From the case study, identify at least three nursing diagnoses and develop a mini care plan for Miss Torres, including nursing interventions and expected outcomes.

3. Research the facilities available in your own community through which a client like Miss Torres might find needed services and suggest ways in which they could help her.

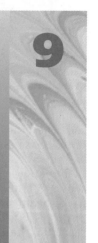

CHAPTER 9

Activity, Rest, and Sleep

Shirley Rose Tyson, RN, MA, EdD

CHAPTER OUTLINE

OBJECTIVES

After completing this chapter, the reader should be able to:

1. Develop an exercise program for older adults.
2. Teach a classmate the nursing measures that help prevent complications associated with immobility.
3. Teach an older client interventions to diminish the risk of falling.
4. Evaluate the interactions between drugs and sleep in older adults.
5. Formulate safe and effective measures to promote healthy sleep in older adults.

KEY TERMS

assistive devices
circadian rhythm
gait
iatrogenesis
immobility
sleep apnea

Interest in health promotion, wellness, and physical and mental fitness has soared in the United States in recent years. Video tapes, magazines, and professional literature abound with information on optimal nutrition, physical fitness, and healthy lifestyles. *Healthy People 2000* (U.S. DHHS, 1990) emphasizes goals of health promotion and disease prevention. With a focus on wellness, health care professionals are in a unique position to influence others to seek physical fitness at any age across the life span. A wellness focus, rather than a problem focus, can motivate an older adult to strive for the highest possible level of wellness. *Wellness* is described by Stolte (1996) as a process that is continually evolving to higher and higher levels of functioning. Therefore, wellness can be achieved by older adults even in the presence of some illness.

In this chapter the discussion centers on activity, rest, and sleep in older adults. The caring nurse needs to understand these areas to provide information, support, and assistance to those in need of such interventions. Activity, rest, and sleep are healthy, normal, cyclic components of daily living. Physical activity, mobility, and exercise—indeed, movement of any kind—are important to older adults. Activity contributes to the maintenance of full functional levels and can slow the rate of loss in those whose health and function are declining.

All body systems—especially the musculoskeletal, cardiovascular, metabolic, and nervous systems—benefit from physical activity, with maximized function viewed as a desirable outcome. Mental activity maintains the brain's ability to function and is reflected as alertness. By keeping physically and mentally fit, an older adult can minimize any physical and mental losses that may accompany aging. Mobility relates to ease of movement and promotes participation in self-care. Self-care, social support, and a healthy environment promote health and wellness.

Rest and relaxation contribute to healthy functioning of the older adult. Sleep, which occupies approximately one third of the average person's life, is considered to have a restorative value and to encompass areas such as physical and mental repair, biological rhythms, hormonal activity, and a sense of well-being. Sleep is a universal need of all humans, across the life span, throughout life.

Impaired physical mobility can result in poor health, especially for older adults, and precipitate negative consequences. Sleep patterns may be affected by age, leading to complaints about the quality and quantity of sleep. The majority of older adults remain mobile, involved in activities and participating in areas in which they have an interest. Such people maintain a lifestyle that supports a balance among mobility, exercise, rest, and sleep.

■ AGE-RELATED CHANGES

The musculoskeletal system consists of bones, muscles, and joints, as well as the supportive structures that make maintaining an upright position possible (see Chapter 16). As people age, the number of those individuals with limitations of activity and mobility increases. Older adults experience a decrease in the number of muscle cells and in muscle strength; beyond the age of 50 years, there is no new bone growth and a gradual bone loss occurs. However, if exercise has been part of an individual's lifestyle, there will be less change in the amount of bone loss and muscle strength.

Osteoporosis is a disease characterized by loss of calcium from the bones. As calcium is resorbed from the bones, the bones become increasingly porous and brittle and thus more susceptible to fractures, particularly of the long bones and vertebrae. A contributory cause is the bone loss associated with menopause; it occurs in 30% of postmenopausal females. Osteoporosis is also seen in men older than 60.

The most common disorder affecting joints is *osteoarthritis*, a chronic degenerative condition beginning in mid life and progressing with old age. It is the most common type of arthritis, affecting most people to some degree by the age of 75 years. Arthritis is probably the most common disorder of the musculoskeletal system in older adults. For other examples of activity-related disorders, see the discussions related to body systems in Unit V, Physiological Challenges of Aging.

Aging can contribute to changes in the components of sleep structure and in its distribution. Sleep-wake and rest-activity cycles may become dissociated as a person ages. Age-related changes also impact the sleep cycle, in that nighttime sleep becomes lighter, more fragmented, and shorter. Many older adults who consider themselves healthy are otherwise bothered by some aspect of their sleep pattern. Some sleep changes should be expected with aging, and older adults need to be taught that sleep habits can be modified to obtain the sleep they need.

▮ ACTIVITY AND EXERCISE

Activity is a normal part of daily living and has an important role in preventing disease, enhancing well being, and reducing disability. It may also preserve the ability to perform important everyday tasks despite the progressive loss of muscle mass associated with aging. Activity is a treatment intervention for older adults, limiting disability and loss of function and preventing recurrence of other conditions.

Exercise is a type of physical activity defined as a "planned, structured, and repetitive bodily movement done to improve or maintain one or more components of physical fitness" (Jones and Jones, 1997). As chronological age increases, exercise can help maintain and enhance functional ability. With the increasing life expectancy of individuals in our society, more and more people are discovering that their quality of life can be greatly improved by exercise.

Exercise increases muscle strength and coordination, contributing to the ability to perform activities of daily living. Even the prescription of minimal exercise can have great impact on sedentary older adults with increased benefits in physical and psychological areas. Physical benefits include

- Decreased glucose tolerance levels
- Decreased cholesterol levels
- Improvement of balance
- Reduction of falls
- Improvement of body tone
- Increase in and improvement in the quantity and quality of sleep
- Improvement in appetite, eating, and digestion
- Improvement in circulation

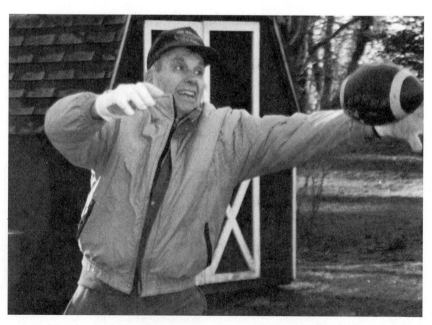

Many older adults enjoy sports into their later years.

Psychological benefits include

- Increased socialization, interaction, and recreational activity with others
- Increased self-esteem and ego strength
- Increased independence
- Increased sense of well-being and positive mood
- Reduction in stress
- Improved self-image
- Improved cognitive functioning

Because the goals of exercise include building muscle tissue and tone, decreasing fat, and controlling weight, exercise is highly recommended to improve the health of sedentary and/or overweight individuals. Any form of exercise can be performed by older adults; however, the preferred type is some form of aerobic activity combined with use of the large-muscle groups (e.g., swimming, brisk walking, cycling). Water exercises in a swimming pool are particularly therapeutic for individuals who may not be able to participate in other activities because they are sensitive to impact or have limited mobility. Older adults with arthritis, painful joints, weak leg muscles, or chronic knee and back problems can move more easily in water. Simple stretching exercises that follow

Wellness

"Regular exercise has many active benefits: improved heart and lung function, lowered heart attack risk, increased energy, improved concentration, raised spirits, and relief from anxiety."

normal body movement may be initiated and maintained on a daily basis. Regular exercise, at least three times per week for a period of 30 minutes, is recommended.

After a complete assessment of the older client, an exercise program can be initiated by the nurse and other health team members that is specifically tailored to the client. Such an intervention treats existing problems and prevents potential ones that could arise from prolonged inactivity. Box 9–1 presents a set of guidelines for such an exercise program.

IMMOBILITY

Immobility is the making of a part or limb immovable. Limitation of mobility, or even com-

---

Box 9-1 GUIDELINES FOR AN EXERCISE PROGRAM FOR OLDER ADULTS

- A physical examination must be undertaken to assess health conditions before an exercise program is started.
- Initiate a program that fits the needs of the individual based on assessed strengths, weaknesses, and interests.
- A fitness training program using aerobic exercise should be specific to the needs of each individual.
- Active exercise should begin with a "warm-up" period to prepare joints and muscles. "Warm-up" includes range of motion and gentle stretching.
- Begin exercise in areas where there is least discomfort and move to areas where discomfort is greater.
- Determine the training heart rate (individuals should check their pulse rate) and evaluate during exercise to ensure the rate is within a safe range.
- Exercise can be done in a seated position while watching television, conversing, or reading. Arm, leg, and foot circling, deep breathing, and arm raising are examples.
- Encourage walking, swimming, and stationary bicycling.
- Advise that exercise on awakening loosens stiff joints.
- Exercise body joints through normal range of motion several times a day.
- At the end of active exercise, there should be a "cool-down" period ending with range of motion, stretching, and relaxing to prevent syncope.

TABLE 9–1. Relationship of Aging, Impaired Mobility, and Effects of Exercise

Body Systems	Effects of Exercise	Consequences of Impaired Mobility	Effects of Aging
Musculoskeletal			
Strength	Increase	Decrease	Decrease
Endurance	Increase	Decrease	Decrease
Flexibility	Increase	Decrease	Decrease
Range of motion	Increase	Decrease	Decrease
Lean bone mass	Increase	Decrease	Decrease
Cardiovascular			
Blood pressure	Same or decrease	Orthostatic hypertension	Increase
Cardiac output	Increase	Decrease	Decrease
Maximal heart rate	Increase	Decrease	Decrease
Risk of thrombosis	Decrease	Increase	Increase
Respiratory			
Functional capacity	Increase	Decrease	Decrease
Depth of respiration	Increase	Decrease	Decrease
Rate of respiration	Increase	Decrease	Decrease
Metabolic			
Basal metabolic rate	Increase	Decrease	Decrease
Gastrointestinal			
Elimination	Increase	Decrease	Decrease
Digestion	Increase	Decrease	Decrease
Urinary			
Drainage	Increase	Decrease	Decrease
Risk of renal calculi	Decrease	Increase	Increase

plete **immobility**, in individuals older than age 65 years can be directly related to arthritis, hypertension, cardiac disease, visual and hearing impairments, impairments of the hips and lower extremities, and fear of falling. Immobility is a problem that must be aggressively addressed by health care professionals because inactivity can cause premature death.

In older adults, disturbances in maintaining activity typically are a result of illness, medication, functional limitations, or lack of accessibility to resources. Many health care professionals in institutionalized settings accept stereotypical notions of older adults, who may be inactive or debilitated as a result of the aging process. It is important to realize that the resident's muscle strength can be lost each week that muscles are resting completely, and each day of bed rest increases the workload of an already compromised heart. Aggressive intervention to arrest, minimize, and treat existing mobility limitation while preventing future

problems associated with functional capacity is within the realm of gerontological nursing care. Consequences of impaired mobility, effects of exercise, and effects of aging on body systems are presented in Table 9–1.

Some older adults rely on **assistive devices** such as canes, walkers, and wheelchairs. These individuals may be confronting a psychological issue of fear of falling and injury. Health teaching and environmental manipulation can bring about increased awareness of safety and protection for older adults, making them more comfortable in initiating and participating in mobility.

Assessing Functional Mobility/Ability

Functional abilities and areas of limitation must be noted before an appropriate plan of care can be developed and implemented. Table 9–2 presents the factors involved in assessment of functional ability in older adults.

TABLE 9–2. Assessment of Functional Mobility/Ability

Physical
Normal mobility
Body alignment
Balance
Coordination of body movements
Gait
Range of motion
Assistive devices
History of falls
Any paralysis
Complications of immobility related to body systems

Psychosocial
Personality changes
Anxiety
Disorientation/confusion
Changes in role perception
Changes in self-concept
Perceived changes in sexuality
Hostility
Withdrawal
Dependency

Cognitive
Decreased motivation
Decreased problem-solving ability
Perceptual changes

Social
Socioeconomic status
Ability to care for self
Availability of resources
Interaction with others
Assistance from others

Environmental
Safety
Comfort
Removal of hazards

psychosocial, cognitive, and environmental aspects (see the following sections)
- Diagnostic tests such as radiographs and laboratory work
- Observation of the older adult's mobility status

PHYSICAL ASSESSMENT

Perhaps most important to mobility are the questions relating to physical assessment of the older client. The following can elicit pertinent information:

1. Do you have the mobility you need to get up and move about?
2. Are you experiencing any change in the way you are used to walking or moving about? If so, exactly what are the changes?
3. Are you having any difficulty getting out of bed on arising?
4. Are you having any difficulty rising from a seated position?
5. Are you having any difficulty getting into and out of the bathtub?
6. Do you require assistance in bathing, dressing, or toileting?
7. Are you able to clean your house, do laundry, shop for groceries?
8. Are you able to walk up and down stairs?
9. Are you able to go outside of your home?
10. Do you drive a car or use public transportation?
11. Do you use any assistive device such as a cane or walker? If so, when did you begin to use this device?
12. How often do you now use this device? Please demonstrate how you use the device.
13. Do you have pain on a regular basis? What medications do you take?
14. Have you experienced any falls recently? If you have, can you describe what happened?

PSYCHOSOCIAL ASSESSMENT

A psychosocial assessment is crucial to an older adult's mobility status, in that self-image can be impacted by immobility. It is also important to assess whether the older adult is motivated by self or others. Here are some pertinent questions:

1. At this time, do you consider yourself healthy?

Interviews, questionnaires, and a checklist, in addition to a collateral history from a spouse or children of the older adult, can provide valuable assessment information. Multidisciplinary assessment with an emphasis on functional abilities is a basis for practice in caring for older adults. It is essential to understand the implications brought about by impairment to develop appropriate plans of care. Data should include the following:

- A history taken from the older adult and family members
- A functional assessment including physical,

2. Have there been any changes in your life within the past year that could contribute to your mobility status?
3. Are you able to accomplish activities that you were once able to?
4. Are you able to accomplish activities that you would like to do?
5. If not, do you have any assistance from family, friends, or neighbors?
6. Who gives you support? Family, church, doctor, dentist, neighbor? Can you talk with them when needed?
7. Can you describe what is a typical day for you?
8. Can you describe your lifestyle?
9. Do you have a fear of falling?
10. Can we discuss ways to assist you in the prevention of falls?

ENVIRONMENTAL ASSESSMENT

An integral part of functional assessment is environmental assessment. The disability that can be a handicap in one environment may not be in another, or, it may be for one person but not for another in the same environment. This is referred to as *person-environment congruence* and means the suitability and appropriateness of a specific environment for a specific person. The following is a useful checklist of items necessary for the safe functioning of an ambulatory adult.

1. Adequate lighting with minimal glare (for entry way, on stairs, reading); a night light should be placed in the bedroom, bathroom, and hallways.
2. Pathways should be clear of clutter, and entanglement risk should be minimized (e.g., to get to the telephone or open the door).
3. Supportive hand rails for stairs and in bathrooms. Grab bars should be placed in the shower with a hand-held shower and shower stool. Bars should also be placed in appropriate places for getting in and out of the bathtub and arising from the toilet.
4. Smoke detectors should be installed wherever necessary.
5. Heating and cooling systems should be operating safely.
6. Hot water temperature should be regulated appropriately.
7. Kitchen safety should be ensured.
8. If indicated, safety in hallway, foyer, lobby, and elevator should be a priority.
9. Easy access to objects on closet shelves in bedrooms or kitchen, without standing on tiptoe or chair or stool.
10. Removal of scatter or throw rugs. All carpeting should be tacked down to floor.

In addition to these assessment topics, we briefly mention the following:

1. Cognitive assessment identifies the older adults' mental status. If a person is not cognitively alert, directions cannot be followed nor health teaching accomplished.
2. Social assessment can reveal problems in acquiring resources, the ability to purchase assistive devices, and health care insurance coverage for devices needed by older adults. In addition, the need for assistance and services to meet physical and medical requirements can be identified.

A thorough functional assessment can identify risk factors of nutrition, dentition, obesity, substance abuse, use of medications, and numbers of medications prescribed. Other factors such as ability for activities of daily living, mobility skills, excretory functions, communication skills, and musculoskeletal and cognitive status can also be assessed. Periodic assessment is important, because performance can improve or decline or deteriorate over time, necessitating changes in treatment or interventions. There are several instruments available to assess functional status, determining the older adult's ability to remain independent in the community.

INSTRUMENTS IN THE ASSESSMENT PROCESS

A number of instruments have been established to assist in the assessment process of older adults:

W e l l n e s s

"Falls can be prevented by maintaining a safe environment. This can include installing hand rails and night lights, removing throw rugs, and placing nonslip mats in bathtubs."

1. The OARS (Older American Resource and Services Center Instrument) is one example of a standardized measurement of basic and instrumental activities of daily living. The OARS provides clinical information for assessing needs and planning interventions (Fillenbaum, 1988).
2. The Katz Index of Activities of Daily Living (Katz et al., 1963)
3. The Lawton Scale for Instrumental Activities of Daily Living. Basic activities of daily living include eating; mobility; transfer to and from bed; transfer to and from equipment, chair, and toilet; continence; bathing; and dressing. Instrumental activities of daily living include housekeeping, laundry, cooking, grocery shopping, finances, transportation, medication, and telephone activities, which the older adult may have difficulty in performing (Lawton and Brody, 1969).
4. The Geriatric Depression Scale (depression is common in older adults)
5. Mental status assessment tools including the Mini-Mental State Examination (Folstein et al., 1975) to assess cognitive status
6. The physical examination questionnaire. Interpretation of test results and scoring allow the health care professional to evaluate abilities and problems with function in each area. Answers to questions can also identify support systems available to the older adult. Results of the functional assessment can assist in planning interventions specific to each patient's abilities, the need for assistance, and the promotion of rehabilitation for abilities that have changed. Treatment, referrals, and rehabilitation for specific alterations should be implemented as soon as possible to prevent further decline.

The Omnibus Reconciliation Act of 1987 (OBRA) is very specific with respect to policies related to comprehensive assessment, maintenance of functional abilities, use of chemical and physical restraints, and drug therapy in long-term care facilities. These policies directly impact gerontological nursing care as they relate to primary and secondary prevention of disability (Marek et al., 1996).

Results of comprehensive assessment can indicate the need for assistive devices, the need for supervision or assistance, and the need for a specially equipped wheelchair, automobile, or artificial limbs. There may also be a need for homemaker services, attendant care, Meals on Wheels, volunteer help, and visitors. Other interventions include support groups with remotivation, reality and counseling focus, advocacy for disabled individuals, and coordination of various agencies and resources.

Assistive devices for ambulation include the following:

- Cane (adjustable, single or quadripod)
- Crutches (available in different lengths)
- Walker

It is the nurse's responsibility to observe whether the older adult is using the assistive device correctly. If this is not so, correct usage should be taught with return demonstration by the individual. If an older adult is able to ambulate, a wheelchair should not be offered. In many long-term care settings, wheelchairs are utilized as transportation. If at all possible, mobility should be encouraged, enhanced, and rewarded because of its physical and psychological gains.

Falls: Hazards to Mobility

This section focuses on falling, which is the hazard with the highest incidence in hospital geriatric units, nursing homes, and other facilities for older adults. However, there are many hazards to mobility, including the following:

- Reduced range of motion of joints
- Loss of muscle strength
- Cardiovascular deterioration
- Metabolic imbalance
- Decrease in gastrointestinal, urinary, and respiratory function
- Iatrogenic factors of bed rest, restrictive movement, restraints, catheters, intravenous fluids, suction
- Medications
- Lack of knowledge regarding available resources
- Psychologically traumatic experiences
- Sociocultural behaviors of role reversal and power relationships
- Lack or absence of social networks
- Cognitive deficits
- Lack of knowledge regarding the benefits of mobility

From this list it is clear that not only physical but also psychological and social factors underlie the occurrence of accidents among older adults. Certainly the continuing debate about whether older adults should be allowed to continue driving a car without regular testing is an example of a complex issue related to the listed factors.

Because immobility is a common problem for institutionalized older adults, nurses in such settings need to work to prevent the onset or progression of chronic illnesses and to avoid the risk of **iatrogenesis,** a term used to describe the creation of additional problems or complications resulting from treatment by a health care professional. Individuals older than age 65 years should be assessed annually to determine hazards to mobility and risk of falling. For those older adults who remain in their homes, a home assessment should be made to identify possible hazards.

Some older adults experience impaired strength, with accompanying problems in mobility, balance, and endurance. If unattended, these problems can lead to serious falls, admissions in long-term care institutions, and consequent loss of independence. Mobility limitation ranges from the need to use special equipment to total dependence on others for movement. Physical frailty and injuries from falls are not the inevitable outcome of aging but are problems for which there are available options and viable solutions.

Because falls are the most prevalent cause of injury in older individuals, and given the dire consequences associated with them, health care professionals must focus on their prevention in all care settings. Thirty to 50 percent of older adults experience at least one fall per year. Falls increase with advancing age, occurring predominantly in women 75 years and older and often in the homes of older adults (Suzuki et al., 1997).

Falls can be classified (Hornbook et al., 1994) as

- Near falls, in which balance is lost but recovered before hitting the floor
- Injury falls, which result in some type of injury
- Medical care falls, which require medical care (including emergency care)
- Fracture falls
- Hospitalized falls, which require a report of the fall's consequences

A fall may be influenced by intrinsic and extrinsic factors. *Intrinsic factors* include normal age-related changes such as decrease in visual acuity, changes in balance and *gait* (manner of walking), and increased body sway. *Extrinsic factors,* or environmental hazards, include poor lighting, thick carpeting, polished floors, sliding mats, stairs, toilet and bathtubs not equipped with grab bars, unsafe footwear, and unstable furniture.

The highest incidence of falls is noted in the 80- to 89-year age group. In the community, women fall more frequently than men, but in the institutionalized setting there is equal distribution of falls between men and women (Tideiksaar, 1994). Common factors that increase the risk for falls include

- History of previous falls
- Increased age
- Gait problems
- Sensory impairment
- Muscle weakness
- Cerebrovascular disease
- Urinary and bladder dysfunction

Substance abuse, polypharmacy, psychoactive drugs, psychosocial issues of loss, social isolation, loneliness, and depression also contribute to increased risk for falls. Physical restraints deny freedom of movement and chemical restraints (drug therapy) slow movement, both of which can contribute to falls.

Because responsibility for prevention of falls rests with all health care providers, preventive measures should include assessment of sensorimotor changes that are associated with risk for falls and assessment of institution and home settings. Patient teaching with recommendations to patient and family regarding environmental hazards should help decrease the incidence of falls in this vulnerable age group. Home assessment for fall hazards should be conducted in every room in the home with emphasis on the bathroom, kitchen, and bedroom. Interior stairs, tables, stools, hand rails, and lighting and exterior steps, walkways, hand rails, and lighting are very important parts of assessment in a fall prevention program. The fall assessment guide of Box 9–2 assists health care professionals in planning and interventions in the hospital, nursing home, or community setting.

Interventions include structuring a safe environment, teaching clients how to fall to prevent more serious injuries, a restraint-free environment, good maintenance of devices used for mobility, and regular physical and environ-

Box 9-2 FALL ASSESSMENT GUIDE

- Thorough physical examination to assess medical problems
- History that specifically addresses falling episodes
- Assess for fall phobia (Tideiksaar, 1994), which is an abnormal fear of falling, characterized by restriction of activities and use of assistive devices
- Neurological assessment
- Balance and gait assessment
- Musculoskeletal function
- Cognitive status
- Functional status
- Environmental assessment
- Mobility status
- Physical status
- Use of prescribed and over-the-counter medications
- Use of alcohol

mental assessments. Environmental modifications of the home and institution can be a major therapeutic tool in fall prevention.

The physical assessment should examine vision, blood pressure, cardiovascular condition, and the Romberg and sternal push test. The following observations should be part of the examination (Tideiksaar 1994):

1. Sit and rise from a chair
2. Walk and turn around
3. Climb and descend stairs
4. Bend down and pick up an object
5. Reach up arms while standing on tiptoe

Prevention management should emphasize

- Treating the underlying disease or condition
- Eliminating the medications that could present a problem with mobility
- Modifying living environments to compensate for mobility dysfunction.

Older adults will continue to fall, owing to the aging process and concomitant illnesses, unless steps such as a fall prevention program are taken to reduce falls. A fall prevention program such as that in Box 9–3 should be designed by multidisciplinary health team members. Such a program will benefit not only older adults but also health care personnel whose responsibility it is to prevent falls. Identification of intrinsic and extrinsic factors with accompanying interventions offers viable solutions in preventing or reducing the majority of such incidents. A fall history taken from the older adult and family members is critical to the program.

CASE STUDY

Peso Losado, an 81-year-old widower, visits the nurse-managed community clinic complaining of chronic fatigue. A nurse is assigned to him and conducts a thorough assessment.

Box 9-3 FALL PREVENTION PROGRAM

- Take a fall history (know why, when, and where the person fell).
- Understand medical, psychological, and social etiology of falls.
- Take a team approach toward fall management.
- Perform an environmental assessment for fall hazards.
- Design a fall management plan.
- Work with a multidisciplinary team to implement fall prevention.
- Design a fall research study.

History. Mr. Losado considers himself relatively healthy and has been for most of his life. During the past 7 years he has been treated for hypertension. He is alert and responsive and understands the reason for the antihypertensive medication, its dosage, and effects. Mr. Losado has lost about 8 pounds recently and complains of fatigue "all the time" that seems to be unrelated to any specific activity.

Functional Assessment. Mr. Losado is independent in all of the basic activities of daily living, although he is experiencing some changes in mobility. He walks with a cane and has difficulty with stairs. Twice he has fallen—once last month while arising from the chair to answer the doorbell and again 2 days ago on the way to the bathroom during the night. His married daughter, who lives upstairs, assists with many of the instrumental activities of daily living. Sometimes he accompanies her to do the grocery shopping, participating in the activity, paying for his groceries himself, and enjoying the outdoors. On Wednesdays and Sundays, Mr. Losado goes to his daughter's for dinner and meets with his grandchildren and son-in-law. Mr. Losado cooks for himself, but recently this activity has diminished owing to the fatigue. He gets out of the house to attend church weekly, attend the clinic, visit a friend who lives nearby, and occasionally go to the supermarket for small items. Because of the fatigue, he is curtailing his activities. He has given up driving and takes the bus that stops in front of his home. Currently he is afraid of falling and calls on his daughter or her teenaged children whenever he needs assistance.

Psychosocial Assessment. Widowed for 10 years, Mr. Losado has a daughter who is married with three teenage children and lives upstairs in this two-family home. His daughter and grandchildren are willing to offer help at any time, although the daughter has full-time employment and the children are busy in school. Until recently, Mr. Losado was a fairly active person in church and in the senior center. His income is more than adequate for his needs. He has no history of mental illness or depression, although he states that lately he feels "down at times." His score on the Geriatric Depression Scale is good. If his recent impairment in mobility status were to continue, there would be a decline in social relationships, but his daughter and her family will continue to participate in his care, if necessary, for as long as he needs it.

Cognitive Assessment. Mr. Losado does not seem to have any memory impairment after testing on the Mini-Mental State Examination for memory and the Short Blessed Test of Orientation—Memory—Concentration (Katzman, 1983), which is a quick screening test for identifying cognitive impairment. (Evaluation of cognitive impairment is important because some causes are reversible , such as those from medications, nutritional deficiencies, thyroid problems, and other medical causes. Physical assessment determines alterations that could indicate disease. For a complete review of physical assessment, see Chapter 2.)

Findings. Mr. Losado's blood pressure is 120/80 mm Hg. He has lower-extremity weakness and arthritis of the knees, which causes pain at times. The cane he uses was purchased at the neighborhood drug store and is too high for his height. His skin is dry and flaky. Mr. Losado is experiencing the first signs of frailty as his mobility function declines. Immediate intervention can prevent his developing complications of poor nutrition, medical problems, injury as a result of his physical frailty, depression, and isolation.

The following recommendations are designed for Mr. Losado as part of nursing intervention to keep him active, alert, and productive for as long as possible.

Potential for Alteration in Nutrition. If Mr. Losado's nutrition does not improve, he is at risk for nutritional deficiency. Many older adults who live alone do not wish to cook and eat alone. Referral to Meals on Wheels for some meals through the week is a possible intervention; in addition, some meals in his daughter's home would improve his nutrition and also provide socialization. Also, visiting the senior center as often as possible would supplement meals and provide social interaction. Adding vitamin and mineral supplements to the diet is also a desired implementation.

Potential for Falling. Mr. Losado has several risks for falling such as arthritis, lower-extremity weakness, and ill-fitting assistive device (cane). He would benefit from a regular exercise program for muscle strengthening, a cane that is an appropriate fit, and observation to see whether there is correct usage. The cane would offer support and remove some stress from Mr. Losado's arthritic knees, preventing inflammation and pain. A rehabilitation therapist or nurse can teach leg exercises of flexing and extending, reminders about getting up slowly, and how to use the cane on arising. Grab bars should be installed in a bathroom around the toilet, bathtub, and shower to assist his ambulation. Night lights should be placed wherever appropriate for assistance when needed during the night for bathroom use. If he continues to fall with no evident reason, further evaluation is indicated.

Potential for Social Isolation. Mr. Losado may continue normal activities with interventions and treatment of the above problems, which will increase his socialization and improve self-esteem and mood. He could benefit from community activities such as adult day care and senior centers, many of which provide socialization, meals, supervision, exercise programs, transportation, discussion sessions, and recreational activities.

REST AND RELAXATION

Rest and sleep contribute to wellness. All humans require rest and sleep to function physically and mentally. There should be adequate rest, relaxation, and sleep periods during each 24-hour day to maintain a healthy pattern of each.

Regular activity promotes rest and relaxation. Throughout the day, older adults require greater amounts of rest that are just as important to promoting health as are the periods of activity. To maintain a healthy pattern of rest and sleep, most older adults require 7 to 8 hours of sleep. Rest is as necessary to a person's healthy functioning as is activity. Obstacles to rest should be identified and eliminated. Rest equalizes metabolic capacity and demand. However, because a person is "resting" does not necessarily indicate relaxation for that person.

Older adults have negotiated many stresses by virtue of their longevity. Acute stress with appropriate intervention often produces no harm, but chronic stress with no recovery from interventions can have a deleterious effect on the body. Stress management, healthy lifestyles, and relaxation techniques can be used as interventions.

Relaxation techniques for older adults can include

- Meditation and prayer
- Relaxation exercises including yoga, qigong, and tai chi
- Music
- Guided imagery
- Relaxing bath or shower
- Exercise such as swimming, walking, bicycling

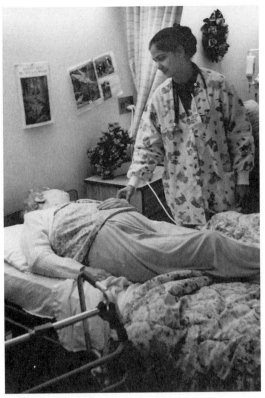

In inpatient settings, it is necessary to check on sleeping patients regularly.

- Travel
- A hobby that provides pleasure
- Table games with others such as cards, Scrabble, and bingo
- Art work, painting
- Sharing and spending time with others

Relaxation activities can be solo (involving the person only) or with others (social interaction). They should be selected for the person's interests, abilities, and lifestyles and promote relaxation.

SLEEP

Although recuperative and integrative, sleep can be a major health issue for many older adults, who commonly report disturbed or inadequate sleep. Sleep is a complex, active process that follows a pattern of well-defined cycles. There are two major kinds of sleep: Non–rapid eye movement (NREM) and rapid eye movement (REM), which alternate throughout the night with an average cycle of 90 minutes each in healthy adults.

Caring

❝*The caring nurse needs to understand activity, rest, and sleep in older adults to provide information, support, and assistance to those in need of such interventions.*❞

There are four stages of NREM sleep:

- Stage I is the lightest level of sleep during which a person can be easily aroused.
- Stage II is deeper than the previous stage but light enough for easy arousal; a deeper stage of relaxation is reached and some eye movement can be observed through closed lids.
- Stage III is progressively deeper. Muscles are relaxed, it is more difficult to be awakened, and temperature and heart rate are reduced.
- Stage IV is the deepest level, where restorative sleep takes place. Body functions are reduced. Insufficient amount of this stage can lead to emotional dysfunction.

During REM sleep, one dreams and may awaken with a feeling of having a restless night. It is during REM sleep that problems may be solved and perspectives gained about troublesome issues. Nonessential data taken in during the day are discarded and essential data needing to be saved are categorized and integrated into the brain's storage system. REM periods lengthen and alternate with NREM stages II and III. Four to six REM periods occur nightly, accounting for 20% to 25% of all sleep. REM sleep restores the body mentally and psychologically, and deep sleep restores it physically.

Almost all commonly used hypnotics and sedatives as well as alcohol interfere with REM sleep.

The role of the nurse—whether in home, acute care, community, or long-term care—includes assessment and facilitation of sleep. Comprehensive assessments of the quality and quantity of sleep achieved, and accurate diagnosis of sleep disturbances with accompanying appropriate management strategies, are an important challenge to nurses working with older adults because sleep is of utmost importance to all humans Box 9–4. The questions posed in the sleep history questionnaire of Box 9–5 will become part of the assessment.

Factors Influencing Sleep

Sleep concerns reported by older adults regarding quality and quantity of sleep usually result from individual and environmental factors. Sleep dissatisfaction is often the result of interaction between individual characteristics such as anxiety and emotional discomfort and characteristics of the sociocultural environment. These may be classified as

- *Intrinsic factors* (pain, bodily discomfort, nocturia)
- *Extrinsic factors*, which derive from social conditions and from the environment as noise, poor air quality, room temperature, a comfortable place to sleep, seasonal changes, light exposure, diet, living habits, and medications

For many individuals, changes in the sleep-wake pattern occur over the life span (Floyd,

---

Box 9-4   ASSESSMENT OF SLEEP PATTERN ALTERATION IN OLDER ADULTS

- Obtain a sleep history taken from the older adults, family, or caregiver.
- Perform a complete physical examination to elicit impairment in vision, hearing, or touch sensation and to evaluate body systems.
- Perform a cognitive assessment to identify if there is any organicity.
- Order diagnostic tests such as a polysomnogram, which would involve multiple measurements obtained by placing electrodes in specific areas during sleep to obtain data regarding brain waves tracing variations in brain electric force, eye movements, and muscle tension.
- Order other tests (if any) to be performed in a sleep laboratory.
- Request observations of sleep patterns by sleep specialist.

Box 9-5   SLEEP HISTORY QUESTIONNAIRE

1. How much sleep do you get?
2. Are you having trouble sleeping? If so:
3. How long have you been experiencing this?
4. Do you get up early?
5. Do you stay up late?
6. Do you have difficulty falling asleep?
7. Is there a fragmented sleep pattern?
8. Do you have nightmares or night terrors?
9. Is the sleep unrefreshing?
10. Is the sleep interrupted by awakening to go to the bathroom?
11. Have there been any significant changes in your life within the past 6 months? Any medical or stress-related problems?
12. Can you describe a typical night's sleep?
13. Is there use of prescription, over-the-counter drugs, or alcohol to obtain sleep?
14. On awakening, do you have leg cramps, chest or abdominal pain, shortness of breath, or a need to go to the bathroom?
15. Is the environment conducive to sleep?
16. Is there excessive caffeine intake?
17. Is there much fluid intake in the evening hours?
18. What is your normal diet?

1993); however, there are older adults who report no sleep problems. It is not clear why sleep-pattern disturbances affect some and not others in the age 65 and older group.

Nurses should be aware of the factors that influence sleep patterns of older adults. Recommendations should be made for a search for several types of interventions to treat sleep problems on an individual basis.

Sleep Disorders in the Older Adult

According to the *Diagnostic and Statistical Manual of Mental Disorders* (American Psychiatric Association, 1994), the diagnosis of a sleep disorder is made only if the problem exceeds 1 month in duration. Many factors contribute to sleep disruption; Box 9–6 lists some common ones. These should not be taken lightly, because

Box 9-6   FACTORS CONTRIBUTING TO SLEEP DISRUPTION

1. Loneliness caused by loss of partners, friends, or relatives
2. Hospitalization or institutionalization in long-term care
3. Extended travel
4. Changes in lifestyle or residence
5. Prescribed medications
6. Diuretics administered late in the afternoon
7. Over-the-counter medications
8. Medical or psychiatric illness
9. Poor sleep habits
10. Primary sleep disorder
11. Other stressful life events

lack of sleep can lead to fatigue, irritability, daytime napping, and some memory and emotional problems (Schultz and Videbeck, 1994).

Additional factors that may impact or be impacted by sleep disorders are the lives of family members, caregivers, nursing facility residents, and hospital staff—particularly nursing staff during evening and nighttime hours. Sleep disorders that cause distress and discomfort should be assessed and not dismissed as "normal aging changes." Dementia can cause an inversion of the day-night sleep pattern with daytime sleep and nocturnal wakefulness.

Sleep disorders involve a decreased amount of sleep, sleeping at times other than the desired time, feeling unrefreshed on awakening in spite of the amount of sleep obtained, frequent awakenings, and early morning arousal. Sleep disorders are usually associated with pathology, and it is the nurse to whom the problem of sleep disorders is most frequently directed.

INSOMNIA

Insomnia is the inability to sleep or having one's sleep prematurely ended. Insomnia leads the list of sleep disturbances in older adults and is a symptom of many illnesses. Many determinants such as physical or psychological disorders, **circadian rhythm** disturbances (pertaining to the 24-hour day), poor sleep environments, poor sleep habits, or substance abuse contribute to insomnia (see Boxes 9–6 and 9–7).

There are three types of insomnia:

1. *Transient insomnia,* which lasts a few days, usually corrects itself. Stress, anxiety, and lifestyle changes are contributing factors. Once the stress is removed or adjustment made to changes, the insomnia is usually corrected.
2. *Short-term insomnia,* which may last up to 3 weeks. Loss of a loved one, other personal losses, and health concerns are common causes. Intervention by appropriate health care professionals is required to treat the problem. Counseling and psychotherapy are options, as are pharmacological and nonpharmacological (Box 9–8) agents.
3. *Long-term insomnia* lasts for an indefinite time. The etiology is often unclear because the insomnia is usually secondary; if underlying causes are identified through careful assessment and subsequently treated, the insomnia may be reversed.

Education is essential in the management of insomnia. Staff and clients should know about normal changes in sleep patterns that occur with increasing age.

HYPERSOMNIA

Hypersomnia is excessive sleeping, classified as a disturbance in the sleep-wake cycle. Excessive daytime somnolence may be caused by lack of sleep at night, boredom, depression, dementia, polypharmacy, or a physical condition. This increased sleeping for pathological amounts of time is outside the normal range and requires careful history taking and assessment as well as prompt diagnosis and treatment. Hypersomnia can be disabling; when severe, patients find it

---

Box 9-7 COMMONLY PRESCRIBED MEDICATIONS THAT MAY CAUSE INSOMNIA

- Ranitidine (Zantac) for ulcers
- Alprazolam (Xanax) for nervous disorders
- Diltiazem (Cardizem) for heart disorders
- Nifedipine (Procardia, Adalat) for heart disorders

Box 9-8 **NONPHARMACOLOGICAL INTERVENTIONS FOR HEALTHY SLEEP**

1. Maintain usual bedtime routine.
2. Keep interruptions during the night to a minimum or remove them altogether.
3. Decrease environmental noises.
4. Avoid alcohol.
5. Avoid smoking in the evening because nicotine is a stimulant.
6. Avoid caffeine-containing foods, beverages, and medications after lunch.
7. Take a warm relaxing bath or shower before bedtime.
8. Participate in a daily exercise program.
9. Engage in some type of relaxation techniques before bedtime. Some suggestions are reading, massage, meditation, imagery, soothing music, deep breathing exercises, walking, and gentle exercise.
10. Keep to a routine schedule of arising, daily activities, rest, and bedtime.
11. Avoid strenuous activity to within 2 hours of bedtime.
12. Make the bed and sleep environment as comfortable and conducive to sleep as possible.
13. Avoid heavy evening meals; herbal tea or other hot drink before bedtime may promote sleep.
14. Restrict fluids in the evening before retiring to reduce the frequency of awakening to go to the bathroom.
15. Tryptophan (an essential amino acid and a precursor to serotonin) plays a role in sleep regulation and is found naturally in milk, dairy products, and animal and fish protein

difficult to remain awake (DeBenedetto et al., 1991). Excessive daytime somnolence is a complaint of many older adults, especially if they are inactive, as may be the case in an institutionalized setting.

SLEEP APNEA

Sleep apnea is a primary sleep disorder characterized by periods of sleep-associated cessation of breathing called *apneas*. Apneas are compensatory mechanisms, in that when the individual awakens the apneic episodes terminate. Although it occurs in one third of all people older than age 65, most are unaware of its existence.

Individuals with sleep apnea often complain of morning headaches, depression, behavior changes, loud snoring, memory loss, or choking during sleep. Significant breathing problems occur during sleep, resulting in disturbed sleep during the night and excessive daytime sleepiness. Often individuals are unaware of the irregular breathing patterns that have pre-

vented their restful sleep. Sleep apnea is a serious medical condition associated with hypertension, heart disease, and stroke, and it can result in death.

There are two major types of sleep apnea: central and obstructive. *Central apnea*, which occurs more often, occurs when both air flow and respiratory efforts are absent. *Obstructive apnea*, the more dangerous type, has more repetitive episodes of upper-airway obstruction in which respiratory efforts persist although air flow through the nose and mouth is absent. Complete cessation of breathing for more than 10 seconds during sleep occurs, whereas diaphragmatic efforts persist to overcome the obstruction. As a result, profuse oxygen desaturation occurs, leading to cardiac arrhythmia and other life-threatening sequelae that sometimes result in sudden death. Approximately 80% of individuals with obstructive sleep apnea have hypertension and a high amount of body fat (Miceli, 1996). Symptomatology includes

- Loud snoring
- Excessive daytime sleepiness
- Headaches

- Morning fatigue caused by broken sleep with frequent arousals
- Nocturia
- Depression, anxiety
- Cognitive impairment on awakening

Evaluation by a physician trained in sleep disorders includes

- Overnight polysomnography
- Oximetry or sleep latency testing

Because disordered breathing increases with age (Morin, 1993), sedatives, hypnotics, and alcohol should be avoided; their use appears to worsen obstructive sleep apnea.

Interventions include surgical removal of tonsillar tissue or other surgery to relieve upper airway obstruction or wearing a collar around the neck to prevent neck flexion and relieve airway obstruction. Cessation of smoking, use of medications like progesterone, and use of pacemakers to stimulate contraction of the diaphragm are recommended. If the individual is obese, weight reduction should be initiated. A mask worn over the nose during sleep with continuous flow of air powered by a compressor can alleviate the apnea. Sleeping on one's side or in a prone position, continuous positive airway pressure (CPAP), tracheostomy, or medications are additional interventions for obstructive sleep apnea (Miceli, 1996). The nurse can teach the older adult to retire and to awaken at the same time every day (if necessary use an alarm clock) and can discourage daytime napping.

If apnea occurs for prolonged periods:

- Awaken the older adult and turn on side; if supine, turn onto stomach.
- Monitor blood pressure.
- Monitor heart rate and regularity.
- If CPAP is applied, ensure correct application.

C a r i n g

❝ The caring nurse can work with the older adult and/or family members in assessing, planning, implementing, and evaluating the older adult's sleep pattern and sleep environment, thus contributing to improvement in sleep.❞

SLEEP-RELATED RESPIRATORY DISTURBANCE

Sleep-disordered breathing has been observed to occur among healthy older adults in the absence of disease. Snoring has been shown to increase with age. Family members may be the only ones reporting a history of snoring because the snoring older adult may be unaware of the disruption.

Restless leg syndrome and periodic leg movements in sleep are much more common in older adults than sleep-related respiratory disorders. Contributing causes may be

- Diseases of the spine
- Degenerative joint disease
- Peripheral vascular disease
- Iron-deficiency anemia

Restless leg syndrome (a type of periodic leg movement) appears to be more common with advancing age. Leg twitching or discomfort is exacerbated with rest and relieved with movement. Diagnosis is made by history and polysomnography.

Because the environment can positively or negatively influence the quality and amount of sleep a person receives, an environmental assessment for sleep should be part of the overall assessment and history taking (Box 9–9).

Medications and Sleep

Unsatisfactory sleep is a common complaint for older adults, with 45% reporting some degree of insomnia. A significant number use hypnotics on an occasional or regular basis. There are some prescribed medications that interfere with the sleep pattern (see Box 9–7); however, these medications are often needed for daily functioning.

To avoid drug interactions, physicians should become more informed about the risks and benefits of prescribed medications and the number and types being taken by an individual. The lowest possible dosage of any medication should be prescribed for the shortest time period possible. As the population ages, this becomes a great responsibility of health care professionals.

The physiological, pathophysiological, and sociogenic effects of aging place older patients

Box 9-9   ENVIRONMENTAL ASSESSMENT FOR SLEEP

Hospital and nursing home can have serious effects on sleep
Noise vs. silence
Light (bright or dim, glare, uneven levels of illumination) vs. darkness
Comfortable bed vs. uncomfortable, unfamiliar bed
Unfamiliarity of environment
Fear of the unknown
Physical discomfort or pain
Use of equipment for medical/surgical procedures (e.g., oxygen mask, intravenous line)
Awakened often for treatment, medications, and procedures

at greater risk for pharmacokinetic and pharmacodynamic interactions. Additionally, adverse effects of possible addiction, rebound insomnia, nightmares, or daytime drowsiness outweigh the benefits of sleeping medication.

The most common pharmacological treatments for sleep disorders are sedatives, which promote sleep by relaxing the individual, and hypnotics, which actively induce sleep. The goal of drug therapy is to help the individual to sleep on a short-term basis, while other nondrug strategies are being tried. Hypnotics with shorter half-lives are recommended to avoid daytime drowsiness and gait instability. Administration should be before and not at bedtime. Drug metabolism and excretion are slower in this age group, contributing to build-up over time, resulting in carryover effects into daytime hours.

Over-the-counter medications are often used by older adults. Because dependence occurs so quickly, some authorities take the position that sedatives or hypnotics should be administered intermittently (not every night but every other night), resulting in fewer withdrawal effects.

Sleep medications are often perceived by nurses as well as patients to be the most effective sleep intervention, although more appropriate interventions relating to the cause of the problem might be implemented. Use of sleep medications in the hospital can continue adversely into use at home. In the long-term care setting, sleeping medications must be carefully monitored. These medications should not be used over extended periods of time because of possible adverse effects.

Although most orders are on an as-needed basis, it is the nurse who makes the decision to medicate. Nonpharmacological interventions can be recommended, suggested, or implemented for older adults with sleep pattern disturbances (see Box 9–8). Health teaching provides older adults with knowledge about age-related changes. This understanding makes it less likely for them to request sleeping medications and more likely to use safe and effective measures to promote sleep. Nursing intervention can help older adults to practice good sleep habits and achieve healthy sleep instead of "drugged sleep."

Sleep logs or documentation may be kept by patients to outline their sleep patterns. Sleep records, a sleep history, physical examination, and psychiatric evaluation are methods used to arrive at an appropriate diagnosis. Individuals suspected of having sleep apnea and other sleep problems should be referred to a sleep disorders center or sleep clinic for further assessment and evaluation by polygraphic monitoring of physiological variables during sleep.

Nursing interventions in acute or long-term care settings should be directed toward providing optimal treatment while being aware of the older adult's needs. They should be taught about medications that can cause insomnia (see Box 9–7). Late life insomnia can be effectively treated with nonpharmacological interventions (see Box 9–8). The nurse should also teach the hazards of over-the-counter drugs for sleep; many have serious side effects, including

- Bradycardia
- Blurred vision
- Disorientation
- Delirium

Many older adults do not consider over-the-counter agents to be drugs and may not volunteer information on their usage. Almost all commonly used hypnotics, sedatives, and alcohol interfere with REM sleep.

External environments should be adjusted. Regular follow-up reassessment should be scheduled. Goals include achieving a more healthful lifestyle conducive to sleep and minimal use with gradual withdrawal of hypnotics for those on short-term medication support and those who have taken these drugs for long periods. Discussion with older adults will reveal whether there is compliance and avoid misuse of drugs.

Summary

All adults can benefit from preventive health techniques. The goal of prevention in old age is to maximize quality of life by minimizing physical and emotional suffering, loss of function, and development of dependence.

Mobility problems in older populations are common. They are the result of pathological processes and are not normal aspects of aging. If problems go untreated, further functional decline will result. Immobility is harmful. Intervention to prevent complications will contribute to quality and quantity of life for most older adults.

A careful history and physical examination narrows the differential diagnosis of sleep disorders. There are many nonpharmacological interventions that the caring nurse may teach or implement that can contribute to healthy sleep for older adults. Evaluation of the home environment should be individualized to meet the older adult's need for sleep. Sleep deprivation is harmful. In the long-term care setting, the nurse may have to be innovative in designing a sleep-conducive milieu for the older adult.

Many older adults live alone, where safety and security are often the cause for anxiety and worry. These issues may impact sleep. In addition, sensory changes of temperature regulation and impairment in vision or hearing are other factors that detract from or disrupt sleep. The caring nurse can work with the older adult and/or family members in assessing, planning, implementing, and evaluating an older adult's sleep patterns and sleep environment, thus contributing to improvement in sleep.

REFERENCES

American Psychiatric Association. (1994). Diagnostic and Statistical Manual of Mental Disorders. 4th ed. Washington, D.C.: American Psychiatric Association.

DeBenedetto M, Cuda D, Leante W. (1991). Diurnal hypersomnolence and chronic snoring: An epidemiological study. Acta Otorhinolaryngol Ital 11(6):579–586.

Fillenbaum G. (1988). Multidimensional Functional Assessment of Older Adults. The Duke Older Americans Resources and Services Procedures. Hillsdale NJ: Laurence Erlbaum Associates. (This is the resource for the OARS Assessment Tool).

Floyd J. (1993). The use of a cross-method triangulation in the study of sleep concerns in healthy adults. J Adv Nurs Sci 16(2):70–80.

Folstein M, Folstein S, McHugh P. (1975). Mini-Mental State: A practical method for grading the cognitive state of patients for the clinician. J Psychiatr Res 12:189–198.

Hornbrook M, Stevens V, Wingfield D, et al. (1994). Preventing falls among community-dwelling older persons: Results from a randomized trial. Gerontologist 34(1):16–23.

Jones J, Jones K. (1997). Promoting physical activity in the senior years. J Gerontol Nurs 23(7):41–48.

Katz S, Ford A, Moskowitz R, et al. (1963). Studies of illness in the aged: The index of ADL: A standardized measure of physiological and psychological function. JAMA 185:914–915.

Katzman R. (1983). Validation of a short orientation memory-concentration test of cognitive impairment. Am J Psychiatry 140:734–739.

Lawton MP, Brody EM. (1969). Assessment of older people: Self-maintaining and instrumental activities of daily living. Gerontologist 9:179–186.

Marek K, Rant, M, Fagin C, Krejci J. (1996). OBRA '87: Has it resulted in positive change in nursing homes? J Gerontol Nurs 22(12):32–39.

Miceli D. (1996). Sleep and activity. In Lueckenotte A, ed. Gerontological Nursing. St. Louis: CV Mosby.

Morin C, Kowatch R, Barry T, Walton E. (1993). Late life insomnia can be effectively treated with non-pharmacological interventions. J Consultation Clin Psychiatry 61(1):137–146.

Pfeiffer E, ed. (1978). Multidimensional Functional Assessment: The OARS Methodology. 2nd ed. Durham, NC: Duke University Press.

Schultz J, Videbeck S. (1994). Sleep disturbances. In Manual of Psychiatric Nursing Care Plans. 4th ed. Philadelphia: JB Lippincott.

Stolte K. (1996). Wellness: Nursing Diagnosis for Health Promotion. Philadelphia: JB Lippincott.

Suzuki M, Shimamoto Y, Kawamura I, Takahasi H. (1997). Does gender make a difference in the risk of falls? A Japanese study. J Gerontol Nurs 23(1):41–48.

Tideiksaar R. (1994). Falls and dysmobility: Epidemiology, causes, consequences, evaluation, and prevention. Nursing Care for the Elderly: Clinical/Practical Issues for the 90s. Conference, Mt. Sinai Medical Center, New York, June 10, 1994.

U.S. Department of Health and Human Services Public Health Service. (1990). Healthy People 2000: National Health Promotion and Disease Prevention Objectives. DHHS publication No. (PHS) 91-50212. Washington, DC: U.S. Government Printing Office.

SUGGESTED READING

Drugary M. (1997). Breaking the silence: A health promotion approach to osteoporosis. J Gerontol Nurs 23(6):36–43.

Galindo-Ciocon D, Ciocon J, Galindo D. (1995). Gait training and falls in the elderly. J Gerontol Nurs 21(6):10–17.

Rush K, Ouellet L. (1997). Mobility aids and the elderly client. J Gerontol Nurs 23(1):7–15.

Ryan J, Spellbring A. (1996). Implementing strategies to decrease risk of falls in older women. J Gerontol Nurs 22(12):25–31.

Schaller K. (1996). Tai chi chih: An exercise option for older adults. J Gerontol Nurs 22(10):13–17.

CRITICAL THINKING EXERCISES

Lee Wong, a 79-year-old Chinese American widower, walks to the senior center each day for lunch. Mr. Wong needs the assistance of a cane to ambulate. Twice in the past 10 days Mr. Wong has stumbled while at the senior center, and once he actually fell to the floor but with no adverse effect. Mr. Wong lives in a second-floor, three-room apartment with his grandson, his grandson's wife, and their six school-age children. Every member of the family has a job, so that Mr. Wong is often home alone even after school is dismissed for the day.

As a nurse on the staff of the senior center, you call at Mr. Wong's home. The old building is somewhat derelict, with a broken tread on the stair leading to the second floor. In the apartment itself, the cord of an electric rice cooker snakes across the floor because there is only one outlet in the room used as a kitchen. The plumbing is worn out, and Mr. Wong says sometimes only a trickle of cold water is available for the family's use. There is no refrigerator, and a few items of food are stored on the fire escape outside the window. Because of the crowded conditions there are no chairs, and Mr. Wong spends much of his time sitting on the cot where he sleeps at night. Mr. Wong is proud of his family's efforts to get ahead and states that he understands why he is alone so much.

1. In which areas of Mr. Wong's life is it reasonable to assume you can intervene? Identify at least three nursing diagnoses for Mr. Wong and develop a mini care plan for him, including interventions and expected outcomes.
2. Do an environmental assessment and plan ways to approach the Wong family about making the home setting safer for their eldest member.
3. Cite other community resources that could be brought in to help Mr. Wong and his family. Keep in mind the cultural differences that may be involved and be aware of the need to preserve the self-image of each member of the family.

CHAPTER 10

Personal Safety:
Pharmacologic, Physical, Social

Carol Sue Holtz, RN, PhD

CHAPTER OUTLINE

OBJECTIVES

After completing this chapter, the reader should be able to:

1. Take a history of an older adult's current medications, including both prescription and over-the-counter drugs, analyze potential interactions, and recommend modifications if necessary.
2. Create a checklist for evaluating an older adult's risk (if any) while driving an automobile and indicate when reexamination for a license would be advisable.
3. Compare and contrast the types of restraints and the situations in which they may or may not be necessary.
4. Teach a classmate the signs of substance abuse and the nursing interventions related to them.
5. Assess an older adult for signs of physical or emotional abuse and suggest interventions for each of them.

KEY TERMS

chemical dependency
polypharmacy
recovery
substance abuse

Today's older adults are leading active lives that might astonish their grandparents. Adults in their 60, 70s, and even 80s are participating in sports competitions. A former president of the United States jumps from an airplane, fulfilling a dream held since the World War II. Travel brochures lure older adults to wander the globe, curiously soaking up experiences in faraway places. Whereas some people retire at the traditional age of 65, or earlier, many others continue to participate in the work force, in some cases starting their own business after being retired from corporate positions. Indeed, corporations are taking another look at traditional retirement practices, and the federal government is likely to raise the age of eligibility for Social Security to reflect the realities of an aging work force.

At the same time, as people age they become more vulnerable to physical risks than when they were younger. Moreover, although many older adults are in excellent physical and psychological health, others experience some changes that can pose a challenge to their safety. Physiological changes resulting from the aging process eventually affect everyone to some degree. Changes in vision, hearing, strength, and gait stability can cause older adults to be more accident prone (see Chapter 8). In addition, some older adults have to deal with changes arising from acute and chronic diseases that pose serious threats to their personal safety. There are a number of factors, sometimes associated with aging, that can reduce mobility and cognitive functioning:

- Multiple illnesses or disorders, particularly when accompanied by pain
- Polypharmacy, prescribed and/or over-the-counter (OTC) drugs
- Depression regarding changes in role function or loss of friends and loved ones
- Decreased financial resources, sometimes leading to poor nutrition or social isolation
- Disability

When problems of alcohol and drug abuse arise, they are often the result of the older person's struggle to cope with unwanted physical, psychological, and social changes. Education for health in the later years is a potent antidote for this kind of despair. Some older adults do experience alterations in their cognitive functioning and become unable to use sound judgment; they may be confused, forgetful, easily distracted, anxious, or agitated. This chapter takes a look at some of the issues that can cause potential or actual alterations in the physical or psychological safety of older people. The information provided can be used by nurses in a variety of settings to educate older clients so that they can participate in the full range of activities desired by most older adults.

W e l l n e s s

"Older adults concerned with wellness sometimes question medical prescriptions that seem to duplicate other medications already being taken."

MEDICATIONS

Adults older than 65 years of age comprise about 12% of the population, yet they consume over 30% of all prescription and 40% of all OTC medications. Some older adults may be taking as many as 5 to 10 different prescribed medications, with concomitant risks of adverse interactions; this situation is often referred to as **polypharmacy.** Some of this polypharmacy is due to the increased susceptibility of older adults to chronic and acute illnesses (Kelley, 1996), but it represents a danger that often goes unaddressed.

Another risk factor is that drug reactions can result from *normal* therapeutic dosages in older adults. This may be the result of age-related changes in the body's receptors to a medication and also changes in its absorption, distribution, metabolism, and excretion. Adverse drug reactions are two and one-half times greater in people older than 60 years of age. Drug-related hospitalizations are more common in older adults.

Incorrect self-administration of medications is another cause of drug reactions. Omission of medications, taking another person's prescription, misuse of OTC medications, and medication errors are common causes of drug-related problems in older adults (Stoehr, 1995).

Medications for older clients should be prescribed in light of the anatomical and physiological changes of aging, and with the increased awareness for potential toxicity or adverse reactions. The overall effects of a medication depend on the response of the body and the target organ sensitivity. Various anatomical and physiological changes that occur with normal aging can potentially affect absorption of medications. Decreases in secretion of hydrochloric acid, in the mucosal surface area of the small intestine, and in blood flow within the small intestine (approximately 40% less) contribute to decreased drug absorption in older adults. The distribution, metabolism, and clearance of a medication all change with advancing age.

The liver and the kidney are two organs through which most drugs are excreted. The period of time for excretion increases as blood flow to the liver, kidney function, and gastrointestinal motility decrease with age. See Table 10–1 for examples of commonly prescribed medications that can affect metabolism, excretion, liver and kidney function, and gastrointestinal motility.

Adverse drug reactions may cause confusion, nausea, loss of balance, a change in bowel patterns, or sedation. It is helpful if patients are first given low doses of medications when they have potential for a reaction. Health caregivers need to elicit information about all OTC medications being taken by their patients. Medication schedules should be made as simple as possible, with doses once or twice daily when feasible. All patients should learn about the benefits and side effects of their medications and the consequences of noncompliance (Chutka, Evans, Fleming, and Mikkelson, 1995).

The normal process of aging can render a person less tolerant of medications. Consider the following (Chutka, Evans, Fleming, and Mikkelson, 1995):

- The older body contains less total body fluid, which can result in higher blood levels of water-soluble medications.

TABLE 10–1. Possible Effects of Commonly Prescribed Medications

Reduced metabolism from decreased liver blood flow	Analgesics
	  Meperidine (Demerol)
	  Morphine
	Antidepressants (tricyclics)
	  Amitriptyline (Elavil)
	  Desipramine (Norpramin)
	  Nortriptyline (Aventyl)

Reduced elimination from decreased kidney function	ACE inhibitors
	  Captopril (Capoten)
	  Lisinopril (Zestril)
	Antiarrhythmics
	  Digoxin (Lanoxin)
	  Disopyramide (Norpace)
	  Procainamide (Pronestyl)
	Antihypertensives
	  Clonidine (Catapress)
	  Methyldopa (Aldomet)

Constipation from decreased gastrointestinal motility	Antacids
	  Aluminum compounds
	Anticholinergics
	  Atropine
	Antihistamines
	  Benadryl (Diphenhydramine)

- Increased adipose tissue can result in a greater accumulation of fat-soluble medications. Decreased secretions in the gastrointestinal tract can result in a slight reduction in drug absorption.
- Reduced liver size and liver metabolism can result in slower metabolism and a longer half-life of some medications.
- Reduced number of nephrons in the kidneys can result in slower glomerular filtration rate and creatinine clearance, which may lead to a slower elimination of some medications.
- Decreased albumin concentration may cause delayed distribution and higher concentration of some medications.
- Drier oral mucosa can cause difficulty in swallowing medications.
- Decreased muscle mass can cause difficulty in absorbing the usual adult intramuscular medication doses.
- Reduced circulation to the bowel and vagina can cause prolonged melting time for suppositories.

Self-administration of medications is a problem for many older adults. Poor eyesight may produce inability to differentiate various medication labels and containers and their direction labels, and the swallowing of tablets or capsules may be difficult with dry oral mucosa. Injectable medications may be difficult to administer because of reduction in muscle mass, especially in the extremities. Using suppositories may be a problem for those with poor vision, because of the need for unwrapping. If the person is arthritic, the dexterity needed for taking medications may be lacking. For older adults who are on limited budgets, costs of medications may be a major problem. The older adult may choose not to have the prescription filled, borrow leftover medications from others, use an older outdated supply, or stretch the prescription by skipping doses (Chutka, Evans, Fleming, and Mikkelson, 1995).

Poor vision can interfere with the reading of prescription labels, dosage instructions, and directions for opening containers. More than 3 million older adults are visually impaired, and 1 million are legally blind in both eyes. Many visually impaired elderly live alone, are responsible for taking their own medications on a specific schedule, and take a variety of medications for coexisting conditions. Poor compliance with medical regimens may be the result of decreased vision and impaired cognition that causes an inability to follow a complicated drug regimen. Nurses need to spend time with the client to talk about the proper way of taking medication and to determine whether the client can take medications as directed (Kelley, 1996).

Age-Related Changes in Adapting to Selected Medications

A general knowledge of age-related changes in adapting to medications is essential for nurses and other health care professionals. Here are some common pharmaceutical groupings and the changes generally experienced by older adults for whom they are prescribed (Chutka, Evans, Fleming, and Mikkelson, 1995):

1. *Anticoagulants.* Most data suggest that lower dosage is required for older adults.
2. *Antihypertensives.* Aging is associated with abnormal baroreceptor response to hypotension and reduction in peripheral venous tone, which can result in orthostatic hypotension in older adults who are not on medication; antihypertensive drug use increases this risk.
3. *Antibiotics.* Several antibiotics (e.g., the penicillins, vancomycin, the aminoglycosides) are excreted by the kidney, but most antibiotics have a large margin of safety and aging usually is not associated with significant changes.
4. *Diuretics.* As many as 45% of the hospitalized elderly use diuretics. Renal clearance is decreased with age, and problems can include dehydration, hypotension, and electrolyte imbalance (especially hypokalemia).
5. *Nonsteroidal antiinflammatory drugs (NSAIDs).* These medications, while useful, are associated with significant problems (e.g., bleeding, hepatic and renal toxicity) in older adults.
6. *Sedatives, antipsychotics, and antidepressives.* Aging is sometimes associated with a decline in intellectual responsiveness and percep-

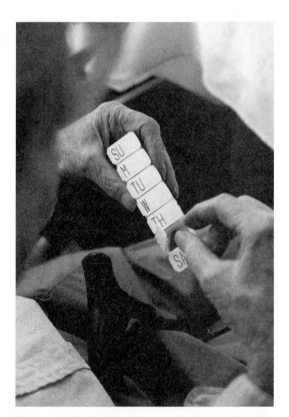

When an individual is taking a number of medications, using a compartmented dispenser can help with accurate compliance.

tion, as well as impaired learning ability and memory; thus, sedative hypnotic drugs may lead to adverse central nervous system reactions in older adults. Some older adults have a paradoxical agitation when taking barbiturates.

7. *Analgesics.* The rate of distribution of morphine and meperidine (Demerol) is slower in older adults; no significant changes occur with acetaminophen in aging clients.

Adverse Reactions

Special attention to adverse reactions or signs of toxicity is necessary when nurses are dealing with older adults. Adverse reactions include the following (Stolley et al., 1991):

- Slurred speech
- Change in mental functioning
- Change in gait
- Insomnia or drowsiness
- Visual changes
- Alterations in hearing (eighth cranial nerve damage)
- Seizures
- Tremors
- Irritability
- Dry mouth
- Constipation
- Blurred vision
- Urinary retention
- Headache
- Restlessness

Side effects to medications seen in the elderly may also include anorexia, confusion, indigestion, fatigue, or anxiety. Undernutrition, seen in a portion of the older adult population, may affect drug metabolism, action, and excretion.

It is important that nurses have the flexibility within physicians' orders to make judgments regarding when to administer medications pro re nata (p.r.n.), when to withhold medications, when to follow up when a client refuses an order, when to question the correctness of orders, and when to request new or modified orders.

Many elderly patients have problems with swallowing because of disease, cognitive impairment, dry mucous membranes, or poor positioning. Nurses can sometimes increase compliance by crushing tablets and mixing them with food or fluids; however, not all medica-

tions can be handled in that way. Medications may be administered in liquid rather than tablet form if swallowing is difficult. Good routine oral hygiene is also imperative (Matteson, McConnell, and Linton, 1997).

Digitalis toxicity is one of the most common medication reactions in the elderly. Common signs (Stolley et al., 1991) include:

- Gastrointestinal disturbances (nausea, vomiting, anorexia, diarrhea)
- Central nervous system malfunction (headache, weakness, apathy, visual disturbances)
- Cardiac problems (ventricular tachycardia, premature ventricular contractions, and bradycardia)

Tardive dyskinesia—a syndrome that includes hyperkinetic involuntary movements of the mouth, lips, and tongue—is a serious side effect of antipsychotic medications, especially in older adults. Drooling, chewing, sucking, or smacking of the lips may occur (Stolley et al., 1991).

Wellness

66*Because sensitivity to heat or cold gradually increases with age, many older adults grow accustomed to monitoring their own comfort levels.*99

EXCESSIVE HEAT OR COLD

Physiological as well as behavioral changes contribute to the increased vulnerability of older adults to excessive heat or cold. Physiological problems may include diminished sensory perception, impairment of thermoregulatory capacity, and reduced ability to judge the thermal environment accurately. In addition, prescription drugs can interfere with the body's ability to sustain temperature. Behavioral changes may include trying to save money on heating and electric bills by choosing not to turn on heating or air conditioning systems when needed. Some older adults live in housing that was constructed before modern insulation became available, and the lack of adequate insulation allows loss of hot or cool air through cracks and leaks (Macey and Schneider, 1993).

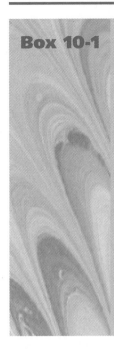

Box 10-1   FACTORS CONTRIBUTING TO INCREASED VULNERABILITY TO COLD

- Failure to sense cold
- Impaired shivering to generate heat
- Peripheral vascular constriction
- Medications
- Decreased activity
- Insufficient clothing
- Inadequate heating systems
- Unwillingness to use heat because of high cost
- Lack of subcutaneous fat
- Failure to respond behaviorally to protect oneself against cold
- Failure of metabolic rate to rise in response to cold
- Conditions that decrease heat production such as anemia, starvation, and hypothyroidism
- Conditions that increase heat loss such as burns or open wounds
- Conditions that impair thermoregulation such as tranquilizers, sedatives, antidepressants, vasoactive drugs, and alcohol

Data from Ebersole P, Hess P. (1998).Toward Healthy Aging. St. Louis: CV Mosby; and Worfolk J. (1997). Keep frail elders warm. Geriatr Nurs 18(1):7–11.

Hypothermia, or excessive cold, is described as a state of low body temperature in which the rectal temperature is 35°C (95°F) or below (Worfolk, 1997). Pathological causes of hypothermia in older adults include infections, cerebrovascular diseases, alcoholism, diabetes, or general confusion. Problems with cold temperature in older adults usually arise when indoor temperatures fall to between 50°F and 65°F (Box 10–1).

Excessive cold not only lowers body temperature, causing hypothermia, but also injures cells, causing frostbite. Frostbite, which results from exposure to extreme cold, occurs in body areas most frequently exposed, such as the nose, cheeks, ears, fingers, and toes (Ebersole and Hess, 1998; Worfolk, 1997). In a study by Macey and Schneider (1993) of 3326 older adults aged 60 years or older, data showed that older men were more likely to suffer death from excessive cold and older women were more likely to die of the effects of excessive heat. In addition, minority older adults and those living in nonurban areas were more likely to suffer death from temperature-related causes.

Hyperthermia, or excessive heat, is caused by the inability to rid the body of heat by radiation, convection, and sweat evaporation. Three types of reactions to heat may occur:

1. *Heat cramps*—severe pain in arms or legs as a result of the loss of sodium chloride in perspiration
2. *Heat exhaustion*—a vasomotor collapse, accompanied by faintness, weakness, and moist skin with a pale or ashen appearance
3. *Heat stroke (sunstroke)*—caused by failure of the perspiration-regulating mechanism during a prolonged exposure to heat and characterized by dry, hot, flushed skin, faintness, dizziness, fever, or unconsciousness (Ebersole and Hess, 1998; Worfolk, 1997). Intervention strategies for thermal changes in heat and cold are seen in Box 10–2.

DRIVING

"Driving is a complex activity that requires that individuals have a high level of physical and cognitive ability to avoid accidents and injury to themselves and others" (Elias et al., 1994). Carr (1993) asks, "When is it time for the older driver to hang up the car keys?" Clearly, many older adults are able to continue driving safely throughout their lifetime. In the United States, being able to drive is essential to both mobility and autonomy. Although other forms of transportation are available in some areas, the automobile still remains far and away the most

Box 10-2   INTERVENTION STRATEGIES FOR THERMAL CHANGE

Excessive Heat

1. Discourage heavy physical activity and provide more rest periods.
2. Teach wearing light-colored, lightweight cotton clothes to reduce sweating.
3. Encourage a diet high in carbohydrates and low in protein; increase fluids and salt.
4. Use air conditioners or fans (75°F is ideal for older adults).
5. Use community shelters, where available.
6. Watch for cessation of sweating, indicating a heat stroke.
7. Place a distressed client in recumbent position.
8. Transport client immediately to an emergency medical center if unconscious or displaying an excessive temperature.

Excessive Cold

1. Encourage physical activity.
2. Encourage client to wear warm clothing, including socks and cap at night.
3. Discourage alcohol consumption (it lowers body temperature by vasodilation).
4. Keep room between 68°F and 70°F.
5. Take temperature as needed. Older adults with rectal temperatures below 95°F need immediate attention.
6. Warm hands and feet and cover client with a warm blanket.
7. Encourage a warm tub bath, water temperature not exceeding 104°F to 108°F.
8. Give client warm liquids if conscious.

Data from Ebersole P, Hess P. (1998). Toward Healthy Aging. St. Louis: CV Mosby; Worfolk J. (1997). Keep frail elders warm. Geriatr Nurs 18(1):7–11.

desired method of transportation, and the automobile is the major source of transportation for people older than 65 years of age in the United States. Yet, older drivers may have special problems not found in younger people, including decreased motor skills and poor hearing and vision. In addition, older adults may be taking medications that impair perception and reaction to stimuli (Kelley, 1996). Older adults must deal with many losses, such as declining health and the loss of loved ones, and losing the ability to drive because of poor health will be perceived as yet another loss. So it is essential that testing of sensorimotor skills be done thoroughly and accurately before considering the withdrawal of a person's driving privileges.

A number of skills are necessary for a person to be a safe driver. First, adequate perception, which includes vision and hearing, is necessary. The person with corrected visual acuity less than 20/40 should see an ophthalmologist for further evaluation and treatment, including testing of visual fields. Hearing also needs to be evaluated, but hearing impairments do not generally represent as high a risk as visual problems. Other conditions that can impair driving ability include the following (Carr, 1993):

- Musculoskeletal deformities may restrict range of motion in the neck. Improvement for viewing the road can be enhanced by using pillows and wide-angled rear-view mirrors.
- Sensory neuropathy can impair use of foot controls.
- Cognitive disorders can seriously affect an older adult's driving skills. Problems such as syncope, seizures, dizziness, or hypoglycemic reactions are among the acute medical conditions that can affect safe driving.
- Any condition that could potentially result in an impairment in consciousness should be identified in evaluating the older adult's con-

tinuing ability to drive safely. State laws require that people with seizure disorders be seizure free for 6 to 12 months before resumption of driving.

- Chronic diseases such as dementia, stroke, and Parkinson's disease can impair driving ability. Impairments in joint function arising from arthritis should be evaluated for safe driving potential.
- Medications (e.g., antihistamines, ophthalmic medications, skeletal muscle relaxers, antihypertensives, antipsychotics, analgesics, barbiturates, hypnotics, and narcotics) can also impair safe driving.

Older drivers often drive slowly to compensate for declining sensorimotor skills, and they may fail to yield because of decreased attentiveness to road signs. It is often necessary for family members to assess whether an older relative remains a safe driver, but the recommendation that a person cease driving may carry more authority if it comes from a physician, nurse, or other health care worker. Some states require physicians to inform motor vehicle departments if a person has the potential for losing consciousness or is unable to safely manipulate an automobile because of physical, emotional, or cognitive reasons. Many states are now addressing the concern of reissuing a driver's license, especially for those older than 70 years of age (Carr, 1993).

Drivers older than age 60 have lower accident rates than those younger than 30, but accidents tend to increase after age 75. After age 85, older drivers have 4 times the number of accidents of those who are 50 to 59 and, when involved in accidents, are 15 times more likely to die as are drivers in their 40s (Rigdon, 1995).

Unfortunately, little effort has been made to develop a car that will help older adults to drive more safely. Research at General Motors Corporation reveals that vehicle designers face several barriers in designing a car to meet the needs of the aging driver. Car designers and engineers often lack knowledge about aging, are susceptible to negative stereotyping of older adults, and lack data from applied research to develop a car specifically adapted to meet their needs. The issue of withholding driving privileges from an older adult will continue to be a thorny one in the United States in view of society's dependence on the automobile (Carr, 1993).

FALLS

Educating older clients in prevention of falls is one of the most important areas of teaching for

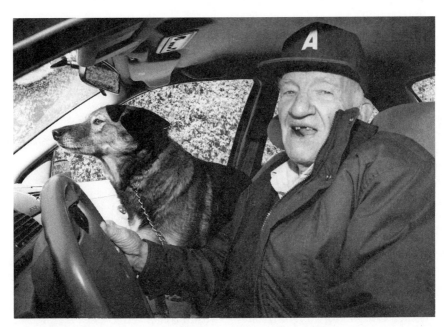

Although many older adults continue to be safe drivers, it is prudent for them to seek testing on a periodic basis.

this age group (see also Chapter 9). Multiple falls, with subsequent injuries, are more prevalent among those older than age 75 and are the second leading cause of accidental death in that age group. Home safety is of special concern because the majority of older adults live in their own home and spend more time there as they age (Watzke and Smith, 1994). A disproportionate number of older adults who report to hospital emergency departments have had accidents that involve (1) stairs and floor coverings, (2) beds, (3) bathtubs and showers, and (4) step stools or ladders. Bathtubs and step ladders were ranked by this group as the most problematic. Difficulties with cognitive processes such as perception, attention, risk taking, and use of sedatives play an important role in accidents of the elderly (Miller, 1995; Watzke and Smith, 1994).

Injuries resulting from falls may have serious consequences that require hospitalization and nursing home admission. Commodore (1995) states that 70% of all fall-related deaths in the United States occur in the oldest population group. Complications of falls include fractures, pneumonia, sepsis, dehydration, heart failure, and skin ulcers. Twenty-five percent of those older than 70, and 35% of those older than 80, fall annually; and 50% of those falls are repeated.

Fear of falling is a common problem that often results in self-imposed reductions in mobility and social interaction. After a fall, families of the older adult often become overprotective and tend to restrict the person's autonomy. Older adults who experience falls are often characterized by poor health and have greater difficulty with activities of daily living (Commodore, 1995; Miller, 1995). Factors in the environment that contribute to falls include

- Slippery floors and bathtubs
- Lack of grab bars
- Low toilet seats
- High beds

Health issues related to falls can include

- Hypotension
- A history of falls
- Dizziness
- Dysrhythmias
- Pain
- Alcohol use

Ross (1991) and Commodore (1995) state that a fall frequently initiates a deterioration in

health. Conversely, a deterioration in health may result in a fall. Dementias, poorly controlled diabetes, and strokes may alter an older person's judgment. Side effects and interactions from medications may also contribute to the risk of falls. Whatever the precipitating factor, close observation by the nurse after a fall is necessary to monitor for untoward developments in an older adult client. Many falls result from poor judgment—of the client, the family, the nursing staff, or others. Also a significant number of falls occur during elimination. For many older adults, the desire to remain continent is a stimulus that gets them out of bed, but they may need assistance. Nurses need to teach and reinforce safety practices.

Observation of the older adult who is under medication is essential if safety is to be maintained. Older clients metabolize medications more slowly than younger clients, and a normal dose may result in impaired abilities. Alcohol consumption increases the risk of falls. Many medications cause hypotension, which can lead to a fall. These medications include

- Ganglion blockers
- Sympatholytics
- Methyldopa
- Oral diuretics
- Phenothiazines
- Antihistamines
- Tricyclic antidepressants
- Diazepam
- Barbiturates
- Anticholinergics
- Digoxin

Blood pressures should be taken in reclining, sitting, and standing positions at prescribed intervals until assessment can determine that the patient is out of danger of orthostatic hypotension.

Nursing Interventions

Ross (1991) and Miller (1995) state that nurses must identify which patients are at risk for falls. Nursing interventions for preventing falls in the older adult inpatient population include performing an admission assessment, repeated every 8 hours, for cognitive, sensory, and motor function. If the patient demonstrates no deficits in cognition, sensation, or mobility, the health caregiver can ensure that the call bell is within reach, the bed is lowered, and the wheels of the bed and wheelchair are locked as appropriate. If problems are noted during assessment, the nurse needs to alert all caregivers to the potential for falling, put special identification bands on the patient and above the bed, and offer assistance for all toileting and transfers. All falls should be reported and documented in a progress note on the medical records, and special incident reports should be completed (Brady et al., 1993). Commodore (1995) suggests that nurses teach clients and their families to identify risks, to assess the environment, and to make necessary adjustments and adaptations for decreasing accident risks.

RESTRAINTS

The increase in injuries from falls related to restraints has led health care providers to reevaluate the use of restraints, and a movement toward untying the elderly is growing in the United States (see Chapter 4). After the passage of the Omnibus Reconciliation Act of 1987, the Joint Commission on Accreditation of Hospitals provided guidelines restricting the use of physical restraints.

The use of restraints, however, is still common. Eighteen to 22 percent of hospitalized patients 65 and older are restrained. Patients who are confused, who use poor judgment, or who exhibit behavioral problems are those most likely to be restrained. Physical restraints have been defended on the ground that they protect the patient from harm, especially from falling. Yet the use of restraints involves numerous risks, direct or indirect. Such risks include hyperthermia, new-onset bladder and bowel incontinence, new pressure ulcers, increased nosocomial infections, severe nerve injuries, joint contractures, and even death by strangulation (Mion and Strumpf, 1994).

Use of restraints has become a moral dilemma because every patient's need for autonomy and dignity must be weighed against the older adult's increased risk of falls with subsequent injuries. Nurses can use the following measures as alternatives to restraints (Bryant and Fernald, 1997; Commodore, 1995):

- Alarm systems with ankle or wrist bracelets
- Bed or wheelchair alarms
- More personnel for observation
- Locked doors
- Creative furniture arrangements
- Education for the patient and family
- Lower beds

- Fall management programs
- Adaptive equipment such as grab bars, hand rails, side rails, and bath chairs and rails

Patients unable to maintain a sitting posture because of poor trunk muscle strength are sometimes restrained in a chair, but other alternatives can be used. A reclining chair with a modified leg lift maintains the patient's center of gravity in the chair. With the help of adaptive cushions, an upright position can be maintained without restraints (Mion and Strumpf, 1994).

Caring

"Side rails and restraints are used only at the request of the patient or when all other interventions for safety have been exhausted."

According to Cruz, Abdul-Hamid, and Heater (1997), all nursing units should provide a restraint resources manual containing the following:

- A letter from an authoritative person encouraging a change
- A handout on risks/benefits of restraints
- A hospital restraint policy and related procedures
- A completed sample of documentation form
- A quality improvement monitor
- A review of problem behaviors with alternatives and expected outcomes
- A list of case studies with solutions
- A manufacturer's handout on restraint products
- A reference list and selected articles
- A patient care plan

If a client needs restraints, the following must be charted (Aiken, 1995):

1. Alternatives used before restraints
2. Reason for restraint (describe client behavior and type of restraint used)
3. Verbal or written orders for restraint
4. Time and date when restraint was applied
5. Times when restraint was monitored
6. Client response to restraint
7. Hospital policy and procedure regarding how often a client must be checked and released from restraints

8. Care given when client is released from re-straints
9. Assessment for
   - Skin integrity
   - Circulation
   - Respiratory status
   - Client's verbal response

C a r i n g

"*The nurse needs to alert all caregivers to the potential for falling, put special identification bands on the patient and above the bed, and offer assistance for all toileting and transfers.***"**

SIDE RAILS

A side rail is a restraint when it restricts freedom of movement by preventing a client from getting out of bed regardless of whether the client is able to do so safely. A physician's order is necessary when side rails are used to restrict freedom of movement, but a side rail is not a restraint when clients choose to use them, such as in helping to get up, turn in bed, or prevent falls. If clients cannot make their preferences known, then family should be consulted. Clients can be considered low risk if side rails are not necessary but are used because of the person's preference. A moderate-risk client may be one who has the desire to get out of bed unassisted but lacks the ability to do so safely. Because this client needs either side rails or an alternate safety protection, the side rails are considered a restraint and need a physician's order. The high-risk client is one who needs side rails to restrict movement because there are no alternatives, the alternatives have failed, or the benefits of side rail use outweigh the disadvantages. When the nurse is considering a change in side rail use, the client's risk when getting into and out of bed must be assessed. If a decision by client and/or family members to lower side rails is made, a gradual process can be initiated (Donius and Rader, 1994; Miller, 1995).

In April 1992 the Health Care Financing Administration identified side rails as restraints in some situations and requested that long-term facilities address the issue. Side rails need careful consideration because they may have negative consequences, such as the following (Donius and Rader, 1994; Miller, 1995):

- Increasing the distance of falls from the bed
- Obstructing vision
- Separating the care receiver from the caregiver
- Creating noise
- Causing trauma if the client strikes the side rails or becomes entangled in them
- Dislodging tubes when raising or lowering them
- Creating a sense of being trapped

Whedon and Shedd (1989) reviewed 35 non–research- and research-based articles addressing prediction and prevention of patient falls. They state that when a nurse needs to use interventions, it is not possible or appropriate to choose all of the interventions. Box 10–3 presents Whedon and Shedd's list of possible interventions. Box 10–4 is a guide to the physical assessment of older adults who may be at risk for falls.

▪ SUBSTANCE ABUSE

The *Diagnostic and Statistical Manual of Mental Disorders* (American Psychiatric Association, 1994) defines **substance abuse** as continued use despite persistent or recurrent social, occupational, psychological, or physical problems (American Psychiatric Association, 1994).

Alcohol Abuse

For older adults, alcoholism can be related to "(a) loss of control over the timing and amount consumed, (b) development of tolerance, and (c) interference with the completion of occupational and social obligations" (Mackel, Sheehy, and Badger, 1994). Alcohol abuse is a significant problem in older adults, occurring in 18% to 20% of older adult patients in general hospitals, 28% in psychiatric hospitals, and up to 40% in nursing homes. Although liver

Box 10-3 NURSING INTERVENTIONS FOR FALLS

Assessment and Planning

- Assess patients to identify risk for falls.
- Develop a standardized nursing care plan or individualize nursing care plans for patients at risk for falling.
- Assess effects of medications that would place patients at risk for falling.
- Identify high-risk patients with colored tags (on armband, Kardex, medical record, above bed, on call bell, and on patient's door).
- Reassess risk levels at certain time intervals after admission.
- Identify risk factors on nursing care plan and during change-of-shift report.
- Reevaluate the nursing care plan after a fall.

Interventions

- Ensure that patients wear properly fitting shoes or slippers with nonskid soles and avoid loose, trailing clothing, and ensure that tubes and drains do not interfere with safe ambulation of the patient.
- Toilet patient before administering sedation and/or give bedpan or urinal every 4 hours.
- Place disoriented patients in rooms near the nurse's station and keep confused and high-risk patients sitting up during the day near the nurse's station or where they can be watched.
- Maintain close supervision of confused patients and/or encourage use of family members/sitters to stay with them.
- Increase frequency of rounds and plan them to meet patient's needs, not nurse's needs.
- Deal with confused, agitated patients with reality therapy, behavior modification, and TLC.
- Reassess staffing patterns during high-risk time of the day.
- Never cluster all staff members together at report.
- Clean eyeglasses of patients regularly.
- Restrict use of flurazepam (Dalmane); use chloral hydrate (fewer side effects).
- Keep bed in low position except when giving care.
- Keep call light, water, urinal, bedpan, and tissues within easy reach of patient; place items at appropriate side of bed.
- Arrange furniture and objects so that they are not obstacles.
- Use dim light at night.
- Raise side rails of beds and stretchers.
- Lock wheels on bed, wheelchairs, stretchers, and commodes.
- Wipe up all foods and fluids from the floor immediately; post large visible signs of wet floor; do not polish floor.
- Place hold bars in bathrooms and hallways.
- Install nonskid surfaces on floor of bathrooms.
- Use shower chairs.
- Use half side rails to prevent climbing over rails.
- Be alert for equipment needing maintenance (carpet, floor, lights).
- Raise height of seats.
- Use audiovisual monitoring to observe restless patients.
- Check tips of canes, walkers, crutches for presence of nonskid covers.
- Close doors to reduce noise.
- Keep intercom open from patient's room to nurse's station.
- Use floor-level lighting.
- Develop "safe" furniture for patients.

Continued

Box 10-3 NURSING INTERVENTIONS FOR FALLS *(Continued)*

Patient Education

- Teach patients safe use of hospital equipment (wheelchairs, crutches, walkers).
- Identify patients with orthostatic hypotension risks and teach them to rise slowly from a lying or sitting position, to dangle feet before walking, and to perform ankle pumping in a sitting position before walking.
- Inform patients and families of high-risk-for-fall status.
- Familiarize patients with surroundings after admission.
- Encourage physical fitness, muscle building, and movement therapy.
- Caution patients against bending the head sharply backward.
- Instruct patients to lean only on heavy, stable objects.
- Instruct patients with sensory or motor deficits to call before going to the bathroom or ambulating.
- Instruct patients not to turn on their heel.
- Reinterview/instruct patient after fall.
- Instruct patient to void at bedtime and regularly during waking hours.
- Instruct patient not to wear loose shoes.
- Caution patients to open doors and go around corners slowly.
- Never expect a patient with memory problems to remember; always repeat information.
- Present safety education classes.

Staff Education

- Present fall-prevention workshops or inservices (include information on physical changes with aging and medicines with side effects that may cause falling).
- Instruct physicians on appropriate patient activity orders.

Adapted from Whedon M, Shedd P. (1989). Prediction and prevention of patient falls. Image 21(2):108–114.

metabolism of alcohol does not decrease with age, liver size and blood flow decrease by 30%. The central nervous system of the older adult is more sensitive to the sedative effects of alcohol, especially in those with preexisting brain disease such as dementia or cerebrovascular disease. The older adult may attempt to self-treat through alcohol such conditions as self-neglect, contusions, malnutrition, depression, falls, urinary incontinence, diarrhea, and a general "failure to thrive" problem. In addition, the lifestyle of some elderly people fosters drinking because they live alone, are retired, and may become lonely and depressed (Egbert, 1993; Hoffman, 1995).

Alcoholism has many adverse affects on the elderly, causing problems such as liver disease,

cerebellar degeneration, peripheral neuropathy, peptic ulcers, gastritis, and drug reactions. Cognitive functioning decreases with alcohol-related brain injuries. Alcoholic dementia is a specific, irreversible dementia associated with alcoholism that is identified in the older adult population. Detoxification in older adults may necessitate hospitalization and take a week or more. Therapy includes use of thiamine, multiple vitamins, and fluids and, if needed, lor-azepam (Ativan) or oxazepam (Serax), the drugs of choice (Egbert, 1993; Hoffman, 1995).

Diagnosis of alcoholism in older adults is more difficult than in others because older adults have physiologic changes in the metabolism of alcohol as well as many nonspecific

Box 10-4 PHYSICAL ASSESSMENT OF THE ELDERLY AND NURSING INTERVENTIONS FOR PREVENTION OF FALLS

Sensory Changes

Vision
- Use proper corrective eyeglasses that are cleaned regularly.
- Treat cataracts, glaucoma, or macular degeneration.

Hearing
- Use hearing aids.
- Remove impacted cerumen.

Touch
- Teach client awareness to lack of sensitivity (protection of hands and feet in hot or cold environment).

Cardiovascular Changes
- Treat cardiac dysrhythmias and blood pressure and orthostatic changes.

Musculoskeletal Changes

Mobility
- Teach exercises to improve muscle tone, strength, endurance, and flexibility.

Gait
Balance

Neurological Changes

Tremors
- Give medical treatment if appropriate.

Gait
Balance

Urological Changes

Incontinence
- Arrange toileting schedules.

Use of Diuretics
- Maintain nutrition and fluids.

Benign Prostatic Hypertrophy
- Watch diuretic medication schedule.

Foot Disorders/Deformities
- Remove bunions, calluses.
- Wear well-fitting shoes (low heeled and nonskid).

Nutritional Changes

Anemia
Malnutrition
Fluid and Electrolyte Imbalance
- Maintain proper fluid and electrolyte balance.

Continued

Box 10-4   PHYSICAL ASSESSMENT OF THE ELDERLY AND NURSING
INTERVENTIONS FOR PREVENTION OF FALLS (Continued)

Acute Illness
- Treat infections.
- Monitor mental status changes.

Psychosocial Changes
- Monitor and treat (if appropriate):
  Confusion
  Depression
  Anxiety
  Agitation
  Fear of falling

Drug Use
- Monitor number of over-the-counter drugs.
- Monitor alcohol use.
- Observe for interactions and side effects, such as orthostatic hypotension, dizziness, or change in mental status.

Environmental
- Inspect or discuss home health hazards inside and outside the home.

Fall History
- Record events leading up to fall(s), following fall(s), injuries from fall(s).

Adapted from Miller J. (1995). Falling and the elderly. In Stanley M, Beare P, eds. Gerontological Nursing. Philadelphia: FA Davis.

signs or symptoms. The amount of alcohol consumed is a particularly unreliable measure in older adults because the quantity consumed may be no more than what was tolerated with no problems at a younger age. Ingested alcohol becomes part of the total body fluids and, because of the decreased body fluids of older adults, creates a greater overall concentration of alcohol than a younger person would have with the same amount of alcohol ingestion (Egbert, 1993). Alcohol and drug interactions are a serious potential problem in the older person. Alcohol enhances acetaminophen toxicity, even with normal doses—an effect potentiated by the age-related decrease in acetaminophen clearance. Aging also enhances the central nervous system effects of opiates, and alcohol consumption acutely decreases opiate clearance, compounding opiate toxicity (Egbert, 1993; Hoffman, 1995).

Alcoholism may be related to organic brain syndrome and cause symptoms such as confusion, short-term memory loss, and decreased verbal ability. With 3 to 4 weeks of abstinence, these problems can disappear. Alcoholic dementia, discussed earlier, is a severe and irreversible problem. Symptoms include short- and long-term memory deficits, aphasia, and apraxia (Egbert, 1993; Hoffman, 1995).

A chemical abuse program for older adults is described by Lindblom and associates (1992). The Elders Health Program was initiated by the departments of social work and geriatric medicine at an urban general hospital as a project to address the chemical dependency needs of the elderly. The identification phase consisted of (1) questionnaires such as the CAGE and the Manitoba Drug Screening Dependency Screen, (2) a physician assessment, and (3) a social assessment. The intervention was "a systematic approach involving a social network of chemically dependent elderly people to encourage change" (Lindblom et al., 1992). The older adults worked on recognizing the dependency, identifying the negative consequences and complications, and observing enabling and co-dependency behaviors. Some of the assessment criteria for chemical dependency included signs such as drowsiness, withdrawal, isolation, poor appetite, falls, and changes in daily habits; history of misuse or abuse of drugs; and a medical or drinking history. The authors believe that ageism has prevented the development of treatment programs for chemical dependency designed for older adults and, in their study, have attempted to show that older adults have a network that can be used to help clients accept the need to change.

NURSING IMPLICATIONS

Alcoholism in older adults increases the chances of falls and other accidents, causing problems especially for those who live alone. Nutritional deficiencies, which result from lack of good eating habits or changes in food absorption and metabolism, contribute to a poor nutritional status for older adult drinkers. Alcohol can compromise the immune system, causing higher vulnerability for infections, and can cause problems with the ability to sleep well. In addition, alcoholism can enhance cardiovascular and gastrointestinal problems (Mackel, Sheehy, and Badger, 1994).

A complete assessment of the older client is necessary to detect alcohol abuse. This assessment should include a history of falls and other accidents, the presence of acute-onset dementia, nutritional deficiencies, and any

Wellness

"Increased public awareness of substance abuse can lead older adults to consult health care professionals about their appropriate levels of alcohol or medication."

change in the social situation. The patient may self-report alcohol use. A depression and nutritional screening and a complete physical evaluation including a complete blood cell count and laboratory evaluation of aspartate aminotransferase, alanine aminotransferase, serum albumin, uric acid, high-density lipoprotein, transferrin, ferritin, and blood alcohol levels is part of an alcohol-abuse protocol workup (Mackel, Sheehy, and Badger, 1994). After detection or confirmation of alcohol problems the patient will need treatment, which can include hospitalization. Cessation of drinking, treatment of withdrawal, and rehabilitation are necessary. Good nutrition, fluids, and vitamins, especially thiamine, are included (Mackel, Sheehy, and Badger, 1994). Box 10–5 lists the warning signs of alcohol abuse.

Chemical Abuse

Chemical dependency is a prolonged habitual reliance on a substance that has a negative im-

---

Box 10-5 RECOGNIZING WARNING SIGNS OF ALCOHOL ABUSE

1. Increasing intolerance of the effects of alcohol (the person needs to drink more and more to obtain and maintain the desired effect).
2. Irresponsibility, such as missed appointments or broken promises.
3. Inattention to personal grooming.
4. Poor judgment.
5. Frequent falls, bruises or fractures, for which the person seeks no treatment.
6. Recurrent blackouts accompanied by temporary memory loss.
7. Hidden alcohol supply at home, workplace or car.
8. Hand tremor when sober.
9. Unexplained weight loss.
10. Insomnia.
11. Facial puffiness.

Bartlett J. (1995). Living Longer and Better with Health Problems. Springhouse, PA: Springhouse.

pact on physical health and may also mask symptoms of other serious diseases. Chemical dependency has the potential to cause a variety of other problems, including withdrawal from family and friends, development of depression, and anxiety or sleep disturbances. The term *dependency* can also connote the ongoing use of substances beyond their efficient, beneficial effect or in spite of significant negative consequences or side effects. Recovery from chemical dependency can occur only when chemical use is discontinued and recovery begins. **Recovery** is an active developmental process with predictable stages (Barnea and Teichman, 1994).

Substance abuse in older adults is a hidden problem in the United States. In this country only 2% of those older than age 50 use marijuana, compared with 56% of young people, and less that 4% of patients older than 60 are treated for addiction to opiates. Few older adults intentionally abuse illegal drugs; drug use is usually associated with various developmental pressures characteristic of young people. Because these pressures are moderated in adulthood, substance abusers either die early or grow out of their addictive behaviors. Some older adults who were addicted in youth continue to use drugs into old age. It is possible that in the coming decades there will be an increase in the extent of drug use among older adults because of the rise in life expectancy, the increase and extent of use in the general population, and the increase in the number of middle-age applicants for drug treatment, particularly methadone maintenance (Barnea and Teichman, 1994).

W e l l n e s s

66*Older adults participate in Neighborhood Watch and other programs that are designed to protect people both in their homes and on the streets.*99

The most significant factor in substance abuse among older adults is the older person's lack of knowledge (or erroneous information) regarding the appropriate use of a medication and its possible adverse effects. Factors relating to biological aging (e.g., impairment of memory, decline in vision or hearing, heightened sensitivity to chemical substances) affect both dosages and side effects. In addition, older adults face age-related problems that must be handled. These include loss of social status as a result of retirement, loneliness and social isolation as a result of the death of spouse or close friends, decline in self-image and self-esteem, and rise in anxiety and depression. The use of psychoactive substances can become one of the means of coping with these problems. Older men tend to misuse all psychoactive substances, except for psychotropic drugs, more than women do. Many older adults become drug dependent easily. Sleeping pills and antidepressants can interact with each other, producing further complications. Because of the high toxic potential of psychoactive substances, they can be used for suicide. Barbiturates are the most prevalent means of suicide among the aged (Barnea and Teichman, 1994).

■ CRIME

Crime is of particular concern to many older people. Special programs that provide safety information, escort services, or victim counseling have been established in many communities. It is important that nurses working in the community be aware of crime issues and be prepared to help their clients cope with them. Federal programs, through the Law Enforcement Assistance Administration, assist elderly crime victims. The Office of Community Victim Assistance Programs offers crime prevention advice and victim assistance (Watson, 1991).

Criminal victimization of older adults is common, and research indicates that rates are even higher than reported, especially among poor and minority older adults. In contrast, middle- and upper-middle-class older adults from the dominant population tend to trust police and believe that police will offer assistance. Factors associated with underreporting include minority group membership, low socioeconomic status, belief that law-enforcement officers will do nothing, fear of reprisal, and shame. Robbery and purse snatching in public places are the leading offenses against minority older adults. Young unemployed males 15 to 24 years of age are among the most frequent perpetrators of crime against older adults. Older people are also disproportionately represented among the victims of homicide and suicide within the home (Watson, 1991).

The incidence of poverty among African

Americans and Hispanic Americans has been higher than for those of the dominant culture and, as a consequence, older members of these subcultures have fewer choices of residence. Living in low-income areas that are home to large numbers of school dropouts and unemployed people increases many older adults' chances of becoming the targets of crime. Many older adults go shopping without an escort and are at risk of robbery and assault, particularly at night. Self-defense, or an attempt to escape from a violent act, is normal behavior for most adults, but older people, sometimes with diminished cognitive and motor abilities, may be unable to flee or repel an assailant.

Aside from actual victimization, many older adults have a continual fear of crime. Such fear in people older than age 70 may lead to a self-imposed house arrest, because they believe that poor police protection makes going out even in daylight a risky undertaking. Unfortunately, self-confinement is not foolproof and will not necessarily safeguard older adults from an invasion of the home, nor from victimization by a caregiver. Elder abuse occurs most frequently within the home by a family member or nonfamily caregiver (Watson, 1991).

Some suggestions for decreasing crime perpetrated on the elderly are as follows (adapted from Ebersole and Hess, 1998). In public:

1. Organize a buddy system. (Neighbors watch out for each other, and go out in pairs or groups to the laundry, grocery, and shopping areas.)
2. Avoid wearing fancy clothes or jewelry in public.
3. Go out in daylight, especially if you must go alone.
4. Carry a cane or umbrella as a defensive weapon.
5. Wear a small police whistle around your neck.
6. Never carry large amounts of money with you.
7. Use a "fanny pack" or money belt under clothes when carrying valuables, rather than a purse or wallet.
8. Don't attach an identification tag to a key.
9. Get a trained dog and take it along when going for walks.

At home:

1. Get deadbolt locks and a door peephole.
2. Don't open the door for a stranger. Ask for identification before admitting anyone.
3. Never tell anyone that you're alone.
4. Lock all windows.
5. Keep all valuables in the bank safety deposit box, with a minimum in the home.
6. Don't give any information to strangers on the telephone.
7. Keep a loud-barking dog in the house.
8. Never send or give money to strangers from unknown organizations/charities.

Caring

66*Caring nurses are always alert to signs of physical or emotional abuse as they assess new and ongoing clients.***99**

ELDER ABUSE

Elder abuse and neglect are serious underreported and underdetected phenomena in the United States that affect thousands of older adults every year. About 1 million people older than age 65 experience some form of abuse or neglect. Reporting laws vary from state to state, yet most laws reflect one or more of the following categories:

- Physical abuse
- Neglect
- Exploitation
- Abandonment
- Psychological abuse

Physical abuse is defined as the act of battery or assault. *Neglect* is defined as unreasonable withholding of some goods or services necessary for physical or mental health. *Exploitation* denoted taking advantage of a person for personal or financial benefits. *Abandonment* is the desertion or withdrawal of care with no provision for alternate care. *Psychological abuse* refers to unreasonable verbal abuse or hostile behavior.

The possible causes of abuse of older adults include the following:

- Degree of dependency overwhelms the caregiver to the extent that hostile and aggressive behavior emerges
- Neglect that may occur when an older caregiver can no longer keep up with the dependency needs of the client
- Psychopathology of the abuser, who may be

mentally ill, on drugs, intoxicated, or mentally retarded and cannot control behavior
- Family violence—stressed caregiver

> ## Caring
>
> **"*The nurse must assess, evaluate, and sometimes intervene to change the environment of older adults to provide the safest possible situation.*"**

Clinical Manifestations

Nurses and other caregivers must be alert to the clinical manifestations of abuse. In some states they are required to report such signs to the authorities. Clinical manifestations of abuse include the following:

1. Unexplained bruises and welts on face, lips, mouth, torso, back, buttocks, or thighs, in various stages of healing, clustered forming regular patterns, reflecting the shape of the article used to inflict, and regular absence such as on weekends or vacation
2. Unexplained burns
   - Especially on soles, palms, back, or buttocks
   - Immersion burn (socklike or glovelike, doughnut-shaped); burns on buttocks or genitalia
   - Patterned like electric burner or iron
   - Rope burns on arms, neck, or torso
3. Unexplained fractures in various stages of healing
4. Unexplained lacerations or abrasions to mouth, lips, gums, eyes, or genitalia

The following are some manifestations of physical neglect:

- Constant hunger
- Poor hygiene
- Inappropriate dress
- Lack of supervision especially in dangerous activities or long periods of time
- Consistent fatigue or listlessness
- Unattended physical problems
- Abandonment

Manifestations of sexual abuse include the following:

- Difficulty in walking or sitting

- Torn, stained, or bloody underwear
- Bruises, pain, or itching in the genital area

Emotional maltreatment may be indicated by the following:

- Habit disorder (sucking, biting, rocking)
- Conduct disorder (antisocial, destructive)
- Neurotic traits (sleep or speech disorders)
- Neurotic reactions (hysteria, obsession, compulsion, phobias, hypochondria)

Nursing Interventions

Nursing interventions when abuse is suspected or identified can include (Fulmer, 1995; Hansen, 1996)

- Detect as soon as possible.
- Contact social service agencies, hospital emergency department, or police department.
- Assess in an emergency department of a hospital.
- Ask questions tactfully.
- Educate staff and community to be aware of elder abuse.
- Develop new ways to assist caregivers to cope with stress and physical exhaustion of caregivers.
- Provide physical treatment of wounds.
- Suggest change in living arrangements.
- Reestablish trust.

Summary

This chapter addresses the safety issues of the elderly. Because of the physiological and psychological changes that come with age, problems such as crime, accidents, driving, falls, intolerance to excessive heat or cold, difficulties with medications, and elder abuse are common safety issues for the older adult population.

Society often does not want to believe that older adults, just like the young or middle-aged, may have problems with alcohol or drugs that need to be identified and treated. Problems with alcohol and drug abuse are frequently unexplored by health care professionals, yet they are important concerns for the clients and their families.

To provide the safest possible situation for the clients, nurses must assess, evaluate, and sometimes intervene to change the environment of older adults, whether they reside in the community or in a long-term facility. Personal safety is not only an individual but also a societal concern that is reflected in the various laws, both state and federal, that relate to it.

RESOURCES

Alcoholics Anonymous World Services
475 Riverside Drive
New York, NY 10163
(212) 870-3400

Al-Anon
P.O. Box 862, Midtown Station
New York, NY 10018
(800) 356-9996

American Association of Retired Persons
Domestic Maltreatment of the Elderly: Toward Prevention—Some Do's and Don't's. (1990). Washington, DC: AARP

National Council on Alcoholism and Drug Dependence
12 W. 21st Street
New York, NY 10010
(800) NCA-CALL

National Safety Council
444 North Michigan Avenue
Chicago, IL 60611
(800) 621-7619 ext 6900

National Center on Elder Abuse
810 First St. N.E., Suite 500
Washington, DC 20002-4267
(202) 682-2470; Fax (201) 289-6555

NCEA assists interested organizations and individuals in their efforts against elder abuse, neglect, and exploitation by conducting training workshops, producing newsletters, operating an informational clearinghouse, engaging in research, and developing and disseminating technical reports of national value.

Adult Protective Services
In most jurisdictions, adult protective services, the area agency on aging, or the county department of social services is designated as the agency to receive and investigate allegations of elder abuse and neglect. If the investigators find abuse or neglect, they make arrangements for services to help protect the victim.

National and State Information
Often people who want to help older relatives or friends do not live near them. Long-distance caregivers can call a nationwide toll-free eldercare locator number (1-800-677-1116) to locate services in the community in which the older adult lives. In addition, some states have established a statewide toll-free number to provide centralized aging services information for residents of their state.

State Elder Abuse Hotlines
Many states have instituted a 24-hour toll-free number for receiving reports of abuse. Calls are confidential.

Local Enforcement
Local police, sheriff's offices, and prosecuting attorneys may investigate and prosecute abuse. In states whose statutes make elder abuse a crime, there may be a requirement to report suspected abuse to a law enforcement agency.

REFERENCES

Aiken T. (1995) Legal issues affecting the elderly. In Stanley M, Beare P, eds. Gerontological Nursing. Philadelphia: FA Davis.

American Psychiatric Association. (1994). Diagnostic and Statistical Manual of Mental Disorders. 4th ed. Washington, DC: American Psychiatric Association.

Barnea Z, Teichman M. (1994). Substance misuse and abuse among the elderly: Implications for social work intervention. J Gerontol Soc Work 21(3/4):133–148.

Bartlett J. (1995). Living Longer and Better with Health Problems. Springhouse, PA: Springhouse.

Brady R, Chester F, Pierce L, et al. (1993). Geriatric falls: Prevention strategies for the staff. J Gerontol Nurs 19(9):26–32.

Bryant H, Fernald L. (1997). Nursing knowledge and use of restraint alternatives: Acute and chronic care. Geriatr Nurs 18(2):57–60.

Carr D. (1993). Assessing older drivers for physical and cognitive impairment. Geriatrics 48(5):46–51.

Chutka S, Evans J, Fleming K, Mikkelson K. (1995). Drug prescribing for elderly patients. Mayo Clin Proc 70:685–693.

Commodore D. (1995). Falls in the elderly population: A look at incidence, risks, healthcare costs, and preventive strategies. Rehabil Nurs 20(2):84–89.

Cruz V, Abdul-Hamid M, Heater B. (1997). Reducing restraints in an acute care setting: Phase I. J Gerontol Nurs 23(2):31–40.

Donius M, Rader J. (1994). Use of side rails: Rethinking a standard of practice. J Gerontol Nurs 20(11):23–27.

Ebersole P, Hess P. (1998). Toward Healthy Aging. St. Louis: CV Mosby.

Egbert A. (1993). The older alcoholic: Recognizing the subtle clinical clues. Geriatrics 48(7):63–69.

Elias J, Winn F, Elias M. (1994). Introduction: The aging driver phenomenon. Aging Res 20:1–2.

Fulmer T. (1996) Elderly maltreatment. In Stanley M, Beare P, eds. Gerontological Nursing. Philadelphia: FA Davis.

Hansen C. (1996). Instant Nursing Assessment: Gerontologic. Albany, NY: Delmar.

Hoffman A. (1995). Alcoholic problems in elder persons. In Stanley M, Beare P, eds. Gerontological Nursing. Philadelphia: FA Davis.

Kelley M. (1996). Medications and the visually impaired elderly. Geriatr Nurs 17(2):60–62.

Lindblom L, Kostyk D, Tabisz E, et al: (1992). Chemical abuse in the elderly: An intervention program for the elderly. J Gerontol Nurs 18(4):6–14.

Macey S, Schneider D. (1993). Deaths from excessive heat and excessive cold among the elderly. Gerontologist 33(4):497–499.

Mackel C, Sheehy, Badger T. (1994). The challenge of detection and management of alcohol abuse among elders. Clin Nurse Specialist 8(3):128–135.

Matteson MA, McConnell ES, Linton, AD. 1997. Gerontological Nursing. 2nd ed. Philadelphia, WB Saunders.

Miller J. (1995). Falling and the elderly. In Stanley M, Beare P, eds. Gerontological Nursing. Philadelphia: FA Davis.

Mion L, Strumpf N. (1994). Use of physical restraints in the hospital setting: Implications for the nurse. Geriatric Nursing 15(3):127–131.

Rigdon J. (1995, October 29). Older drivers pose growing risks on roads. The Wall Street Journal, pp A1, A8.

Ross J. (1991). Iatrogenesis in the elderly. Contributors to falls. J Gerontol Nurs 17(9):19–23.

Stoehr G. (1995). Pharmacology and the elderly. In Stanley M, Beare P, eds. Gerontological Nursing. Philadelphia: FA Davis.

Stolley J, Buckwalter K, Fjordbak, Bush S. (1991). Iatrogenesis in the elderly: Drug-related problems. J Gerontol Nurs 17(9):12–17.

Watson W. (Fall/Winter 1991). Ethnicity, crime, and aging: Risk factors and adaptation. Generations 53–57.

Watzke J, Smith D. (1994). Concern for and knowledge of safety hazards among older people: Implications for research and prevention. Exp Aging Res 20:177–188.

Whedon M, Shedd P. (1989). Prediction and prevention of patient falls. Image 21(2):108–114.

Worfolk J. (1997). Keep frail elders warm. Geriatr Nurs 18(1):7–11.

CRITICAL THINKING EXERCISES

Angelina Benedetti, an 88-year-old woman, has alterations in visual perception due to normal aging. Her last eye examination was 2 1/2 years ago. She is currently taking a total of seven different prescription medications prescribed by three different physicians for her heart disease and hypertension. In addition, she also takes one or two over-the-counter drugs whenever the need arises. Mrs. Benedetti lives with her 56-year-old daughter in a two-bedroom apartment. During the past 6 months, Mrs. Benedetti was brought to the local hospital emergency department by her daughter on eight occasions for bruises on her arms, nose, knees, and feet. Mrs. Benedetti states that she is constantly falling at home and it seems to be getting worse.

1. Consider Mrs. Benedetti's accident history and decide what further information is necessary for a thorough assessment. Is there reason to suspect that Mrs. Benedetti is the victim of abuse? If so, what action should you take using your own community's standards. Specify at least three nursing diagnoses with related appropriate nursing interventions.

Tariq Hassam, a 79-year-old man, lives in a city housing project where crime is increasing rapidly. In good weather Mr. Hassam enjoys walking to the nearby park with some of the other men in the building. Recently, several of the residents of the project have been robbed in their apartments and one was mugged in the park. Now Mr. Hassam is afraid to be alone in his apartment and even more frightened to walk outside.

2. How can Mr. Hassam increase his level of safety both within his apartment and when he leaves the building? What is available in your own community to address these issues? What personal and social responses need to be made to ensure Mr. Hassam's safety day to day.

Pedro Allende, a 91-year-old man who resides in a nursing home, recently began roaming around his room at night and fell, breaking his leg. Mr. Allende's physician wrote an order for restraints, but his family is greatly opposed to tying him up in his bed or chair.

3. Prepare to discuss specific alternatives to restraints with both Mr. Allende and his family. If alternatives have been tried and have failed, address the issues of legality and safety in the use of restraints for Mr. Allende.

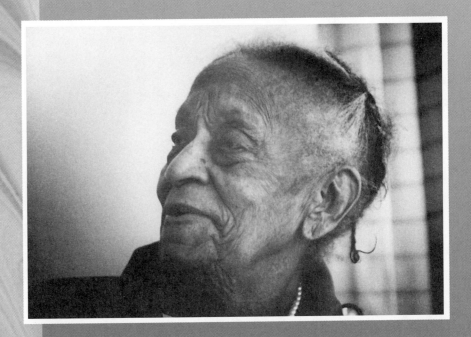

Supporting Wellness in Diverse Settings

CHAPTER 11

Community Health Care:

Health Promotion and Community Living

Annette Bairan, PhD, RN, CS, FNP

CHAPTER OUTLINE

OBJECTIVES

After completing this chapter, the reader should be able to:

1. Write a teaching plan for promoting health and wellness to clients who are (a) living independently, (b) in assisted living, or (c) in a nursing home.
2. Teach a class of older adults six coping skills designed to help them gain access to community services.
3. Differentiate among the following: (a) senior centers and nursing centers; (b) adult daycare and home health care; (c) lay caregivers and parish nursing.
4. Identify ECHO housing and accessory apartments in your own community. Are they legal in your locale?
5. Formulate five nursing interventions for a client whose caregiver is experiencing high stress levels.

KEY TERMS

assisted living
block nursing
continuing care retirement communities (CCRCs)
elder cottage housing opportunity (ECHO)
hospice
integrated community living
lifecare
parish nursing
qigong
residential care facilities (RCFs)
single-room occupancy (SRO) housing

Community health care of older adults is a broad concept encompassing the health and care of older adults in a variety of community living and service arrangements. The focus of this chapter is on individuals who are living in the community, beginning with healthy older adults living independently and progressing to older adults with some deficits in functioning who are dependent and living in various accommodative settings. Emphasis is on health promotion among community-dwelling older adults and the nurse's roles and interventions in assisting older adults in health promotion activities. This emphasis is carried throughout the continuum of living arrangements. Finally, there is a discussion of the evolving types of community living arrangements and health care services for our growing aged population.

■ HEALTHY OLDER ADULTS

Community-dwelling older adults are for the most part relatively healthy people. Although many older adults have at least one or more chronic health conditions, the majority of older adults tend to rate their overall health status subjectively as good, very good, or excellent. Eighty-five to 88 percent of a random sample of older adults reported that they function without any significant restrictions on their activities of daily living (Thorson, 1995). Many are not yet retired and are productive workers contributing to the economy. As of 1996, the first baby boomers began turning 50 years of age. This upcoming cohort of older adults will be better educated, better off financially, and healthier than past cohorts of older adults.

Many baby boomers have taken exercise and nutrition more seriously than previous generations, and we may well see a more positive image of aging with these trendsetters.

Negative images of aging and older people may have more to do with a personal fear of aging and death rather than the real state of affairs. One study by Ghent-Fuller (1996) explored the experiences of healthy older adults regarding the anticipation of death of self in later life. The participants reported an ongoing process of "creating readiness" and "achieving purpose" related to their death. They also reported five spheres of being: internal being, relationships with others, existence in the world as a solitary person and as part of humankind, and existence after death. By understanding this anticipation of death, nurses can better assist older adults in planning for death emotionally, spiritually, and legally (such as explaining and assisting with living wills, advance directives, and durable powers of attorney for health care). (For more about death and dying, see Chapter 25.)

W e l l n e s s

"Health-promoting behaviors are more likely to occur in older adults who participate in self-care activities and have a positive self-concept."

Health Promotion

Health promotion activities are ones that tend to enhance health status, often indirectly reducing the risk of various diseases. This enhanced health status, or sense of well-being, is not only beneficial to older adults directly but also benefits the community economically and socially. Older adults are valuable resources to the communities in which they live: they provide assistance to others of all ages—related and unrelated (Kincade et al., 1996). Often health promotion focuses on lifestyle modification in terms of exercise, good nutrition, stress reduction, and avoidance of alcohol, drugs, and tobacco. These lifestyle changes are easily advised but are often difficult to carry out. As to which older adults will be more likely to participate in health promotion activities, Padula (1997) found the following variables to be predictors: relationship quality, perceived health, education, internal health locus of control, and social support.

LIFESTYLE MODIFICATION

Pender (1996) offers some experiential and behavioral processes for lifestyle change. *Experiential processes* for change are more internally focused and include consciousness raising, self-reevaluation (self-confrontation), and cognitive restructuring (rational emotive therapy). For example, cognitive restructuring is based on the belief that we tend to evaluate a situation and our ability to cope with it, and these two evaluations determine our response to the situation, positive or negative. It is not so much the situation as it is our internal self-statements and our emotions associated with these statements; therefore, if we can assist older adults to recognize their negative self-statements ("I will always be overweight," "I can never stop smoking") and help them correct this negative pattern of thinking, we will be assisting them to modify their lifestyle to one that is healthier.

Behavioral processes focus on behavioral change directly and include reinforcement (reward) management, modeling, counterconditioning, and stimulus control (Pender, 1996). For instance, stimulus control is based on the belief that changing the events that precede a behavior (e.g., smoking) can decrease or eliminate negative behavior (the smoking) and increase positive behavior. Cues that trigger the behavior are manipulated (restricted, eliminated, or expanded) so as to produce the desired behavior. An example of cue elimination for the smoker would be sitting in the no-smoking area with the nonsmokers. These strategies would be helpful in assisting older adults (and ourselves) in changing behaviors that are detrimental to health.

In addition to using traditional nursing texts and journal articles to find health promotion strategies, nurses could also use the Nursing Interventions Classification (NIC) resource (McCloskey and Bulechek, 1996). All six domains may be applicable concerning lifestyle modifications; however, health promotion grows readily out of the behavioral domain, which includes the classes of behavior therapy, cognitive therapy, communication enhancement, coping assistance, patient education, and psychological comfort promotion. For example, cognitive restructuring is broken down into specific interventions, such as assisting the person to understand that irrational self-statements can prevent the desired behavior. Why not attempt to use this resource in promoting health care with older adults?

NUTRITION AND EXERCISE

Nutrition is positively associated with good health and longevity. Additionally, nutrition is important in maintaining vigor and well-being and in treating many health problems (e.g., diabetes mellitus, which is the sixth leading cause of death in older adults). Physical changes associated with aging—such as the decreases in physical activity, lean body mass, intracellular water, and intestinal absorption—may change the need for various nutrients. Caloric needs are lower for older adults, with the average recommended caloric intake as follows (Pender, 1996):

- Moderately active women, aged 51 to 75, 1800 calories (1600 calories if older than age 75)
- Moderately active men, aged 51 to 75, 2400 calories (2050 calories if older than age 75)

There is controversy regarding these values; some people believe they are too restrictive for older adults, and acceptable levels may be somewhat higher. It could be argued, however, that lower caloric intake is beneficial based on research that diet restriction in laboratory animals retards aging and increases their maximum life span (Masoro, 1992), and it is the only nutritional intervention that has been found to do so.

For older adults who are obese, nurses need to counsel them as to ways to increase their physical activity and change their eating patterns over the long term. Not only is obesity a health risk for coronary artery disease, certain types of cancer, diabetes, and social disability, but various popular fad diets often result in "yo-yo" dieting (cycles of losing and gaining weight), which is thought to be harmful to one's health. (Byproducts of fat metabolism in the blood may be deposited in the lining of blood vessels and may also be harmful to various organs.)

Water is necessary for all people, but especially for older adults. The sensation of thirst is often diminished in older adults, so that they may neglect to drink sufficient quantities of water (i.e., 1.5 L/24 h). Intracellular water declines with age and loss of muscle, and renal function diminishes, making water balance harder to maintain. The outcome may be dehydration—the most common cause of fluid and electrolyte imbalances in older adults (Chernoff, 1994).

Recommendations concerning dietary fat of older adults are the same as those for young and middle-aged adults—total fat intake should be less than 30% of total calories with decreased amounts of saturated fat and cholesterol. As for carbohydrates, older adults should increase their intake of complex carbohydrates to at least 55% of their total calories. This increase of carbohydrates will likely result in increased intake of vitamins, minerals, and fiber as well. There is little evidence to support mineral deficiencies in most older adults, but the majority of free-living older adults are deficient in vitamin D intake (Mahan and Escott-Stump, 1996). Calcium supplementation of 1000 to 1500 mg/d is recommended for postmenopausal women (Levenson and Bockman, 1994).

Some older adults alter their diet in negative ways; for example, they skip meals or reduce the amount eaten, they eat a very limited variety of food (which limits coverage of the basic food groups), or they drink insufficient amounts of water. Older adults have a greater incidence of gastrointestinal problems that can interfere with appetite, digestion, and absorption of nutrients, chewing and swallowing problems, gastroesophageal reflux disease, hiatal hernias, indigestion, constipation, and so forth. Nurses need to assess for these conditions and intervene to promote the nutritional status of older adults.

Poor nutrition may arise in older adults for reasons beyond the physical; psychological and sociocultural factors also influence eating. Loss of loved ones and friends, loss of mobility and independence, loss of financial security, diminution of self-worth—these are some of the losses that some of the old-old can experience, resulting in various forms of suffering, such as loneliness, grief, depression, and giving up the will to live. After loss of a loved one, some older adults (especially if living alone) are too depressed to purchase and prepare balanced meals, much less eat the food alone. Eating is very much a social activity in our culture, and for people accustomed to dining with others, eating alone is often done only to satisfy

hunger. In one study of nutritional health-seeking behavior in older adults, the authors found this behavior to be composed of two factors—avoiding and seeking nutrition (Quinn et al., 1997). Predictors of both nutritional health factors were economic resources, self-discipline, and enthusiasm. Interventions were recommended for older adults with the risk factors of advanced age, male gender, and low economic resources. (For more detailed information on nutrition in older adults, refer to Chapter 7.)

Exercise becomes more important with age because it can slow, stop, or even reverse physical decline. Strength training can nearly eliminate loss of muscle, which is a major physical characteristic of aging. Muscle strength declines rapidly in the old-old population and is a significant risk factor for falls among older adults. Falls often result in fractures in older adults, which increase morbidity and mortality that reflect unnecessary human suffering and tremendous economic loss for the nation as a whole. Yet exercise can reduce the risk of falls and fractures in older adults (Fiatarone, 1994). A single session of aerobic exercise can produce calm, lower blood pressure, and reduce stress response even hours afterward; regular exercise has even more lasting effects. Yet Travis and associates (1996) discovered that older adults who walked in malls were more motivated to walk because of the associated social relationships than for the physical effects of health promotion and disease prevention.

Much of the literature states that older adults should see their physician before starting an exercise program, although we know that a sedentary lifestyle is a greater health risk than the risk of someone's dying from a heart attack during exercise. The conservative approach would be to advise older adults to visit their health care provider if they have not had a physical examination during the past 2 years or they have one of the following risk factor for coronary disease: hypertension, smoking, diabetes, obesity, family history of early heart attacks, high levels of low-density lipoprotein cholesterol, or low levels of high-density lipoproteins.

Booth and Tseng (1995) want physicians to prescribe exercise more often. They have developed a simple table that shows the ages at which exercise should be promoted to prevent or treat various diseases. The table pictures five conditions that exercise helps to prevent *or treat* in all ages, 1 to 100; these conditions are coronary heart disease, depression, hypertension, obesity, and osteoporosis. Exercise also helps to prevent stroke in all ages and helps treat rheumatoid arthritis in ages 60 to 100. Nurses need to counsel older adults on the benefits of exercise.

COPING AND ADAPTATION

Another approach to enhancing health promotion in older adults is to teach coping and adaptation strategies and skills. These skills may encompass many specific interventions: stress reduction; hope therapy; strengthening social support systems; increasing socialization; relaxation and leisure activities; and humor. Nurses are known for their good communication skills and are usually adept at assessing a person's perception of events, everyday coping and problem-solving skills, and social support systems. On the basis of this assessment, the nurse may have the opportunity to teach new and more effective coping skills, such as assertiveness training, listening skills, identifying and prioritizing alternative solutions, and so forth.

Support groups are a method of coping that some older adults use; these groups are composed of people in similar situations or crises who are willing to support one another. Members expect to be accepted and understood and to receive suggestions that help solve their problems. It has been estimated that 7.5 million adults participated in a support group in the early 1990s (Lieberman and Snowden, 1993). An aging-parents support group that I co-led is composed, somewhat surprisingly, of young-old individuals who are caring for their old-old parents. The feedback from group members has been very positive, and a camaraderie has developed among the leaders and the regular members that has carried over into strong outside social ties.

Stress Reduction

Stress may be the result of major life events or just hassles but, amazingly, hassles are often better predictors of stress than major life events. In a study by Lamborn (1996), hassles were the best predictor of depression in healthy older adults. Unanticipated life events (e.g., an unexpected death) are generally more stressful than anticipated events, and the same event can produce different consequences for different people (from high levels of stress to virtually no stress). Saliency of the event is one major factor; for example, a pianist with disabling arthritis of the hands would likely be more stressed by the condition than the ordinary individual. Some older adults may redefine stressful situations as opportunities for growth or may use positive comparisons for encouragement (e.g., comparing themselves to people their own age).

More people are turning to alternative means of reducing stress such as meditation, biofeedback, hypnotherapy, guided imagery, hypnosis, massage, yoga, qigong, and herbs. **Qigong** (pronounced she-gong) is a combination of movement, meditation, and breath regulation that enhances the flow of vital energy in the body (Burton Goldberg Group, 1995). It is practiced every day by about 200 million people, and it is part of the health care programs in most Chinese hospitals. Qigong is reported to reduce stress, increase resistance to disease, and increase circulation. Meditation not only relaxes and helps to relieve stress, anxiety, and pain but also has been helpful with drug addiction. Biofeedback is used to gain control over involuntary functions such as brain waves, blood pressure, and pulse. In the cost-conscious climate of health care today, more people are looking at alternatives to traditional medicine and finding them to be cost effective, prevention conscious, and, in many instances, assistive of self-healing.

Meaning of Life and Spirituality

We all have our own interpretation of the meaning of life, whether we are conscious of it or not. Older adults, especially the old-old, often review their life in terms of interpretation and meaning. This life-review process can be a positive type of catharsis that brings about a time of reflection about life and our place in it; it may also stimulate the need to complete any unfinished business (e.g., clearing up old misunderstandings and rifts). In general, after some rationalizing and suppressing, life reviews are positive experiences (Thorson, 1995).

Spirituality involves the search for meaning in life and the belief in a higher power (Wilson and Kneisl, 1996). Spiritual health is the development of an individual's spiritual nature to its fullest, including learning how to love and forgive and to experience joy, happiness, hope, and peace. It is also part of the holistic practice of nursing—one of the three central aspects of mind, body, and spirit. The ability to fulfill one's unique potential (self-actualization) and that of others also contributes to spiritual health. Spirituality may be a significant variable in physical and mental health, especially for older adults. The North American Nursing Diagnosis Association (NANDA) (1994) defines spiritual distress as "disruption in the life principle which pervades a person's entire being and which integrates and transcends one's biological and psychosocial nature." Factors that contribute to spiritual distress include

- Increased awareness of aging
- Chronic pain and suffering
- Disability
- Anger toward a higher power
- Challenged values and beliefs

There are many characteristics that could indicate spiritual distress:

- Alterations in behavior (anger, hostility, crying, withdrawal)
- Sleep problems
- Questions about meaning of life
- Conflict about beliefs and/or relationships with the higher power
- Being unable to participate in the usual religious practices

Forbes (1994) developed a structured interview guide to be used with the Spiritual Well-Being Scale, which measures one's relationship with God and satisfaction with life.

Spirituality is not the same as religiosity; spirituality is broader and may or may not include religion, whereas *religiosity* refers to the behaviors associated with spiritual beliefs such as various rituals and participation (attending church, synagogue, mosque, or temple; prayer; reading holy texts; baptism, confirmation, bar and bas mitzvahs).

W e l l n e s s

66*Interventions for hope instillation include assisting older adults to identify areas in which they can have hope, teaching them new coping skills, assisting them to expand their spirituality, and offering them guided life review or reminiscence.*99

According to Pender (1996), nurses should assess the following areas of spirituality:

- Relationship with a higher being (including beliefs, rituals, and participation)
- Relationship with self (life goals, hope, priorities, and spiritual growth)
- Relationships with others (openness to others, concern for others, and respect for others)

Some older adults are in a state of spiritual health; others are in spiritual distress. According to Strickland (1996), ministering to people's spirit by listening to the other person's experiences is caring, transpersonal, and healing. These exchanges can be healing to both the client and the nurse.

Hope and Optimism

Hope and optimism are attitudes that enhance health. Most people have heard of a terminally ill person who lived past the expected time of death, seemingly because of a desire to be alive for some great event such as a marriage, graduation, or birth of a family member, or even a holiday observance, only to die immediately afterward. Also, one hears about the power of optimism, or positive thinking, to effect change. *Hope* is defined as the wish for something with the expectation of its fulfillment.

Although there seems to be scant discussion of hope in the nursing literature (relative to its importance), there is discussion of its opposite—hopelessness. NANDA (1994) lists *hopelessness* as a nursing diagnosis, defining it as the state in which a person perceives limited or no alternatives to a situation and cannot mobilize the necessary energy to attend to it. Hopelessness is a salient feature of major depression, and older adults are at risk for depression. The many losses that some older adults experience (especially the old-old and the poor) can lead to hopelessness. A study by Karns (1996) found that a sample of community-dwelling older adults who attended a senior center had a high level of hope, as measured by the Miller Hope Scale. Having hope is often related to the ability to find meaning in life and to spirituality. Interventions for hope instillation include assisting older adults to identify areas in which they can have hope, teaching them new coping mechanisms, assisting them to expand their spirituality, and offering them guided life review or reminiscence (McCloskey and Bulechek, 1996).

Depression seems to be the antithesis of hope, and yet depression is relatively common among older adults. But it often goes unrecognized by health care providers. Dalton and Busch (1995) studied homebound older adults and their home health nurses' ability to recognize depression among them. Although 27.5% of the older adults were found to be depressed, the nurses recognized depression in less than half of that group, and none of the nurses documented any depression-related nursing diagnosis.

Optimism, or a positive attitude, seems to be a character trait of some people. Most of us have known a person who seems to be optimistic in all situations. Caring nurses intervene to build optimism in their older adult clients.

Humor

Norman Cousins (1976) believed that laughter is the best medicine. He reported that he laughed his health problems away after nearly dying in the hospital while undergoing traditional medical care for a degenerative spinal condition. Cousins checked himself out of the hospital and into a hotel and then treated himself by watching old movie comedies. Humor is generally acknowledged to be a commonly used coping strategy that also stimulates the immune system.

Nurses can use humor as a therapeutic strategy to enhance the well-being of older adults. In the Nursing Interventions Classification (NIC), humor is used to "establish relationships, relieve tension, release anger, facilitate learning, or cope with painful feelings" (McCloskey and Bulechek, 1996). Some appropriate interventions include assessing the type of humor the person appreciates, making available different sources of humor, monitoring the person's response, and avoiding content to which the person is sensitive.

Social Support

Social networks refer to the systems of family and friends with whom older adults interact and have some form of social bond. Informal social supports refer to the support obtained from these networks—for example, emotional support, instrumental aid (assistance with specific tasks), informational support, and affirmation (to affirm one's strengths and potentials) (Pender, 1996). The following social support systems are relevant to the health of older adults: natural (family), peer, organized religious (church), organized caregiving professionals, and organized lay support groups (mutual help). Maintenance of social support is one of the important variables of later life; social support has a positive influence on a person's well-being and is a mediator or buffer against stress, whereas low levels of social support are associated with health problems and even death (Williams and Chesney, 1993).

To age successfully, older adults need to maintain primary relationships with significant others. Contrary to popular belief, most older adults maintain frequent contact with their families. Although extended family and close friends are important, research suggests that primarily it is the nuclear family that people turn to when in need (Thorson, 1995). The strongest bonds in social networks are family ones, and these bonds can provide support when the older adult needs it. For older adults who do not have family bonds or for whom they are ineffective, isolation or institutionalization is not uncommon. Even for those older adults who do have families, there is a chance that they may outlive their families. Future sources of social support for older adults will likely be dampened by their increased numbers and the associated increase in the prevalence of chronic disease, the smaller size of families, and the high rate of divorce. Nevertheless, informal support networks will continue to have great significance for older adults.

Nurses need to assess the older adult's desires and perceptions concerning social support before planning interventions. It may be that an older adult values autonomy and independence more than social support. If the older adult does want social support in terms of services or relationships, the nurse needs to assess for adequacy and availability of existing social support systems. Additionally, the nurse must assess the person's social networks—the size (number of people), composition (family or friends), geographic proximity, homogeneity (shared characteristics), strength of the bonds, and density (number of relationships) (Pender, 1996). Social networks and support may be the main reason for living (raison d'être) for some older adults, especially the old-old and the poor.

Autonomy and Independence

Autonomy here refers to the degree of control a person has over decision-making and other activities without interference. Autonomy is highly valued by the dominant culture of our society, and thus most older adults value it, especially when they become disabled and dependent—and even more so if they become institutionalized. However, in some of the subcultures of our society there is less value placed on autonomy, and it is necessary to be sensitive to these differences.

Autonomy is relevant to the issue of health care for older adults because some health care providers continue to treat older adults, especially those with physical or cognitive disabilities, in paternalistic ways. To educate ourselves about the meaning of autonomy, perhaps each person in the class could imagine playing the role of a disabled older adult who can no longer care for himself or herself and therefore must be admitted to a nursing home. The class member would pretend to live in the facility for a few days and nights, with few personal possessions, little-to-no privacy (a roommate), little personal space, and restrictions on when and what to eat, when and where one can go, and when one must go to bed, bathe, and dress. Do you get the idea? To experience lack of autonomy is to value it more.

Some older adults seem to value autonomy and independence over life itself; witness the number of stories in which an older person, alone in his or her home, physically disabled to the point of being unsafe, still refuses to be moved into any institutionalized living arrangement. We, as nurses, must be attentive to autonomy needs of older adults and to possible solutions. Informing and counseling families of older adults about available community resources is a place to begin.

> ### W e l l n e s s
>
> 66*The great majority of older adults age in place; they do not move to retirement communities or specialized health care facilities.*99

Leisure

Most Americans can expect to spend about one third of their lives in leisure. Leisure is positively associated with high levels of life satisfaction and morale. Many older adults enjoy creative arts, educational experiences, travel, or volunteering, with most pursuing the same type of leisure activities in their later years. Leisure activities and programs can help to fill the void that sometimes exists after various role losses associated with retirement from work and changes in family. Besides producing rest, relaxation, and diversion, leisure activities contribute to better physical and mental health and enhance self-esteem, confidence, and feelings of social integration.

Leisure education has been shown to positively affect the health and well-being of older adults (Mahon and Searle, 1994). Adult education is a major source of recreation and enrichment for older adults. Elderhostel is an educational program for older adults that offers short-term courses on college campuses on every continent of the world. It now serves more than 250,000 older adults a year at 1500 institutions (Thorson, 1995). Elderhostel has proven to be a great way to combine travel and educational enrichment for older adults.

Prevention of Illness and Injury

Prevention of illness and injury can be partly accomplished by health promotion activities such as those just mentioned. In addition, some well-known behaviors help to prevent illness and injury; these include avoiding people with contagious diseases, avoiding environmental (water, soil, and air) pollutants, avoiding dangerous occupations and hobbies, and wearing protective equipment (e.g., seat belts, bicycle helmets, ear plugs, sunscreen lotion, sunglasses).

FALLS

Injury is a leading cause of disability in older adults, and the most common causes are falls, motor vehicle accidents, and fires or burns. The leading cause of accidental death in the home is falls, with the majority involving people older than 65 years (Smith and Maurer, 1995). The risk of falls greatly increases with advancing age. Extrinsic causes of falls in older

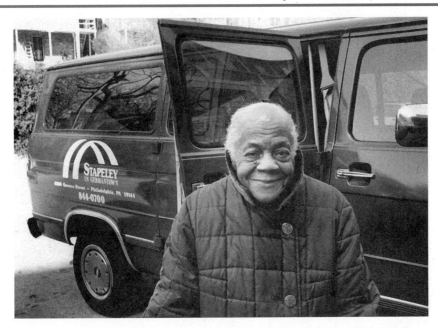

Many senior centers provide van service for clients who participate in day programs.

adults include poor lighting, slippery rugs or floor, low toilet seats without grab bars, showers and tubs without grab bars, and stairs without rails. Nurses are knowledgeable in this area and can intervene by teaching about these hazards and how to prevent or solve them. Also, nurses who visit clients' homes as part of their nursing functions have the opportunity to directly assess the environment and give counsel on the spot.

Intrinsic causes of falls could be a lack of balance, vertigo or syncope, muscle or joint weakness or impairment, impaired vision, cognitive impairment, acute or chronic diseases, postural hypotension, and medication use. Yet studies have shown that strengthening lower-extremity muscles, improving joint flexibility, and balance training can benefit older adults' gait or balance (Fiatarone et al., 1994). Nurses can make important contributions toward the health of older adults by assessing and intervening in the areas of risks (e.g., teaching muscle-strengthening exercises).

Connell and Wolf (1997) examined the environment and behaviors associated with falls and near-falls of older adults. They identified several patterns: collisions in the dark, not avoiding hazards, preoccupation, slippery floor coverings, excessive environmental demands, and habitual and inappropriate envi-

ronmental use. Another study found that falls could be reduced by improving postural stability by enhancing alertness and attention among older adults (Topp, Estes, Dayhoff, and Suhrheinrich, 1997). Nurses can assess older adults for a lack of alertness and attention during transferring activities and ambulation and teach methods of maintaining alertness and attention during these activities. (For more about falls, see Chapters 9 and 10.)

IMMUNIZATIONS

Older adults, especially those with chronic medical disorders, are at increased risk for complications from influenza infections (Report of the U.S. Preventive Services Task Force, 1996). *Annual influenza vaccine* is recommended for all people aged 65 and older, and *pneumococcal vaccine* is recommended for all people aged 65 and older who are immuno-competent. During the 10 influenza epidemics from 1972–1973 to 1990–1991, in excess of 20,000 deaths were reported for each. Over 90% of these deaths due to pneumonia and influenza were in people aged 65 and older. Therefore, it is very important that nurses continue to remind older adults about the importance of getting the influenza and pneumococcal vaccines. Additionally, older adults (like other adults) need to get periodic tetanus and diphtheria toxoid booster injections.

■ COMMUNITY LIVING

Older adults live in or visit daily a variety of community settings. The main categories include

- Integrated community living
- Various types of retirement communities
- Assisted living and board-and-care homes
- Senior centers
- Adult daycare centers
- Individual homes or apartments in which home health care is delivered
- Undomiciled settings such as shelters and streets
- Other evolving forms of settings

Integrated Community Living

Most older adults live in their own home, most in the United States own their home, and most want to stay in their own home. The great majority of older adults age in place; they do not move to retirement communities. They are, as far as living arrangements are concerned, integrated into the community (*heterogeneous by age*) rather than being segregated by age (*homogeneous by age*). Although these older adults in integrated community living are naturally experiencing some (usually gradual) decline in physical health and function as they age, in general *there is little or no decline in social and psychological functions* (Palmore, 1995). Many older adults act, feel, and think like middle-aged adults. These older adults are validating the activity theory (see Chapter 1) by being active and retaining roles and statuses from middle age. This theory holds that the happy older adult is an active older person.

Most older adults need health care only occasionally; they are performing self-care. Participants in self-care activities have a better self-concept, which tends to reinforce health-promoting behaviors (Kreidler et al., 1994). Self-care practices increase the probability that older adults will maintain their functional independence longer. Nurses must assess older adults for their ability, desire, and readiness to perform self-care in all areas before assisting them (and removing the opportunity for self-

care). For those older adults who are ill, nurses need to assist them to find meaning in their illness, because older adults who have found meaning in their illness experience increased motivation for performing self-care activities (Baker and Stern, 1994).

Nurses have always made important contributions to the health care of older adults, regardless of where older adults are domiciled. Now, in the midst of tremendous upheaval in health care policy and financing, the locus of health care is moving from acute care settings to health care settings in the community. Nurses who have worked only in acute care settings will need to accommodate to this shift by learning new roles and skills that are more applicable to community health nursing. This community shift in nursing education and practice will also entail a renewed emphasis on sociocultural, economic, and political aspects of community and family nursing. And, because about 95% of older adults are living in community settings at any one time, this renewal of community health nursing will encompass health care of older adults.

C a r i n g

❝*In every health care setting there is an opportunity for nurses to insist on the highest possible standards of service.***❞**

Retirement Communities

Retirement communities for older adults exist in a variety of forms, sizes, and places—some with full social and health services and some with few or no services. Most retirement communities belong to one of the following types: (a) retirement new towns, (b) retirement villages, (c) retirement subdivisions, (d) retirement residences, and (e) continuing care retirement centers (CCRCs).

Why do older adults choose to move to retirement communities from their middle-years residences, why do they choose one type of retirement community over the other, and why do some move out of state and others not? Many older adults move simply because they have the money to do so and they desire to move. To move takes money, so that older adult movers are generally upper-middle-class and upper-class people who have the resources to buy another home. Money again determines which type of retirement community is chosen. When making decisions about moving, older adults consider the location of the housing (region of country, rural or urban); the housing itself (type and scale); the amenities, activities, and services available; security; price; and the characteristics of the residents (age, health status, religion, and socioeconomic status). Older adults who select expensive retirement communities tend to be young-old adults with high incomes who are in relatively good health and desire a leisure lifestyle.

Most of the moves made by older adults occur within their same county of residence, but when they do move out of state, the majority move south or west, with Florida being the state with the biggest gain and the highest percentage of people aged 65 and older (Thorson, 1995). When older adults do move out of state, they are generally healthy and move in their early years of retirement. Some of them will move back to their native state when they are in their 70s or 80s (return migration). Older adults who return to their native states are often in poor health and/or widowed and they are moving to be close to an adult child (caregiver).

The number of community-dwelling older adults who live alone has increased dramatically during the past few decades. Often the ability to live alone is associated with being independent and having a high quality of life, but there are some older adults living alone who are in poverty, socially isolated, and in poor health. Using a representative sample of community-dwelling adults aged 70 or over, Davis and colleagues (1997) found that adults who live alone or who change from living with someone to living alone do not experience increased mortality; but living with someone other than a spouse may be associated with higher mortality.

RETIREMENT TOWNS, VILLAGES, AND SUBDIVISIONS

Retirement new towns are large, self-sufficient communities with all major services and recreation. They usually consist of single-family houses, condominiums, and cooperatives; an example of such a new town is Sun City, Arizona. *Retirement villages* are smaller than towns, generally not planned to be self-sufficient, but often located near a full range of services. *Retirement subdivisions* are located in a city, often with limited support services, so they use services offered by the community. They usually consist of single-family houses or mobile homes.

Towns and villages are communities in and of themselves; therefore, health care is usually integrated within them as it is in nonretirement communities. But retirement communities generally have more of a focus on health care than do nonretirement communities. This focus is in response to the characteristics of most of their residents (i.e., a population with more chronic health disorders and more disability and frailty).

As with other vulnerable population groups, nurses can have a significant impact on older adults in these communities. Health promotion and disease and injury prevention are mainstays of nursing and can be effectively implemented with these older groups through education. In addition to primary care, secondary care of these older adults would involve screening and early casefinding of common disorders, referring and collaborating with other health care professionals, assisting with medications and treatments, and assessing and monitoring disease conditions. Tertiary care would involve rehabilitation nursing in the forms of education about the disease or disability and its treatments, prevention of further disability, and how to adapt to any disability.

RETIREMENT RESIDENCES

Freestanding retirement residences usually offer supportive environments for independent older adults in the form of single high-rise buildings. These facilities generally offer communal meals, housekeeping, recreation, transportation, and security. The services of a nurse or nursing clinic may or may not be part of the rental package, but comprehensive medical care is not provided. To qualify for admission, residents must be a certain age (for example, older than 55 or 60) and be able to care for themselves. Some residences, however, do offer assisted living options that are designed for residents who need greater assistance.

In these retirement residences, nurses have much to offer in terms of health promotion and disease and injury prevention. A sample of nursing activities for such older, independent adults includes

- Nutrition, exercise, and safety education
- Assessment of health status
- Psychosocial support and counseling
- Monitoring of chronic diseases and associated treatments
- Anticipatory guidance in terms of the last developmental stage and its associated tasks

Nurses serve as advocates for residents and can serve as liaison with families and community agencies.

Some retirement residences have a clinic on site that can serve exclusively as a nursing center. These nursing centers may be hubs of activity, with older adults seeking advice and counsel from the nurse and socializing during the process and with nurses teaching health promotion, illness and injury prevention, and self-care. Residents of one retirement high-rise reported that they needed and valued the services of the nursing center located in the building, and the nursing services contributed positively to their health (Scott and Moneyham, 1995).

CONTINUING CARE RETIREMENT COMMUNITIES

Continuing care retirement communities (CCRCs) integrate three levels of housing: independent living, assisted living, and skilled nursing facilities. This community arrangement may be purchased or rented, guaranteeing shelter and full services, although the monthly fee will differ with the level or type of care being utilized by the resident. The advantage is that an individual can truly age in place; that is, a person can move in and remain until death, never having to move out into another facility. This is accomplished by moving among the three levels according to the person's current health care needs.

Another version of CCRCs is termed *lifecare*. **Lifecare** facilities are similar to CCRCs with one exception: the older adult enters by purchasing a unit (paying an entrance fee), then paying a monthly service charge—but this monthly amount never varies whatever the level of care required by the resident. For ex-

ample, if an individual has to move from independent living to the nursing home, the monthly charge remains the same and care is guaranteed until death. With lifecare, the resident is able to age in place and have peace of mind, knowing that monthly fees will not vary with the level of care needed. The main disadvantage of lifecare is cost; entrance fees are very expensive. Higgins (1992) states that there is a shift away from the advance-fee type of CCRCs toward the fee-for-service type on the part of the providers and the users. Yet Somers (1993) sees lifecare as a viable option for long-term care of older adults, especially in the absence of a long-term care policy for our nation. Lifecare offers a guarantee of housing and health care for its participants that emphasizes high quality and compassion.

The typical independent resident of a CCRC is a white woman, age 82, who is widowed, divorced, or never married (Netting and Wilson, 1991). One study found that the majority (75%) of the residents of a CCRC depended on others in the CCRC for social activity, and the well residents tended to assist and support the frail ones (Stacey-Konnert and Pynoos, 1992). The authors concluded that living in a CCRC helped residents to maintain their social networks as they aged.

Assisted Living and Board-and-Care Homes

Assisted living is one of the fastest growing types of housing for older people. The term *assisted living* is often used interchangeably with *personal care*, especially if the personal care unit is part of a larger retirement community. The American Association of Retired Persons (AARP) commissioned a study entitled Assisted Living in the United States: A New Paradigm for Residential Care for Frail Older Persons? conducted by Kane and Wilson (1993). For the study, the authors defined *assisted living* as

> . . . *any group residential program that is not licensed as a nursing home, that provides personal care to persons with need for assistance in the activities of daily living (ADL), and that can respond to unscheduled needs for assistance that might arise (Kane and Wilson, 1993, p. xi).*

As a type of supportive housing, assisted living can enhance independent living for frail older adults. Assisted living services usually include meals, personal care services (assistance with bathing, dressing, and undressing), assistance with medication management, housekeeping, social activities, transportation, security, and 24-hour responsibility for the resident. Services typically available can be classed as personal care, nursing, case management, and hotel-type services.

The design and furnishings of assisted living facilities are more residential than institutional, giving the place a homey atmosphere of private space within a communal setting. Being able to have and control one's own personal space and have input into decisions about lifestyle and care are major advantages to this type of supportive housing, which enhances the autonomy of the residents. Residents of these settings vary in their need for assistance from those with minimal needs to those who are almost nursing home certifiable (Kane and Wilson, 1993). The typical residents tend to be more disabled than the group that was targeted for assisted living.

Board-and-care homes, or **residential care facilities (RCFs)**, house almost 1 million older adults nationally (Rogg and Rogg, 1995). (To make it confusing, additional names are used: personal care, assisted living, adult foster care, adult congregate living, domiciliary care, community care, sheltered care, and supervised care.) They are run by homeowners who provide meals, laundry, and housekeeping for older adults. Quality varies from excellent to substandard, with some people charging that residents have limited opportunities for exercise, recreation, community participation, and activities that are challenging and prepare them for resumed independent living.

Nurses serving these facilities can perform the same functions as those performed for independent residents in retirement residences and for dependent residents in skilled nursing facilities. Many of these homes probably utilize licensed practical nurses (LPNs) and nursing assistants, so that registered nurses (RNs) would assume more administrative and case management functions. In addition, nurses should conduct or coordinate individualized assessments, with subsequent planning, inter-

vention, and evaluation to manage actual and potential problems associated with functional and organic conditions. A study of Oregon's assisted living settings with a sample of 947 showed that nursing needs or procedures ranged from medication management (75%), wheelchair or walker dependent functions (54%), behavior management services (40%), and protective oversight for safety (30%) (Kane and Wilson, 1993).

Senior Centers

Senior centers are an important means of assisting older adults to remain socially and physically active. They are open, at no charge, to people older than 60 years of age who can care for themselves. Transportation may be provided; congregate meals are usually offered for a minimal price; and various activities and recreation are offered, including trips, crafts, classes, speakers, music, singing, dancing, exercise, and games. In some cases, health screening, education, and primary care services are offered. Ralston (1991) reported that data on participation rates for minority older adults are not complete, yet Sabin (1993) found a higher frequency of use of senior centers by older, less educated, nonwhite older adults versus younger, better educated, white older adults. Frequency of attendance was higher for the socially active senior rather than the isolated one. But there is diversity in terms of who attends the center, the number and type of programs offered, and the size of the staff, resources, and facility.

The nurse's role is multifaceted in the senior center, just as in other settings. Health promotion and preventive activities are paramount, with education being the major thrust. Besides education about physical parameters such as nutrition, exercise, and safety, psychosocial education and counseling are important. Older adults are in the last stage of life, and some experience the resurgence of past conflicts and issues. These people often feel the need to reach some degree of resolution and find meaning in their lives, and nurses can offer emotional support and empathy. Nurses also can assess for the need for other types of professional help, as in the situation of clinical depression, and can make appropriate referrals. (Elderly white men have the highest rate of suicide among people of other ages, gender, or ethnic groups.)

Adult Daycare

Adult daycare centers are often seen as life-savers to many older adults and their care-givers. The centers give respite to caregivers and time to caregivers who work out of the home, often provide care that caregivers are not capable of providing, and offer a social out-let to the older person. Besides providing relief to caregivers, the centers also strive to maintain or improve the functional abilities of older people, to improve their quality of life, and to delay institutionalization (Miller, 1995).

W e l l n e s s

"Older adults who live alone can be helped to avoid isolation through education about the social and transportation resources of their community."

Some studies have documented the prevalent belief of positive outcomes in terms of client and family satisfaction (Scott, 1993), but one study found no difference in health outcomes between clients in adult day health care and those in "customary care" (nursing homes and home care) (Rothman, Hedrick, Bulcroft, and Erdly, 1993). Another study found that community-based long-term care (adult day health care, home nursing, home aide care, and hospice) did not increase survival or slow the rate of functional deterioration in the clients (Weissert and Hedrick, 1994).

Adult daycare centers are seen as alternatives to institutionalization, providing 8 hours of care a day for 5 days a week for adults with mental and/or physical impairments. Many centers have a sliding fee scale, and some costs may be covered by Medicare. The centers usually provide nursing care, personal care, social services, meals, transportation, and recreational opportunities. The level of nursing care provided often depends on the resources of the center. Examples of nursing care include

- Assessments
- Administration of medication
- Wound dressing
- Range-of-motion exercises
- Monitoring the physical environment
- Counseling
- Teaching
- Coordination of services
- Referrals
- Psychosocial support
- Advocacy
- Monitoring health problems

A nurse may also serve as the administrator of the center.

Home Health Care

Home health care is the most rapidly growing component of the health care industry, although most of the growth has been in the for-profit freestanding and hospital-based home health agencies (General Accounting Office, 1992). In fact, the traditional nonprofit agencies, such as the visiting nurse associations and government agencies, declined in number. Many factors have influenced this growth in home health, one being the increase in the number of older adults in our population. Not only have the number of older adults increased dramatically, but the old-old (aged 85 and older) is the fastest growing segment of the older population.

Another factor in the growth of home health care is public policy regarding health care for the elderly. Hospitals have discharged patients "quicker and sicker" in response to the method of Medicare reimbursement using diagnostic-related groups (DRGs) of disease classification. This change from *retrospective payment* (actual cost of care) to *prospective payment* (a fixed rate) was instituted by the government to reduce the enormous rise in health care costs. It appears that DRGs did help to control the rise in hospital costs, but they also brought about a decrease in the average length of stay of Medicare patients, returning older adults to their homes quicker and sicker than before. Home health care, especially privately owned agencies, responded by expanding to meet the needs of older adults in their homes.

The growth of medical technology is another factor influencing home health growth. Patients are now being discharged from the hospital to their homes with ventilators, total parenteral nutrition, chemotherapy, antibiotics, and peripherally inserted central catheters. The transfer of complex medical technology into the home setting has resulted in specialty home health agencies who hire nurses with the associated expertise to care for clients utilizing these various technologies.

Besides the aging of America, other demographic changes are influencing the growth of home health care. The size of families (number of children) is decreasing so that there will likely be fewer adult children to care for the elderly in the future, and these children will be older when they are needed to care for their parents (Clemen-Stone, Eigsti, and McGuire, 1995). Because women have longer life expectancies than men, there is an increased likelihood that older women will not have spousal caregivers when they are in need. The increasing rates of divorce and remarriage will surely affect future caregiving by some degree, owing to changes in the bonds of affection and obligation between adult children and their parents and stepparents.

HOME HEALTH CARE NURSING

Home health care is not new to public health nursing. In fact, *visiting nursing* (or district nursing) was the forerunner of public health nursing in the United States in the 1800s. Public health nurses focused on caring for the sick in their homes and also preventing disease and promoting health. In public health nursing in the 1930s, emphasis on caring for groups of people (versus individuals) began to emerge (Smith and Maurer, 1995). Now the terms *public health nurse* and *community health nurse* are used interchangeably as meaning the synthesis of nursing and public health practice applied to population groups.

Home health nursing is defined by the American Nurses' Association (ANA) (1992, p. 5) as a "synthesis of community health nursing and selected technical skills from other specialty nursing practices." In this instance, the specialty of focus is gerontological nursing. In 1986, the ANA developed standards for home health nursing practice; since then, the ANA has described the scope of home health nursing practice and developed a new certification in home health care at the generalist's level of practice. Within the *Standards of Home Health Nursing Practice* by ANA (1986), all home health services are planned, organized, and carried out by a professional nurse at the master's level of education with experiences in community health and administration. Besides focusing on the nursing process, theory, professional development, research, and ethics, the *Standards* also emphasizes continuity of care (discharge planning, case management, and coordination of services) and interdisciplinary collaboration (liaison role).

Home health care is often the deciding factor in preventing nursing home placement of older adults. Basic services covered by Medicare include skilled nursing; physical, occupational and speech therapy; social work; home health aide services; nutritional counseling; and medical supplies and equipment (Miller, 1995). Medicare requires that patients be homebound and have a need for intermittent skilled care and that the care must be ordered by a physician. (Medicare does not cover custodial care or housekeeping and food service needs.)

Home health nurses (HHNs) serve the client and family in a variety of roles: caregiver, teacher, supporter, case manager, advocate, counselor, advisor, and respite. Some responsibilities of the HHN include

- Assessing, planning, and evaluating the effectiveness of services
- Assessing and modifying the environment for convenience, comfort, and safety
- Coordinating care with other health care providers
- Monitoring family health, especially the caregiver's
- Increasing self-care capacity of clients
- Providing a link with other community resources
- Educating the family about reimbursement benefits

HHNs often have to emphasize different nursing abilities from those of hospital nurses. First, HHNs lack the immediate accessibility to other professionals and to resources like those available to hospital nurses, so HHNs must have a certain degree of security with their own competencies to effectively practice this role with its independent nature. Second, HHNs have to know how to deal with more social and cultural subtleties, especially if the family is of a different ethnic, religious, and/or cultural group from that of the nurse. (Of course, hospital nurses also encounter these differences, but they do so within their "own" territory, the hospital.) HHNs encounter the client and family in their own familiar surroundings, where client and family have more control over interactions, decisions, and nursing care choices. Third, HHNs also have to be very creative in improvising and adapting procedures within the home environment. Just to find a place for the nursing bag may be problematic in some small homes. Necessary supplies may be lacking if, for example, a sterile dressing becomes contaminated. Some hospital nurses are attracted to home health because of the day hours, only to find that they have less control over client behaviors and compliance and/or they miss the comfort of backup personnel and equipment.

Another factor that HHNs must consider during home visits is safety for themselves. Kendra and associates (1996) reported that home health care staff identified the following as risk factors in home visiting: geographical location, high crime rate, inappropriate behaviors of clients or others in the home, infectious diseases, and evening assignments. How did they try to solve these risk factors? The solutions included personal protective equipment, escorts, buddy systems, preplanning of visits, and safety programs.

The use of nurses as case managers or care managers in community health is not a new practice; public health and visiting nurses were coordinating resources for clients in their homes in the early 1900s. Case management is and has been a process consisting principally of client assessment and the provision, coordination, and monitoring of services. The new context for viewing the role of case manager is as part of a community-wide system to address the fragmentation and costliness of the provision of health care for at-risk older adults. Case management is needed not only in an attempt to reduce the cost of health care but also to coordinate health care for older adults across the continuum of care settings.

Caring

"Prevention of illness and injury through safety assessments and education regarding immunizations is a vital part of nursing care."

Case or care management is essential for comprehensive health care of elderly in all settings. Case management is similar to the nursing process in that it is a problem-solving process—one whose primary functions are to assess the health care needs of the client and family within their environment, coordinate needed resources and services to meet these needs, and then continually monitor the client's and family's progress toward optimum health (ANA, 1986). As case managers, nurses use their knowledge of physical, psychosocial, and environmental assessment; normal aging; disease processes; medications; treatments; health promotion; disease prevention; community resources; communication; teaching; coordination; collaboration; and caring. Nurses may perform case management services for the elderly in many settings, such as home health, adult daycare, health maintenance organizations, nursing clinics, senior centers, retirement communities, assisted living homes, and hospitals.

LAY CAREGIVERS

Another very important aspect of home health is the lay caregiver, who is often present or close by the client. The voluminous gerontological literature on caregiving generally focuses on the burdensome nature of the role (caregiver burden). Some sources discuss the positive outcomes of caregiving, but generally the discussion centers on the negative. The majority of caregivers of older adults are women—71.5% of the 2.2 million (Stoller, 1993). These caregivers are very important, not only for the family and client in terms of social and psychological support and physical care of the older adult but also for society: caregivers alleviate some of the economic burden of our nation's health care costs.

The HHN needs to focus on the caregiver *along with* the client, that is, to remember to include the client whenever possible in the whole nursing process—especially when any decisions need to be made about care. However, if the client is unable to participate in the decision-making process, then generally the family member who is the primary caregiver becomes the one with whom the HHN works in planning and implementing care for the client.

Hospice Care

Hospice care has grown rapidly in recent years. Factors associated with this growth include the aging of our population, the increase in medical technology, the spiraling health care costs, and the desire of some consumers to have more control over their health care. Hospice home care is a specialized type of home care. Hospice care is more a philosophy of care than a place of care; **hospice** was designed to give palliative care to terminally ill clients and their families in both home and inpatient institutions. In addition to physical care such as pain relief and symptom management, hospice focuses on the psychological, social, and spiritual needs of the client and families, helping the client to die with dignity, and assisting the family with the grieving process. In hospice care, one of the three main diagnoses of home care clients is cancer (Clemen-Stone et al., 1995). The slow progression of cancer often results in more home care for older adults with cancer than for older adults with other diseases. It takes a very knowledgeable, skilled, and caring nurse to effectively assess and manage all the complex variables in caring for a dying client and grieving family.

Presently, Medicare covers hospice home care for the same services given in home health care, with the additional coverage of outpatient drugs for pain relief and symptom management; short-term inpatient care, including respite care; counseling; and homemaker services. (There is a small co-insurance fee for outpatient drugs and inpatient respite care.)

The ANA (1987) developed standards for the practice of hospice nursing in 1987. These standards are similar to those of home health nursing in that they emphasize interdisciplinary collaboration and continuity of care in addition to the common core of the nursing process, theory, research, ethics, and professional development.

Undomiciled Settings

Homelessness is very complex and varied in its social, psychological, and physical manifestations, and in its causes and effects. This complexity is often reflected in controversies over the definition of homelessness, the number of homeless, and causes versus effects. People may be classed as homeless if they have no place to stay (i.e., outdoors all the time or in places not designated for shelter), if they sleep in emergency shelters, or if they live in cheap hotels, motels, or rooming houses (Smith and Maurer, 1995). Causes of homelessness among older adults may be related to the decline in number of available **single-room occupancy (SRO) housing** and the refurbishing of inner cities.

In the early 1900s, older white men made up the largest group of homeless, and often their situation was associated with alcoholism and mental illness. Today the demographics of homelessness have changed, even though men still represent the largest group. Older adults (aged 50 and older) represent about one fifth of the overall homeless population (Cohen et al., 1997), but, although this proportion of homeless older adults is less than previous years, the absolute number of older adults has increased.

Most homeless older adults appear older than their stated age. This premature aging is most likely associated with the harsh environments in which the homeless live—the cold, heat, rain, violence and threat of violence, and lack of shelter and accommodations—which often lead to hypothermia, hyperthermia, trauma, fear, infections and other illnesses, infestations, malnutrition, sleep deprivation, substance abuse, and/or accidents. Common acute physical disorders among the elderly homeless are minor upper respiratory tract infections, trauma, and minor skin disorders. Common chronic physical disorders are hypertension, cardiac disorders, peripheral vascular disease, gastrointestinal disorders, and eye disorders. Substance abuse is a major problem among the homeless, with alcohol being the drug of choice, although this can vary by region of country. Older homeless adults are more vulnerable than the younger homeless and live in fear of violence.

In a sample of 900 homeless individuals in St. Louis, DeMallie and colleagues (1997) found that 13% of the 600 men and 3% of the 300 women were aged 50 and older. The older adults in the sample were characterized by more men, more whites, poorer health, lower incomes, and more lifetime alcohol use than were the younger adults. The authors concluded that older homeless adults have differ-

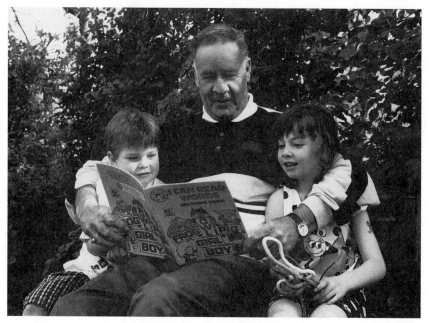

Older adults who live with children and their families can provide affectionate attention and learning enrichment to grandchildren.

ent vulnerabilities to homelessness than do the younger group. The needs of the older homeless adults include care for medical and psychiatric problems and substance abuse.

The nurse's roles in caring for older homeless people include all the roles that the nurse fulfills in caring for older adults in the community plus the roles that nurses assume when caring for the homeless. These roles vary by setting (shelters, clinics, health departments, churches), the nurse's capabilities, focus of care (primary, secondary, or tertiary), and the degree of assistance provided by other health care professionals. Nurses need to be cognizant of the complexity of environmental hazards and insults to the homeless elderly. Nurses have a unique opportunity to collaborate with many other community groups, and with the homeless themselves, in pursuing goals such as adequate housing, health care, and socioeconomic services for the homeless. Nurses need to advocate for the homeless by working with public and private agencies, professional nursing organizations, and governmental groups such as legislators, municipal councils, boards of health, and even members of Congress to improve the welfare of the homeless.

EVOLVING TYPES OF COMMUNITY SERVICES

The leading edge in living arrangements for older adults can be viewed in the advertisements of developers. Splendid architectural creations against tropical or desert landscapes are graced with smiling, healthy-looking older adult couples walking arm-in-arm, dancing, or playing golf. This dream world will come true for a few older adults, but, just as in earlier life, the majority will not have the money to afford such luxurious accommodations. Some will continue to age "in place" in their home of many years.

Aging in Place

NURSING CENTERS

With the majority of older adults aging in place, the types of health care delivery systems that will have more impact on them include home health care (discussed previously), nursing centers, parish nursing, and block nursing. Nursing centers have also been called community nursing organizations, nursing clinics, and community nursing centers. These centers give older adults direct access to nursing services, and nurses are accountable and responsible for the care. More nursing centers will become freestanding in the community; they will be run by advanced practice nurses in independent practice who are master's-prepared certified specialists in gerontological, community, family, or adult nursing. These entrepreneurs will hire other nurses (and even physicians) to assist them in caring for older adults in the community. Nursing centers focus more often on wellness, health promotion, and disease and injury prevention—covering nutrition, physical fitness, stress reduction, health education, health screening, counseling, and so forth. But nurses also diagnose and treat clients. With direct reimbursement to advanced practice nurses likely to increase, centers will very likely increase in number to serve not only the traditionally underserved portions of the elderly population, such as the homeless and those in poverty, but also those middle-class older adults who have medical care through Medicare but are still in need of the type of services that usually only nurses deliver.

PARISH NURSING

Parish nursing began in the late 1960s in the United States when churches started to employ nurses to provide holistic and preventive care to members of the congregation. The nurse or nurses hold a formal position within a church that is designed to minister to the members' physical, emotional, and spiritual needs. Parish nurses are giving primary and secondary health care to congregations that are large and small, rural and urban, and of various ages and faiths (Schank, Weis, and Matheus, 1996). The nurse's roles include educator, counselor, liaison, referral resource, advocate, collaborator, case finder, as well as change agent and leader.

Similar to community health nurses in schools and the workplace, the parish nurse serves a somewhat captive population. This fact is advantageous to many of the roles of the parish nurse, especially that of health educator. Older people often feel that they are in a trusting environment, whether they are in the parish facilities or homebound and being served by visits from members. This positive, supportive environment is a great asset to the parish nurse in promoting various healthy activities. An additional asset is that the nurse has the support and assistance of the minister and staff.

BLOCK NURSING

Block nursing may be one of the future trends in community health nursing. Originally, **block nursing** involved a nurse giving nursing care to people living on the same block as the nurse according to need rather than ability to pay. This innovative nursing model can allow older adults to remain in their homes even though they are not totally independent. One study found that 85% of the people served by block nursing would have been institutionalized if they had not received this nursing care, and the cost of the care was 25% less than that of custodial care in a nursing home (Jamieson, 1990). Various federal agencies and private organizations have funded some block nursing programs.

SHARED HOUSING

Many older adults who are aging in place need maintenance jobs done around the house or in the yard, and some live in fear of burglars or other violence. One solution to these concerns is shared housing, in which the homeowner rents a room to another person in return for home maintenance or other needed tasks, companionship, or rental income. Among older adults, shared housing usually involves an older homeowner with extra room who needs assistance with household tasks, needs the income, and/or feels safer with someone else in the home. Housemate-matching services have arisen to accommodate these people; nursing arrangements can also arise to accommodate these older adults in the community. Community nursing centers with associated home visiting services is a prime example, and these centers could help to serve other older adults living in other community arrangements.

ACCESSORY APARTMENTS AND ECHO HOUSING

Other types of evolving living arrangements for older adults include accessory apartments and **elder cottage housing opportunity (ECHO)** housing. *Accessory apartments* ("mother-in-law" apartments) are those created from existing single family homes into separate living space with a separate entrance, kitchen, bath, living, and sleeping areas. Often the adult child of aging parents will invite the parents to live in an accessory apartment; this gives the older adults privacy, independence, and the knowledge that their son or daughter is nearby in case of need. ECHO housing is a small, freestanding, factory-built temporary housing unit that is often erected next to the home of an adult child. (They are popular in England and Australia; other names are "granny flats" and "kangaroo housing".) They have the same advantages as do the accessory apartments: privacy and independence for both parties and proximity and convenience in case of need. Older adults in these community housing arrangements have access to community-focused nursing services just as do others in the same community.

Summary

Community health care of older adults is provided in a variety of community living and service arrangements. As the population ages, it is essential that first priority be given to wellness and health promotion. Nurses are in a unique position to teach many of the interventions that can protect the health of a community's older adults throughout the life span. A wide array of options includes interpersonal skills, social skills, disease and accident prevention measures, and care of the body through nutrition and exercise.

Most older adults will choose to remain "in place," living in their own homes until the end of life. Some older adults who remain healthy will opt for retirement communities where daily life is geared to the interests and capabilities of older adults. Others will be faced with a degree of dependency that arises from minor to severe disorders or disabilities, and there are facilities of many types to serve this population. Options for these older adults include continuing care retirement communities, assisted living, and board and care, among others. Nurses need to be current about the resources of their own community to help older adult clients make informed choices about their final years.

REFERENCES

American Nurses' Association. (1986). Standards of Home Care Nursing Practice. Kansas City, MO: ANA.

American Nurses' Association. (1987). Standards of and Scope of Hospice Nursing Practice. Kansas City, MO: ANA.

American Nurses' Association. (1992). A Statement on the Scope of Home Health Nursing Practice. Kansas City, MO: ANA.

Baker C, Stern P. (1994). Finding meaning in chronic illness as the key to self-care. Canad J Nurs 25:23–36.

Booth FW, Tseng MD. (1995). American needs to exercise for health. Med Sci Sports Med 27(3):462–465.

Burton Goldberg Group. (1995). Alternative Medicine. Fife, WA: Future Medicine.

Chernoff R. (1994). Thirst and fluid requirements. Nutr Rev 52(8 part II):S3.

Clemen-Stone S, Eigsti DG, McGuire SL. (1995). Comprehensive Community Health Nursing: Family, Aggregate, and Community Practice. 4th ed. St. Louis: CV Mosby.

Cohen CI, Ramirez M, Teresi J, et al. (1997). Predictors of becoming redomiciled among older homeless women. Gerontologist 37:67–74.

Connell BR, Wolf SL. (1997). Environmental and behavioral circumstances associated with falls at home among healthy elderly individuals. Arch Phys Med Rehabil 78(2):179–186.

Cousins N. (1976). Anatomy of an Illness. New York: WW Norton.

Dalton JR, Busch KD. (1995). Depression: The missing diagnosis in the elderly. Home Healthcare Nurse 13(5):31–35.

Davis MA, Moritz DJ, Neuhaus JM, et al. (1997). Living arrangements, changes in living arrangements, and survival among community dwelling older adults. Am J Public Health 87:371–377.

DeMallie DA, North CS, Smith EM. (1997). Psychiatric disorders among the homeless: A comparison of older and younger groups. Gerontologist 37:61–66.

Fiatarone MA, O'Neill EF, Ryan ND, et al. (1994). Exercise training and nutritional supplementation for physical frailty in very elderly people. N Engl J Med 330:1769.

Forbes E. (1994). Spirituality, aging, and the community-dwelling caregiver and care recipient. Geriatr Nurs 15(6):297–301.

General Accounting Office. (1992). (Report to the Chairman, Subcommittee on Health and Long-Term Care, Select Committee on Aging, House of Representatives), Medicare: Rationale for Higher Payments for Hospital-Based Home Health Agencies. Washington, DC: U.S. Government Printing Office.

Ghent-Fuller JB. (1996). The experience of anticipating death of self in healthy later life. Dissertation Abstracts. (University Microfilm No. AAIMM15009; Print index reference: MAI 35-03:0687).

Higgins DP. (1992). Continuum of care retirement facilities: Perspectives on advance fee arrangements. Special Issue: Aging in Place: Evolving Approaches in Theory and Practice. J Housing Elderly 10:77–92.

Jamieson MK. (1990). Block nursing: Practicing autonomous professional nursing in the community. Nurs Health Care 11:250–253.

Kane RA, Wilson KB. (1993). Assisted Living in the United States: A New Paradigm for Residential Care for Frail Older Persons? Washington, DC: American Association of Retired Persons.

Karns EL. (1996). A study of hope in a group of community-dwelling older adults. Dissertation Abstracts. (University Microfilms No. AAl1383076; Print index reference: MAl 35-03: 0792.)

Kendra MA, Weiker A, Simon S, et al. (1996). Safety concerns affecting delivery of home health care. Public Health Nurs 13(2):83–89.

Kincade JE, Rabiner DJ, Bernard SL, et al. (1996). Older adults as a community resource: Results from the National Survey of Self-Care and Aging. Gerontologist 36(4):474–482.

Kriedler KC, Campbell J, Lanik G, et al. (1994). A nursing center's use of change theory as a model. J Gerontol Nurs 20:25–30.

Lamborn R. (1996). Coping strategies and development of depressive symptomatology in community residing elderly. Dissertation Abstracts. (University Microfilm No. AAl9708087; Print index reference: DAl 57-10B:6580.)

Levenson D, Bockman R. (1994). A review of calcium preparations. Nutr Rev 52:221.

Lieberman M, Snowden L. (1993). Problems in assessing prevalence and membership characteristics of self-help group participants. J Appl Behav Sci 29(2):166–180.

Mahan LK, Escott-Stump L. (1996). Krause's Food, Nutrition, & Diet Therapy. 9th ed. Philadelphia: WB Saunders.

Mahon MJ, Searle MR. (1994). Leisure education: Its effect on older adults. J Phys Ed Recreation Dance 65(4):36–41.

Masoro EJ. (1992). Retardation of aging processes by nutritional means. Ann NY Acad Sci 673:29–35.

McCloskey JC, Bulechek GM. (Eds.). (1996). Nursing Interventions Classification (NIC). 2nd ed. St. Louis: CV Mosby.

Miller CA. (1995). Nursing of Older Adults: Theory and Practice. 2nd ed. Philadelphia: JB Lippincott.

Netting FE, Wilson CC. (1991). Accommodation and relocation decision making in continuing care retirement communities. Health Soc Work 16:266–273.

North American Nursing Diagnosis Association. (1994). Nursing Diagnoses: Definitions and Classification, 1995–1996. Philadelphia: NANDA.

Padula CA. (1997). Predictors of participation in health promotion activities by elderly couples. J Fam Nurs 3(1):88–106.

Palmore E. (1995). Duke Longitudinal Studies. In Maddox GL, ed. Encyclopedia of Aging. 2nd ed., pp. 295–297. New York: Springer.

Pender NJ. (1996). Health Promotion in Nursing Practice. Stamford, CT: Appleton & Lange.

Quinn ME, Johnson MA, Poon LW, et al. (1997). Factors of nutritional health-seeking behaviors: Findings from the Georgia Centenarian Study. J Aging Health 9(1):90–104.

Ralston PA. (1991). Senior centers and minority elders: A critical review. Gerontologist 31:325–331.

Report of the U.S. Preventive Services Task Force. (1996). Guide to Clinical Preventive Services. 2nd ed. Baltimore: Williams & Wilkins.

Rogg CS, Rogg OK. (1995). Georgia Senior Resource Guide. Atlanta: Care Solutions.

Rothman ML, Hedrick SC, Bulcroft K, Erdly WW. (1993). Effects of VA adult day health care on health outcomes and satisfaction with care. Med Care 31(Suppl 9):SS38–SS49.

Sabin EP. (1993). Frequency of senior center use: A preliminary test of two models of senior center participation. J Gerontol Soc Work 20:97–114.

Schank MJ, Weis D, Matheus R. (1996). Parish nursing: Ministry of healing. Geriatr Nurs 17(1):11–13.

Scott CB, Moneyham L. (1995). Perceptions of senior residents about a community-based nursing center. Image J Nurs Scholarship 27(3):181–186.

Scott EB. (1993). Circular victimization in the caregiving relationship. West J Nurs Res 15:230–245.

Smith CM, Maurer FA. (1995). Community Health Nursing: Theory and Practice. Philadelphia: WB Saunders.

Somers AR. (1993). "Lifecare": A viable option for long-term care for the elderly. J Am Geriatr Soc 41:188–191.

Stacey-Konnert C, Pynoos J. (1992). Friendship and social networks in a continuing care retirement community. J Appl Gerontol 11:298–313.

Stoller EP. (1993). Gender and the organization of lay health care: A socialist-feminist perspective. J Aging Stud 7:151–170.

Strickland D. (1996). Applying Watson's theory for caring among elders. J Gerontol Nurs 22(7):6–11.

Thorson JA. (1995). Aging in a Changing Society. Belmont, CA: Wadsworth.

Topp R, Estes PK, Dayhoff N, Suhrheinrich J. (1997). Postural control and strength and mood among older adults. Appl Nurs Res 10(1):11–18.

Travis SS, Duncan HH, McAuley WJ. (1996). Mall walking: An effective mental health intervention for older adults. J Psychosoc Nurs Ment Health Serv 34(8):36–40.

Weissert WG, Hedrick SC. (1994). Lessons learned from research on effects of community-based long-term care. J Am Geriatr Soc 42:348–353.

Williams RB, Chesney MA. (1993). Psychosocial factors and prognosis in established coronary artery disease: The need for research on interventions. JAMA 270:1860–1861.

Wilson HS, Kneisl CR. (1996). Psychiatric Nursing. 5th ed. Menlo Park, CA: Addison-Wesley.

CRITICAL THINKING EXERCISES

Joseph O'Malley, age 78, is a retired state employee whose wife died a year ago. Mr. O'Malley has continued to live in the family home, although the complications of his diabetes are becoming more serious. Circulatory problems in his legs make it difficult for him to perform activities of daily living, and a home health care nurse has been calling on him each day. Mr. O'Malley's three children live in other states, and he has refused to leave the house he shared with his late wife to join any of his children's families. Before his activity was curtailed by the problems with his legs, Mr. O'Malley walked to a nearby senior center each day, where he would chat with a number of old friends from the neighborhood. Two of these friends drop by his house occasionally now that he no longer goes to the center. The nurse assesses Mr. O'Malley's living arrangement and notes that his surroundings are no longer neat and clean, his clothes are untidy and sometimes odoriferous, and his meals when alone are lacking in variety and nutritious value. Mr. O'Malley insists that he is satisfied with the present situation.

1. What immediate interventions can the nurse take to improve Mr. O'Malley's health and safety?
2. What services are available in your own community that could help Mr. O'Malley to improve his daily life?
3. Looking ahead, create a plan that is designed to provide for Mr. O'Malley's needs if he is no longer able to live on his own. Take into account his advancing diabetes and his need for socialization.

CHAPTER 12

Acute Health Care

Annette Bairan, PhD, RNCS, FNP

CHAPTER OUTLINE

OBJECTIVES

After completing this chapter, the reader should be able to:

1. Conduct a panel discussion on the meaning and manifestations of ageism and involve the class in suggesting ways to counter ageism in self and others.
2. Describe the steps to be taken in orienting an older adult patient who is being admitted to the hospital.
3. Formulate three interventions for each of the "common problems" discussed in this chapter.
4. Discuss the reason for beginning discharge planning at the time of admission and specify five elements that must be considered when planning a patient's discharge. What is the disadvantage in beginning this planning at the outset?

KEY TERMS

ageism
continuity of care
discharge planning
iatrogenic
incontinence
minimum data set (MDS)
nosocomial infections
subacute care

Acute health care of older adults is generally delivered in a hospital, currently the most common acute care health delivery setting. Emergency departments function as primary care units for many older adults (and others), and the majority of patients admitted to general hospitals are older adults. The greater number of admissions for this age cohort arises in part because older adults as a group have a tendency toward reduced physiological reserves and depressed immune functions, which place them at greater risk for some types of illnesses and injuries, and they are also more likely to exhibit chronic health conditions with acute episodes.

Older adults admitted to hospitals are generally sicker than younger patients, and older adults are admitted more often and stay about twice as long, with managed care and prospective payment systems influencing their health care more and more (Fillit, 1994). Shortened stays have resulted in discharging every age group "quicker and sicker," with the more vulnerable patients (such as frail older adults) being more at risk for complications and other negative outcomes.

Hospitals are not always beneficial places for older persons. Creditor (1993) found that, in spite of successful treatment in hospitals, older persons with chronic illnesses show a functional decline, and nosocomial infections are becoming more common and more serious, especially for older patients. Others report that one-third to one-half percent of hospitalized patients lose function for reasons not related to their primary diagnosis (Inouye et al., 1993).

Hospitals are starting to improve services to older adults and to look for nurses who have gerontological education and expertise. Yet the majority of nurses who work in hospitals have little or no formal nursing education in the specialized care of older adults, and very few undergraduate nursing programs offer a required course in gerontological nursing (Hogstel and Cox, 1995). Nurses can fulfill many professional roles in the management of older adults in acute care settings (see Chapter 26). In addition to the direct caregiver role, there is a need for managers and administrators, consultants, researchers, teachers, and advanced practice nurses.

◼ OLDER ADULTS IN ACUTE CARE SETTINGS

When older adults are seen in the emergency department or admitted to the hospital, their emotions may range from relief (as symptoms are alleviated) to anxiety and high levels of stress. For those who have maintained health and vigor well into their young-old years, the need for hospital care may be an unexpected and unwelcome assault on their sense of autonomy and their perception of self. The middle-old may have lost friends with terminal illnesses who spent their last days in a hospital and so for them a hospital stay may have come to be associated with the end of life. Either of these groups, but especially the old-old—the frail elderly—may experience one or more of the following when hospitalized:

- Anxiety
- Fright
- Depression
- Confusion
- Disorientation
- Agitation

Being older and having been in the hospital during the past year are two of several characteristics that are associated with increased risk of nursing home placement and subsequent death (Wolinsky, Callahan, Fitzgerald, and Johnson, 1992).

Being alone and isolated from familiar faces and surroundings induces feelings of helplessness and dependency and can even lead to despair and alienation. Confusion and disorientation may follow, as the older adult's delicately balanced physiological homeostasis is disrupted. Nurses need to be sensitive to the psychological and emotional responses of hospitalized older adults to intervene successfully in their recovery process.

Confronting Ageism

Some nurses may have negative feelings about older adults. **Ageism,** discrimination based on a person's age, is still present in our society. The youthful beauty and vigor promoted daily by advertising and the media have turned our attention away from the mature beauty, serenity, and wisdom that are the hallmarks of successful aging. In addition, many people (including nurses) are uncomfortable when faced with aging because it reminds them of their own mortality. Nurses who carry such negative associations can have a detrimental effect on the older adults in their care that may be both subtle and unconscious.

Sulman and colleagues (1996) reported that hospital staff regarded long stays in the hospital by older adults (who were waiting to be transferred to long-term care) as "inappropriate" because they no longer needed acute care services. This attitude obviously interferes with quality nursing care. Hudson and Sexton (1996) found that older adults rated physical comfort and psychosocial activities higher than nurses did, whereas nurses rated *discharge planning* higher. Clearly, there is room for a reevaluation of the nurse/patient relationship in acute care settings, with attention focused on the individual patient and on the interventions that will bring about the highest levels of outcomes for every patient.

Orientation and Assessment

When admitting a patient to an acute care unit, nurses can intervene in a number of ways to alleviate the anxieties that accompany admission to a hospital for most older adults. A first step is to orient both the patient and family members or friends to the physical surroundings: the room with its furnishings, equipment, and toilet facilities; the degree to which these things are shared with another patient; and the room's placement relative to the nurses' station and public rooms (e.g., lounge, rest rooms). Second, it is important to explain the routines of the unit, the personnel who may be entering the room and what their functions are, the procedure and the situations in which

to seek assistance, and the answers to the patient's questions. When you work in a hospital every day it is easy to forget that the hospital setting is both foreign and intimidating to those who are unfamiliar with it, especially when they are ill or injured. Intervening to point out the supportive nature of the surroundings can have a positive impact on the outcome of the older adult patient's stay in the hospital.

ASSESSMENT TOOLS

Admission of the acute-care patient is always accompanied by assessment. There are many assessment tools from which to choose; some are comprehensive, whereas others assess only one area such as mental status. The nurse should choose one that is adequate for the type and scope of assessment needed in the work setting and one that accommodates the nursing framework. Assessment tools may be classified into functional, physical, psychosocial, spiritual, or combined parts (although sometimes the word *functional* encompasses biological, psychological, and social domains). Areas that may be covered are adaptation, mobility, medication, sleep and rest, skin, sensory perception, nutrition, digestion, elimination, metabolic factors, sexual concerns, cognition/perception, self-image, roles, and spiritual concerns (Loftis and Glover, 1993).

C a r i n g

"Ask patients how they would like to have their needs met. 'How can we help?' brings about patients' participation in decision-making."

Comprehensive geriatric assessment is performed by a multidisciplinary team that assesses physical, mental, social, and economic areas of older adults. The assumption of this type of assessment is that older adults (especially the frail old-old) often have complex, interrelated problems that can be better evaluated by a multidisciplinary team.

Physical health of older adults can be assessed by the Cumulative Illness Rating Scale, the Health Index, and the Sickness Impact Profile (Matteson, McConnell, and Linton, 1997). Functional status can be assessed by the Katz Index of ADLs (activities of daily living), the PULSES Profile, the Barthel Index, the Rapid Disability Rating Scale-2, and the Physical Performance Test. Functional scales measure ADLs and IADLs (instrumental activities of daily living such as shopping, preparing meals, housekeeping, transportation, laundry, and ability to handle medicines and finances). Social functioning measures social networks and social supports and can be assessed by the Social Resource Scale and the Social Dysfunction Rating Scale.

CONDUCTING THE ASSESSMENT

At the beginning of the assessment, the nurse should be sure to introduce herself or himself, if this wasn't done previously, and explain what is going to be done. Also, patients should be asked how they are feeling and if they are having any problems. A caring and concerned attitude will readily elicit information from the patient and help in establishing rapport. By listening and observing carefully during the assessment, the nurse can determine a lot about patients' abilities: communication skills, sensory/perceptual acuities, movement and balance, grooming, posture, body language, and skin and even about how the patient interacts with family or friends. Patients can be asked how they would like to have their needs met. "How can we help?" brings about patients' participation in decision-making. Allowing the patient to be in control as much as possible demonstrates that you respect the patient as an autonomous individual. If deficits are detected, the nurse's role is to become an advocate and provide support.

Next in the assessment process, any screening tests that are needed are completed. Then the patient is interviewed to obtain a personal history on significant areas such as activity, exercise, nutrition, sleep, rest, elimination, cognition, perception, sexuality, coping, values, and relationships. Last, an objective assessment of these areas is conducted, documenting all of the findings.

If the patient has been admitted to the hospital from a long-term care setting, the **Minimum Data Set (MDS)** assessment should be requested from the other setting. This is a comprehensive standardized assessment tool used to assess residents in nursing facilities (Matteson, McConnell, and Linton, 1997). It is one part of the Resident Assessment Instrument; the other part is the Resident Assessment Protocols (RAP), which provide recommendations for assessing and intervening in problem areas. Most nursing facilities use the MDS because it is mandatory for reimbursement from Medicare and Medicaid. Use of the MDS not only saves time for the nurse and the patient but should also greatly enhance **continuity of care.** The main categories of the MDS are cognitive, communication/hearing, vision, activity, and mood/behavior patterns; psychosocial well-being; physical functioning/structural problems; continence; diseases; health conditions; oral/nutritional/dental status; skin; medications; and special treatments. After completing the assessment, it is necessary to keep it updated.

Many adults older than age 75 years who are admitted to the hospital are physically frail in addition to having an acute or chronic condition. Yet research has demonstrated that physical frailty in many older adults is preventable and treatable. For instance, Schulz and Williamson (1993) found that physical frailty is not all physical: patients' and families' *perceptions* of causes and consequences of physical frailty partly determine the success of interventions. Older adults' perceptions influence their motivation and commitment to perform the interventions (desired behaviors) and even shape their expectations of what the future holds.

■ COMMON PROBLEMS

Falls and Restraints

Falls are a common problem for older adults, both in the community and in the hospital (see also Chapters 9 and 10). In the hospital setting, the most common accident among older adults is a fall. Serious injuries can result from falls, leading to morbidity and even mortality. Hip fractures are common; 20% of persons who fracture a hip will die within a year. Those who survive have considerable morbidity. Even after hospitalization *and recovery*, about 85% will experience a decrease in mobility 6 months after the fracture (Marottoli, Berkman, and Coonery, 1992).

The risk of falling increases with age, and older women are more likely to suffer serious injury because of their vulnerability for osteoporosis. Factors that are associated with falling can be intrinsic, such as age-related changes in vision, muscle strength, and balance; chronic diseases affecting gait, balance, or judgment; orthostatic hypotension; bed rest; and drug reactions. Factors may also be extrinsic, such as elevated beds, poor lighting, slippery floor surfaces, unfamiliar environment, and obstacles in the way of walking.

Wellness

"Research has demonstrated that physical frailty in many older adults is preventable and treatable."

Falls are often preventable, a significant consideration in caring for older adults. Risk factors that need to be assessed and intervened for include

- Advanced age
- Multiple illnesses
- Weakness
- Disorientation or confusion
- Agitation
- Visual problems
- Communication problems
- Room at a distance from the nurses' station

The patient should be monitored as often as possible—at least every 30 minutes and more often if judged to be necessary. Additional interventions include

- Provide for adequate lighting.
- Remove any obstacles in the way of walking.
- Clean up spills immediately.
- Offer bathroom assistance frequently to the incontinent patient.
- Explain how to call for assistance.
- Keep the bed in low position with side rails up (if approved).
- Teach family and volunteers how to assist the patient.
- Provide nonskid shoes.
- Elevate the toilet seat if low.
- Remind the patient to use grab bars in the tub and by the toilet.
- Remind the patient to use the walker or cane when walking.

Although restraints are sometimes used to prevent falls and wandering in older patients, their use is controversial. It is estimated that more than 500,000 patients are physically restrained daily in U.S. hospitals and nursing homes, and most of these are older adults (Strumpf, Evans, and Schwartz, 1990). As nurses, we know why restraints are used—to manage behaviors that may injure the patient or others—and we also know that restraints can cause morbidity and mortality. Examples include accidental strangulation, increased agitation and aggressiveness, feelings of lack of control, increased rate of nosocomial infections, and pressure sores (Matthiesen, Lamb, McCann, et al., 1996). Matthiesen and associates (1996) surveyed nursing staff about their knowledge, practice, and attitudes regarding physical restraints and found that the education of nursing staff and frequency of contact with older patients could not ensure nursing competency regarding the use of restraints. They believe that staff need nursing role models to assist them to solve problems about restraints and to seek alternatives.

Often families of hospitalized older adults have misconceptions about the use of restraints, and they often are not included in education about restraints (Kanski, Janelli, Jones, and Kennedy, 1996). Kanski and others (1996) surveyed 30 restrained patients on medical-surgical units in a general hospital (family members or guardians answered for 25 of the patients). The researchers found that nearly half of the individuals did not know that a patient has a right to refuse to be restrained and that family members have a right to be part of the decision-making process. Also, about half of the family members were not notified about their relative being restrained. The implications are clear: nurses need to educate family members and patients about the reasons for using restraints, the alternatives available, the length of time they will be needed, and the potential risks associated with restraint use. Nurses also need to check the patient frequently, remove the restraints often, use them only when prescribed, and document all actions.

Another study by Bryant and Fernald (1997) compared acute care nurses with chronic care nurses as to their knowledge and use of alternatives to restraints; the finding was that chronic care nurses used fewer restraints and more alternatives. Acute care nurses reported that they often could not use alternatives because of the patient's serious condition and the need for the use of invasive equipment. Box 12–1 presents alternatives to restraint use.

Adverse Drug Reactions

Multiple medications taken by older adults is a major health issue because older adults are at greater risk for adverse effects of drugs than others (Lee, 1996). Age-related changes, health problems, and polypharmacy can translate into harmful drug reactions. Chapter 10 looked at the dangers of polypharmacy for the older adult who is living in the community. The older adult who is hospitalized is perhaps at greater risk for adverse interactions of multiple medications, but an alert nurse has the responsibility to intervene and advocate for the overmedicated patient.

Age-related changes may affect the absorption, distribution, metabolism, and excretion of medications, thereby resulting in unexpected increases or decreases in the action of the drug. Age-related changes in the gastrointestinal tract are usually not sufficient to interfere with absorption of drugs from the oral route, but distribution of drugs may be affected by decreased total body water, decreased albumin level, decreased cardiac output, and increased adipose tissue relative to lean body mass. For example, decreased albumin can interfere with drugs that are bound and transported by albumin in the bloodstream, with the result that more of the unbound or free form of the drug is found in the plasma. This allows relatively more unbound drug to interact at receptor sites and increases the effect of the drug.

Metabolism of drugs may be affected in older adults, whose age-related changes may include a decrease in the size, blood flow, and enzymatic activity of the liver, where most drug metabolism occurs. This, too, can lead to increased drug concentrations in the plasma. Excretion of drugs by the kidneys is probably the most common problem area in older adults. Renal blood flow and glomerular filtration rate are reduced in older adults, which may result in an increased concentration, even to toxic levels, of the drug in the plasma. These age-related changes have led some health care providers to prescribe lower doses for older adults, following the rubric "Start low and go slow."

Older adults have more chronic diseases than others; this can increase the complexity of drug therapy exponentially. Medications prescribed for one condition can result in adverse effects because another condition is present.

Box 12-1 ## ALTERNATIVES TO THE USE OF RESTRAINTS

Pain relief and other comfort measures
Reality orientation
Pet therapy
Music therapy
Therapeutic touch
Reminiscence
Behavior modification
Companionship
Crafts
Active listening
Placing patient near nursing station
Beds in low position
Call light being accessible
Regular routine
Defusing agitated behavior
Diversional activities
One-to-one supervision

Sometimes the drug regimens are ordered by different providers who do not know the other medications the patient is taking. Nurses need to be vigilant in monitoring patients' medication regimens, not only observing their responses to the various medications but also detecting and preventing possible interactions.

Another potential problem in medicating older adults is the possibility that patients will take their own medicines, which they brought to the hospital from home. Hospital policy may prohibit them from bringing in medicines, but some patients still do so. And some will take their prescribed medicines in addition to the ones being administered to them. Some will take over-the-counter drugs also. The implication is that drug interactions may develop that cannot possibly be predicted or prevented. So older patients should be asked what drugs they are taking at home; or, if they have been transferred from a nursing facility, the MDS can be checked for medications. Then they can be asked if they brought any medicines with them, and the hospital policy regarding having and taking their own medications can be reviewed.

Caring

"Ask your older patients what medications they are taking at home and if they brought any with them; then review hospital policy regarding having and taking their own medications."

Confusion

Confusion is a significant sign in older adults because it may be the only sign of serious illness. Causes of confusion in older adults can be classified as neurological, cardiovascular, pulmonary, metabolic, drug intoxication, nutritional deficiencies, environmental, and psychological (Ignatavicius, Worman, and Mishler, 1995). Specific examples include Alzheimer's disease, cerebrovascular accidents, congestive heart failure, dysrhythmias, pneumonia, hypoventilation, fluid volume deficit, hypoglycemia, hyperglycemia, adverse drug reactions, unfamiliar environment, sensory deprivation, sensory overload, depression, anxiety, pain, and fatigue.

An acute state of confusion is called *delirium*. Delirium is often seen in hospitals and other settings that are unfamiliar to the person. The patient may attempt to climb out of bed, pull out intravenous cannulas, or become agitated, incoherent, and disoriented. Delirium is usually short term and reversible. Dementia, on the other hand, is chronic, slow, and characterized by progressive cognitive decline. Both conditions can be related to confusion. It is important that the nurse intervene when patients present with delirium—first to prevent injury, second to assess for probable cause, and third to treat or remove it. There are multiple causes of delirium, some of which include infections, medications, and surgery, as well as circulatory, renal, and pulmonary disorders.

Caring

"The caring nurse knows that if staff do not wash hands between attending to patients, the probability of nosocomial infections rises exponentially."

Miller and associates (1996) studied acute confusion among older surgical patients on an orthopedic/trauma unit. They found that acute confusion was a significant problem among the older patients, impairing the patients' ability to localize, interpret, and communicate discomfort to the nurses. Self-reports of discomfort were found to be unreliable as indicators of discomfort among the patients studied. Therefore, the authors recommend that acute confusion be a priority for intervention among nurses who are giving care to older surgical patients.

Nurses must direct interventions toward the presenting behavior of the acutely confused patient (e.g., disorientation) and try to discover the cause of this reversible condition, because removing the cause (when possible) often results in dramatic improvement. If the cause is environmental, such as unfamiliarity with surroundings or sensory overload in a critical care unit, then using the nursing process results in a goal of familiarizing the patient with the surroundings or reducing the sensory stimulation surrounding the patient. Confusion can cause great apprehension and fear, so it is important to give emotional support not only to the patient but also to the family. Nurses must explain the presenting symptoms and the possible causes to the family, tell them about the plan of action, and involve them in decisions as much as possible.

Incontinence

Urinary **incontinence** is the major reason for institutionalization of older adults. Many families perceive this event to be the deciding factor in discontinuing home care and placing the older person in a nursing facility. It is a very stigmatized condition, although television advertisements are now showing attractive old (or even middle-aged) women who can still socialize with friends while wearing a particular brand of disposable undergarment. Although the problem of incontinence affects men as well as women, television has not yet dared to suggest a similar solution for males. Some people believe that urinary incontinence is a normal part of aging. This, along with the stigma, results in its being one of the most underreported health problems.

More than 10 million adults in the United States are incontinent of urine. The psychosocial distress is great, and the cost is estimated to be over $10 billion annually (Ignatavicius et al., 1995). The many causes include neurological, urological, metabolic, and psychological disorders and various medications. Some specific causes of urinary incontinence include mental status changes such as confusion and delirium, cognitive deficits, depression, immobility, restraints, prostatic obstruction, urinary infections, cystocele, and rectocele.

Urinary incontinence is common in older medical and surgical patients, especially the frail old-old, who may have multiple system disorders. Thorough assessment is needed to determine the possible cause of the incontinence so that interventions can be directed toward it. Examples of interventions for incontinence include changing medication regimens, treating depression, treating urinary infections, removing restraints, and assisting with mobility to the bathroom. Additional interventions include Kegel exercises, limiting fluids a couple of hours before bedtime, scheduling diuretics at times more suited for patient's activities, keeping a record of intake and output, limiting bladder irritants (coffee, tea, and colas),

explaining the cause of incontinence and its treatments, and offering psychological support for a distressing condition.

Depression

Depression should be of major concern to all people who care for older adults. It is one of the most common complaints of older adults and is the leading cause of suicide in this age cohort. Major (or clinical) depression is different from the "blues" that all of us feel at times, and, amazingly, major depression is often undetected by health care providers. A survey of 149 registered nurses found that the nurses had a good knowledge base of the symptoms of geriatric depression—identifying the traditional symptoms *and* two other behaviors: irritability and blaming others (Proffitt, Augspurger, and Byrne, 1996). Nevertheless, the nurses reported that they were not assessing their patients for depression even though they had the knowledge base to do so.

Major depression is defined as having five or more of the following symptoms during a 2-week period (and at least one of the symptoms is depressed mood or loss of interest or pleasure) (American Psychiatric Association, 1994):

- Depressed mood most all day every day
- Decreased interest or pleasure in nearly all activities most of nearly every day
- Weight gain or loss
- Insomnia or hypersomnia
- Psychomotor agitation or retardation nearly every day
- Fatigue
- Feelings of worthlessness
- Difficulty in thinking or concentrating
- Recurrent thoughts of death

Of these symptoms, older adults are more likely to present with loss of interest or pleasure, loss of weight, insomnia, and fatigue (Blazer, 1993).

Major depression is hard to diagnose in older adults because some of the symptoms may be misperceived as part of normal aging. For example, consider insomnia. Older adults report more difficulty with getting to sleep, sleeping, early awakenings, and sleep being broken up into segments. Many older adults tend to attribute their fatigue to getting older, chronic disease, or to inactivity; fatigue could be due to the latter two factors but also to depression.

Wellness

"*Allowing the older adult patient to be in control as much as possible demonstrates that you respect the patient as an autonomous individual.***"**

Older adults sometimes experience memory loss or difficulty concentrating and are diagnosed as having some type of dementia, when in fact they are suffering from major depression, a treatable "copycat" diagnosis that, when missed, could result in institutionalization of the individual. This underscores the importance of nurses' assessing closely for the symptoms of depression during all their interactions with older patients. These observations can assist in more accurate diagnosis and spare the older patient and family much suffering and expense.

Nosocomial Infections

Infections are a major cause of death in hospitalized older adults. Decline in immune function is considered a hallmark of biological aging, and the result of this immune system aging is increased susceptibility to infection. Therefore, all health care providers need to be very diligent in preventing the spread of infections to hospitalized older adults. **Nosocomial infections** refer to those infections that were contracted in the health care setting that were not present at the time of admission of the patient—infections the patient acquired from health care providers or staff, other patients, or possibly visitors.

Hospitals house acutely ill patients who carry microorganisms that may be resistant to drug therapy. This increases the probability of hospital-acquired infections for all patients, especially old-old patients or those who have depressed immune systems. If staff do not wash their hands between attending to patients, the probability of nosocomial infections rises exponentially. A nosocomial infection acquired from treatments or procedures is termed **iatro-**

genic illness (which literally means physician induced). For example, insertion of indwelling urinary catheters may result in a bladder infection; insertion of an endotracheal tube may contribute to a respiratory tract infection; or insertion of intravenous catheters may cause thrombophlebitis. Nurses must use all precautions possible to prevent the spread of infections from patient to patient and to prevent infections due to inserting and maintaining invasive equipment.

Malnutrition and Dehydration

Some of the older patients in the hospital are malnourished. Factors that predispose older adults to malnutrition can be classed as social, psychological, and physical. Examples include poverty, social isolation, grief, depression, dementia, alcoholism, functional impairments, poor dentition, and difficulty chewing. These factors usually lead to a decrease in dietary intake, which, over a period of time, leads to malnutrition.

Wellness

"*Nurses can help older patients find a renewed sense of hope and security necessary for reaching optimal functioning and recovery.***"**

Nursing assessment should include observations of what the patient eats and how much. Good nutrition is essential for good health, yet in hospital settings patients may be placed on food and fluid restrictions (nothing by mouth, NPO) for relatively long periods of time before surgery or diagnostic procedures. Hospital food is often not appealing to patients, and some have decreased appetites anyway. Pain, discomfort, and bed rest all add to the problem. The nurse should ask about food preferences and try to incorporate them into the diet. The environment where the individual eats should be made as bright and cheerful as possible. (For more about nutrition, see Chapter 7.)

Dehydration is the most common cause of fluid and electrolyte imbalances in older adults (Chernoff, 1994). With aging, the thirst sensation is often decreased so that older adults may not consume adequate amounts of water. Also, intracellular water declines with age and with the loss of muscle tissue. Renal function also declines, which makes water balance harder to maintain. Nurses should be cognizant of these factors so as to monitor intake and output in older patients and intervene before they become dehydrated. Also, skin turgor may not be a reliable indicator of dehydration in older adults because aging is associated with decreased turgor.

Armstrong-Esther and colleagues (1996) found in one study that nurses' knowledge was inadequate concerning the fluid needs of older adults and the signs and symptoms of dehydration. All of the older patients received less than the recommended amount of daily fluid (2000—2500 mL), and patients who were cognitively impaired, incontinent, and dependent received less fluid intake than others.

Immobility Complications

Most nurses have a thorough knowledge of immobility complications. For older adults, the risks of immobility are greater than for other adults because of age-related changes as well as changes associated with chronic and acute conditions. For example, some older women are at risk for fractures due to osteoporosis, and immobilized frail and very old adults are at high risk for pneumonia, which is a common cause of death among older adults. Some chronic diseases tend to immobilize older adults because the diseases interfere with activity. (Severe congestive heart failure and chronic obstructive lung disease interfere with adequate gas exchange in the lungs.) Restraints are a common cause of immobility in older adults. Other causes are bed side rails, lack of staff to assist patients, cognitive impairments, major depression, and pain on movement. Nursing interventions include encouraging movement, passive and active range of motion, exercises (in bed, in chair, or standing), and ambulation.

◼ DISCHARGE PLANNING AND CAREGIVER CONCERNS

Discharge planning is more crucial than ever, with length of stay decreasing for all ages and categories of conditions, and with more sur-

geries being done on an outpatient basis. Today, **discharge planning** needs to begin on admission because of these shortened stays, so nurses must begin assessment of the patient's functional abilities and limitations as soon as possible. Placing older patients in appropriate settings after hospital discharge continues to be problematic, especially for long-term care. Social workers are good resources for placement problems and perform the placement role in many hospitals. When patients return home, home health care visits may be limited, and family members may be burdened by caregiving without adequate support or respite. Nurses can use discharge planning assessment tools to better determine appropriate post-hospital placement. An example is the Blaylock Discharge Planning Risk Assessment Screen (Blaylock and Cason, 1992).

Coordination of community services before discharge is necessary for continuity of care, especially because many patients are now discharged with complex equipment and materials that require complicated procedures to care for them.

Studies have shown that coordination of care, advocacy, and greater knowledge of older adults are keys to narrowing service gaps between acute care settings and home (Dugan and Mosel, 1992). In addition, more family members are performing the caregiver role, which has opened up a large area of study and concern in terms of how the role affects the caregiver, the care receiver, and other family members, and how these family dynamics impact our society in general. Short-term respite care is being used to relieve family caregiver burden and allow the older adult to remain in the community longer; some even suggest that hospital-based respite may be a viable option. Chang and others compared groups of older adults in respite, acute care, and living in the community (Chang, Karuza, Katz, and Klingensmith, 1992). They concluded that hospital-based respite resulted in a slight benefit for the chronically ill older group over the other two groups, even though iatrogenic illness and aggressive treatment are still potential risks.

People of all ages desire respect, dignity, and control of their environments, but older adults are especially vulnerable in these areas because of the losses they often experience as they age. It is essential that older adult patients be involved in both planning and interventions. In addition, families should be included in both planning and giving care to their older member. "In understanding patients and their life contexts and formulating treatment partnerships with them and their families, we can help older patients find a renewed sense of hope and security necessary for reaching optimal functioning and recovery" (Cutillo-Schmitter, Rovner, Shmuely, and Bawduniak, 1996). Families are often informal caregivers at home and thus can offer the psychosocial and moral support much needed by the older person when in the acute care setting. Families can be the link to the outside world, one strong enough to lead the patient to say internally "I am not here to die but to recuperate and return home."

Wellness

"It is essential that older adult patients be involved in both planning and interventions."

Finally, the process of caring for an older adult patient in an acute care setting should be multidisciplinary whenever feasible. The wide array of disciplines represented within an acute care facility is one of its greatest assets. For older adults, who may be admitted with more than one diagnosis or with an acute problem that is unrelated or only partly related to one or more chronic conditions, the ready availability of a variety of specialists is a major asset. With the cooperation of several different types of health care professionals, the most beneficial treatment plan can be created. Rehabilitation units are especially adept at bringing together a team of physical and occupational therapists, social workers, and others to work with nurses in assessing and treating older adults.

EMERGENCY CARE

Emergencies among older adults can be caused by chronic or acute diseases or conditions, accidents (especially falls), attempted suicide, dehydration, thermal challenges (frostbite, heatstroke), or any of the myriad causes that apply to all age groups. Emergencies may also result from disruption or failure of any organ system (e.g., cardiovascular, respiratory, neurologic). For older adults, emergencies are made more serious by the following factors:

- Age-related changes that increase older adults' vulnerability to diseases and injuries
- Different presentations of symptoms compared with other age cohorts (e.g., less fever, pain)
- Treating and stabilizing difficulties arising from their altered response patterns

In general, nurses need to treat presenting signs and symptoms (e.g., shock, hemorrhage, seizure, fracture, pain) and continuously monitor for clues to the causes of the condition, especially in light of the often atypical presentations that older adults demonstrate. Psychosocial and emotional support are very important to the older patients and their families, so nurses need to assess these areas, in addition to eliciting older adults' description of the presenting problem. Older adults' perceptions and understanding of illnesses can influence their motivation and commitment to better health and can also improve their coping abilities (Schulz and Williamson, 1993). Some studies have found that repeated utilization of emergency departments by older adults is reduced by intervening and referring those with mental and social health needs to appropriate services in the hospital and community (McCoy, Kipp, and Ahern, 1992).

Caring

"An alert nurse has the responsibility to intervene and advocate for the overmedicated patient."

SUBACUTE CARE

"**Subacute care** has emerged as an alternative for many seriously ill, but medically stable patients who still require highly skilled nursing/rehabilitative care and technologically advanced therapies" (Integrated Health Services, Inc. [IHS], 1993). Integrated Health Services subacute care is practiced in the medical specialty unit (MSU); this care alternative is intended to be a high-tech/high-touch environment—a "mini-hospital." Patients in subacute care no longer need the acute services of the hospital but still need skilled nursing or rehabilitative care and technologically advanced therapies. Subacute care provides many of the same services that hospitals offer but at a lower cost, typically ranging from 20% to 60% less than comparable hospital care. The cost savings is purported to be the result of not having to maintain other associated services such as operating suites and emergency departments. Acute care nurses staff subacute units with direction by board-certified specialist physicians. Patients are offered a "more comforting environment" that "de-institutionalizes" medical care with high staff-to-patient ratios (IHS, Inc., 1993).

Subacute care is offered to all age groups, and the specialties are increasing from general rehabilitation to wound, renal, pulmonary, pain, oncology, cardiac, surgical, Alzheimer's, orthopedics, neurology, and infectious disease management. Because subacute care simulates acute care nursing, the same assessments and interventions apply in this setting as in the hospital. More time for teaching and psychosocial support for the patient and family is possible in these settings when the staff-to-patient ratio is adequate.

Subacute care settings may be the wave of the future in gerontological health care. Yet one gerontological nurse informed me that she believed subacute care to be mainly a marketing strategy to make more money from Medicare. In Georgia, subacute units are licensed under nursing homes and the state health planning agency has no separate certificate of need for subacute care (B. Kurtz, personal communication, November 21, 1996).

Summary

Older adults who are admitted to acute care facilities such as hospitals have many of the same concerns as patients of all ages, but especially in later years they are vulnerable to issues of ageism, loss of autonomy, declining physiological reserves, and depressed immune functions. Nurses can ameliorate some of these factors by being sensitive to the uniqueness of the individual patient and by completing a thorough orientation and assessment.

Many nursing interventions are aimed at providing comfort and ease of mind, protecting the patient from physical harm, monitoring medications, preventing nosocomial in-fections, ensuring adequate nutrition, and supporting the self-image that undergirds the patient's ability to get well. Nurses work with the patient, the family, and other health care professionals to produce the best possible outcome for the older adult who is hospitalized. Acute care nurses can make significant contributions to the well-being of America's older population by caring for them when they are most vulnerable.

REFERENCES

American Psychiatric Association. (1994). Diagnostic and Statistical Manual of Mental Disorders, Fourth Edition (DSM-IV). Washington, DC: APA.

Armstrong-Esther CA, Browne KD, Armstrong-Esther DC, Sander L. (1996). The institutionalized elderly: Dry to the bone! Int J Nurs Stud 33:619–628.

Bryant H, Fernald L. (1997). Nursing knowledge and use of restraint alternatives: Acute and chronic care. Geriatr Nurs 18:57–60.

Blaylock A, Cason C. (1992). Discharge planning: Predicting patients' needs. J Gerontol Nurs 18(7):5–10.

Blazer DG. (1993). Depression in Later Life. 2nd ed. St. Louis: CV Mosby.

Chang JI, Karuza J, Katz RR, Klingensmith K. (1992). Patient outcomes in hospital-based respite: A study of potential risks and benefits. J Am Board Family Pract 5(5):475–481.

Chernoff R. (1994). Thirst and fluid requirements. Nutr Rev 52(Suppl.):S3–S5.

Creditor MC. (1993). Hazards of hospitalization of the elderly. Ann Intern Med 118(3):219–223.

Cutillo-Schmitter TA, Rovner B, Shmuely Y, Bawduniak I. (1996). Formulating treatment partnerships with patients and their families: A case study. J Gerontol Nurs 22(6):23–36.

Dugan J, Mosel L. (1992). Patients in acute care settings: Which health-care services are provided? J Gerontol Nurs 18(7):31–36.

Fillit H. (1994). Challenges for acute care geriatric inpatient units under the present Medicare Prospective Payment System. J Am Geriatr Soc 42:553–558.

Hogstel MO, Cox M. (1995). Hospital resources for care of acutely ill older persons. J Gerontol Nurs 21(11):25–31.

Hudson KA, Sexton DL. (1996). Perceptions about nursing care: Comparing elders' and nurses' priorities. J Gerontol Nurs 22(12):41–46.

Ignatavicius DD, Workman ML, Mishler MA. (1995). Medical-Surgical Nursing: A Nursing Process Approach. 2nd ed. Philadelphia: WB Saunders.

Inouye SK, Wagner DR, Acampora D, et al. (1993). A controlled trial of a nursing-centered intervention in hospitalized elderly medical patients: The Yale geriatric care program. J Am Geriatr Soc 41(12):1353–1360.

Integrated Health Services, Inc. (1993). Subacute Care: Tomorrow's Healthcare Today (brochure). Owings Mills, MD: Integrated Health Services, Inc.

Kanski GW, Janelli LM, Jones HM, Kennedy MC. (1996). Family reactions to restraints in an acute care setting. J Gerontol Nurs 22(6):17–22.

Lee M. (1996). Drugs and the elderly: Do you know the risks? Am J Nurs 96(7):24–32.

Loftis PA, Glover TL. (1993). Decision Making in Gerontologic Nursing. St. Louis: CV Mosby.

Marottoli RA, Berkman LF, Cooney LM. (1992). Decline in physical function following hip fracture. J Am Geriatr Soc 40:861–866.

Matteson MS, McConnell ES, Linton AD. (1997). Gerontological Nursing: Concepts and Practice. 2nd ed. Philadelphia: WB Saunders.

Matthiesen V, Lamb K, McCann J, et al. (1996). Hospital nurses' views about physical restraint use with older patients. J Gerontol Nurs 22(6):8–16.

McCoy HV, Kipp CW, Ahern M. (1992). Reducing older patients' reliance on the emergency department. Soc Work Health Care 17(1):23–37.

Miller J, Moore K, Schofield A, Ng'andu N. (1996). A study of discomfort and confusion among elderly surgical patients. Orthop Nurs 15(6):27–34.

Proffitt C, Augspurger P, Byrne M. (1996). Geriatric depression: A survey of nurses' knowledge and assessment practices. Issues Ment Health Nurs 17(2):123–130.

Schulz R, Williamson GM. (1993). Psychosocial and behavioral dimensions of physical frailty. J Gerontol 48(special issue):39–43.

Strumpf N, Evans L, Schwartz D. (1990). Physical restraint of the elderly. In Chenitz C, Stone S, Salisbury S, eds. The Clinical Practice of Gerontological Nursing, pp 329–344. Philadelphia: WB Saunders.

Sulman J, Rosenthal CJ, Marshall WW, Daciuk J. (1996). Elderly patients in the acute care hospital: Factors associated with long stay and its impact on patients and families. J Gerontol Soc Work 25(3/4):33–52.

Wolinsky FD, Callahan CM, Fitzgerald JF, Johnson RJ. (1992). The risk of nursing home placement and subsequent death among older adults. J Gerontol 47(4):S173–S182.

CRITICAL THINKING EXERCISES

Thelma Steinberg, aged 67, a widow, was admitted to the hospital with acute abdominal distress. Physical assessment and laboratory findings led to a diagnosis of diverticulitis. When medical treatment proved unsuccessful, Mrs. Steinberg underwent surgery for bowel resection. After surgery she was treated for some residual infection. Mrs. Steinberg was restless and refused to eat. She said she was afraid that "the stitches might break." She also refused to get out of bed, for the same reason.

1. Identify three nursing diagnoses for Mrs. Steinberg and create a plan of care with expected outcomes.
2. The hospital has a shortage of beds and there is pressure on the staff to release Mrs. Steinberg. In terms of available services in your own community, identify options available for Mrs. Steinberg and prioritize them.
3. Identify the elements of the MDS for Mrs. Steinberg if she were to be moved to another facility.

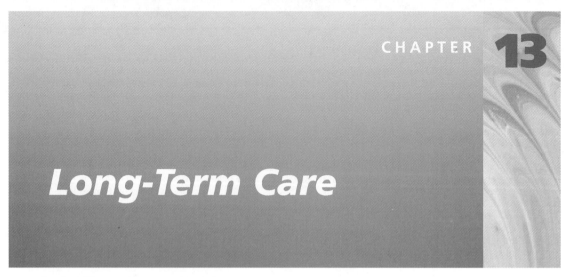

CHAPTER 13

Long-Term Care

Clari Gilbert, RN, BSN, MA

CHAPTER OUTLINE

OBJECTIVES

After completing this chapter, the reader should be able to:

1. Teach a classmate the standards that guide the practice of nursing in a long-term care facility.
2. Compare and contrast long-term care before and after the Omnibus Budget Reconciliation Act of 1987.
3. Describe the actions that are taken by a team conducting surveillance of a long-term facility under the guidelines of the Health Care Financing Administration.
4. Differentiate among the following purveyors of managed care: (a) HMO, (b) IPA, (c) PPO, and (d) Medicare managed care.
5. Discuss the advantages and disadvantages of private long-term care insurance.

advocacy
long-term care
minimum data set (MDS)
Omnibus Budget Reconciliation Act of 1987
resident assessment protocols (RAPs)
resource utilization groups

Long-term care refers to a continuum of services (e.g., preventive, diagnostic, supportive, rehabilitative, maintenance) that are provided over an extended period of time in a variety of community or institutionalized settings. Long-term care originally referred to care in a nursing home (Johnson and Grant, 1985). However, an array of services emerged in the 1960s that, while still available in nursing homes, are now offered in a range from home to hospital-like settings.

The evolution of long-term care has been influenced by many factors. Increasing cost of health care, changes in lifestyle habits, and biomedical advances have all contributed to individuals' living longer with physical impairments and disabling diseases and have created a growing mobile population who resisted the utilization of a less expensive level of care. The long-term care service model is constantly evolving to meet the needs of an evolving population, both on a social and financial level. We are entering the new millennium with an aging, better-educated, and healthier population and a health care system that is about to experience a major overhaul (Ford, 1995).

NURSING MANAGEMENT IN LONG-TERM CARE

Nursing management in long-term care is emerging in an environment that is faced with many challenges—a more frail population, specialized and subacute units, new technologies, and communities with diverse populations. It can no longer be an attitude of "business as usual" but requires one of constant creativity and thought to deal with the expectations of a customer-driven environment. The long-term care delivery system is affecting not only the performance of nursing management but also that of the entire nursing staff, as the phrase "doing more with less" becomes internalized.

Management can be defined as a process, with both interpersonal and technical aspects, through which the objectives of an organization, or that part of it being managed, are accomplished by utilizing human and physical resources and technology. In a majority of long-term care settings, nursing staff make up the largest group of employees with the largest part of the organization's budget and has the greatest amount of public scrutiny, customer expectation, and demand. Therefore, nursing management personnel must be prepared in both technical and interpersonal aspects of management.

The process of management achieves organizational objectives through planning, organizing, directing, and controlling. However, to be a successful manager in long-term care, emphasis must be placed on technical and interpersonal management. *Technical management* is the ability to utilize knowledge in the demonstration of skills. The long-term care manager is a hands-on manager, always ready to show and to teach. Some nurse managers leaving the acute care setting become very disillusioned with management practice in long-term care facilities. Hospitals tend to function in a highly bureaucratic structure where lines of authority are spelled out in detail and policies and procedure manuals are used to inform staff of structure and process. By contrast, in some long-term care settings, bureaucracy is entirely absent, owing to the lack of professional nurses and in-service education. *Interpersonal management* is the ability to establish a work environment where individuals promote team concept and goal achievement. The long-term care manager accomplishes this by being a proponent of positive change, accepting responsibility, and being able to relate to a wide spectrum of people.

THE NURSE ADMINISTRATOR IN LONG-TERM CARE

A nurse administrator in long-term care is a practitioner who upholds the standards of nursing practice, fosters an environment for professional development, promotes educational advancement, and provides for the highest practicable level of care. The person functioning in this role needs to develop a philosophical statement for the department or facility. In developing a philosophical statement, consideration must be given to the needs of both internal and external customers and to the values, goals, and cultural climate of the organization. The statement of philosophy must be specific, operational, and flexible.

The role of the nurse administrator evolves in response to technological advances, fiscal constraints, and changes in the health care delivery system. These changes and constraints are also responsible for the expanded role and expectation of the nurse administrator. The role of the nurse administrator is multifaceted and varies from facility to facility.

Qualifications for a nurse administrator vary from a basic diploma or associate degree with experience to a master's degree, depending on the location (i.e., urban or rural). However, with the current climate in health care, nurse administrators must take the challenge of being better prepared academically to succeed and to advance the practice of nursing in long-term care. With the implementation of a prospective payment system, nurse administrators have greater financial responsibility and must also be prepared in the business aspect of management. Interpersonal and conceptual skills are needed. The ability to relate well to others is paramount, because the administrator's success depends on what is accomplished through others. Conceptual skill enables one to see the overall function of the facility, not only the nursing department, because all parts contribute to the mission of the entire facility. This sometimes means crossing professional boundaries; but with the utilization of good interpersonal skills, collaboration with others can be achieved.

The nurse administrator in long-term care functions under the guidance of gerontological nursing practice standards. In 1969, the first draft of standards for geriatric nursing was presented to the American Nurses' Association. The standards were adopted in 1976 and revised in 1987 (see Chapter 1). These standards guide the nurse administrator in the implementation, evaluation, and supervision of care. In addition to the gerontological standards, nursing models form a conceptual framework for nursing practice.

Models of Care

A *model* is used to facilitate thinking and communication about an object or a concept. Models can be illustrated through schematics, verbal statements, and physical representations. Models enable a person to communicate an abstract concept in concrete terms. Table 13–1 presents several nursing models and the perspectives of the persons who developed them. Despite the fact that these models exist, however, most gerontological nurses still practice based on the conceptual framework learned in their academic settings. Although many models have been refined and expanded with emphasis on ethical principles and nursing knowledge, few have focused on gerontological nursing. The practicing gerontological nurse is wise to continue seeking guidance in applying these conceptual models to a unique population.

Methods

The two most common methods used in implementing care in long-term care settings are *functional nursing,* which is the assignment of care, according to tasks, to various categories of caregivers, and *team nursing,* which involves the assignment of a leader, together with a group of caregivers, who plan and give all care during a shift.

In addition to those two methods, however, there is *primary nursing,* a method of delivering care in which a registered nurse (RN) is responsible and accountable for the care of a resident 24 hours a day. This method is not practiced widely because of the lack of registered nurses in many long-term care facilities. However, at the Center for Nursing and Rehabilitation, a 320-bed nursing facility in Brooklyn, New York, primary nursing was introduced in the late 1980s to the nurses, nursing assistants (CNAs), and residents, and it is ongoing. The benefits of primary nursing to nursing management are increased accountability of staff, increased knowledge of the resident's needs, and increased resident and family satisfaction.

The nursing process forms the basis for the practice of nursing and is included in the definition of nursing in the nurse practice acts of many states. The nursing process involves the utilization of many components, which requires knowledge and skills of the nurse in the

TABLE 13–1. Some Conceptual Models of Nursing

Theorist	Model	Belief
Florence Nightingale	Environmental theory	Physical, psychological, and social environments need to be viewed as interrelated rather than separate and distinct parts.
Hildegard Peplau	Interpersonal process	Interpersonal relationships provide the basis for assisting the client in achieving mature development.
Dorothy Johnson	Behavioral systems	Humans are behavioral systems with multiple subsystems. All parts contribute to the development of the whole.
Lydia Hall	Care, core, cure	The three aspects of nursing interlock and are interrelated, with each aspect changing in size depending on the patient's course of progress.
Martha Rogers	Science of unitary (hu)man	Humans are unified beings who are more than the sum of their parts; they are constantly interacting with the environment.
Dorothea Orem	Self-care	Able individuals care for themselves in the maintenance of life, health, and well-being.
Sister Callista Roy	Adaptation	Humans are adaptive systems and use adaptive responses that promote integrity or wholeness.
Imogene King	Open systems and goal attainment	Humans are open systems who are social, rational, controlling, perceiving, purposeful, and action and time oriented.

management of the older adult. The nursing process can also be used as a problem-solving tool for the nurse manager who is acting as a leader to prevent or resolve problems, as illustrated in Table 13–2.

In addition to the nursing model and method utilized, the nursing process must be considered in evaluating care. Evaluation should utilize the same format as planning. If a plan was developed by a nurse manager, then the evaluation should be by the same person. If a team approach was used, the same approach should be used in evaluating care. The process identifies subjective and objective data and includes the resolution or redefining of the problem or solution.

FEDERAL GUIDELINES

In a long-term care setting, the governing body, known as the board of directors, is a group of individuals who are legally responsible for establishing and implementing policies regarding the management and operation of a nursing facility. A nursing facility must be governed in a manner that enables it to use its resources effectively and efficiently to attain and maintain the highest practicable physical, mental, and psychosocial well-being of its residents. The facility must be in compliance with federal, state, and local laws, as well as regulations, codes, and accepted professional standards and principles that apply to all professionals providing

TABLE 13–2. Leadership Model of the Nursing Process

Comparison of Assignment, Implementation, and Decision Making in the Delivery of Care

ASSIGNMENT

Function	Team
Nurse manager assigns tasks to staff members according to their job descriptions.	Nurse manager assigns staff to a team and a group of residents to the team; team member (nurse) assigns residents and tasks to team members according to job descriptions.

IMPLEMENTATION

Different members of staff perform assigned tasks for a given resident, usually without knowing what others do for that resident.	Each team member does assigned care or tasks for a number of residents; team leader gives care that team member cannot give.

DECISION MAKING

Nurse manager makes most decisions.	Team leader makes most decisions, often based on feedback from team members.

Nursing Process, Requisite Knowledge, and Leader's Role

Components of the Nursing Process	Background Knowledge and Skills Needed	Nurse Leader's Role
Assessment: Collection and analysis of data about patient, leading to accurate identification of problem(s) necessary in making a nursing diagnosis.	Theoretical knowledge of: normal physiology, pathophysiology, psychology, and sociology, including family and cultural beliefs, nursing specialties, and the nursing process. Skills in all communication techniques, systematic observation, inductive and deductive reasoning.	Assign competent caregiver. Facilitate caregiver's efforts. Establish rapport with patient and explain your role. Establish rapport with patient's family and significant others.
Planning: Making decisions about priorities of care, establishing goals, and selecting best nursing actions to achieve desired results, making adaptations as needed.	Above knowledge and skills plus knowledge about nursing theory, skills in performing nursing techniques, using problem-solving techniques, organizational skills, and stating nursing orders clearly and concisely.	Develop a plan of care to meet specific needs of the patient. Promote planning conference with team members to develop plan of care. Lead conference, and facilitate group's work (can delegate conference leadership to another nurse when appropriate). Can assist in the health care team's planning process. Implement effective problem solving.
Intervention: Efficient delivery of nursing care.	All of the above plus skills in supervisory techniques and teaching.	Assign competent caregiver. Give directions effectively. Observe caregiver's performance and patient's reactions. Teach both caregiver and patient.

(*continued*)

TABLE 13–2. Leadership Model of the Nursing Process (*Continued*)		

Nursing Process, Requisite Knowledge, and Leader's Role

Components of the Nursing Process	Background Knowledge and Skills Needed	Nurse Leader's Role
Evaluation: Recognition of change in the patient's condition: Comparison of recognized results with hoped for outcomes. Revision of plan of care. Conference with caregiver; ascertain need for team conference. Determine quality of care.	All of the above plus knowledge about evaluation techniques to be used throughout entire nursing process. Skills in judgmental analysis and measurement techniques. Determining reasons for any deficiencies.	Implement evaluation skills. Compare results to desired outcomes.

Nursing Process and Problem-Solving

Nursing Process	Problem Solving
Assess the patient.	Collect the facts.
Make a nursing diagnosis.	Define the problem.
Plan nursing intervention.	Select the solution.
Implement the plan for nursing intervention.	Implement the selected solution.
Evaluate the outcome of nursing intervention.	Evaluate the effectiveness of solution.

care. The governing body appoints an administrator who is responsible for the management and daily operations of the facility and must be licensed by the state of current practice as a nursing home administrator. The administrator (or executive director) selects a team of professionals to carry out the departmental functions of the facility. Figure 13–1 presents one type of organization for a long-term care facility.

▰ OMNIBUS BUDGET RECONCILIATION ACT (OBRA)

Historical Review

In the 1900s, public facilities were essentially asylums for the poor and chronically ill. The federal and state governments had minimal control over them. Federal involvement began with the enactment of the Social Security Act of 1935. Residents who lived in public facilities were not eligible to receive any of these benefits, providing incentive for the growth of private nursing homes. In 1950, amendments to the act permitted direct payments to health care providers. However, Congress required participating states to adopt licensing stan-

dards for nursing homes. In 1956, the level of federal funding was dramatically increased. The quality of care, however, was criticized in 1959 by a special Senate subcommittee. The committee noted that most nursing homes were substandard, with poorly trained or even untrained staff (Institute of Medicine, 1986). In 1963, the Public Health Service issued the Nursing Home Standard Guide (Fogg, 1994).

The enactment of Medicare and Medicaid in 1965 expanded the authority of the federal Department of Health, Education, and Welfare (DHEW) to set standards for nursing homes. Unfortunately, only a few nursing homes received certification. States were then mandated to set standards for nursing homes under uniform guidelines developed by DHEW. Congress continued to monitor nursing homes closely during the 1970s and attempted many changes, but pressure from various consumer groups resulted in an imposition of a congressional moratorium. In 1983, Health and Human Services contracted with the Institute of Medicine to study federal regulations that might enhance the ability of the system to ensure that residents in long-term care facilities receive satisfactory care. In 1986, the IOM report (*Improving the Quality of Care in*

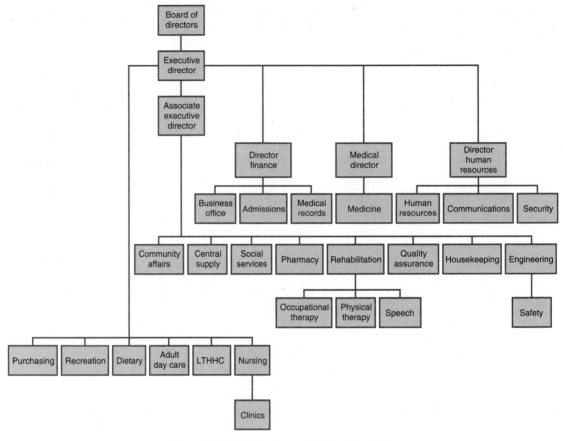

Figure 13–1. Table of organization for CNR.

Nursing Homes) concluded that new regulations were needed that would focus on actual delivery and outcome of care. The report generated much debate among provider associations, government agencies, professional associations, consumers, and community advocates.

On December 22, 1987, Public Law 100-23 was enacted under the name of **Omnibus Budget Reconciliation Act of 1987.** The final law contained three main elements: (1) conditions of participation related to resident care, (2) survey and certification, and (3) enforcement remedies and sanctions. These regulations were published in the *Federal Register* on August 28, 1992 (Fogg, 1994).

Implications for Long-Term Care

Some provisions of OBRA required states to adopt regulations that have changed the face of

long-term care. Elimination of the distinction between skilled and intermediate care facilities brought new challenges to operators and management staff. Mission statements were revisited and revised; new philosophies were formulated.

RESIDENT ASSESSMENT INSTRUMENT (RAI)

The requirements for quality assessment surveys were increased. States were mandated to implement a resident assessment instrument (RAI), which must include specific components established by the Health Care Financing Administration (HCFA). They are (1) the **minimum data set (MDS),** (2) triggers, (3) **resident assessment protocols (RAPs),** and (4) utilization guidelines. The RAI helps the interdisciplinary team to gather definite information on a resident's strengths and needs, which must be addressed in an individual plan of care.

The *MDS* consists of a core set of screening and assessment elements, including definitions and coding categories, that forms the foundation of the comprehensive assessment. Some states have added items to the core MDS that must be completed for each resident when a comprehensive assessment is required (Brown, 1995).

The *triggers* are specific resident responses for one or more of the MDS elements. They identify residents who either have, or are at risk for developing, specific functional problems.

The *RAPs* provide structured problem-oriented frameworks for organizing the MDS information about a resident's health problems or functional status. The information gathered from the MDS and RAPs forms the basis for the plan of care.

The *utilization guidelines* are instructions concerning when and how to use the RAI. The guidelines were published by the HCFA (SOM #272). Resident assessments are required 14 days after admission to a nursing facility, then quarterly, annually, and when a significant change of condition occurs.

NURSE AIDE CERTIFICATION AND TRAINING

Nurse aide training and certification requirements were mandated for all states. Nurse aides must complete at least 75 hours of training and competency evaluation from a state-approved training program to be eligible to take the state's certification examination. Before employment, verification must be obtained from each state's registry in which the nurse aide was employed. Continuing competency must be ensured through annual evaluations and at least 12 hours of in-service education. Recertification is on a biannual basis.

RESIDENT RIGHTS

Rights guaranteed to residents under OBRA can be classified into 10 broad categories:

1. Privacy and confidentiality
2. Medical care and treatment
3. Freedom from abuse and restraint
4. Freedom of association
5. Activities
6. Work
7. Financial affairs
8. Transfer and discharge
9. Grievance and complaints
10. Personal possessions

If a nursing facility fails to promote and protect these rights, it can be denied participation in the Medicare and Medicaid programs.

Wellness

"Nursing management can no longer be an attitude of 'business as usual' but requires constant creativity to deal with the expectations of a customer-driven environment."

Surveillance Process

OBRA 1987 established an "outcome-oriented" approach to the survey process. This was a shift from the previous focus of documentation compliance. The goal, however, is to determine compliance with the required codes for participation in the Medicare and Medicaid program. The survey is conducted by a multidisciplinary team of professionals on a 9- to 15-month cycle, is unannounced, and takes from 3 to 10 days, depending on the size of the facility. The team utilizes observation, record review, and interview to ascertain the facility's compliance with quality of care, resident's rights, physical environment, services provided, and other administrative activities.

The HCFA, a branch of the federal government, contracts with individual states to conduct nursing facilities' surveillance according to procedures set forth by HCFA and the individual state agencies. The team must complete several tasks during the survey process:

1. *Off-site preparation.* It is necessary to review all earlier survey reports of the facility, complaint investigations, and correspondence before arriving at the facility.
2. *Entrance conference.* The team leader meets with facility representatives to inform them of the process.
3. *Orientation tour.* The team tours the facility, identifying potential patterns of noncompliance for thorough investigation.
4. *Resident sampling.* Team members obtain a sample of interviewable and noninterviewable residents for quality-of-care assessment.

5. *Environmental assessment.* The team observes the physical environment to determine its impact on resident outcomes.

6. *Quality-of-care assessment.* Team members observe the overall performance of the facility's staff to determine that the care provided enables the residents to reach highest practicable physical, mental, or psychosocial well-being.

7. *Individual and group residents' rights interviews.* The team interviews residents, family members, or legal representatives to determine the facility's respect for their rights.

8. *Dietary services assessment.* The team observes dietary services to ensure nutritional content and that the service is conducive to quality of life.

9. *Information analysis and decision-making.* The team goes off site to assimilate its data to determine compliance.

10. *Exit conference.* The team leader presents the facility representatives with the results of the survey and gives the facility the opportunity to discuss findings and supply additional information if necessary.

A formal written statement indicating the findings and/or deficiencies is given to the administrator and a copy sent to HCFA by the state agency within a time frame specified by the state. Once the official results are received, a plan of correction is submitted (if necessary). If a deficiency is found, depending on its scope and severity, penalties can range from monetary fines to termination from the Medicare and Medicaid programs.

■ JOINT COMMISSION ON ACCREDITATION OF HEALTHCARE ORGANIZATIONS (JCAHO)

The Joint Commission on Accreditation of Healthcare Organizations (JCAHO), an independent, not-for-profit organization dedicated to improving the quality of care in organized health settings, was founded in 1951. Its major functions include developing organizational standards, awarding accreditation decisions, and providing education and consultation to health care organizations. The JCAHO has been providing accreditation to long-term care organizations since 1966. Its purpose is to encourage quality care and enhance public confidence. In addition, the organization gets the opportunity to demonstrate to residents and families its commitment to provide quality services. The revision of the long-term care standards in 1996 was a significant milestone. It completed the transition from focusing on capability to that of actual performance of the clinical and organizational functions that impact resident care (JCAHO, 1996).

The standards are organized in a framework that envisions the organization as an integrated system. There are 11 functional areas that are divided into two sections: resident-focused functions and organization functions. The Joint Commission has integrated a performance measurement system called ORYX into the accreditation process. The goal of the ORYX initiative is to establish a data-driven continuous survey process that will serve as a stimulus for health care organizations to examine their processes of care and take action to improve care.

Beginning in March 1998, accredited organizations must have selected at least two clinical measures to address 20 percent of the patient population. These clinical measures will be monitored by Joint Commission–approved measurement systems in which the organization has enrolled. The information collected will be transmitted to the Joint Commission on a quarterly basis and will be reviewed and analyzed for the organization's performance.

The JCAHO accreditation decision is based on how well an organization complies with the 517 long-term care standards. The levels of compliance are

- Substantial compliance
- Significant compliance
- Partial compliance
- Minimal compliance
- Noncompliance

The types of accreditation decision are

- Accreditation with commendation
- Accreditation
- Conditional accreditation
- Provisional accreditation
- Nonaccredited

An accreditation is valid for 3 years.

RESOURCE UTILIZATION GROUPS

Resource utilization groups (RUGs) is a patient classification system that groups patients based on activities of daily living needs, certain diagnoses, and the time utilized for care by the clinical staff. It is a hierarchical system comprising a number of groups, each of which has a specific index that determines the payment rate for the classification. This payment system enables a nursing facility to know in advance what its given reimbursement rate will be for a given period. Each patient is assessed by registered nurses who are state-certified assessors, utilizing a form called a *patient review instrument (PRI)*. All the residents are assessed and discharges reported twice annually on a schedule that is dictated by the state regulatory body. A revised case mix index is compiled and payment rates are adjusted by the state regulatory body retroactive to the first of the month in which the assessment was performed.

Impact on Long-Term Care

The increased number of "sicker" patients in hospitals has posed a tremendous financial burden on the Medicare and Medicaid systems because of the high percentage of older adults who could not be discharged. Before RUGs, the reimbursement rate for each resident was constant regardless of needs; therefore, most nursing homes did not admit older adults with a high level of medical or nursing needs. The nursing home environment was known for "custodial care."

The RUGs are to long-term care what DRGs are to the acute care setting. The systems impacted each other in a way that fostered partnerships and linkages between the nursing facility and the hospital. Incentives and disincentives were built into the prospective payment system to encourage the admission of older adults to the skilled-needs nursing facility and the discharge to the community of older adults with less-skilled needs. The higher the case mix, the greater the reimbursement. The nursing administrator in the long-term care environment was now faced with new challenges, from adjusting staffing patterns to increasing the knowledge base of the nurses and certified nurse aides.

Implications for Nursing

The RUGs impacted heavily on nursing and its functions. Approximately 75% of the categories relied heavily on nurses and their interventions. Nurse administrators were faced with making financial decisions that impacted the entire facility. The RUGs methodology is well into its senior years, and various strategies have been developed: the creation of special-care units for high and low RUG categories, different staffing configurations to meet the needs of the unit design, increased focus on staff education, increased computerization, the coming together of the nurse administrator and the finance director, and the entry of the nurse administrator into the boardroom.

SOURCES OF REIMBURSEMENT FOR SERVICES

Medicare

Medicare is a federal health insurance program for adults older than 65 years of age, as well as for people younger than 65 who have certain disabilities. It is administered by the HCFA of the U.S. Department of Health and Human Services. The Social Security Adminis-

> ## *Wellness*
>
> **"***A nursing facility must be governed in a manner that enables it to use its resources effectively and efficiently to attain and maintain the highest practicable physical, mental, and psychosocial well-being of its residents.***"**

tration provides information and handles enrollment. There are two separate parts: Part A, hospital insurance, is financed through part of the Social Security (FICA) tax paid by all workers and their employers; Part B, medical insurance, is optional and is offered to all beneficiaries when they become entitled to Part A coverage. It may also be purchased by most adults older than 65 years of age who do not qualify for premium-free Part A coverage.

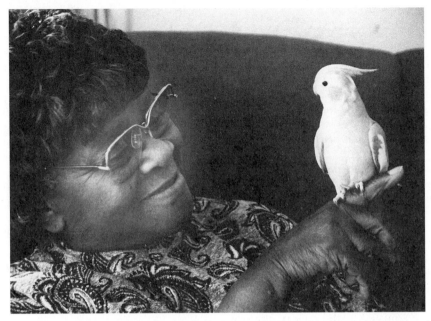

More and more long-term care facilities are introducing pet therapy. Pets brought to "visit" are a source of pleasure and stimulation that is much anticipated by residents.

Medicaid

Medicaid is a federal-state program that was established by Congress in 1965. It pays medical bills for poor older adults, disabled people, and families with dependent children who cannot afford the cost of medical or health care services. Each state has its own eligibility standards, with special requirements for nursing facility residents. A great difference exists for single individuals and married couples.

Eligibility for benefits require an income and asset (resource) test. Income and assets may not exceed a prescribed amount. The process involves total disclosure of all finances, and any attempt to defraud the program can result in penalties. Some older adults fail to apply for Medicaid, their reasons including fear of losing assets, lack of trust, and not fully understanding the process (Congressional Budget Office, 1992).

The Social Security Act, as amended by OBRA 1993, provided for a "look back" period of 36 months before the date of application for Medicaid benefits. This review is to check for transfer or disposal of assets. The look-back period for transfer of assets into trusts is 60 months (Fogg, 1994).

Veterans Administration Benefits

The Veterans Administration (VA) provides care and services for some veterans and their dependents in more than 150 hospitals, many nursing facilities, and various outpatient clinics throughout the United States. Many older adults may be eligible for medical benefits on the basis of their military service and can receive care elsewhere free of charge if unable to pay.

Some VA facilities provide long-term care. In other regions, contractual arrangements are forged with non-VA facilities to provide care and services for veterans and their dependents. State governments and some municipalities also have offices devoted to administering veteran programs and assisting veterans in filing for claims for VA and other federal benefits. VA medical center admission offices are the immediate source of information regarding medical care eligibility (Veterans Administration, Office of Public Affairs, 1995).

Long-Term Care Insurance

Increased medical costs over the past decade have caused older adults to become increasingly conscious of the need for long-term care insurance. Some older adults have experienced total loss of savings with a single illness. A number of insurance companies have advertised "nursing home insurance" as protection against losing all one's savings. However, a number of state insurance commissioners and consumer groups have questioned the validity of some policies. Therefore, the older adult should be cautious and seek legal assistance before investing in a long-term care policy.

Bruce C. Vladeck, head of the HCFA, in responding to a task force report on long-term care financing, stated, "While private long-term care insurance can provide a mechanism for some families to protect their assets, analysis of the last 20 years revealed that private long-term care insurance cannot provide savings for the public sector." He further stated that the real issue is not how to privatize long-term care expenses but how to meet the growing demand for long-term care with constrained public funds (*Nursing Home Regulations Bulletin*, 1997).

Managed Care

Managed care is a broad approach to controlling costs by arranging for care at predetermined or discounted rates. Managed-care plans vary in form, function, and quality. The best plans offer comprehensive care. However, caution must be taken, because the type of plan one chooses can affect out-of-pocket costs, the choice of physician, and the number of physician visits.

HEALTH MAINTENANCE ORGANIZATIONS (HMOs)

Health maintenance organizations (HMOs) were developed as an alternative to other health care systems. In 1973, the United States Congress passed the HMO Act as a means to help control costs. This act financed the development of Kaiser-Permanente medical program in California. Similar programs have since developed in locations across the country. A person insured by an HMO is funded solely for use of long-term care facilities that have contracted with the HMO. The care and services provided are also monitored by the HMO's case manager.

INDEPENDENT PRACTICE ASSOCIATIONS (IPAs)

In an independent practice association, physicians in private practice form an association and then contract with HMOs. This arrangement allows the HMO to expand its client base.

PREFERRED PROVIDER ORGANIZATIONS (PPOs)

The preferred provider organization consists of a network of independent physicians and hospitals that contract with managed-care companies to provide care at discounted rates. The care is not as tightly coordinated as that provided by an HMO, because clients can choose to see physicians outside the network by paying an additional cost.

MEDICARE MANAGED CARE

These plans often provide more comprehensive coverage than traditional Medicare. Although one continues to pay the usual Medicare Part B premium, the costs are generally lower than traditional Medicare as long as the patient follows plan rules. Because there are several managed-care plans, older adults must seek advice from health care professionals, their physicians, and family members.

ADVOCACY IN LONG-TERM CARE

Advocacy is the art of working with or on behalf of an individual or system to bring about positive change. The gerontological nurse has a strong duty of advocacy in caring for the older adult. The American Nurses' Association code of nurses dictates the responsibility of the nurse to be an advocate. The nurse is to take appropriate action if instances of incompetence by any member of the health care team or health care system places the rights of the person in "jeopardy." This obligation comes from the ethical principles of *beneficence* and *nonmaleficence,* as discussed in Chapter 3. This duty extends to populations at risk, and gerontological nurses will be challenged daily toward beneficence when working with the older adult. The belief that making choices about health is a fundamental human right is the motivating factor for the nurse in empowering the older adult. Ethical dilemmas arise when people are unable or unwilling to make choices (Taylor, Lillis, and LeMone, 1993).

Caring

❝*The long-term care nurse manager is a hands-on manager, always ready to show and to teach.***❞**

Advocacy requires knowledge, commitment, and accountability. The gerontological nurse has a responsibility to be informed of issues that affect nurses, patients, and the community at large. The issues arising from health care reform present opportunities to participate in informational sessions and forums, to educate the older adult, and to promote the advocacy role of the nurse.

POLICY AND POLITICS

The 1965 Older Americans Act mandated greater independence among adults age 60 and older. Its programs provide social, health-related, and advocacy needs through a consortia that spans federal, state, local, and private organizations. In 1973, amendments to the act included opportunities for more comprehensive and coordinated systems for the delivery of services. The act also provides for an advocacy role through legal assistance and ombudsman services, administered by individual states through the Administration of Aging.

The ombudsman program is a significant part of the act, providing help and information to older adults, their families, and friends regarding long-term care facilities and policies that govern them. The ombudsman visits nursing facilities, receives and investigates complaints, and refers serious violations of standards to state health departments for action.

HEALTH CARE REFORMS

The issue of health care reform has been a concern at the federal level for over a decade. Many recommendations have been made toward change; however, the cost:benefit ratio to those running for office often overrules the need for reform. Many states thus began the process of exploring reforms for themselves. The Clinton Administration actively embraced the challenge and released a draft plan based on six basic principles: security, simplicity, savings, choice, quality, and responsibility. Leaders from both parties have stated that they are united by mutual goals of increasing health care access and reducing costs. President Clinton assured the public that Congress would enact, and he would sign into law, a health care reform package by the end of 1994.

One of the major changes in the administration's long-term care proposal was a new focus on home and community-based services. This new benefit would have been available to all individuals with functional impairments in three or more activities of daily living or severe cognitive impairments, irrespective of age or income.

The 1994 election, however, triggered a "revolution" in the way long-term care policy issues are discussed and debated. Innovations in regulations and service design resulting from years of public policy, scientific and technological advances, and policy development were called into question (Wettle, 1995). Long-term care is on the brink of major changes, focusing on a continuum of care.

The American Association of Homes and Services for the Aging has advocated a continuum of care since it was founded in 1961. The economics of care, increasing consumer knowledge, and the demand for choices are now making a continuum possible. Nursing homes are no longer the only option. Senior housing facilities, adult daycare centers, home care programs, and senior centers are some alternatives. Assisted living is emerging as a new care model and an alternative to nursing home care (Goldberg, 1995).

Caring

"The gerontological nurse has a strong duty of advocacy in caring for the older adult."

Some providers are accepting the challenges by expanding their services, creating niches, partnering with other providers, and forming alliances to be able to provide a network of services. Long-term care nurses now have the opportunity to market their services as experts in both care and case management.

Summary

The significant revisions of Medicare and Medicaid statutes brought about by OBRA 1987 have changed the face of long-term care and brought about new approaches to caring for the older adult. As people live longer and longer, a more frail population of older adults has brought new demands and challenges to care providers. Nurse managers need to be-

gin to utilize existing models of gerontological care in the delivery of care to this unique population. As the economics of care impact long-term policies, nurses must grasp the opportunities for leadership based on their gerontological expertise, history of advocacy, and dedication to caring.

REFERENCES

Brown D. (1995). Minimum Data Set, Version 2: User's Manual. Natick, MA: Eliot Press.

Chin PL, Jacobs M. (1991). Theory and Nursing: A Systematic Approach. 3rd ed. St. Louis: CV Mosby.

Congressional Budget Office. (1992). Factors Contributing to the Growth of the Medicare/Medicaid Program. Washington, DC: Government Printing Office.

Fogg RJ. (1994). Nursing Home Regulations. New York: Thompson Publishing Group.

Ford AB. (1995). Long-Term Care: A New Model. New York: Springer.

Goldberg S. (1995). Where have nursing homes been? Where are they going? Generations 19(4):78.

Institute of Medicine. (1986). Improving the Quality of Care in Nursing Homes. Washington, DC: National Academy Press.

Johnson C, Grant AL. (1985). The Nursing Home in American Society. Baltimore: Johns Hopkins University Press.

Joint Commission on Accreditation of Healthcare Organizations. (1996). Long-Term Care Standards Manual. Oakbrook Terrace, IL: JCAHO.

Kron T, Gray A. (1987). The Management of Patient Care. Philadelphia: WB Saunders.

Orem D. (1991). Nursing Concepts of Practice. 4th ed. St. Louis: Mosby–Year Book.

Staab AS, Fernell-Lyles M. (1990). Manual of Geriatric Nursing. Chicago: Scott, Foresman.

Taylor C, Lillis C, LeMone P. (1993). Fundamentals of Nursing. 2nd ed. Philadelphia: JB Lippincott.

Veterans Administration, Office of Public Affairs. (1995). Federal Benefits for Veterans and Dependents. Washington, DC: U.S. Government Printing Office.

Wettle T. (1995). The nursing home: Are these the golden years? Generations 19(4):5.

CRITICAL THINKING EXERCISES

Obtain a copy of the OBRA 1987 regulations that were published in the *Federal Register* on August 28, 1992, and become familiar with them. Then, visit a local nursing facility and observe how these regulations are implemented. Describe the nursing model of care that is prac-

ticed. Is it consistent throughout the facility? Try to interview two members of the nursing management team. What are their qualifications? Compare their interpersonal and conceptual skills. Report back to the class on your findings.

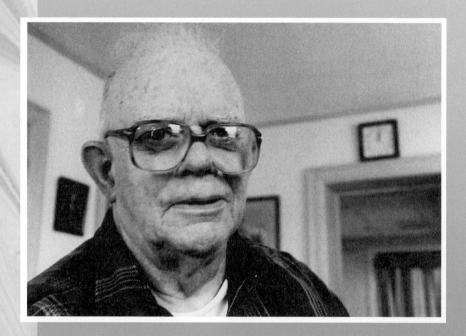

Physiological Challenges of Aging

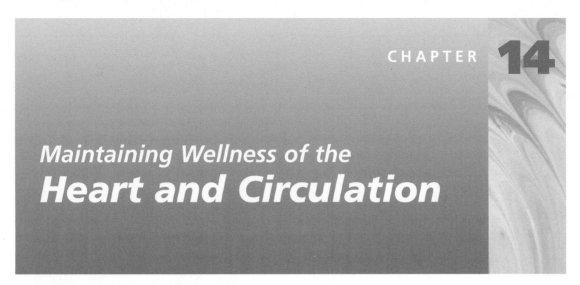

CHAPTER 14

Maintaining Wellness of the
Heart and Circulation

Mary Kipple, RN, MSN

CHAPTER OUTLINE

OBJECTIVES

After completing this chapter, the reader should be able to:

1. Teach a classmate how to inspect, palpate, and auscultate an older adult who is having chest pain.
2. Specify the signs and symptoms of congestive heart failure and contrast them to those of myocardial infarction.
3. Compare and contrast right ventricular and left ventricular failure.
4. Write a teaching plan for a patient who is being discharged after having sustained a myocardial infarction.
5. Interview a patient with cardiac disease and identify five nursing diagnoses for which you then write a nursing intervention.

angina
dysrhythmias
ischemia
myocardial infarction (MI)
stroke

Cardiac nursing demands an arsenal of information and skills to meet the health care needs of a mature adult. Knowledge regarding disease processes, complication intervention, medications, diet therapy, and ancillary resources provides a cornerstone in the base of care. Therapeutic communication, palpation, inspection, and auscultation round out the quality characteristics possessed by the registered nurse. This chapter is designed to assist the nurse in obtaining knowledge and skills associated with older adults who have been diagnosed with cardiac problems. To begin, normal age-related findings found in the older adult must be identified.

▮ HEALTH TEACHING

Cardiac health is one of the central issues of preventive medicine, and the media have been used with relative effectiveness to get information to as many people as possible. In addition, community health care providers disseminate information about maintaining a healthy heart from such varied platforms as community health fairs, public schools, places of employment, club and fraternal meetings, and universities and colleges. Care of the heart is a mainstream area of interest and concern. Teaching topics include the following:

- Promotion of aerobic exercise and workout patterns to fit a wide range of lifestyles, physical modifications, and interests
- Diet therapy, including balanced meal preparation, low-fat choices, and ethnic variations
- Function of cholesterol and triglyceride levels (these increase with age)
- Prevention or cessation of smoking
- Hazards of obesity
- Signs and symptoms of heart/circulation problems

- Identification of family-based illnesses (genetic disorders need early diagnosis, e.g., diabetes, hypertension)

Encouragement and praise by the health care team, especially the nurse, in conjunction with the client's enhanced understanding about the lifestyle adaptations that support cardiac health go a long way to ensure continued and improved healthy cardiac practices.

Education for the individual who has developed a cardiovascular problem is very different in pace from the preventive adaptations that can occur in small increments over the life span and allow for gradual incorporation of the skills into the person's health habits. Conversely, postdiagnosis tutorial sessions for the cardiac patient emphasize a rapid, radical modification of the habits of a lifetime. It is important to be aware that this requirement of abrupt change often results in the patient's having feelings of denial, resentment, and anger. These feelings must be recognized and addressed by both the patient and the educator before learning can take place. Remember, learning is an individualistic art that everyone practices throughout the life span by executing visual, auditory, and kinesthetic (hands-on) actions that are unique to each man, woman, and child.

Before developing a teaching plan for an older adult with a cardiac or circulatory problem, the nurse must identify the following learning skills:

- What is the educational background of the person?
- What is the individual's current mental status?
- Does the older adult have any impairments that will impede participation in teaching?
- Is the person cooperative and eager to follow the instructions?
- Are resources available to assist the older adult in carrying out the teaching plan effectively?

After assessment of the older adult's readiness, the nurse must consider what is to be taught and how the older adult is to be given the information. Return-demonstrations, or scenario play, followed by question-and-answer periods are the most widely used methods employed by health care personnel. It is important to teach the material in short time periods. Question the client periodically to ascertain the need for a break or for clarification of material that has already been presented. Nurses can teach in a nonthreatening manner by being adaptable to individual learning needs. In conjunction with cardiac care, information on medication administration, post–myocardial infarction (MI) care, dietary modification, pain control, overall safety, oxygen safety, infection, and sexuality should be supplied.

C a r i n g

❝Nurses can teach in a nonthreatening manner by being adaptable to individual learning needs.❞

After reviewing the following teaching guidelines, identify points of reference that can be incorporated into the assessment:

1. Cardiac medications (Staab and Hodges, 1996):
   - Take medications the same time every day.
   - Do not skip or double dose.
   - Take medications (except nitroglycerin) with food.
   - Take pulse daily if taking digitalis.
   - Report adverse reactions to physician immediately.
   - Know route of medication, whether sublingually or orally.
   - Do not take any over-the-counter medication without first getting approval from physician.
   - Know drug interactions with other prescribed medications.
   - Know overdosing and underdosing complications.
2. After an MI (Gleeson, 1991):
   - Know signs and symptoms of angina and how to treat.
   - Know when to report angina to physician.
   - Know activity level appropriate for client.
   - Provide emotional support to client and family in dealing with anxiety and changes in diet, exercise, and overall lifestyle.
3. Dietary modifications:
   - Explain low-fat and low-salt dietary restrictions.
   - Discuss calorie counts to maintain proper weight.
   - Suggest a workable diet the client can adhere to in view of finances, cultural/eth-

nic preferences, living conditions, and abilities to procure and fix food.
   - Explain a diet rich in vitamins and iron that can be achieved by the fixed-income older adult.
4. Pain (Herr, 1992):
   - Know prescribed medication, including route, and how often it can be taken.
   - Discuss severity of pain, duration, and location.
   - Advise on alternative measures in alleviating pain.
5. Safety factors (Jech, 1992):
   - Educate about storing of medication in proper receptacle.
   - Develop procedure for calling for assistance.
   - Advise to change position slowly, with adequate time to recover from dizziness or lightheadedness.
   - Keep list of medications, doctors, and disease states that can be found in an emergency.
   - Monitor initial exercise activities for appropriate usage.
6. Oxygen safety:
   - Insist on no smoking in area of oxygen.
   - Avoid flammable products around oxygen.
   - Use mask and prongs appropriately.
7. Infection:
   - Know signs and symptoms of infection.
   - Discuss safety factors for outside institution.
   - Monitor and prevent skin tears or breakdown.
8. Sexuality (Billhorn, 1994):
   - Help the older adult to express needs regarding sex and sexuality.
   - Instruct in ways the older adult with cardiac disease can have a sexual relationship.

▆ AGE-RELATED CHANGES

Age-related changes are those physiological deviations that occur in all people throughout the life span. To better understand the changes, they are divided into three categories: musculature and valve alterations, conductive pathway disturbances, and vascular system modifications.

Musculature and Valve Alterations

Brought about by poor dietary and exercise habits, alterations of the musculature and the valves of the heart take several forms. As accumulation of excess fat surrounds the heart, workload and efficiency of the heart are compromised. Excessive connective tissue production and enlargement of myocytes (myocardial cells), thicken the endocardium (Phipps et al., 1995) and lessen the pump's efficiency. Left ventricular muscle mass thickens by 30% (Miller, 1995). When the muscle mass becomes more dense, there is a slowing of the conduction pathway. Additional stimuli are required to initiate the pumping action but decreased myocardial contractility ensues, with cardiac output restricted (Polanski and Tatro, 1996). As the blood volume swells within the left ventricle, compensatory measures are taken by the heart. First, the left ventricle enlarges to accommodate the static blood volume. Second, blood flow reverses in a backflow manner until the whole body is compromised. Enlargement of the ventricle does not correct the problem; rather, it worsens the plight of the individual by impeding the contractility of the ailing heart even further.

Rigidity and thickening of the mitral and aortic valve leaflets produce two different phenomena: stenosis and prolapse of the valves. "Floppy" or prolapsed valves develop from insufficient amounts of collagen. Prolapsed mitral and aortic valves allow for a backflow of blood to take place, which thereby decreases the cardiac output. Stenotic or rigid valves are unable to close properly from too much collagen. Leaking or "oozing" of blood through the mitral and aortic valves prevails, with diminished cardiac output as a major consequence.

Conductive Pathway Disturbances

Myocardial irritability is attributed to the lack of stimulation induced by calcification of the conduction pathway or insufficient numbers of pacemaker cells. Ectopic beats and heart block occur when the conduction pattern deviates from the normal pathway (see Fig. 14–1). Electrocardiograms performed on older cardiac clients show an increase in the PR, QRS, and QT intervals. Broadening of these segments is attributed to calcification (Carnevali and Patrick, 1993).

Fibroplasia of the sinoatrial node makes for an inability of the heart rate to elevate during exercise, emotional, or physical *stress* (Staab and Hodges, 1996). When the heart lacks the ability to fluctuate, cardiac output is stalemated.

Vascular System Modifications

The ability to dilate or constrict blood vessels permits the body to regulate blood pressure. Deficits take place in the baroreceptors and the arteries themselves. Postural hypotension develops when the baroreceptors found in the aortic arch and carotid sinus become thickened (Staab and Hodges, 1996). Stiffness and rigidity of the arterial system prevent the arteries from compensating, by stretching or constricting, to regulate blood pressure. Arterial equalization is diminished by 50% (Staab and Hodges, 1996).

◼ GUIDELINES SPECIFIC TO ASSESSING CARDIOVASCULAR PROBLEMS IN OLDER ADULTS

The Interview

A good interview always begins with a demonstration of genuine interest in the client. After the introductions, the first step in assessing the older adult's cardiovascular condition is to ask for a general description of current symptoms. Because cardiac trauma is emergent, it is imperative to elicit information quickly. The following is a list of common cardiac symptoms and associated questions:

1. *Pain* is the most frequent complaint. Where is the pain located? How long does the pain last? Describe the type of pain. Does pain come before or after an activity, or during rest? How long has the client had this type of pain? Medications currently being taken for the pain, effectiveness, and time of last dose? Nonpharmacological methods of alleviating pain and their effectiveness?
2. *Shortness of breath* is the second most frequent complaint. When does this occur? How long does it last? When did it start? Does the client have a history of breathing

problems (e.g., chronic obstructive pulmonary disease, allergies)? Does the client require oxygen or high-Fowler's position to breathe? What medications are currently being taken, and when was the last dose?

3. *Edema* is seen in the client with chronic circulation problems. When did the client notice the edema? Where is the edema located? Is the edema pitting? What diet does the client currently follow? Does the client have hypertension? What medications are currently being taken for edema, and when was the last dose?

4. *Fatigue* is seen in clients with circulation problems and MI. Can the client perform activities of daily living (ADLs)? When does fatigue occur? How does the client describe fatigue and its effect on lifestyle?

5. *Dysrhythmias.* Does client feel heart racing? Does the client feel the heart is about to "jump out" of his or her chest? Has the client fainted recently? Why? What medications are currently being taken, and are they effective?

6. *Aching or tenderness in calves of legs.* Is there a circulation problem with possible complications of emboli? When did this occur? Is there bruising or redness of legs? Is there tenderness in the area? Can the client stand for short periods of time without pain? Can weight be borne on the affected leg? What medication is currently being taken and when was the last dose?

It is obvious, from the previous symptomatic questions, that the second most important question of the brief health history is to ask the client about the medication regimen. In most cases, the older adult will have medications written down or will describe them either by drug action or by color and shape of the medication. The nurse should be sure to ask the client how long the medication has been prescribed and check to see if all the prescription and over-the-counter medications taken by the client are compatible. Box 14-1 lists some of the more commonly prescribed drugs associated with cardiac disease.

Advanced directives and living will stipulations are asked about during the initial brief health history interview and should be updated or changed as the client wishes. As a health care professional, the nurse needs to be aware of the client's desires regarding lifesaving measures. One should be sure to document and adhere to the directives.

Physical Assessment

Physical assessment of the cardiovascular system requires inspection, auscultation, and palpation skills. The nurse should note all changes during the initial interview and repeat the assessment process whenever deemed necessary.

Caring

"Encouragement and praise by the nurse, coupled with teaching the client about the lifestyle adaptations that support cardiac health, go a long way to ensure healthy cardiac practices."

INSPECTION

In executing this phase of the physical assessment, nurses make use of their discriminatory olfactory sense and visual prowess in obtaining the needed data. When inspecting the older cardiac client, the nurse should look for the following:

- *Ecchymoses,* old or fresh? Circumference of the lesion(s)? Location of the ecchymoses?
- Is the *skin* mottled, flushed, or cyanotic? To test for cardioinsufficiency, instruct the client to elevate both legs at a 60-degree angle for 60 seconds, then have the client assume a sitting position with legs dangling. If the client demonstrates pallor in the feet with a slow return of color, mottling, or cyanosis in the feet, circulation is impeded (Lueckenotte, 1994). *Note:* A cyanotic effect can also be caused by a compromised thermoregulation process sometimes found in older adults.
- Presence of *surgical scars* in the region. How old is the scar? Condition of the incision? Signs of infection? Color and smell of any exudate?
- *Jugular vein distention,* observed when client is standing or head of bed is elevated 45 degrees. An abnormal finding indicates congestive heart failure or pericarditis.
- Is *edema* present? Where? *Note:* Ask the client how long edema has been present, and does edema diminish when extremities are elevated over a short period of time?
- *Dyspnea,* use of accessory muscles on inspiration. Does the client have orthopnea or exertional dyspnea?

Box 14-1   MEDICATIONS COMMONLY ASSOCIATED WITH CARDIAC DISEASE

Antihypertensive Drugs
Diuretics
THIAZIDE TYPE
Chlorothiazide (Diuril)
Hydrochlorothiazide (Hydrodiuril)

LOOP TYPE
Bumetanide (Bumex)
Ethacrynic acid (Edecrin)
Furosemide (Lasix)

POTASSIUM TYPE
Spironolactone (Aldactone)

Beta Blockers
Atenolol (Tenormin)
Metaprolol tartrate (Lopressor)
Nadolol (Corgard)
Propranolol (Inderal)
Sotalol (Betapace)

Alpha Antagonists
Prazosin (Minipress)

Central Acting
Clonidine (Catapres)
Guanabenz acetate (Wytensin)
Methyldopa (Aldomet)

ACE Inhibitors
Captopril (Capoten)
Enalapril maleate (Vasotec)
Fosinopril (Monopril)

Calcium Channel Blockers
Diltiazem (Cardizem)
Nifedipine (Procardia)
Verapamil (Calan)

Others
Hydralazine (Apresoline)

Dysrhythmics
Atropine
Bretylium (Bretylol)

Digoxin (Lanoxin)
Disopyramide (Norpace)
Esmolol (Brevibloc)
Lidocaine (Xylocaine)
Procainamide (Procan/Pronestyl)
Quinidine gluconate (Quinaglute)
Verapamil (Calan/Isoptin)

Anginals and Vasodilators
Nitrates
Isosorbide dinitrate (Isordil)
Isosorbide mononitrate (Imdur)
Nitroglycerin (Nitrostat, Nitro-Bid/
    Transderm/Nitro-Dur [cream])

Beta Blockers
Atenolol (Tenormin)
Metaprolol tartrate (Lopressor)
Nadolol (Corgard)
Propranolol (Inderal)
Sotalol (Betapace)

Calcium Channel Blockers
Diltiazem (Cardizem)
Nifedipine (Procardia)
Verapamil (Calan/Isoptin)

Anemias
Iron Salts
Cyanocobalamin (Vitamin B_{12})
Epoetin alpha (Epogen)
Ferrous fumarate (Femiron)
Ferrous sulfate (Feosol)
Folic acid
Iron dextran (INFeD)

Clot Busters
Dipyridamole (Persantine)
Heparin
Streptokinase (Streptase)
Urokinase (Abbokinase)
Warfarin (Coumadin)

- Color, consistency, and smell of *sputum*. If abnormal, when did this begin?
- Does client require *oxygen*? Oxygen setting? Use of extra pillows or high-Fowler's position?

- Is the client alert and *oriented* to time, place, and person?
- What is the color and amount of the client's *urine*? How many milliliters of urine are produced in an hour? In 4 hours? What is the

last 24-hour intake and output? *Note:* Decreased urinary output may indicate circulatory insufficiency or severe hypothermia (Miller, 1995).

PALPATION

The next step in cardiac physical assessment is palpation. Location of palpation, as well as questions the nurse should address, is as follows:

- Is there a *pulse deficit* between the apical pulse and the extremity? *Note:* Older adults may exhibit a pulse deficit between the apical pulse and extremities as a consequence of blockage.
- Are the *pulses* bounding, thready, or absent with the client in a supine position? Compare the pedal, posterior tibial, radial, and carotid pulses. Are the pulses regular in rhythm? *Note:* Do not palpate the carotids simultaneously or massage the carotid! What is the severity or grade of presentable edema? *Note:* In ascertaining the progression of abdominal edema, abdominal measurements should be obtained daily.
- Are *veins* in the legs tortuous? *Note:* Arteries and veins lose elasticity throughout the life span, creating a knotty sensation palpated on the venous system of the extremities. The nurse should not massage or palpate the legs of a client with questionable thrombus; instead, Homan's test should be performed.

AUSCULTATION

Auscultation will necessitate the use of a stethoscope. Both the bell and diaphragm are to be used.

- Does the client have a cough?
- Do you hear adventitious lungs sounds?
- What are the heart sounds? Normal S1 and S2 sounds can best be heard with the diaphragm. S1 signifies the closure of the atrial valves (tricuspid and mitral). The tricuspid valve is best auscultated at the fifth intercostal space closest to the left side of the sternum. Mitral valve auscultation is accomplished by listening to the apex of the heart. An apical pulse is counted over a 1-minute duration. Attention should be paid to rate and regularity.

S2 signifies the closure of the ventricles or aortic and pulmonic valves. The aortic valve is best heard at the client's right side, at the second intercostal space adjacent to the pulmonic valve. Any sound heard other than these two are adventitious and are best heard using the bell of the stethoscope. Documentation of the heart sounds should include location and a description of any adventitious sound.

Grading Heart Murmurs

The loudness of the murmur is assessed on auscultation. A grade I murmur is very faint to auscultate. Grade III murmurs are moderately loud. Grade IV murmurs are loud, grade V are very loud, and grade VI are extremely loud (Polanski and Tatro, 1996). *Note:* Conditions that can hamper the nurse in completing the task of auscultation include an increase in the anteroposterior diameter of the rib cage and a rigidity generated by the calcification of the intercostal cartilage. These conditions set up a barrier in which the heart sounds are either muffled or nonexistent. Placement of the stethoscope directly on the client's skin should ameliorate the situation. Providing a quiet environment during the examination will also assist the nurse in better auscultation.

> ### C a r i n g
> *"Practical application of care mapping requires the nurse to be realistic in identifying nursing diagnoses and planning interventions with outcomes that the client can achieve."*

Diagnostic Tests

NONINVASIVE TESTING

1. *Chest radiography:* allows visualization of size and contour of the heart. Enlargement or displacement of the heart, and presence of abdominal aortic aneurysm, can be seen on a radiograph.
2. *Computed tomography:* surveys for left ventricular wall motion, cardiac tumors, myocardial infarction, aortic dissection, and aneurysm (Beare and Meyers, 1994).

TABLE 14–1. Diagnostic Tests Associated with Cardiac Disease

Lab Test Ordered	Elevated Level	Below Normal Level
Complete blood cell count		
1. Red blood cell count	Congestive heart failure	Endocarditis
2. Hematocrit	Hypovolemic shock	Anemia
3. White blood cell count	Infective endocarditis	No cardiac problems
		Thrombus
		Disseminated intravascular coagulation
Prothrombin time and partial thromboplastin time		
Fibrinogen		
Enzyme studies for myocardial infarction (MI)		
1. CPK-MB	Five times greater within 6 h of MI	Back to normal 48–72 h
2. Lactate dehydrogenase	MI	Returns to normal within 72 h
3. Aspartate aminotransferase	Hemolytic anemia is three times greater within 24 h of MI	Returns to normal within 11 days
Arterial blood gases	MI	
1. pH	Alkalosis	Acidosis
2. P_{CO_2}	Acidosis (respiratory)	Alkalosis (respiratory)
3. HCO_3	Alkalosis (metabolic)	Acidosis (metabolic)
P_{O_2}	Administration of high dose of oxygen	Hypoxia
Serum folic acid	None	Anemia

3. *Echocardiography:* emits high-frequency sound waves to diagnose congenital heart disease, cardiomyopathies, and intracardiac masses (Beare and Meyers, 1994). Doppler echocardiograms evaluate the direction of blood flow within the heart. Contrast echocardiograms highlight cardiac structure abnormalities.
4. *Electrocardiography* (ECG): Table 14–2 lists the components of the ECG strip. Normal duration of each segment plus indications of each waveform are also inserted into Table 14–2. *Note:* The ECG can only show the electrical current of the heart, not the diastole or systole. To test for actual contraction of the heart, a pulse must be present.

5. *Magnetic resonance imaging:* detects coronary artery disease and cardiac masses.
6. *Ultrasonography:* specific for coronary artery disease, venous occlusion, and venous insufficiency.

INVASIVE TESTING

1. *Cardiac catheterization:* visualizes the coronary arteries and blockage using contrast dye and radiographs.
2. *Central venous pressure:* must be obtained from a central line and measures right atrial pressure. Normal values are 4 to 12 cm H_2O.
3. *Pulmonary capillary wedge pressure:* measures the left ventricle preload or filling pressure. Normal values are 8 to 12 mm Hg.

TABLE 14–2. Components of the Electrocardiogram

Waveform	Normal	Indication
p wave	0.06–0.12 second	Contraction of atria
PR interval	0.12–0.20 second	Sinoatrial to atrioventricular node transmission
QRS complex	0.06–0.10 second	Contraction of ventricles
t wave	0.16 second	Relaxation of ventricles

4. *Thallium stress test:* measures the severity of coronary heart disease by means of injecting thallium contrast medium into the client and having the client exercise on a treadmill to detect ischemia and infarction of cardiac muscle (Lewis and Collier, 1992).
5. *Venography:* identifies thrombus in lower legs by injection of radiopaque dye into the client intravenously. This dye highlights an area of block-age in the affected leg with the use of radiography.

■ COMMON DISORDERS

Cardiovascular disorders are divided into three categories. The first category pays attention to diseases inclusive of the heart musculature, circulation, or conduction pathway. The second category discusses the diseases of the vascular system throughout the body. Congestive heart disease is included in this category because it is a multidimensional disease process that affects the whole body, not just the cardiac system. The third category is devoted to anemias.

Caring

Be sure to ask the client how long the medication has been prescribed and check to see if all the prescription and over-the-counter medications taken by the client are compatible.

Coronary Heart Disease

With coronary heart disease (CAD), blockage of the coronary arteries, or atherosclerosis, may occur suddenly or gradually. Over the life span, arterial walls gradually narrow as a result of plaque buildup. In the majority of cases, excessive fat intake in our diet is the main contributor to "hardening of the arteries" and a gradual narrowing of the wall diameter. *Sudden* blockage of the coronary arteries, by some other form of embolism, occurs occasionally.

Diagnostic tests and findings include

1. Electrocardiography: elevation in the ST segment.
2. Thallium studies: stress testing of the heart by strenuous exercise. Changes in the ECG will be noted; watch for the client to become dyspneic or complain of angina.

3. Cardiac catheterization: visualization of degree and location of blockage.

Angina

In angina, lactic acid production generates chest pain (**angina**) when arterial occlusion deprives the tissue of life-sustaining blood (**ischemia**). Two types of angina exist. Stable angina happens as stress is placed on the heart to increase its circulation during heavy work or exercise. Stopping the exercise or work plus administering nitroglycerin tablets (to dilate the blood vessels) lessens or stops the pain. Unstable angina arises at any time during rest or exercise. This form of angina is more serious and reflects a dire situation of the heart not being able to obtain an adequate supply of blood at any time. Employing the tactics of decreasing exercise and nitroglycerin does not have a positive effect. Clients will complain of amplified pain with no relief from nitroglycerin.

Myocardial Infarction

Eventually, if not treated, the muscle tissue dies (infarction) from lack of oxygen and nutrients. **Myocardial infarction** is the name for death of the heart muscle. Once the muscle has infarcted, that area of the heart ceases to function. The healthy portion of the heart is now required to pull the extra workload, thereby contributing to a future overload on an already compromised heart. Overload on the damaged heart lays the groundwork for a number of signs and symptoms exhibited by the client. Less obvious symptoms identified in the elderly cardiac client are

- *Shortness of breath* influenced by the impaired pumping action of the heart. This exists as an attempt to restore the waning oxygen supply of the body. The older adult may voice "not being able to catch my breath," or the nurse may observe shortness of breath while the client is at rest.
- *Inability to concentrate and/or disorientation.* The client may exhibit inabilities to keep a train of thought during the interview or may become "fuzzy" on important dates. The nurse should evaluate the client's orientation to time, place, and person. *Note:* The sudden onset of disorientation or a lack of concentration may indicate marked cardiac insuffi-

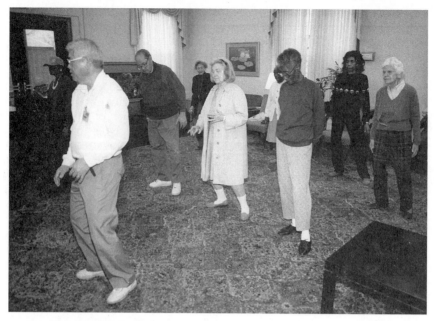

Tai ch'i is a spiritual practice that encompasses physical exercise and stress reduction.

ciency. However, more data gathering is needed to confirm diagnosis. A gradual descent in concentration may indicate noncardiac problems such as hypothermia, dementia, and metabolic disorders, to name a few.

The classic symptoms associated with myocardial infarction disease are listed below:

- The *fear* reaction. The older client may encounter feelings of apprehension, anxiety, and distress, characterized by "an overwhelming sense that something is wrong physically, or of impending death" (Polanski and Tatro, 1996).
- *Pain* is identified by degrees of intensity and location. Chest pain, the most common form of pain, is usually described by the client as being unrelenting heartburn, tightness, or a crushing sensation in the substernal area. Referred pain typically presents in the areas of the jaw, back, or left arm and can occasionally express itself in the right arm or as epigastric pain. Pain severity may be expressed on a continuum ranging from a mild "uncomfortable tightness in the chest" to severe crushing pain (Polanski and Tatro, 1996). An important assessment tool employed by the cardiac nurse involves the database regarding pain severity, location, and duration elicited from the client on admission.

- *Denial* of clinical symptoms deters the medical response time of a client who is experiencing MI. This self-misdiagnosis of symptoms on the older client's part can result in extensive damage to the already-compromised heart. (Refer to the section on health teaching for a discussion of ideas to combat this problem.)
- *Palpitations* suffered by the MI client are tachycardic and result from a decreased circulating blood volume, which is in direct relation to the impaired pumping action of the heart. When the heart becomes ischemic from lack of proper blood flow (CAD, emboli), a message is sent from the heart to increase the rate of contraction or pumping action to compensate for the blood flow deficit, causing the heart to become tachycardic. If the heart muscle deteriorates as a consequence of infarction, the strength of heart muscle contractility is compromised, thereby hampering blood flow. Once more the heart induces tachycardia to meet the blood flow demand. Verbally, the client will define the palpitations as "my heart is racing" or "I feel like my heart is about to jump out of my chest."
- *Weakness, diaphoresis,* and *pallor* will be seen simultaneously. The client complains of

generalized weakness, is pale in color, and is diaphoretic. These three symptoms are associated with a decreased *cardiac output* or blood flow. As cardiac output diminishes, blood is rerouted to the vital organs (the heart, brain, lungs) from the other less-important organs (stomach, liver, spleen, muscles). Without proper nutrients and oxygen, tissues decrease their activities as a conservation tactic.

- *Cardiogenic shock* will occur when 40% or more of the left ventricle is damaged after MI (Phipps et al., 1995). Hypoperfusion presents in these manifestations: systolic blood pressure below 90 mm Hg, tachycardia, cold clammy skin, confusion, and a urinary output less than 20 mL/h. In treating cardiogenic shock the health care team must supply constant intervention to prevent further damage to the heart muscle as well as the other organs of the body.

Diagnostic tests for MI and their findings are

1. Electrocardiography: T wave inversion, widening of the QRS complex, irritability of conduction system, asynchronicity, multifocal beats, arrhythmias.
2. Echocardiography: shows direction of blood flow and deviations.
3. Enzyme studies: initial elevation in CPK-MB, aspartate aminotransferase, and lactate dehydrogenase.
4. Arterial blood gas analysis may show acidosis, either from extended compensated heart disease or if cardiopulmonary resuscitation has been instituted for a prolonged period of time.

Dysrhythmias

As we get older, an increased sensitivity to potassium, sodium, and calcium ions takes place within the heart cells. **Dysrhythmias** (arrhythmias), or irregular heart rhythms, occur. Two arrhythmias common in the older adult are sinus bradycardia and first-degree heart block.

Sinus bradycardia (a heart rate below 50 beats per minute) stems from two major changes in the electrical conduction pathway of the heart: (1) an increase in the density of the ventricle muscle and/or (2) a reduction in pacemaker cells, which causes the pathway to

be stimulated less often. Because the body is receiving less oxygenated blood, clients will complain of syncope and/or fatigue. Treatment modalities for sinus bradycardia may be either chemical or surgical. Use of atropine may stimulate the heart rate for a short period of time until the underlying reason can be identified or until pacemaker insertion.

First degree heart block (Phipps et al., 1995) refers to the conduction delay of the atrioventricular node. Clients are asymptomatic, and treatment is not necessary unless the block is induced by digitalis toxicity, myocardial infarction, or coronary artery disease.

Postural Hypotension

Postural hypotension, also known as orthostatic hypotension, is caused by a sudden change in position rather than a disease state (Staab and Hodges, 1996). The systolic reading will drop over 20 mm Hg when the client is moved to an upright position from a supine position. The client may exhibit signs of tachycardia, dysrhythmias, bradycardia, or lightheadedness.

Hypertension

Isolated systolic hypertension can exacerbate the morbidity and mortality from stroke or cardiovascular disease. A sustained systolic pressure greater than 160 mm Hg is common in the older adult (Beare and Meyers, 1994).

W e l l n e s s

"Requiring a person to make an abrupt change in habits or lifestyle often results in the feelings of denial, resentment, and anger that must be addressed by both the patient and the educator before learning can take place.**"**

Cerebrovascular Accident

Stroke, or cerebrovascular accident (CVA), deprives the brain of blood by forming an embolism, thromboembolism, or hemorrhages within the intracerebral or subarachnoid areas of the brain. Neuromuscular deficiencies become apparent when certain divisions of the brain become ischemic. Poor dietary habits, smoking, diabetes mellitus, and hypertension contribute to this dysfunction by supplying the necessary instrument in embolytic production. Signs and symptoms of stroke include

- *Aphasia,* or loss of comprehension or production of the spoken word and/or written language. The nurse will be unable to understand the words the client is speaking, or the client may be unable to communicate.
- *Dysphasia* refers to an impairment, not loss, of comprehension or production of the spoken word and/or written language.
- *Dysphagia* is inability or difficulty in swallowing. The nurse should institute precautions for aspiration and restrict oral fluids, medications, or food at this time.
- *Sensory loss* is an acute misconception of pain and temperature. Comfort and safety precautions should be implemented at the time of admission.
- *Motor loss* involves hemiplegia, quadriplegia, or paralysis of only one side of the body, depending on where the infarction is located.
- *Behavioral changes* occur such as underestimation of personal abilities, inappropriate laughter, or crying. The client may have an opposite personality from prestroke behavior.
- *Impaired memory* or poor concentration may occur. The client lacks the ability to remember new surroundings or people (Christ and Hohloch, 1993).

Transient ischemic attacks, also known as mini strokes, are evanescent in nature with varying neuromuscular function deficits. Occurring among people 65 years and older, these attacks serve as a warning sign of impending CVA.

Diagnostic tests and findings are

1. Computed tomography: differentiates between an infarction and hemorrhagic stroke.
2. Magnetic resonance imaging: locates bleeding within the brain.
3. Carotid studies:
   - Doppler studies show decreased perfusion to the brain.
   - Ultrasonography highlights decreased blood flow to the brain.

Congestive Heart Failure

Congestive heart failure (CHF), by no means a disease that affects only the heart, is a plethora of symptoms influencing all major body systems. This disease may isolate only the right side of the heart or shunt from the left to the right side, with the left-to-right shunt being the most threatening.

In the *right-sided heart failure,* focus is placed on the accumulation of fluid throughout the body. It is evidenced by generalized edema and ascites. Distended neck veins are prominent on inspection, owing to the excess fluid being stored in the body's tissues. Tachycardia is established by the heart in a quest to siphon off the excess fluid that is being pumped through the cardiovascular system. As the disease progresses, symptoms become more severe.

Symptoms of *left-sided heart failure* involve the pulmonary system dramatically and are more oppressive than right-sided failure:

- *Tachycardia* is maintained during left-sided failure for the reasons just stated. Auscultation of the heart may elicit an S3 sound. This adventitious heart sound is best heard with the bell of the stethoscope at the apex of the heart. It will sound immediately after the S2 sound. Electrocardiographic tracings observed by the nurse will show a heart rate above 100 beats per minute. The client may complain of "fluttering" or say "my heart is racing." Palpation of the radial pulse may or may not be possible, depending on the rate.
- *Tachypnea,* established in an attempt to combat air hunger, is exhibited when alveolar sacs fill with fluid; this prohibits oxygenation and leads to oxygen depletion. Crackles within the lung fields are prevalent and may be auscultated with or without the use of a stethoscope. The nurse should watch accessory muscle utilization and circumoral pallor or bluish nail beds.
- Other symptoms include *weight gain, fatigue,* and *level of consciousness changes.* All result from the excessive fluid accumulation.

Progression of this disease leads to enlargement of the heart from overextension in response to excess fluid and an increased workload. Overextension of the ventricle muscle will eventually elicit a poor cardiac output that is compromised by a weakened muscle. To observe progression of edema, the nurse should weigh the client daily to check for fluid buildup. This will require an accurate daily record of intake and output of fluids for the client. Signs of decreased cardiac output are measured by surveying the client's level of consciousness and ability to complete ADLs successfully.

Diagnostic tests and findings for *right ventricular failure* are

1. Central venous pressure: elevation above 12 cm H_2O is noted.
2. Echocardiography: the right side of the heart is increased in size.
3. Electrocardiography: tracings will demonstrate changes in the P wave (Lewis and Collier, 1992).

Diagnostic tests and findings for *left ventricular failure* are

1. Pulmonary capillary wedge pressure: rate ranges between 25 and 30 mm Hg.
2. Echocardiography: left ventricle is enlarged.
3. Electrocardiography: abnormalities in QRS complex and ST segment will be found.
4. Chest radiography: fluid is evident in the pleural spaces.
5. Arterial blood gas analysis: respiratory acidosis is noted in the acute stage. If state is chronic, compensation will occur.

Abdominal Aortic Aneurysm

Most commonly present in men between 60 and 70 years of age, an abdominal aortic aneurysm is asymptomatic unless the aneurysm is enlarging or rupturing. Often, the diagnosis of aneurysm is found by chance during other diagnostic procedures or when the client complains of a pulsation in the abdomen when reclining.

Diagnostic tests include

1. Abdominal palpation during regular examination.
2. Studies of the abdominal region.

Arteriosclerosis Obliterans

Men between the ages of 60 and 80 years who have a history of cigarette smoking, hypertension, and hyperlipidemia have a higher inci-

dence of developing chronic arterial occlusion (Lewis and Collier, 1992). The client will complain of pain in the lower extremities while exercising or, as the disease progresses, pain while resting. Nocturnal foot pain may also be present. On physical assessment, the nurse will note pallor and coolness in the lower extremities when elevated and redness in the extremity when dangled. The appearance of the skin will be shiny and glossy. Palpation of the pedal, popliteal, and femoral pulses reveals that they are diminished or absent.

Diagnostic tests and findings are

1. Doppler ultrasonography: weak pulses are picked up that cannot be palpated.
2. Angiography: the occlusion is located, and the percentage the blockage entails is evident.

Thrombophlebitis

Thrombophlebitis may develop in older clients with a history of CHF, MI, prolonged immobility, and anemias (Lewis and Collier, 1992). Emboli are the most serious complication of thrombophebitis. Depending on the severity and location of the embolus, the client will voice distinct complaints. In superficial thrombophlebitis, the client may present with tenderness, redness, and warmth at the affected site. Palpation of the area will result in rigid, stiff veins (Lewis and Collier, 1992). Clients who have a deep-vein thrombus may develop no signs and symptoms, or edema, pain, and tenderness on palpation may be present.

Diagnostic tests and findings are

1. Prothrombin time and partial thromboplastin time: studies are markedly elevated.
2. Venography: tests will show location and size of clot.

Iron-Deficiency Anemia

Iron-deficiency anemia is a condition generated from a decrease in red blood cell production (Wold, 1993). In the older client, this anemia is most often diet-induced. Achlorhydria exists in 30% to 40% of older adults (Beare and Myers, 1994). Clinical signs and symptoms present in mild to moderate cases of iron-deficiency anemia include disorientation and confusion. The nurse needs to beware of diag-

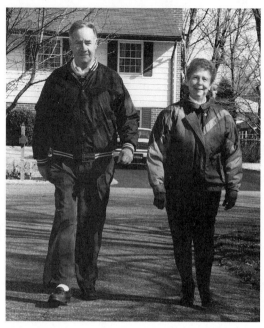

Many older adults walk daily, both for enjoyment and to build strong hearts.

nosing the client as having dementia until laboratory work can substantiate that mental status is not anemia induced. Other signs and symptoms the client may demonstrate include glossitis, pallor, tachycardia, stomatitis, fatigue, weakness, and shortness of breath.

Anemia of Chronic Disease

Developing over a long period of time, anemia of chronic disease is characterized by a low serum iron level, which is associated with infections, inflammatory diseases, cancer, and chronic renal failure. Treatment is limited to periodic transfusions of packed red blood cells.

▮ NURSING INTERVENTIONS

Practical application of care mapping requires the nurse to be realistic in identifying nursing diagnoses and planning interventions with outcomes that the client can achieve. Owing to the prevalence of multiple health problems in older adults, the efficacy of some interventions may be limited. Interventions will be presented to the client and family by the nurse and auxiliary team members. Some potential interventions are included here under the subheadings of activity, psychosocial, elimination, cardiac function, and safety. Actual and potential complications (diagnoses) appear in italic. Causative factors are in parentheses, with interventions listed under their respective diagnoses. Teaching concerns are enclosed by brackets.

Activity Issues

1. *Activity Intolerance*
   (CAD, CHF, pain, fear, medications, bed rest, anemia, vascular disease)
   Supplemental oxygen; [teach oxygen safety]; isometric exercises to evolve into independent exercise; outline exactly what client can and cannot do in form of exercise; praise compliance with regimen.
2. *Impaired physical mobility*
   (Stroke, MI, CAD, vascular disease, and anemias)
   [Teach safety tips related to mobility constraints; teach rehabilitation techniques to family and client]; allow client to ventilate frustration and fears regarding immobility.

Cardiac Function

1. *Altered cardiac output*
   (CAD, MI, dysrhythmias, and CHF)
   Bed rest; decrease stress level; [teach relaxation techniques; teach what client is allowed to do on routine basis]; assist with ADLs.
2. *Altered tissue perfusion*
   (Calcification of arteries, CAD, stroke, MI, CHF, hypertension, and immobility);

[teach limitations of activities]; supplemental oxygen; passive/active range of motion exercises; assist with ADLs; turn schedule if appropriate.

3. *Pain*
(Ischemia, from vascular disease, anemia, CAD, and MI; surgery, for CAD and vascular disease; and infarction, from stroke and MI)

Psychosocial Issues

1. *Altered family process*
(Role changes in family, hospitalization, and financial woes)
[teach family and client about disease process and treatment modalities]; allow for visitation of family members; direct family members to ancillary personnel for questions regarding role changes and finances.

2. *Altered health maintenance*
(From independent to dependent care recipient, disability, decreased sensorium, sudden changes in home environment)
Individualize home to client's needs; acquire suppliers of rehabilitative equipment for family; allow client to make some decisions on routine care; [teach skills needed to regain independence]; listen to client voice concerns over health maintenance.

3. *Altered thought process*
(Medications, stroke, electrolyte imbalances, ICU syndrome,* and other disease states)
Provide frequent orientation to time, place, and person; monitor electrolytes; provide for adequate rest cycles, working clock, and calendar in room; [teach relaxation techniques]; maintain client's nightly routine; monitor sleep periods for restlessness or abnormal sleep patterns; and schedule tests or laboratory studies in

early evening or late afternoon if possible.

4. *Anxiety*
(Hospitalization, disease process, financial concerns, and self-image disturbances)
[Teach about disease process, treatment course of action, diagnostic tests requested]; provide support personnel in allaying monetary fears and changes in person, family, and lifestyle.

5. *Disturbance in self-concept*
(Role changes, fear of unknown, and lifestyle changes)
Encourage client to ventilate feelings and fears to nurse or chaplain; reassure client and family members by [teaching new role concepts and disease process alterations]; compliment family members and cardiac client on attempting and succeeding in role changes and lifestyle changes.

6. *Fear*
(Disease process, hospitalization, finances, the unknown, procedures)
Allow for expression of fears; [teach disease process, testing procedures, and outcomes]; repeat teaching as needed; encourage family visitation where appropriate; supply chaplain or mental health services when requested.

7. *Grieving*
(Loss of self-concept, physical constraints of disease, and lifestyle changes)

8. *Ineffective coping of individual or family*
(Knowledge deficit of hospitalization or role changes)
Allow family to participate in care; answer questions family or client may have regarding care; [teach family and client about care and disease process].

9. *Nonadherence*
(Fear, knowledge deficit, religious beliefs)
[Teach disease process, limitations, and outcomes]; seek assistance from clergy/staff/physician/administra-

---

*Patients become agitated and hallucinate due to decreased amount of "sleep" time resulting from all interruptions and machine noises. It is transient when the patient is allowed to sleep undisturbed.

tion; listen to reasons for nonconformity. *Note:* The nurse *must* respect and adhere to the wishes of the client. Remember the nurse is the client's advocate in health care.

10. *Powerlessness*

(Hospitalization, knowledge deficit, age of client). Until the 1990s, consumers of health care did not display assertiveness in seeking out, obtaining, or receiving services. The population did not question the physician or other health care members but left all decisions to the medical community. Today's consumer is expected to become involved in health care decisions but may hesitate because of a lack of self-esteem or confidence.

[Teach disease process, diagnostic tests, and changes in lifestyle]; provide for frequent question and answer sessions; allow client to assist in care as much as possible; anticipate questions or concerns the older adult may have regarding disease process or care facility; do not appear rushed in answering questions; praise the mature adult in seeking out knowledge pertaining to disease state.

11. *Perceptual alterations*

(Stroke, aging, medications, hospitalization, MI, vascular disease, fear, fatigue, and angina)

[Teach safety tips and limitations]; allow for verbalization of concerns; compliment client on a job well done.

12. *Sexual dysfunction*

(Stroke, angina, MI, fear, knowledge deficit)

Provide an environment of understanding and professionalism when teaching; [teach alternative methods]; anticipate anxiety and reluctance to participate in discussion.

Elimination Issues

1. *Altered nutrition: less or more than body requirements*

(CAD, MI, and lifestyle changes)

[Teach dietary standards for health maintenance]. *Note:* Pay heed to financial costs and living conditions in as-

sisting the client with food acquisition and preparation. Do not take away all food likes and dislikes in menu preparation; incorporate some of the food likes into the menu periodically. Remember, older adults lose tastebuds and prefer sweet and salty foods.

2. *Altered patterns in urinary elimination*

(Bed rest, anxiety, medications, stroke, changes in bladder capacity, sphincter control [Hogstel and Nelson, 1992])

Provide privacy for elimination; maintain routine for elimination; maintain accurate intake and output; [teach monitoring techniques for intake; and output]; [teach importance of maintaining adequate intake]; procure list of preferred liquids; [teach signs and symptoms of edema, signs and symptoms of dehydration, and Kegel exercises].

3. *Constipation*

(Medications, diet insufficiency, prolonged bed rest, and diminished fluid intake [Hogstel and Nelson, 1992])

Increase fiber and fluid in diet; encourage activity if not contraindicated; provide elimination to follow normal home routine; [teach dietary enhancement of fluid and fiber]. *Note:* Inquire if client engages in the use of enemas, suppositories, or laxative compounds on a daily basis for regular elimination.

4. *Fluid volume deficit or excess*

(Nausea, vomiting, increased salt intake, decreased/increased intake)

Accurate intake and output; weigh daily; dietary salt modification; [teach low sodium diet, and recording of intake and output].

Safety Issues

1. *Risk for infection*

(Invasive procedures, poor nutrition, poor circulation, frailty, immunosuppressive medications, and anemias)

Maintain technique during sterile procedures; improve dietary standards; keep skin intact; [teach proper handwashing techniques to staff, client, and client's family]; monitor vital signs and laboratory work for signs of infection; and correct universal precautions.

2. *Risk for injury*

(Unsteady gait, poor eyesight and hearing, decreased sensation in extremities, and unfamiliar surroundings)

[Teach safety tips for ambulation appliances]; [teach safety equipment in room (call bells, "panic button," nurse call system); furnish ample lighting]; and [teach medication safety].

3. *Impaired skin integrity*

(Bed rest, skin fragility, and invasive procedures)

Frequently observe skin health and integrity; keep clothing and client clean and dry; institute turn schedule if client unable to turn self; [teach passive/active exercise every day]; increase fluids; and increase intake of protein and calories if skin integrity is compromised (White et al., 1994).

4. *Knowledge deficit*

(Disease process, changes in lifestyle, and limitations of disease)

[Teach the client and family to make informed decisions]; praise the family and older adult frequently for correct information and procurement of new skills or knowledge; allow for question and answer periods.

Summary

The older adult brings a wealth of knowledge and life experiences to the health care facility on admission. These experiences need to be vocalized by the client so that the health care professional will understand and appreciate where the older adult has been and what goals the client has for health care. In review, the older adult client with heart disease requires the use of all assessment tools currently being employed for the adult client. Evidenced by the numerous diagnoses needed to care for the cardiac client, specialization in *gerontics* (nursing care of the elderly) requires the health care professional to acquire competency in all aspects of older adult health care. New technological advances in areas such as pharmacology, rehabilitation, and nutrition, to name a few, will advance the nurse to new levels of service regarding the aging client in the immediate future.

RESOURCES

American Heart Association
7272 Greenville Avenue
Dallas, TX 75231-4596
(800) 242-8721
www.amhrt.org

Cholesterol, Genetics, & Heart Disease Institute
1875 S. Grant Street, Suite 700
San Mateo, CA 94402
(800) heart-89
www.heartdisease.org

United Seniors Health Cooperative
1331 H. Street, NW, Suite 500
Washington, DC 20005-4706
(202) 393-6222
www.ushc-online.org

National Women's Resource Center
5255 Loughboro Road NW
Washington, DC 20016
(202) 537-4015
www.healthywomen.org

NOAH (New York Online Access to Health)
555 W. 57th Street, 16 Floor
New York, NY 10019
(212) 541-0340
www.noah.cuny.edu

American Holistic Health Association
PO Box 17400
Anaheim, CA 92817-7400
(714) 779-6152
www.ahha@healthy.net

Heart to Heart Volunteers
PO Box 16
Escondido, CA 92033
www.csusm.edu

National Heart, Lung, & Blood Institute
National Institutes of Health
Bethesda, MD 20892
(800) 575-well
www.nih.gov

Heart Information Network
Center for Cardiovascular Education
New Providence, NJ
www.heartinfo.com

REFERENCES

Beare P, Meyers J. (1994). Principles and Practice of Adult Health Nursing. 2nd ed. St. Louis: CV Mosby.

Billhorn D. (March/April 1994). Sexuality and the chronically ill older adult. Geriatr Nurs 15(2):106–108.

Carnevali D, Patrick M. (1993). Nursing management for the elderly. 3rd ed. Philadelphia: JB Lippincott.

Christ MA, Hohloch F. (1993). A Study and Learning Tool: Gerontologic Nursing. Springhouse, PA: Springhouse.

Corbett J. (1996). Laboratory Tests and Procedures with Nursing Diagnoses. 4th ed. Stamford, CT: Appleton & Lange.

Gleeson B. (May 1991). After myocardial infarction: How to teach a client in denial. Nurs '91 34(5):48–55.

Freeman Clark JB, Queener SF, Burke Karb V. (1997). Pharmacologic Basis of Nursing Practice. 5th ed. St. Louis: Mosby–Year Book.

Herr K. (January/February 1992). Night leg pain in the elderly. Geriatr Nurs 13(1):13–16.

Hogstel M, Nelson M. (1992). Anticipation and early detection can reduce bowel elimination complications. Geriatr Nurs, 13(1):28–33.

Jech A. (January/February 1992). Preventing falls in the elderly. Geriatr Nurs 13(1):43–44.

Lewis S, Collier I. (1992). Medical-Surgical Nursing: Assessment and Management of Clinical Problems. 3rd ed. St. Louis: CV Mosby.

Lueckenotte A. (1994). Pocket Guide to Gerontologic Assessment. 2nd ed. St. Louis: CV Mosby.

Miller C. (1995). Nursing Care of Older Adults. 2nd ed. Philadelphia: JB Lippincott.

Phipps W, Cassmeyer V, Sands J. Lehman M. (1995). Medical-Surgical Nursing: Concepts and Clinical Practice. 5th ed. St. Louis: CV Mosby.

Polanski A, Tatro S. (1996). Luckmann's Core Principles and Practice of Medical Surgical Nursing. Philadelphia: WB Saunders.

Staab A, Hodges L. (1996). Essentials of Gerontological Nursing: Adaptation to the Aging Process. Philadelphia: JB Lippincott.

White M, Karam S, Cowell B. (1994). Skin tears in frail elders: A practical approach to prevention. Geriatr Nurs 15(2):95-99.

Wold G. (1993). Basic Geriatric Nursing. St. Louis: CV Mosby.

CRITICAL THINKING EXERCISES

1. Design a plan of nursing care for the patient with right-sided congestive heart failure. Incorporate drug therapy into the plan of care.

2. Compare the effects of left-sided and right-sided congestive heart failure within the body.

3. Discuss the signs and symptoms of myocardial ischemia (heart attack). Include laboratory work and drug therapy in the discussion.

4. Develop a plan of care for a patient with infective endocarditis that results in mitral valve stenosis.

5. Develop a preoperative teaching plan for a patient undergoing open heart surgery.

6. List the predisposing factors associated with deep vein thrombosis. Identify which ones are modifiable and which ones are nonmodifiable.

7. Develop a teaching plan for a patient with primary hypertension. Include drug therapy, dietary modifications, exercise therapy, and stress modification.

Maintaining Wellness of the
Lungs and Respiration

Vanessa Jones Briscoe, RN, MSN
Martha A. Badger, MSN, RNCS, GNP
Jacklen Swopes Robinson, MSN, RNCS
Lovely Abraham, MSN, RNCS, GNP
Barbara Diebold Ahlheit, MSN, RNCS

CHAPTER OUTLINE

OBJECTIVES

After completing this chapter, the reader should be able to:

1. Perform a respiratory assessment for the older adult patient with pneumonia.
2. Formulate a plan of care for the older adult who verbalizes the desire to quit smoking.
3. Instruct a group of patients with COPD regarding two common treatment modalities for the disease.
4. Develop four nursing interventions for the older adult patient with COPD.
5. Write four possible nursing diagnoses for the older adult with the following symptoms: chronic cough, dyspnea, fatigue, and chest discomfort.

KEY TERMS

crackles
hyperventilation
rhonchi
wheezes

Adequate respiratory function is essential for life, and it is also essential for *quality* of life. Anything that interferes with breathing demands primary attention and diverts the afflicted individual from ordinary daily activities. Insufficient respiratory health can lead older adults to a life of dependency.

There are many age-related changes that affect respiratory function in old age; however, ventilation and oxygenation usually remain adequate. Unfortunately, our industrialized world has created environmental pollutants such as smoking, air pollution, and carcinogen exposure that take a toll on respiratory function and may contribute to the respiratory problems that individuals experience. These events, coupled with normal age-related changes, place older adults at an increased risk for acute and chronic respiratory disorders.

Respiratory illnesses account for a great deal of both mortality and morbidity in the United States. The economic cost of these diseases is significant. It is estimated that 84.8 million Americans suffer from some form of chronic respiratory disease, costing billions of health care dollars yearly (COPD Facts, 1997).

Coughing, shortness of breath, and dyspnea are symptoms frequently described by patients with respiratory disease. These symptoms often interfere with even the simplest of routine activities (e.g., bathing, dressing, climbing stairs). It is essential, when addressing respiratory health, to obtain not only physical assessment data but also information on environmental elements (e.g., smoking, pollution) to adequately assess the interplay of environmental and age-related effects on the respiratory system.

◼ HEALTH TEACHING

Self-Care

Making people aware of factors that heighten their risk of developing respiratory diseases (e.g., chronic obstructive pulmonary disease [COPD], lung cancer) is the first step toward primary prevention, as well as early detection and treatment. Health teaching for self-care includes information about the following.

1. *Carcinogen exposure.* Exposure to carcinogens usually occurs in the workplace; however, some persons are exposed in their home environment. Exposure to carcinogens accounts for approximately 15% of lung cancer cases (Cleary, Gorenstein, and Omenn, 1996). Common carcinogens include asbestos, radiation, chromium, and radon.

2. *Genetic predisposition.* A positive family history, coupled with the presence of environmental carcinogens, can increase an individual's risk for acquiring certain respiratory diseases. These individuals need to learn to avoid exposure and seek routine physical examinations for early detection of respiratory problems.

3. *Nutrition.* Vitamins are thought to aid in the battle against certain respiratory cancers. Fruits and vegetables rich in beta-carotene and retinol (a form of vitamin A) are believed to be chemoprotective. Some studies have also identified vitamin E and the mineral selenium as having protective properties against lung cancer (Cleary et al., 1996). Increasing these vitamins and minerals in diets may aid in reducing lung cancer rates for some high-risk individuals. Examples of foods high in beta-carotene and retinol are carrots, peaches, apricots, squash, and broccoli. Good sources of vitamin E include brussels sprouts, leafy greens, spinach, whole grains and cereals, and eggs.

4. *Age.* The incidence of respiratory illnesses increases with age. Thus it is important for older adults to protect themselves against acute episodes of influenza and pneumonia, as well as to seek treatment of any chronic respiratory condition. It is recommended that older adults have annual influenza vaccinations and a one-time pneumococcus vaccination with 23-valent pneumococcal vaccine. Individuals with waning immune systems may need revaccination every 6 years (Ely, 1997).

5. *Smoking.* If smoking were eliminated today, so would be most of the respiratory diseases diagnosed in the United States. It has been estimated that smoking accounts for 80% to 90% of cases of COPD and lung cancer. The association between smoking and respira-

tory diseases has been demonstrated beyond a doubt, and every effort should be made to encourage the older adult to "kick" the smoking habit (COPD Facts, 1997).

Kicking the Smoking Habit

More than 70% of smokers claim they want to quit (Hearn, 1996). Studies have indicated that sometimes just a suggestion from a health care provider will encourage the individual to take action. Once the person decides to quit smoking, a plan must be made. It is extremely difficult to kick the smoking habit. The nicotine in cigarettes is highly addictive, both physically and mentally. Clients need to be aware that the physical symptoms of withdrawal usually last 1 to 2 weeks. These symptoms can include anything from headaches and irritability to increased tension, fatigue, increased appetite, and/or coughing. The client is taught that, after quitting, situations will arise that trigger the desire to smoke. In the planning phase, the client needs to address ways to deal with these situations. The plan to stop smoking also needs to include dietary and exercise modifications. There is a tendency to gain weight when smoking is terminated. Food often tastes better, the person tends to eat more, and the metabolism is slower (nicotine speeds up the metabolic rate). Enlisting the help of family and friends can be a great support in kicking the habit. The client can be taught a variety of ways to go about kicking the smoking habit. Many smoking cessation options are available:

1. *Nicotine replacement therapy (NRT)*. Nicotine replacement therapy delivers small, controlled doses of nicotine via a patch, chewing gum, or nasal spray. This helps to wean the smoker off the chemical. Nicotine replacement therapy claims a success rate of 20% to 45% (Rose, 1996).
2. *Scheduling*. With this method, the person weans the body from the dependence on nicotine by cutting back on the number of cigarettes smoked per day. The person smokes a predetermined number of cigarettes per day at equal intervals throughout the day. The number is cut down by one third each week for 4 weeks. Week 5 is quit week. One study found that scheduling is as effective as NRT (Rose, 1996).
3. *Cold turkey*. "Cold turkey" is the prevailing method used to quit smoking in the United States. Anyone who tries this method needs to be aware that the symptoms of nicotine withdrawal are worst when the addictive substance (nicotine) is abruptly stopped. Bearing the physical discomforts is the big challenge for individuals choosing this method. A plan that includes how to deal with the withdrawal symptoms and temptations is a must for individuals going "cold turkey" (Rose, 1996).

■ AGE-RELATED CHANGES

By providing oxygen to the cells for the combustive processes of metabolism and removing carbon dioxide (the waste product of metabolism), the respiratory system constitutes the vital mechanism for gas exchange. The respiratory system is divided into upper and lower tracts; the upper respiratory tract consists of the nose, sinuses, pharynx, and larynx, and the lower respiratory tract consists of the trachea and the lungs. The primary structure involved in gas exchange is the lungs, which undergo various age-related changes throughout life. Box 15–1 lists the ways in which these changes affect all body systems.

W e l l n e s s

"Exposure to carcinogens accounts for approximately 15% of lung cancer cases and can occur in the workplace or at home."

In the aging lung, both inspiration and expiration show a decreased volume. For example, the forced expiratory volume in 1 second decreases by 20 mL annually after 20 years of age (Table 15–1). Aging affects the mechanical aspects of ventilation. Chest-wall compliance decreases because ribs become ossified and joints grow stiffer. The elasticity of the lungs diminishes as the alveoli enlarge and become thinner. Cilia that are usually in constant motion, trapping debris to be expelled in the sputum, show decreased action in the aging lung. There may also be a decreased sense of thirst, resulting in less liquid consumption, which

> ## Box 15-1 AGE-RELATED LUNG CHANGES
>
> Anterior-posterior diameter
> Increased rigidity of chest wall
> Reduced elastic recoil
> Calcification of costal cartilage
> Decreased diaphragm and accessory muscle strength and mass
> Skeletal defects (kyphosis and scoliosis)
> Reduced total lung surface
> Reduced ciliary number and function
> Decreased immune response
> Decreased cough reflex
> Decreased oxygen diffusion capacity
> Decreased Po_2 and Pco_2
> Decreased response receptors to hypoxemia and hypercapnia
> Decreased functional respiratory reserve
> Decreased vital capacity
> Reduced forced expiratory volume
> Increased air trapping with increased residual volume

leads to thicker secretions that are even more difficult to expel. The results of these mechanical, functional changes are increased lung compliance, reduced ventilatory capacity, decreased vital capacity, and increased residual volume. Gas exchange is impaired as the pulmonary capillary network and surface area decrease. Respiratory muscle strength and endurance decrease with age; hence, the older adult will experience a decreased Pao_2 and diminished ventilatory reserve.

GUIDELINES SPECIFIC TO ASSESSING RESPIRATORY PROBLEMS IN OLDER ADULTS

Patients with respiratory disease present with four primary symptoms or chief complaints: dyspnea, cough, increase in secretions or a change in secretion character, and chest discomfort. In evaluating, it is important to consider onset, duration, and character of symptoms. The patient is asked if there are factors that cause the symptom, make it worse, or improve it.

Dyspnea, or difficulty breathing, is a common symptom associated with respiratory disease. In describing this symptom, patients may verbalize feelings of suffocation, lightheadedness, weakness, exhaustion, and panic because they are unable to get their breath.

Cough can be described as chronic or short-term. A chronic (long-term) cough is one that lasts more than 1 month. Both types can cause chest discomfort associated with musculoskeletal pain, fractured ribs, and elevation in blood pressure. A chronic cough can also lead to fatigue and weight loss. As aging occurs, there is a loss of an effective cough reflex. This can lead to aspiration of stomach contents and an increase in susceptibility to aspiration pneumonia.

Sputum production is increased in the patient with chronic bronchitis because of hypertrophy and hyperplasia of the bronchial glands. However, the older adult may be less able to move up these increased secretions because of a decreased number of cilia. It is important to determine the time of day of the increased sputum production and the character and color of the sputum.

Chest discomfort may be described as musculoskeletal pain brought on by frequent coughing spells. Stress fractures of the ribs are occasionally found in patients receiving chronic corticosteroids who experience frequent, violent coughing spells. Signs and symptoms obtained from the respiratory history and physical assessment will provide clues regarding the client's problem. Table 15–2 explains

TABLE 15–1. Pulmonary Function Studies: Lung Volumes and Capacities

Term	Symbol	Normal Amount	Description	Remarks
Tidal volume	TV	500 mL	Amount of air inspired or expired with each normal breath	TV may not vary with disease states
Inspiratory reserve volume	IRV	3300 mL	Maximal amount of air inspired after normal inspiration	
Expiratory reserve volume	ERV	1000 mL	Maximal amount of air that can be forcefully expired after normal expiration	ERV is decreased in restrictive diseases
Residual volume	RV	1200 mL	Amount of air that remains in the lungs after forced expiration	RV may be increased in obstructive diseases
Inspiratory capacity	IC	3800 mL	Amount of air inspired during maximal inspiration and starts at the normal resting expiratory level	IC may be decreased in restrictive diseases
Functional residual capacity	FRC	2200 mL	Expiratory reserve volume plus the residual air in the lungs after normal expiration	FRC may be increased in obstructive diseases
Vital capacity	VC	4800 mL	Maximum amount of air forcibly exhaled after forced maximal inspiration	VC may be decreased in obstructive diseases
Total lung capacity	TLC	6000 mL	Volume to which the lungs can be expanded with the greatest inspiratory effort	TLC may be decreased in restrictive diseases and increased in obstructive diseases

the subjective and objective findings for four frequently noted pathological processes in the elderly: pneumonia, tuberculosis, cancer of the lung, and COPD.

Other systems in the body may affect the lungs. Musculoskeletal defects (e.g., kyphoscoliosis, osteoporosis) may also compromise the aging lung by causing a decreased area for gas exchange. The diaphragm and accessory muscles weaken with age, which leads to less effective cough reflex. There is also a decline in the immune system, making the older adult more susceptible to infection. Seldom do older adults display only one illness. Often they have several persistent and severe illnesses that predispose them to further complications.

Psychosocial changes may also affect the aging client. Increase in respiratory symptoms may interfere with quality of life, promote social isolation, and lead to depression. Frequently, clients seek medical assistance when their symptoms are uncomfortable. These symptoms may include dyspnea, chest discomfort, cough, or increased secretions. Coexisting factors that may further compromise the aging client with respiratory problems include poor nutrition, activity intolerance, and poor immune response.

TABLE 15–2. Symptoms and Physical Findings in Respiratory Diseases Common in the Elderly

Pneumonia	TB	Lung Cancer	COPD
Subjective Symptoms (What the Patient Describes)			
Cough	Weight loss	Weight loss	Cough
Fever (low grade)	Cough	Cough	Increased sputum
Sputum	Weakness	Dyspnea	production
production	Dyspnea	Fatigue	Tachypnea
Confusion	Fever (low grade)		Dyspnea
Dyspnea	Night sweats		
	Hemoptysis		
	Dyspnea		
Objective Symptoms (Findings Observed During the Physical Examination)			
Crackles	Decreased breath	Decreased breath	Wheezing
Fever	sounds	sounds	Decreased breath
Tachypnea	Crackles	Change from	sounds
	Fever	baseline	Crackles
	Hemoptysis	Tachypnea	Tachypnea
		Cough	
		(productive or	
		nonproductive)	
		Fever	

Respiratory Assessment

Respiratory assessment to identify obstructive and/or restrictive disorders of the older adult is no different from that of the younger adult patient. (The disorder is *obstructive* if there are problems with airway resistance, e.g., COPD. It is *restrictive* if there is decrease in chest expansion.) The data obtained, however, may be interpreted differently in light of age-related changes.

CHIEF COMPLAINT

The nurse should begin by obtaining a current respiratory history that includes information regarding current problems and symptoms. It is important to determine the location, quality, severity, and duration of the symptom(s). Also, those factors that the patient believes improve or worsen the problem should be determined.

HISTORY

Along with a complete patient profile, the health history should focus on physical and functional problems. The nurse should note how these problems are affecting the older adult's daily life and living situation. Assessment of current and past medical conditions, inventory of medications and treatments, and determination of any complications with the regimen are indicated. It is also necessary to document the family history and support system, along with the level of the patient's understanding of the disease process and ability to cope with and manage the condition.

VITAL SIGNS

Vital signs include temperature, pulse, respiratory rate, blood pressure, and weight. The quality of respirations as well as the rate is assessed. **Hyperventilation** is an increase in the amount of air entering the alveoli. Older adults seldom have high-grade fevers; thus, the nurse must be suspicious of any low-grade fever. Body weight should always be included in the assessment, along with any recent change from the patient's normal baseline.

PHYSICAL EXAMINATION OF THE CHEST

Inspection. Both the posterior and anterior chest are observed while noting the rate, rhythm, depth, and effort of respiration. Normal inspiration to expiration ratio is 1:2. Abnormal retraction of the interspaces during inspiration may indicate COPD or laryngeal obstruction. The anteroposterior diameter of the chest is normally increased in older adults, but it may be *significantly* increased in the patient with emphysema (barrel chest). Kyphoscoliosis is often seen in older adults secondary to osteoporosis and aging. This condition will distort underlying lungs, making assessment difficult.

Palpation. While palpating the chest wall, the nurse should note any masses and costal or intracostal tenderness.

Auscultation. The patient is asked to breathe deeply through the open mouth as the nurse listens for breath sounds with the stethoscope. Breath sounds are the same in older adults as in younger persons. *Vesicular breath sounds* are heard throughout the chest. They are soft and low pitched, with the expiratory sound shorter in duration than the inspiratory sound. *Bronchial breath sounds* are heard over the large tracheal airways. These sounds are high pitched and loud and have a hollow or harsh quality. *Bronchovesicular sounds* are heard over the center and large airways; they have a tubular or breezy sounding quality. Hyperresonance or dullness can be found over the areas of consolidation.

> ### C a r i n g
>
> **"***Educating the older adult patient and family members about possible medication adversities can assist in achieving therapeutic goals and improve patient outcomes.***"**

Adventitious (abnormal or added) *breath sounds* are of two types, noncontinuous and continuous. Noncontinuous, nonmusical sounds usually heard in late inspiration are called crackles or rhonchi. They may be heard anywhere in the lung. **Crackles** in the bases of the lungs may be a normal finding in the older or bedridden patient; they usually clear with deep breathing or with the use of an incentive spirometer. **Rhonchi** (gurgling sounds) heard during inspiration and expiration are produced by secretions in the trachea and large bronchi. They may be heard in patients with pulmonary edema or in patients who are unable to cough up their secretions. These sounds usually clear if you ask the patient to cough.

Wheezes are continuous musical, high-pitched sounds. They have a whistle or squeak and are usually heard on expiration, but they may also be heard on inspiration. Be alert to changes in breath sounds. Absence of wheezes in a patient who was wheezing earlier, along with decreased breath sounds, may indicate a worsening of overall condition and should be reported immediately.

▬ COMMON DISORDERS

Pneumonia

Pneumonia is an acute inflammatory reaction of the lung parenchyma that is the fifth leading cause of death in the United States. Although it is routinely treated on an outpatient basis, it is one of the top five causes for hospitalization. Pneumonia is usually caused by an infectious agent and is particularly problematic for the older individual with co-existing morbidities. Koivula and colleagues (1994) identified several conditions that place older adults at an increased risk for developing pneumonia. The study concluded that independent risk factors for developing pneumonia were alcoholism, bronchial asthma, immunosuppressive therapies, lung diseases (e.g., COPD, chronic bronchitis), heart diseases, institutionalization, and age (> 70 years). Being knowledgeable about these factors and circumstances will aid in identifying those patients at risk for developing pneumonia.

There are three categories of pneumonia: atypical pneumonia, bacterial pneumonia, and aspiration pneumonia. Atypical pneumonia is often caused by *Legionella pneumophila*, *Mycoplasma pneumoniae*, influenza viruses types A, B, or C, or *Pneumocystis carinii*. Bacterial pneumonias are caused by *Streptococcus pneumoniae*, *Staphylococcus aureus*, *Klebsiella pneumoniae*, *Pseudomonas aeruginosa*, or *Haemophilus influenzae*. Of the three types of pneumonias, most cases are of bacterial origin, with *Streptococcus*

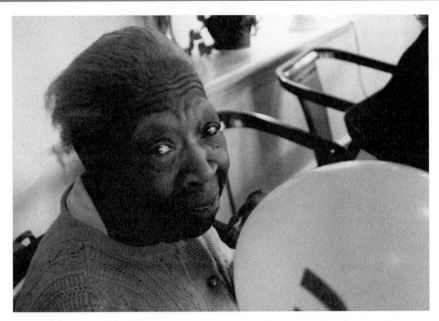

Good pulmonary function is necessary to blow up a balloon.

pneumoniae being the most common infectious agent. Occurring mostly during the winter and spring, bacterial pneumonia has a higher incidence among older adults and persons with chronic diseases (e.g., COPD, congestive heart failure, alcoholism). Aspiration pneumonia is often seen in older adults, particularly those with mechanical problems (e.g., dysphagia, abnormal swallowing reflexes, chronic diseases, debility, or a history of strokes). In this type of pneumonia, there is colonization of bacteria in the posterior pharynges.

Because of age-related changes in the immune system and other comorbidities, the usual symptoms of pneumonias are not generally the client's chief complaints. Cough, fever, pleuritic pain, and sputum production typically seen with a diagnosis of pneumonia are often absent in older adults. Instead, the older individual may present with symptoms characteristic of complications or procession of an existing chronic disease process. Inception may be evidenced by symptoms of confusion, general deterioration, weakness, anorexia, tachycardia, and tachypnea (Smeltzer and Bare, 1996). Because of this different presentation, the diagnosis may be missed and treatment delayed— possibly contributing to the high mortality rate from pneumonia that is seen in older adults.

Diagnosis of pneumonia is confirmed by clinical presentation (fever, leukocytosis, demonstration of infiltrates on chest x-ray films). Infiltrates may not be evidence in dehydrated patients. Laboratory testing will include white blood cell counts, blood cultures, and sputum Gram's stain and culture.

Treatment of pneumonia includes the administration of an appropriate antibiotic for 1 to 3 weeks, depending on the causative organism. Additionally, supportive treatment includes:

- Adequate nutrition
- Increasing fluid intake (be cautious of the risk of fluid overload)
- Adequate rest
- Facilitating sputum production
- Administering oxygen therapy (if not contraindicated because of preexisting conditions such as emphysema)
- Assisting with sufficient pulmonary ventilation (deep breathing and coughing exercises, frequent position changes, and ambulation)

Recommendations for admission to the hospital include the following (Ely, 1997):

1. Unstable vital signs

- Pulse rate less than 50 or over 140 beats per minute
- Blood pressure: systolic less than 90 or over 200 mm Hg; diastolic less than 60 or over 120 mm Hg
- Respiratory rate less than 30 breaths per minute
- Fever over 101°F
2. Hypothermia
3. Azotemia
4. Abnormal blood gases: pH less than 7.3 or more than 7.45; Po_2 less than 60 mm Hg
5. Leukopenia
6. Comorbid illnesses: cancer, diabetes, renal disease, congestive heart failure, COPD
7. Evidence of extrapulmonary involvement
8. Acute impairment of activities of daily living

To reduce or prevent serious complications of pneumonia in high-risk groups, vaccinations against pneumococcal and influenza viral infections are recommended for older adults in general. However, specific groups targeted are residents in long-term care facilities, debilitated patients, and those with cardiovascular disease and chronic diseases of the respiratory system.

Pneumococcal polysaccharide vaccine (PV) is considered by many sources to be safe, efficacious, and cost effective in reducing the incidence of bacteremic pneumococcal illness. However, only about 30% of persons 65 years of age have been vaccinated (CDC, 1995). Pneumococcal polysaccharide vaccine is free to seniors who are enrolled in Medicare Part B and are seeing physicians who accept Medicare payment.

Pulmonary Tuberculosis

The resurgence of tuberculosis (TB) since the mid 1980s is a growing public health problem in the United States, with mortality and morbidity rates rising. It is estimated that older adults will account for 60% to 70% of future TB cases (Mehta and Dutt, 1995). The primary causative agent is *Mycobacterium tuberculosis*. TB is transmitted by inhalation of infectious droplets. When infected persons cough, speak, or sneeze, they spray a contaminated aerosol that may be inhaled by others and deposited in the upper lobes of their lungs.

The incidence of TB has traditionally been higher among the older population because of their waning immune function. However, the population in general has seen an overall increase in the prevalence of TB arising from human immunodeficiency virus activity and the emergence of resistant strains of TB. Other risk factors for TB include malnutrition and poor sanitation. Additionally, the presence of chronic diseases such as diabetes, renal disease, cancer, smoking, and alcoholism, as well as institutionalization, places individuals at an increased risk for acquiring TB (Mehta and Dutt, 1995).

W e l l n e s s

❝*Individuals who have a positive family history, coupled with the presence of environmental carcinogens, need to learn to avoid exposure and seek routine physical examinations for early detection of respiratory problems.***❞**

Pulmonary TB is often insidious. Most patients present with low-grade fever, fatigue, anorexia, weight loss, night sweats, chest pain, and a persistent cough. The cough initially may be nonproductive but may progress to mucopurulent sputum with hemoptysis.

As with other conditions, the manifestation of TB in the elderly may have an atypical presentation, such as unusual behavior and an altered mental status, fever, anorexia, and weight loss. Additionally, the presence of comorbidities and polypharmacy further complicates the diagnosis and treatment of this disease.

A positive skin test does not necessarily mean active disease, but the person may have come in contact with the disease and the immune system responded to it. Purified protein derivative (PPD) is given intradermally (inner aspect of the arm); a positive result is an induration of 10 mm or more after 24 to 72 hours. A questionable reaction is an induration of 5 to 9 mm. This reaction may result from recent infections or partial anergy occurring in the presence of overwhelming TB or from corticosteroid treatment, debilitation, or advanced age. *Anergy* is a reaction of less than 5 mm induration in the presence of infection. This type of reaction may occur in the presence of one of the previously mentioned conditions, but it is more likely to be seen in an older or very ill patient.

For older adults with a negative skin test, two-step PPD testing is recommended. A second skin test (booster) 1 to 2 weeks after the initial test will unmask "true positives," indicating a past or present infection. However, if the result of the second test is also negative, true negativity is established (Mehta and Dutt, 1995). All older adult patients admitted to long-term care facilities should undergo the two-step PPD testing.

Chest radiography is useful in diagnosing TB. At least two thirds of the patients will have pulmonary involvement, particularly of the upper lobes of the lungs (Mehta and Dutt, 1995).

Pulmonary TB is treated primarily with chemotherapeutic agents (antituberculosis agents) for up to 12 months. The most widely used medications are isoniazid, rifampin, streptomycin, ethambutol, and pyrazinamide (Smeltzer and Bare, 1996).

Close monitoring for drug side effects and interactions is essential. Older adults are at risk of developing drug-induced hepatitis when receiving isoniazid. Baseline liver function tests should be obtained before starting therapy and then repeated monthly for 3 months and then at 3-month intervals (Mehta and Dutt, 1995). Streptomycin usually requires lower dosages based on age and renal function. Careful monitoring for hearing and renal impairment is necessary when using this medication. Ethambutol may cause visual impairments (decreased visual acuity, scotoma, and loss of the ability to discriminate red and green colors). Rifampin has been shown to interfere with the action of commonly prescribed medications (digoxin, corticosteroids, anticoagulants, theophylline, and oral hypoglycemics). Isoniazid reduces the anticonvulsant action of phenytoin. Educating the patient and family members about these possible medication adversities can assist in achieving therapeutic goals and improve patient outcomes.

Important prevention and control measures for this fatal communicable disease include routine screenings for TB using the Mantoux test, isolation of persons with active TB until they are noninfectious, and treatment of TB with recommended medications.

Chronic Obstructive Pulmonary Disease

Smoking is the major precipitator of COPD, which is the fifth leading cause of death in the United States. COPD is a general physiological condition that encompasses pulmonary emphysema, chronic bronchitis, and asthma (Celli et al., 1997). Characterized by progressive and irreversible airway obstruction, COPD is not always distinctive clinically and symptoms often overlap. However, their pathological presentation is clearly distinctive.

EMPHYSEMA

Emphysema is characterized by changes in the structure of the alveoli. These changes cause alveoli distention or rupture, which results in inflammation and swelling of the bronchi, excessive mucus production, and loss of lung elasticity, creating an ineffective gas exchange system. By the time symptoms of emphysema develop, pulmonary function is often irreversibly impaired, leaving the patient (usually a former smoker) to suffer progressive disability and reduced life expectancy.

Smoking is the major cause of emphysema. In a small percentage of patients, however, there is a familial predisposition to emphysema associated with deficiency of $alpha_1$-antitrypsin, a nonspecific proteolytic enzyme inhibitor.

Although there are different causes of emphysema, the physical signs and symptoms in each case are similar. Symptoms in emphysema include chronic cough, wheezing, dyspnea (on exertion and at rest), and tachypnea with prolonged exertion. The patient is often thin, with an enlarged anteroposterior diameter of the chest (barrel chest), and is observed using accessory muscles for respiration. Pursed-lip breathing, clubbing digits, hyperresonant chest to percussion, and elevated hemoglobin often complete this clinical picture. Arterial blood gases (ABGs) usually remain normal until very late stages of the disease. These patients are often called "pink puffers" because of their ability to maintain normal arterial oxygen levels and have dyspnea. Pulmonary function tests reveal increased functional residual capacity, residual volume, and total lung capacity and decreased functional ventilatory capacity and forced expiratory volume in 1 second.

CHRONIC BRONCHITIS

Chronic bronchitis is characterized by the presence of a productive cough that persists at least 3 months a year for 2 consecutive years. Excessive mucus production and a chronic cough are the major characteristics of chronic bronchitis; these clinical symptoms result from the overstimulation of the bronchial mucosa by inhaled environmental irritants. Cigarette smoking is the major antagonist; it not only causes inflammation and irritation to the airways but also alters the lungs' immune defenses. The oversecretion and buildup of mucus, in addition to impaired host defenses, creates an excellent environment for bacterial colonization of normally sterile airways, hence subjecting the person to increased risk of respiratory tract infections.

Chronic bronchitis is associated with cor pulmonale (right-sided heart failure), hypoxemia, and polycythemia. Clinical manifestations include productive and persistent cough, exertional dyspnea, cyanosis, peripheral edema, weight gain, crackles, and tachycardia. The ABGs reveal a decreased PaO_2 and increased $PaCO_2$. Pulmonary function tests disclose increased residual volume and functional residual capacity and decreased forced expiratory volume in 1 second.

ASTHMA

Asthma affects about 5% of the population in the United States. Most people are diagnosed in childhood. Although it may be diagnosed in the older adult for the first time, in most cases older adults with asthma have been coping with this chronic condition for most of their lives.

Asthma is a clinical syndrome of dyspnea, wheezing, and cough, characterized by hyperresponsiveness of the trachea and bronchi to a variety of stimuli. Because of its intermittent and reversible nature, asthma differs from other obstructive lung diseases. The asthmatic attack may be induced by certain physical and/or psychological stimuli that cause spasms of bronchial passages, swelling of the bronchial membranes, and increased mucus production within the airways. This, in turn, narrows the airways, restricting the air flow and limiting gas exchange. The asthma attack may be mild or

W e l l n e s s

❝*The association between smoking and respiratory diseases has been demonstrated beyond a doubt, and every effort should be made to encourage the older adult to "kick" the smoking habit (COPD Facts, 1997).***❞**

severe, lasting for minutes or days, and resolves itself spontaneously or because of therapy (Clinical Reference Systems Ltd., 1994; Smeltzer and Bare, 1996).

Diagnosing factors, substances, or circumstances that precipitate the attack can be challenging and require extensive investigative skill. The individual may have some allergen(s) that causes the attack; most are airborne and seasonal. Examples include pollens, molds, dander, and foods. Or, the attacks may be triggered by specific events or conditions such as exercise, respiratory tract infections, or emotions (Clinical Reference Systems Ltd., 1994; Smeltzer and Bare, 1996). It is important to identify the event that stimulates the asthmatic attack and educate the patient regarding ways to avoid the causative agent(s) and get prompt treatment in the event of an attack.

COPD MANAGEMENT

Diagnosis of the type of COPD (emphysema, chronic bronchitis, or asthma) is based on the clinical history and physical examination, pulmonary function tests, ABGs, complete blood cell count, and chest radiography. The goals of treatment for COPD include

- Relieving symptoms (improving oxygenation and decreasing carbon dioxide retention)
- Improving physical and functional status
- Preventing and treating respiratory infections
- Avoiding airway irritants and allergens
- Controlling complications

Smoking cessation, medications (bronchodilators, beta-adrenergic drugs, anticholinergic drugs, corticosteroids, and oxygen), nutrition, and adjunctive therapies form the foundation of effective treatment.

It is critical for the elderly patient with COPD to stop smoking. Smokers who quit, even after decades of smoking, have improved pulmonary perfusion and function and decreased cardiovascular mortality compared with those who continue to smoke. Additionally, smoking cessation will help slow osteoporosis and reduce the risk of hip fractures (Webster and Cain, 1997).

First-line drug therapy for COPD in older adults includes (Webster and Cain, 1997)

- Beta agonists: albuterol (Proventil, Ventolin)
- Metaproterenol sulfate (Alupent, Metaprel)
- Bitolterol mesylate (Tornalate)
- Pirbuterol acetate (Maxair)

These medications stimulate the beta$_2$ receptors in the lungs, resulting in bronchial dilation and increased mucociliary clearance. Usual administration is via inhalation therapy with metered-dose inhalers (MDIs) with a spacer. The result is faster onset of action of the drug with fewer side effects. Older adults are notorious for using improper technique of the MDI. Education and reevaluation of technique is important because proper use of the MDI is essential for reliable delivery of the medication. See Box 15–2 for instructions.

Anticholinergics—ipratropium bromide (Atrovent) and atropine sulfate (Dey-Dose)—are effective bronchodilators and decrease respiratory secretions. These drugs are often used in combination with beta agonists to manage severe COPD (Webster and Cain, 1997).

Theophylline preparations directly relax the smooth muscles of the respiratory tract, producing bronchospastic relief. The result is a decreased dyspnea. The therapeutic range for theophylline is narrow, and older adults frequently fall victim to its many side effects (i.e., nausea, vomiting, shakiness, restlessness, tachycardia, dysrhythmias, and seizures). Theophylline levels are monitored by blood levels to ascertain therapeutic drug levels (10 to 20 mg/dL).

Corticosteroids are useful in reducing airway hyperresponsiveness and inflammation. Inhaled corticosteroids are commonly used to treat chronic asthma. Corticosteroids (inhaled or oral) also appear to enhance the effects of beta agonist medications and are often prescribed as an adjunct for patients with escalating COPD symptoms (Webster and Cain, 1997).

Box 15-2   USING A METERED-DOSE INHALER

It is recommended that an aerosol holding device, such as the AeroChamber, be used with all metered-dose inhalers that do not contain a built-in aerosol holding chamber.

1. Instruct the patient to sit or stand to allow for the best gravity deposition of the aerosol particles.
2. Inspect the aerosol holding device for foreign objects.
3. Insert the inhaler mouthpiece into the holding chamber.
4. Shake the holding chamber with inhaler firmly three or four times.
5. Place the mouthpiece in front of lips.
6. Exhale fully.
7. Spray one puff into holding chamber and immediately begin to inhale slowly until a full breath is taken.
8. Hold your breath for 5 to 10 seconds.
9. Exhale. Wait 1 to 2 minutes and repeat above steps as prescribed by your clinician.

Antibiotics are used to treat recurrent infections in patients with COPD. Antibiotics also reduce the inflammatory response in the airways that often accompanies infections. The choice of antibiotic is based on the infecting organism. Treatment with the drug is usually for 2 weeks. Oxygen therapy in hypoxemia (PaO_2 55 mm Hg or less) patients is the one treatment for COPD proven to reduce morbidity and mortality rates (Adair, 1994). The goal of oxygen therapy is to maintain the PaO_2 between 61 and 70 mm Hg or the SaO_2 between 91% and 94% (Adair, 1994). Continuous home oxygen use may also be indicated when the PaO_2 is between 56 and 59 mm Hg and there are signs of end-organ hypoxemia (cor pulmonale, polycythemia, neuropsychiatric dysfunction, disabling dyspnea, or angina pectoris). Patients will be eligible for Medicare reimbursement with appropriate documentation and supportive information.

Oxygen systems are available in stationary, portable, and ambulatory types. The choice of oxygen source will depend on careful assessment of the patient's needs and resources.

Adequate nutrition is essential for good prognosis in patients with COPD. Malnutrition and weight loss are prevalent among this population. Frequent factors include early satiety associated with dyspnea, gastric irritation from bronchodilators, altered desire for food due to chronic sputum production, and depression. Careful assessment is needed to uncover the underlying problem. Nutritional status should be monitored by routine assessments of weight, laboratory values, serum albumin, transferrin, and total iron-binding capacity; zinc levels are also an important indicator of nutritional status.

Food types are important when counseling patients with COPD. For example, carbohydrate metabolism produces higher amounts of carbon dioxide than does metabolism of lipids or proteins. The malnourished hypercapnic patients may benefit more by increasing calories higher in fats and not carbohydrates. Interventions to improve food intake may include

- Encouraging the patient to eat small, frequent meals
- Measures to prevent fatigue during meals (bronchodilators before meal and periods of rest before meals)

Caring

"Making older adults aware of factors that heighten their risk of developing respiratory diseases is the first step toward primary prevention, early detection, and treatment."

- Instructions to avoid foods that cause bloating
- Eating in an unhurried, relaxed atmosphere

Major nursing diagnoses for patients with COPD include

- Ineffective breathing pattern
- Impaired gas exchange
- Ineffective airway clearance
- Activity intolerance
- Potential for infection (see Boxes 15–3 and 15–4)

Lung Abscess

The elderly person with an impaired cough reflex or difficulty swallowing is at risk for aspirating foreign material and developing a lung abscess. Other at-risk persons include those with central nervous system disorders (e.g., Parkinson's disease, cerebrovascular accidents, seizures), altered mental status, compromised immune function, and respiratory tract infections.

A lung abscess is a localized necrotic lesion that contains purulent material. The lesion collapses and forms a cavity. Most lung abscesses occur because of aspirated material from the nose or mouth. However, an abscess may result secondary to bronchial obstruction, TB, pulmonary embolism, or pneumonia.

Caring

"Caring nurses emphasize adoption of healthy lifestyle behaviors in the treatment of respiratory conditions."

Clinical presentation may resemble other respiratory illnesses and include fever, productive cough, dyspnea, weakness, anorexia, and weight

Box 15-3 COMPLAINTS OF CLIENTS WITH RESPIRATORY PROBLEMS AND RELATED NURSING DIAGNOSES

Client Complaint: Dyspnea
Nursing diagnosis

- Breathing pattern, ineffective
- Activity intolerance
- Nutrition altered: less than body requirement

Client Complaint: Chest Discomfort
Nursing diagnosis

- Gas exchange, impaired
- Breathing pattern, ineffective

Client Complaint: Cough
Nursing diagnosis

- Gas exchange, impaired
- Breathing pattern, ineffective
- Infection, potential for

Client Complaint: Increased and Abnormal Secretions
Nursing diagnosis

- Airway clearance, ineffective
- Gas exchange, impaired
- Nutrition altered: less than body requirement
- Infection, potential for

Additional nursing diagnosis to consider:

- Communication, impaired: verbal alteration in coping

---

loss. Clinical diagnosis is usually confirmed by chest radiography, sputum culture, and bronchoscopy (Smeltzer and Bare, 1996). Treatment will include antibiotics, as well as postural drainage and chest physiotherapy to promote adequate drainage of the abscess. A diet high in protein and calories should be encouraged to facilitate healing in light of the catabolic state and weight loss that often accompany this disease condition (Smeltzer and Bare, 1996).

Lung Cancer

Lung cancer is the second most common cancer in the United States and the leading cause of cancer death for both men and women (Cleary et al., 1996). A major cause of morbidity and mortality in the aging population, carcinoma of the lung can generally be attributed to environmental exposure to carcinogenic agents. Tobacco smoke is often cited as the most lethal car-

cinogenic agent in the maturation of lung cancer; it is directly responsible for at least 90% of all lung cancers (Sethi, 1997). Other carcinogenic agents include air pollution and asbestos exposure. Major campaigns against cigarette smoking have been initiated in recent years. The present older adult population, however, came to maturity when cigarette smoking was considered glamorous rather than hazardous.

The major forms of lung cancer are small cell carcinoma (formerly called oat cell), squa-

Wellness

"Beta-carotene, vitamins A and E, and selenium are thought to protect against carcinogens and can be obtained from fruits and vegetables in a well-balanced diet."

Box 15-4   NURSING INTERVENTIONS FOR NURSING DIAGNOSES RELATED TO CLASSIC RESPIRATORY SYMPTOMS

Breathing Pattern, Ineffective

1. Place in semi-Fowler's position or sitting and leaning on a table.
2. Teach pursed-lip breathing.
3. Provide education regarding control of panic attacks.
4. Evaluate effectiveness of education, medications, and degree of dyspnea.
5. Review relaxation techniques and patient's coping ability.
6. Teach patient to cover mouth and nose when in cold weather to warm inspired air.
7. Inspiratory resistor may be helpful to strengthen the diaphragm.
8. Consult dietary department. Frequent small high-protein meals may be helpful for the patient with muscle wasting.
9. Teach diaphragmatic breathing.
10. Consult occupational therapy for teaching energy conservation techniques.
11. Assess for pain and provide for pain relief.
12. Ambulate as indicated
13. Avoid gas-forming foods.
14. Encourage rest periods between activities.
15. Mechanical ventilation may be necessary if impaired breathing pattern is not corrected.

Gas Exchange, Impaired

1. Determine baseline arterial blood gases.
2. Use oximetry to monitor hemoglobin saturations. Keep saturations at 90% or greater (90% saturation is approximately the equivalent of 50 mm Hg Pao_2).
3. Assess for desaturation.
4. Assess for positional desaturation of oxygen in patients with unilateral pneumonia.
5. Teach the patient proper technique in using an incentive spirometer. Ensure that the patient takes a slow deep breath followed by a 5-second or greater breath hold.
6. Instruct the patient to use the incentive spirometer every 1 to 2 hours while awake.
7. If oxygen is ordered, ensure that the patient uses it continuously. If a facemask is ordered, convert the patient to a nasal cannula during meals.
8. If the patient is stable and oxygen saturations are less than 90% at rest, consider home oxygen therapy. Contact airline or cruise ship for guidelines for traveling with oxygen at least 72 hours before departure.
9. Mechanical ventilation may be indicated if the patient cannot be oxygenated using conventional oxygen therapies.
10. Place the patient in an upright position with the head of the bed elevated.
11. Maintain a patent airway.

Airway Clearance, Ineffective

1. Maintain adequate hydration.
2. Instruct patient in effective coughing.
3. Assess every 2 hours for need to suction if an artificial airway is present.

Box continued on following page

| **Box 15-4** | NURSING INTERVENTIONS FOR NURSING DIAGNOSES RELATED TO CLASSIC RESPIRATORY SYMPTOMS (*CONTINUED*) |

4. Provide humidity for all artificial airways.
5. Consider postural drainage, percussion, and vibration for patients with cystic fibrosis and bronchiectasis.
6. Teach patient correct technique of using a metered-dose inhaler.
7. Provide a reservoir adapter to use with the metered-dose inhaler (i.e., AeroChamber, Inspirese).
8. Provide information regarding smoking cessation.
9. Change patient's position every 2 hours.
10. Splint chest if coughing is painful and consider providing pain relief before coughing effort.
11. Observe for signs of infection.
12. Instruct to avoid bronchial irritants such as smoke or fumes.

Activity Intolerance

1. Provide rest periods between all activities.
2. Patient to rest 30 minutes before meals and 1 hour after meals.
3. Consult occupational therapy department to teach energy conservation techniques and to evaluate for adaptive devices.
4. Consider patient for pulmonary rehabilitation program.
5. Evaluate patient's home arrangements.
6. When exercising, have the patient start with frequent short distances and work up to fewer walks but with a greater distance.
7. Assess sexual health. Make suggestions for enhancing sexual relationship if indicated.
8. Consider handicapped parking permit.
9. Utilize bronchodilator medication 30 minutes before strenuous exercise.

Infection, Potential for

1. Annual flu vaccine unless allergic to eggs.
2. Pneumonia vaccine (usually a once in a lifetime vaccine).
3. Instruct to avoid large crowds and anyone with a suspected virus, infection, or the flu.
4. Encourage medication compliance and provide education regarding medications.
5. Instruct to complete all of the antibiotic prescription.
6. Instruct to seek medical assistance immediately if a respiratory problem or infection is suspected.
7. Teach to cough into a tissue and dispose of it properly.
8. Provide education regarding cleaning of respiratory equipment.
9. Review signs and symptoms of respiratory infection.

mous cell carcinoma (epidermoid), adenocarcinomas, and large cell carcinoma. Males traditionally have a higher incidence of lung cancer, but the rate has increased among females. The increased frequency of smoking among women has produced this predictable increase. Peak incidence for lung cancer is 55 to 65 years of age. The prognosis of lung cancer is often poor because the cancer has metastasized when symptoms are first noticed. Symptoms will depend on the location, tumor size, and degree of obstruction. Most frequently, the patient will complain of a cough (with or without sputum), wheezing, dyspnea, hemoptysis, fatigue, and anorexia. Diagnostic evaluation will often consist of a chest radiograph, sputum sample for cytology, bronchoscopy, lung scans, and biopsy. Treatment may include surgical interventions as well as radiation and/or chemotherapy. The presence of coronary artery disease and pulmonary insufficiency may limit the treatment options for older adults, and surgical intervention will be contraindicated. Treatment of lung cancer is often palliative rather than curative. Less than 10% of individuals with lung cancer are alive 5 years after diagnosis.

Summary

Respiratory problems are common among older adults because of a combination of age-related changes and environmental factors to which they become more susceptible with age. Diagnosis and treatment are often complicated by subtle presentations, comorbidities, and polypharmacy. Many of the interventions implemented for chronic conditions will be evaluated based on relief of the subjective and objective findings. Often intervention will not produce a cure, but frequently symptoms can be minimized.

Education is key to successful management, because most of the care and decision-making will be carried out in the home by the patient or family members. Understanding of the disease process and the numerous treatment modalities will enable the patient to make informed decisions regarding care. Because older adult patients often fall victim to adverse drug reactions and interactions, they must be educated on the mechanisms of action, efficacy, and side effect profiles of their medications. Adoption of healthy lifestyle behaviors cannot be overemphasized when treating respiratory conditions. Smoking cessation is always a goal.

RESOURCES

American Lung Association
1740 Broadway
New York, NY 10019
(212) 245-8000

Asthma and Allergy Foundation of America
19 W. 44th Street
New York, NY 10036
(212) 921-9100

Emphysema Anonymous
P.O. Box 66
Fort Myers, FL 33902
(813) 334-4226
1-800 TRY-TO-STOP (1-800-879-8678)

REFERENCES

Adair N. (1994). Chronic airflow obstruction and respiratory failure. In Harrard WR, Bierman EL, Blass JP, et al., eds. Principles of Geriatric Medicine and Gerontology. New York: McGraw-Hill.

Celli B, Cosentino A, Fiel S, et al. (1997). Step by step through the workup (diagnosing chronic obstructive pulmonary disease). Patient Care 31(2):20.

Centers for Disease Control and Prevention. (1995). Increasing pneumococcal vaccination rates among patients of a national health care alliance—United States, 1993. JAMA 274(17):1333.

Cleary J, Gorenstein L, Omenn G. (1996). Lung cancer: Prevention is the best cure. Patient Care 30(14):34.

Clinical Reference Systems Ltd. (1994). Asthma, p 18. Electronic Collection: A17347496.

COPD Facts. (1996 and 1997). Colorado HealthNet.

Ely, EW. (1997). Pneumonia in the elderly: Diagnostic and therapeutic challenges. Infect Med 14(8):643–654.

Hearn W. (1996). How to quit (smoking cessation: Agency for Health Care Policy and Research report). Am Med News 39(19):29.

Huether SE, McCance KL. (1996). Understanding Pathophysiology. St. Louis: Mosby–Year Book.

Koivula I, Sten M, Makela, Pirjo H. (1994). Risk factors for pneumonia in the elderly. Am J Med 96(4):313.

Mehta JB, Dutt AK. (1995). Tuberculosis in the elderly. Infect Med 12(1):40–46.

Rose R. (1996). How to quit smoking. Weight Watchers Magazine 29(9):38.

Sethi T. (1997). Lung cancer (science, medicine, and the future). BMJ 314:652.

Smeltzer SC, Bare BG. (1996). Brunner and Suddarth's Textbook of Medical-Surgical Nursing. 8th ed. Philadelphia: Lippincott-Raven.

Webster JR, Cain T. (1997). Pulmonary disease. In Cassel CK, Cohen HJ, Larson EB, et al., eds. Geriatric Medicine. 3rd ed. New York: Springer-Verlag.

 CRITICAL THINKING EXERCISES

J. J., an 80-year-old woman, is being seen in the emergency department for exacerbation of her chronic bronchitis. She presents as a thin, poorly nourished, dyspneic woman, She complains of increased coughing spells and states that her sputum is increasing in amount and is

(*continued on following page*)

CRITICAL THINKING EXERCISES (Continued)

yellow. J. J. appears irritable and anxious when she tells you that she has been a pack-a-day smoker for over 40 years. She complains of fatigue and states that she sleeps poorly at night. Her vital signs are BP, 160/90; P, 120; R, 32; and T, 100°F. Wheezing is noted throughout all lung fields and her anterior-posterior diameter is exaggerated. You check J. J.'s ABGs and find the following: pH, 7.25; $Paco_2$, 75; Pao_2, 48; HCO_3, 27 mEq/L; and Sao_2, 80. Oxygen at 2 L/nasal cannula is started. The physician orders for J. J. to be transferred to a medical unit; however, no beds are available. She is treated in the emergency department with intravenous fluids, oxygen, antibiotics, and corticosteroids. Repeat ABGs are pH, 7.35; $Paco_2$, 60; Pao_2, 55; HCO_3, 27 mEq/L; and Sao_2, 86. J. J. is discharged from the emergency department 48 hours later. Discharge orders include low sodium diet as tolerated; activity as tolerated; enalapril (Vasotec), 10 mg PO every morning; Alupent Inhaler, 2 puffs q 6 hours;

ampicillin, 500 mg tid (for 14 days); and prednisone, 60 mg, decreased by10 mg qd times 5 days.

1. What additional information is needed to assess whether J. J. will need home health care?
2. Explain the pathology of chronic bronchitis.
3. Would J. J. benefit from smoking cessation? If so, what would be the benefits?
4. Explain the main purpose of the following classes of drugs in treating COPD: antibiotics, bronchodilators, and corticosteroids.
5. J. J. is observed using the MDI incorrectly. Explain how you would demonstrate proper use of the device.
6. Identify strategies that might improve her caloric intake.
7. What types of prevention measures could this patient take to prevent respiratory exacerbations and complications?

CHAPTER 16

Maintaining Wellness of the
Bones and Muscles

Carol Dennis, DSN, RN

CHAPTER OUTLINE

OBJECTIVES

After completing this chapter, the reader should be able to:

1. Assess the function of the musculoskeletal system.
2. Teach a healthy older adult about the normal age-related changes that occur in the musculoskeletal system with aging.
3. Formulate a definition of *mobility.*
4. Compare and contrast common musculoskeletal disorders that affect mobility of the older adult.
5. Formulate a nursing care plan for an older adult who is experiencing a musculoskeletal disorder.
6. Write a health promotion self-care teaching guide for an older adult client with a musculoskeletal disorder.

KEY TERMS

hematopoiesis
osteoblastic activity
osteoclastic activity
osteotomy
subluxation

The musculoskeletal system, in conjunction with other body systems, is responsible for an individual's mobility and capacity for movement. Mobility, which represents independence, is a necessary component of a person's daily activities throughout the life span. Loss of mobility may be viewed by the older adult as a loss of independence; thus, older adults value highly the ability to remain mobile (Ebersole and Hess, 1998; Miller, 1995). For any age group, loss of independence is a grave concern, and it can be especially so for an older adult, who is at great risk of experiencing serious consequences when loss of independence occurs. Therefore, safety also becomes an issue of high priority in the older adult population (see Chapter 10). Assessment of the musculoskeletal system must include a thorough and careful evaluation of older adults for the normal changes of aging as well as for risk factors related to falls (Miller, 1995).

The musculoskeletal system spans the entire body and provides structure. Bones and muscles working in unity allow an erect stance and a wide array of movements. For physical activity to occur smoothly and effortlessly, all the parts of this system must function together as a unit. The musculoskeletal system is a defense against injury, which carries the risk for permanent disability. It provides support to surrounding tissues and protects body organs and other internal structures. **Hematopoiesis,** [which is] blood cell formation and development, occurs in this system and provides mineral homeostasis (Luckmann, 1997; Marek, 1995; Seidel et al., 1995; Sims et al., 1995).

▉ HEALTH TEACHING

Health teaching about the musculoskeletal system needs to be begun early so that a lifelong pattern of behavior can be established to pre-

vent the development of disease processes later in life. Although not all musculoskeletal conditions and disease processes can be avoided, a healthy lifestyle will lessen their impact. National surveys indicate that girls as young as 10 years old are not consuming the daily recommended amounts of calcium (Lappe and Meyer, 1997). The goal of prevention is to maximize bone mass and minimize bone loss. Older adults who have not had the benefit of earlier health promotion teaching still need the opportunity to become educated about this system. It is never too late to change one's behavior so that a more healthy lifestyle can be achieved. Box 16–1 demonstrates appropriate health promotion teaching related to conditions of the musculoskeletal system that are common to the older adult population. Risk factors that predispose an older individual to the development of musculoskeletal problems are listed in Box 16–2.

▉ AGE-RELATED CHANGES

The normal age-related changes of the musculoskeletal system generally affect mobility. The process of formation and resorption stabilizes the amount of bone mass between 30 and 50 years of age. However, after about age 50, this process becomes unstable and more bone resorption than formation occurs, causing the musculoskeletal system to gradually lose bone mass. This continual resorption removes calcium and eradicates the bone's organic matrix. Both types of bones, *cortical* (composed mostly of long bones) and *trabecular* (found in the vertebral column and flat bones), are affected by aging changes, which can lead to increased porosity, thinning, and even destruction. The initial reduction in bone mass occurs in trabecular bone, predisposing the older adult to the development of compression fractures in the vertebrae. Cortical bone mass decline predisposes the individual to fractures of the femur (Burke, 1997).

Demineralization of bones is a lifelong process, but it occurs at a greater rate in an aging individual than in a young person. Normally, demineralization takes place at about 1% each year for both men and women; however, beginning about the time of menopause

Box 16-1 **HEALTH PROMOTION TEACHING FOR THE MUSCULOSKELETAL SYSTEM**

1. Teach dietary intake of appropriate foods containing calcium (dairy products are the major source of dietary calcium).
2. For those who are not receiving enough calcium through dietary measures, calcium supplementation is necessary. Serial serum calcium levels need to be drawn. Include the appropriate amount to take each day, correct dosing schedule, and any special measures associated with the particular supplement being taken.
3. Encourage an age-appropriate weight-bearing exercise program to increase bone mass and muscle strength.
4. Vitamin D plays a role in calcium absorption and bone metabolism, and exposure to sunlight is necessary for the synthesis of vitamin D. Those who are unable to seek exposure to sunlight at least 15 minutes each day may need to take a multiple vitamin containing vitamin D. Caution older adults not to overexpose themselves to sunlight—15 minutes is adequate.
5. Advise maintenance of ideal body weight to preserve weight-bearing joints.
6. Advise use of proper body mechanics when lifting or moving heavy objects to prevent injury to the spinal column.

the rate increases to about 10% a year for women, increasing the risk of developing osteoporosis (Townsend, 1996). Calcium levels in young adults remain steady within a normal range, but in older adults some of the calcium-regulating mechanisms are either increased or decreased, leading to faulty calcium blood level regulation. The body then pulls calcium from the bones in an effort to maintain adequate blood levels (Burke, 1997). For women, factors affecting calcium loss from bones include estrogen deficiency, calcium malabsorption, lifestyle factors (e.g., inadequate calcium intake, lack of exercise), and genetic history. Some factors besides age that influence demineralization are gender, diet, tobacco use, alcohol intake, activity, and racial background (Sack, 1996).

Loss of muscle mass because of a decline in the number of muscle fibers is significant in

Box 16-2 **RISK FACTORS FOR THE DEVELOPMENT OF MUSCULOSKELETAL PROBLEMS**

- Level of bone mass at maturity
- Gender—being female
- Age
- Diet
- Alcohol intake
- Smoking
- Medications
- Activity
- Being overweight
- Family history
- Lifestyle
- Mobility aids

the aging individual, but it occurs more slowly in men than in women because men usually have more muscle mass than women (Burke, 1997; Sims et al., 1995; Townsend, 1996). There may be a decline in muscle strength for many older adults. The amount of strength lost depends on the muscle group and on muscle group use (Burke, 1997). Sometimes, older adults believe that they should not exercise because they are older and are losing muscle strength; however, lack of exercise actually increases the loss of strength (Burke, 1997). Individuals may lose 30% or more skeletal muscle mass by 80 years of age. Other factors impacting muscle mass are diet, disease, and inactivity (Sack, 1996).

Some age-related changes in the neurological system, such as a progressive decrease in reaction time and a decrease in speed of movement, agility, and endurance, exert an adverse affect on muscle function (Burke, 1997; Seidel et al., 1995). The sense of balance, which is governed by several centers in the brain including the cerebellum, is changed in the older adult (Sims et al., 1995).

Eventually the cartilage in joints erodes, increasing stress on the underlying bone and leading to changes secondary to inflammation and proliferation, which decrease flexibility. Joint mobility in old age is further hampered when collagen fibers replace the elastic synovial tissue and the synovial fluid increases in viscosity (Sack, 1996) (Box 16–3).

Older adults may exhibit the following musculoskeletal disorders: osteoporosis, osteomalacia, Paget's disease, muscle cramps (restless leg syndrome), osteoarthritis, spondylosis, rheumatoid arthritis, gouty arthritis, and fractures.

■ GUIDELINES SPECIFIC TO ASSESSING MUSCULOSKELETAL PROBLEMS IN OLDER ADULTS

Clients should be asked if they are experiencing malaise, weakness, fatigue, and/or sleep disturbance. Joints are assessed for pain and/or stiffness as to duration, location, and character. What makes it better or worse? What level of activity is the client capable of carrying out? What type of daily exercise, if any, is the client capable of performing?

The physical examination involves observation, palpation, and comparison of joints for symmetry, size, shape, color, appearance, temperature, and pain. How much joint mobility is present in the affected joints compared with nonaffected joints? Is there crepitus? Is the individual able to perform activities of daily living (ADLs)? If not, how much and what type of assistance is needed?

When assessing the musculoskeletal system of an older adult, it is expected that there will be a loss of bone density with a decrease in muscle mass, muscle tone, and strength. The range of motion (ROM) is assessed for all joints, as in the assessment of younger individuals. However, it is important to know if the older adult has undergone a hip replacement because clients who have had this type of surgery should not flex the operative hip to 90 degrees, due to the possibility of dislocating the hip; adduction of the operative leg past the midline is to be avoided for the same reason.

Box 16-3   AGE-RELATED CHANGES IN THE MUSCULOSKELETAL SYSTEM

- Decrease in bone and muscle mass
- Demineralization
- Decline in muscle strength
- Progressive decline in reaction time
- Decline in speed of movement
- Decrease in agility
- Decrease in endurance
- Changed sense of balance
- Decreased joint flexibility, joint stiffness and enlargement
- Shortening of spine and loss of height

Joints may be swollen and painful, so gentle handling is necessary. Each vertebral process should be gently palpated. If the older client complains of pain or tenderness and decreased back movement, a compression fracture may be present.

COMMON DISORDERS

Osteoporosis

Osteoporosis, a metabolic bone disease, is an age-related disorder with many causes in which demineralization of the bone occurs, creating decreased bone density and leading to easily fractured bones in individuals 45 years of age and older at the rate of approximately 1.5 million per year (Burke, 1997). The areas of the skeletal system most frequently affected are the radius (wrists), femur (hips), and vertebrae (back). More females than males develop osteoporosis. Osteoporosis is a significant health problem in the United States, costing approximately 6 billion dollars per year; it is the 12th leading cause of death in the United States (Ignatavicius and Bayne, 1991; Lonergan and Harris, 1996).

Bone is a dynamic tissue with continuous formation of new bony tissue (**osteoblastic activity**) and resorption of old bone (**osteoclastic activity**). An individual's bone mass, or density, peaks during the age range of 30 to 35 years; then calcium is lost from both cancellous and cortical bone. After menopause, bone mass rapidly decreases secondary to decreased serum estrogen levels. Forty to 45 percent of an individual's bone density is lost over the life span. One estimate claims that 50% of all women older than 65 show some symptomatology of osteoporosis. Primary osteoporosis is the most common type and is not associated with any underlying pathological cause. Secondary osteoporosis, on the other hand, does have an underlying cause (e.g., hyperparathyroidism, long-term therapy with corticosteroids). When there is an underlying cause, the treatment is directed toward the cause.

In females, the rate of bone density loss is increased for 5 to 8 years after the menopausal year, and this loss is thought to be related to an estrogen deficiency (Burke, 1997). When there is a lack of serum estrogen, calcium is not resorbed. Fractures resulting from postmenopausal osteoporosis are usually compression fractures of the spine. Cortical bone mass is lost more slowly than cancellous bone mass; thus, fractures resulting from this type of loss usually are femoral. The cause of osteoporosis is unknown. However, there are many risk factors that can predispose an individual to the development of osteoporosis (Table 16–1).

Some of these are controllable and some are not. Approximately 20 million females and 5 million males in the United States have osteoporosis (Luckmann, 1997). The individual who is experiencing osteoporosis usually has very few clinical features, and a fractured bone may be the first indication of the problem. Osteoporosis is very often the predisposing factor for fracture development in older adults. In those individuals who are 90 years of age and older, 32% of the women and 17% of the men will suffer at least one hip fracture secondary to osteoporosis. The mortality rate for older adults with hip fractures is greater than 50%, and the disability effects are devastating (Sands, 1995).

Wellness

❝It is never too late to change one's behavior so that a more healthy lifestyle can be achieved.❞

Osteoporosis may be referred to as the "silent disease" because bone loss occurs but symptoms do not. The older adult may experience severe and unremitting back pain secondary to collapsed vertebrae. As vertebrae collapse, older adults often lose height. On observation, a stooped posture, kyphosis, and a waddling gait may be noted. Diagnosis is based on laboratory findings, including dual-energy x-ray absorptiometry, a method of testing that provides a precise measurement of bone density. The client is exposed to radiation for a shorter period of time when this method is used. Other, older methods of testing for bone density include single-photon absorptiometry and quantitative computed tomography (Sack, 1996). A urine specimen may show an elevated calcium level while the serum calcium level remains within normal limits. A serum specimen checked for Gla-protein (osteocalcin) will demonstrate an elevation (Luckmann, 1997).

TABLE 16–1. Risk Factors for Osteoporosis

Common Characteristics	Expression
White race	Females after menopause
Body build	Thin, lean, little exercise (obese individuals store estrogen in body tissues that can be used as needed to maintain serum levels)
Exercise	With exercise there is decreased resorption and increased new bone formation
Mobility	Immobility leads to rapid resorption and very little, if any, new bone formation
Dietary factors	A well-balanced diet ensures adequate calcium and vitamin D intake. Individuals need exposure to sunlight for adequate vitamin D, which aids in the metabolism of calcium
Level of bone density when mature	Females have less (about 20% less) bone density than males at maturity
Gender	Occurs more frequently in females than in males
Alcoholism	Regular, excessive intake of alcohol
Medication intake	May interfere with absorption of calcium from the intestine
Disease processes	Some disease processes may cause malabsorption of calcium from the intestine
Caffeine intake	High caffeine intake

Box 16–4 features an overview of general assessment for osteoporosis.

The overall aim of treatment is to retain bone density by inhibiting bone resorption. It is also necessary to prevent complications, such as fractures, and provide comfort and relief from pain. Prevention is the best treatment. Although this condition may not be entirely avoided, certain self-care preventive interventions can be implemented. Older adults, as well as all individuals, should avoid the use of tobacco and excessive alcohol. Older adults have a need for sufficient amounts of calcium in the diet—1000 to 1500 mg/d (Burke, 1997; Luckmann, 1997). A low-impact, weight-bearing exercise program is important.

Drug therapy is the main medical approach to the treatment of osteoporosis. *Estrogen replacement therapy (ERT)*, when begun in the early postmenopausal period, does slow rapid bone density loss and has demonstrated a 50% reduction in fractures (Fleming, 1992). The exact mechanism of action in preventing osteoporosis is not known. This is a long-term treatment modality because discontinuing the estrogen will reactivate the accelerated loss of bone mass. Those density losses that are totally age related are not affected by the use of estrogen. However, there are certain cancer risks of ERT that must be considered for each woman on an individual basis (Burke, 1997). Although the risk of developing uterine or breast cancer is very small, it is also a real concern; this can be offset somewhat by the concurrent addition of a form of progesterone. When both estrogen and progesterone are given, the combination is referred to as *hormone replacement therapy (HRT)*.

Calcium supplementation in the treatment of osteoporosis prevents bone resorption by stimulation of the parathyroid gland (Luckmann, 1997). Calcium will not increase bone mass or prevent a fracture from occurring. It will, however, aid osteoblastic activity in forming new bone. The postmenopausal women needs about 1500 mg of calcium each day. The average American adult diet, however, is deficient in meeting this calcium requirement. Various calcium preparations are listed in Box 16–5.

Each dose of calcium supplement must be taken either with or after a meal because any interaction with hydrochloric acid affects calcium absorption. Calcium supplements should be taken with a full glass of water to lessen the possibility of developing stones or hypercal-

Box 16-4   ASSESSMENT OVERVIEW FOR OSTEOPOROSIS

History
Age, gender
Presenting problem
Reason for seeking medical attention now

Risk Factors
Ethnic background
Frame size
Nutritional factors
Lifestyle patterns (sedentary, tobacco use, alcohol consumption, caffeine intake)
Disease processes
Medication history

Observations
Posture
Height (changes)
Spinal deformities

Pain
Location
Quality
Duration

Laboratory Findings
Urine calcium
Serum calcium and Gla-protein

Adapted from Luckmann J. (1997). Saunders Manual of Nursing Care. Philadelphia: WB Saunders.

cemia. Vitamin D is necessary for calcium absorption and may be contained in the calcium preparation; if not, a multiple vitamin is generally advisable (Sands, 1995).

Other medications used in the treatment of osteoporosis include calcitonin, sodium fluoride, and etidronate (Didronel). Calcitonin decreases osteoclastic activity, bone breakdown, and (due to analgesic effects) pain from osteoporotic fractures (Luckmann, 1997). Nausea

Box 16-5   CALCIUM SUPPLEMENTS (% ELEMENTAL CALCIUM)

Calcium carbonate (40%, preferred)
Calcium phosphate (31%)
Calcium lactate (13%)
Calcium gluconate (9%)

Adapted from Sands JK. (1995). Human sexuality. In Phipps WJ, Cassmeyer VL, Lehman MK, eds. Medical-Surgical Nursing Concepts and Clinical Practice. 5th ed. St. Louis: CV Mosby.

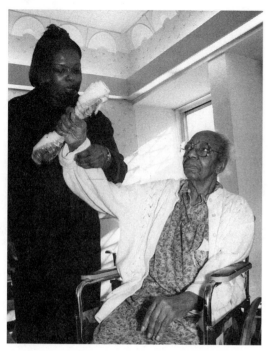

Dumbbells may be used by clients who are chairbound to maintain adequate range of motion in the upper body.

and flushing may be caused by calcitonin, which is destroyed by the gastrointestinal tract; therefore, it must be administered by a parenteral route. This drug should be administered each day by nasal spray, alternating nostrils, or by injection every 1 to 3 days for treatment of osteoporosis (Deglin and Vallerand, 1997). Sodium fluoride, when administered with calcium, regenerates bone density, with best results noted in patients with spinal osteoporosis (Luckmann, 1997). Etidronate suppresses bone resorption and turnover. If a dose is missed, it should be taken only if not close to the time of the next scheduled dose. One should never take a double dose (Deglin and Vallerand, 1997).

A new class of drugs that has been approved for treatment of osteoporosis is the group called *bisphosphonates*, which have antiresorptive properties. The risk of fractured vertebrae in postmenopausal women has been reduced by almost 50% by use of the medication alendronate (Fosamax) (Lappe and Meyer, 1997). Classified as a bone resorption inhibitor, alendronate inhibits osteoclastic activity. This medication actually reverses the progression of os-

teoporosis (Deglin and Vallerand, 1997). See Box 16–6 for nursing interventions related to these medications.

Osteomalacia

Osteomalacia, sometimes called *adult rickets*, is defined as abnormally soft bone tissue secondary to an imbalance in calcium and phosphorus levels that is most often related to an inadequate activation of vitamin D (Lappe and Meyer, 1997). The result is deformity in weight-bearing bones and pathological fractures. This disease process mainly affects women.

Causes of this disease include inadequate intake of vitamin D and inadequate exposure to the sun, which is necessary for vitamin D synthesis. Certain physical conditions, which include primary hypoparathyroidism, renal tubular disorders, pancreatic insufficiency, hepatobiliary disease, and small intestine disease, lead to this disorder by creating malabsorption or by interfering with metabolism of vitamin D.

Clinical features of osteomalacia include generalized demineralization and progressive multiple deformities of the bones—especially of the spine, pelvis, and lower extremities—with progressive muscular weakness. Bowing and bending deformities of the long bones may be seen. Pseudofractures, called Milkman's syndrome, and cyst formation are frequently present. There is persistent skeletal pain, and fractures are common. Widespread decalcification, called Looser's zones, is noted on the radiograph. Serum calcium and phosphorus levels are decreased, with a moderately high alkaline phosphatase level. Biopsy is sometimes used to help with diagnosis (Lappe and Meyer, 1997; Luckmann, 1997).

Paget's Disease (Osteitis Deformans)

Paget's disease is a progressive skeletal disease in which there is abnormally rapid bone resorption and formation. The new bone formation is not replaced at the lines of stress and therefore creates large, malformed bones with poor mineralization. The most frequent areas affected by Paget's disease are the femur, tibia, lower spine, pelvis, and cranium (Lappe and Meyer, 1997; Luckmann, 1997).

The exact cause of Paget's disease is un-

Box 16-6   NURSING INTERVENTIONS RELATED TO THE ADMINISTRATION OF CALCITONIN, ETIDRONATE, AND VITAMIN D PREPARATIONS

Calcitonin

1. Monitor weight
2. Teach client that a flushed feeling may occur that may be minimized by taking the dose in the evening.
3. Check for allergic reactions before administering the first dose.
4. Assess serum electrolyte levels.
5. If on long-term therapy, a medication alert tag (bracelet) should be worn indicating the medication being taken.

Etidronate

1. Monitor serum electrolyte, creatinine, and blood urea nitrogen levels.
2. Provide emotional support because maximum effect may require weeks to months.
3. Teach the client to take the drug on an empty stomach and wait for 90 minutes before eating.
4. Teach client to not take a dose of this medication within 2 hours of drinking milk or milk products, or taking antacids, mineral supplements, or medications high in calcium content, magnesium, iron, or aluminum.

Vitamin D Preparations

1. Monitor serum calcium levels and monitor urine for calcium.
2. Assess for side effects that indicate overdose, ataxia, fatigue, irritability, seizures, somnolence, tinnitus, elevated blood pressure, and gastrointestinal distress or constipation.
3. Do not take over-the-counter prescriptions containing calcium, phosphorus, or vitamin D without obtaining physician's approval.

Fosamax

1. Swallow the pill whole in the morning with a full glass (6–8 oz) of water (not mineral water) at least 30 minutes before taking any other beverage, food, or medication.
2. Remain in an upright position (avoid reclining) for at least 30 minutes and until after eating the first meal of the day.

Instruct client to keep all follow-up appointments with physicians and for laboratory testing.

Adapted from Clark JB, Queener SF, Kalb VB. (1993). Pharmacologic Basis of Nursing Practice. St. Louis: CV Mosby.

known. In the United States, approximately 3 million people older than age 40 years are affected by Paget's disease (Luckmann, 1997). Older adults within the age range of 50 to 70 years are those who most often have Paget's disease. This disease process occurs more commonly in men than women. There is a familial tendency, although no definite hereditary pattern has been identified (Lappe and Meyer, 1977).

Most individuals (90%) with this disease are asymptomatic and may be diagnosed on routine examination by radiography. Bowed legs, barrel-shaped chest (which in advanced cases may affect respiratory and cardiovascular functioning), kyphosis, and an enlarged skull may be noted on observation. Some clients complain of fatigue and intense skeletal pain. Changes in skin temperature may be noted, and the individual may complain of symptoms typical of nerve compression. Levels of serum alkaline phosphatase are elevated. The serum calcium level may be normal or elevated and anemia may be an indication of this disease process. Hydroxyproline, indicative of osteoclastic activity, may be elevated, as measured by a 24-hour urine collection (Lappe and Meyer, 1997). Before the development of symptoms, radiographs show increased bone mass, but after clinical symptoms appear there is a characteristic mosaic appearance seen on the radiograph (Lappe and Meyer, 1997; Luckmann, 1997). Bone scans may be used in the diagnostic process, as well as computed tomography and magnetic resonance imaging. These diagnostic instruments improve visualization of the bone and help determine if the bony lesion is active or inactive.

Many asymptomatic individuals are not treated, whereas those with mild conditions may be treated with antiinflammatory medications and analgesics for bone and joint pain. Agents used to inhibit osteoclastic-mediated bone resorption include calcitonin, etidronate, and mithramycin (Googe and Gerlach, 1992). Mithramycin is used only when an individual does not respond to other treatment. This agent is cytotoxic and may cause such side effects as hepatotoxicity, thrombocytopenia, nephrotoxicity, severe anorexia, and nausea and vomiting (Lappe and Meyer, 1997). Heat therapy, massage, and bracing are other orthopedic measures that may be used to manage pain.

Restless Leg Syndrome

Restless leg syndrome is an idiopathic neurological condition involving irritating crawling, itching, or tingling sensations of the legs while resting. These sensations cause an overwhelming desire to move, which manifests as muscle twitching or myoclonic jerks. These movements are painful and interfere with sleep because they are often worse at night (Reimer, 1997; Parker and Clinton, 1992).

A diagnosis of restless leg syndrome is made when the number of movements is equal to or greater than five per hour of sleep. These sleep interruptions lead to repeated awakenings, causing insomnia and daytime sleepiness (Ebersole and Hess, 1998).

Treatment of this condition consists of administering clonazepam (Klonopin), a benzodiazepine, or baclofen, a skeletal muscle relaxant. These medications decrease the extent of the movements and awakenings. Levodopa-carbidopa (Sinemet), an anti-Parkinson's disease drug and imipramine (Tofranil), a tricyclic antidepressant, act more directly and tend to eradicate the movements. The use of a transcutaneous electrical nerve stimulator (TENS) unit before going to sleep has been found to be helpful in some situations (Reimer, 1997).

Osteoarthritis

A noninflammatory joint disease, osteoarthritis is characterized by a chronic, slowly progressing degeneration and loss of articular cartilage in synovial movable joints. Osteoarthritis was formerly classified as degenerative joint disease, which is an inaccurate classification because there is no biochemical or metabolic degeneration. Osteoarthritis can be classified as primary (or idiopathic) or secondary (Lappe and Meyer, 1997). Primary osteoarthritis has no known cause, is associated with aging, is more common in women, and has been demonstrated to have a genetic basis thought to be an autosomal recessive trait. Secondary osteoarthritis, more common in men, is associated with joint injury or disease process. When only one or two joints are affected, it is described as localized; when three or more joints are involved, it is said to be generalized. Primary osteoarthritis is the most common type of arthritis, and approximately 60 million Americans are affected by this condition. Half of the population has osteoarthritis by 16 years of age. The weight-bearing joints—hips, knees, and spine—are most often affected. Finger joints and the great toe are also frequently affected. Between 50 and 60 years of age, the incidence peaks; in those who are 75 years and older the incidence is as high as 85%, and this group is usually symptomatic. Among the older adult population, osteoarthritis is the number one cause of disability.

The cartilage covering the ends of bones is lost secondary to enzymatic destruction. When this cartilage wears away the ends of the bones rub together, becoming rough and damaging the bony tissue. Cysts and fissures frequently develop within the bone and may leak fluid content of the cyst into the synovial space, causing further joint damage. The joint capsule may become inflamed, due to the breaking off of small pieces of new bone that lodge in the synovial space (Lappe and Meyer, 1997; Luckmann, 1997).

The onset of osteoarthritis is frequently insidious. The typical course of this condition is usually one of periods of discomfort followed by periods that are comparatively symptom free (Sack, 1996). The client with osteoarthritis may complain of aching pain in or around the joint and stiffness with loss of joint motion in the involved joints. With progression of the disease process, the aching pain may be felt during resting periods and during the night. The large, weight-bearing joints are the ones affected, and crepitus may be heard as the bony ends inside the joint rub together. The joints may become enlarged and exhibit obvious deformity that is accompanied by muscle spasms. Heberden nodes and Bouchard nodes develop in the hands because of new bony growth that is depositing in the joint, which causes the joint to swell (joint effusion). Flexion contractures may be seen in the hip joints, while the knees may develop *varus* (turning inward toward the midline of the body) and flexion contractures. The movable spinal joints, the cervical and lumbar areas, exhibit a loss of joint space leading to pain, numbness, and tingling arising from pinching of the spinal nerve. The client may develop a limp due to pain, stiffness, and joint instability if the hips and knees are affected.

Although young clients with primary osteoarthritis usually show normal findings of a complete blood cell count and erythrocyte sedimentation rate, as well as negative results for rheumatoid factor and antinuclear antibody tests, older adults may demonstrate elevations in erythrocyte sedimentation rates as well as small elevations in tests for rheumatoid factor and antinuclear antibody (Sack, 1997). Radiographic examinations typically demonstrate joint space narrowing with minimal soft tissue swelling and normal mineralization. As the disease progresses, sclerosis, marginal osteophyte (bone ridges or spurs) formation, occasional subchondral bony cysts, and joint deformity occur (Googe and Gerlach, 1992b; Sack, 1996). Bone scans are useful in determining which joints are affected. Magnetic resonance imaging helps determine the extent of joint damage. If a sample of synovial fluid is taken to be used to differentiate the diagnosis of osteoarthritis from rheumatoid arthritis, the sample should be clear yellow when osteoarthritis is present and milky, cloudy, or dark yellow if rheumatoid arthritis is present (Luckmann, 1997).

W e l l n e s s

"Older adults are more likely to participate in exercise programs if other older adults with similar problems are participants in the program.**"**

The therapeutic goals are to decrease pain and deformity, increase or maintain joint ROM, and maintain joint function. Osteoarthritis is treated with both nonpharmacological and pharmacological interventions. Nonpharmacological interventions include exercise regimens to maintain ROM and to strengthen muscles, applications of heat and cold, use of relaxation techniques and meditation, massage therapy, biofeedback, and hypnosis. The exercise regimen should ideally be one of low impact that emphasizes isometric exercises (performed without joint motion). The client is encouraged to perform exercise even if mild discomfort is felt, because low levels of exercise are beneficial and may help in relieving the chronic pain of osteoarthritis. Taking a warm shower or applying heat to a painful joint before beginning the exercise program allows the individual to more fully participate by increasing tendon expansion and raising the pain threshold. Water aerobics are helpful for those individuals who are obese or whose disease process is severe. A transcutaneous nerve simulation unit may be useful in controlling the pain. Maintaining the individual's ideal body weight is prescribed. Assistive devices are used as needed to provide safety and to promote independence, and joint protective techniques are used to prevent trauma (Luckmann, 1997; Sack, 1997). When a joint becomes inflamed and acutely painful, it may be rested and protected from movement by placing it in a splint. Skin traction or a cervical collar may be used to decrease pain in the vertebrae. Obese individuals are urged to lose the extra weight (Lappe and Meyer, 1997).

Pharmacological interventions are accomplished with the use of nonsteroidal antiin-

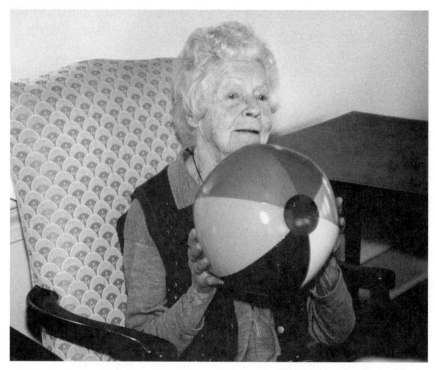

A plastic ball provides safe exercise and the opportunity for interaction.

flammatory drugs (NSAIDs), corticosteroids, and analgesic medications. Nonsteroidal anti-inflammatory drugs are indicated for the relief of mild to moderate pain. Therapeutic effects may not be reached for 2 to 3 weeks after initiating treatment with an NSAID. For those adults who are 65 years or age or older and who are likely to have other chronic conditions, such as hypertension, heart disease, or renal disease, NSAIDs must be used cautiously, employing the lowest dose possible to achieve the therapeutic effect. Because NSAIDs may be irritating to the gastrointestinal tract, it is necessary to administer the medication with food, an antacid, or a histamine-2 receptor antagonist (Pepcid AC) and 8 ounces of water. The client, especially an older adult, should be monitored closely for signs of bleeding (Lappe and Meyer, 1997; Luckmann, 1997; Sack, 1996).

Some clients who experience unrelenting joint pain require a corticosteroid injection directly into the painful joint for relief. These injections usually provide prolonged relief and are, therefore, administered only once or twice per year. Larger joints can utilize a more powerful drug than can smaller joints (Sack, 1996). Results are generally noted in about 48 hours.

Mild analgesics (salicylates) are administered to relieve mild to moderate pain. Narcotics are not used because of the chronicity of osteoarthritis. Enteric-coated aspirin is given because it has a less irritating effect on the gastrointestinal tract and because of its antiinflammatory properties. Acetaminophen is also sometimes used when an individual is unable to tolerate the high doses of aspirin; however, acetaminophen does not have antiinflammatory properties (Luckmann, 1997).

When conservative medical approaches for the management of osteoarthritis are no longer effective in controlling pain and preserving joint motion, surgical interventions are considered. Conservative surgical interventions are considered first. An **osteotomy** is performed to realign a joint and to decrease joint strain by removal of a section of bone (Lappe and Meyer, 1997; Marek et al., 1995). This type of surgery is commonly performed on the legs for correction of *valgus* (knock-knee) and *varus* (bowleg) (Lappe and Meyer, 1997). This surgical approach is considered for those who are not appropriate for a total joint replacement. For example, the very young, the very active, and those who are obese are not good candidates for total joint replacement surgery (Luckmann, 1997). Fusion of a joint is called *arthrodesis* and is conducted with the intent of pain relief and joint stability. This surgical approach is considered when the joint cannot be reconstructed (Lappe and Meyer, 1997), for those whose disease process is too advanced to have an osteotomy, and for those who are too young or too active for a total joint replacement. Arthroscopic surgery is implemented to debride or remove bits of cartilage or bone (Marek et al., 1995).

More progressive surgical interventions are undertaken only when considered imperative. Arthroplasty is the total replacement of a joint. Hips and knees are the joints most frequently replaced. An arthroplasty is performed to restore joint motion and function to the muscles and ligaments and to create a new joint. An arthroplastic procedure is indicated when the joint has become painful and disabled and is no longer responding to more conservative interventions. The prosthetic devices used in arthroplasty surgeries were designed for older adults and for those who live a more sedentary lifestyle (Lappe and Meyer, 1997; Googe and Gerlach, 1992a).

The risk of complications developing after a total hip arthroplasty is a concern of the entire health care team. Some of these complications are rare but are definite threats to the client. Peroneal nerve damage may occur, arising from nerve compression. Hemorrhage and hematoma formation may be seen when there is major resection of tissues and when there is extensive revision of the hip. Because osteomyelitis is so difficult to treat, infections are a major concern. Thromboembolism development after hip arthroplasty is the most common and most serious complication (Lappe and Meyer, 1997). Fat (released from bone marrow) embolism is the type of embolus most often noted after a total hip arthroplasty and is evidenced by a sudden onset of dyspnea, restlessness, agitation, confusion, and stupor. Other clinical features include tachypnea, tachycardia, fever, hypoxemia, and elevated sedimentation rate. These symptoms occur within 24 to 48 hours postoperatively and are likely to be fatal. More than half of the deaths after hip arthroplasty are due to embolism. The operative leg should be maintained in an abducted, slightly externally rotated position for at least 6 weeks postoperatively and maybe for an even longer period of time. To remind the client to maintain this leg position, a wedge-shaped pillow is placed between the legs and is attached around the back of each leg with a Velcro tab. Dislocation and **subluxation** can occur without careful attention to prevention of these complications. Dislocation, when it occurs, is usually noted within a 6-week postoperative period. Sometimes there is a discrepancy in leg length postoperatively. Other long-term postsurgical complications include fractures, nonunion of the bone, loosening of the prosthetic components, and infection (Lappe and Meyer, 1997).

Caring

"Older adults may require special instruction charts or written instructions to help reinforce the learning experience.**"**

Disabling pain, secondary to the osteoarthritic condition, with decreased ROM may affect an individual's functional ability to provide self-care. When functional ability and self-care are impacted, then self-esteem is lowered. The older adult who is experiencing this functional loss may fear losing independence as well. Sometimes this fear becomes reality when the disability progresses. Contractures may develop in the affected joint(s), creating a loss of joint function and further impinging on the individual's independent status.

Spondylosis

Spondylosis is a vertebral ankylosis, a fusion of a vertebral area of the spine causing immobility and consolidation of a joint or joints due to disease, injury, or surgical procedures. Spondylosis causes stenosis of the cervical spinal canal, which produces a chronic compression of the spinal cord and leads to degeneration of the intervertebral disks (Sagar, 1996). The effects are generally noted in the lumbosacral area and may be evidenced as a nonspecific complaint ("clumsy feet" or "legs gave way") (Ebersole and Hess, 1998). The client may demonstrate a spastic gait using small, stiff steps with a narrow base of support (Sagar, 1996). Deep tendon reflexes may be increased, with Babinski signs. The individual may complain of muscle cramps and appear to be leaning to one side (Luckmann, 1997). A definitive diagnosis may be reached with the aid of imaging techniques, including magnetic resonance imaging or computed tomography.

Conservative treatment is implemented first, and if these interventions do not improve the condition, more aggressive intervention is considered (Sagar, 1996). Conservative interventions include those used in treatment of a client experiencing low back pain. The goal of these measures is to place as little strain as possible on the lower back, thereby preventing pain (Carson, 1997). Cervical spinal surgery may be indicated when all other interventions have lost their effect. Surgery may prevent the progression of the symptoms but may not reverse spinal cord damage that has already occurred; therefore, indication for performing this type of surgery for this condition is controversial (Sagar, 1996).

Rheumatoid Arthritis

Rheumatoid arthritis is a chronic systemic inflammatory disorder primarily involving the connective tissues and the synovial membranes of the joints. The cause of rheumatoid arthritis remains unknown. Theories of etiology consider autoimmune, genetic, and viral factors. It usually affects the body symmetrically and typically is a polyarthritis. Rheumatoid arthritis affects females three times more than males (Luckmann, 1997; Meyer, 1997; Sack, 1996). More than 3 million Americans have the diagnosis of rheumatoid arthritis. For those adults 65 years and older, the prevalence of rheumatoid arthritis increases to approximately 10%, and women and men are equally affected (Meyer, 1997). It is believed that an infectious agent may trigger onset of the disease and that rheumatoid arthritis may be exacerbated by fatigue and/or emotional distress (Luckmann, 1997).

Rheumatoid arthritis may develop insidiously, over a period of weeks to months; or its appearance may be explosive, with a sudden manifestation over a short period of time. The client may complain of localized symptoms such as painful, red, swollen, tender, and stiff joints with decreased mobility. Joints feel warm and spongy to palpation. Common systemic symptoms include anorexia, weight loss, fatigue, malaise, and low-grade fever. Subcutaneous nodules may develop over bony prominences. Joint stiffness in the morning that lasts up to 1 hour is frequent and indicates articular inflammation.

The erythrocyte sedimentation rate is increased when the disease is active. Other laboratory values that indicate widespread inflammation include a normocytic, normochromic anemia, as evidenced by a hematocrit reading and thrombocytosis. Blood samples show the presence of antinuclear antibody. Serum samples show rheumatoid factor to be present in about 80% of clients who have rheumatoid arthritis, although this does not provide a definitive diagnosis for the disease. Older adults who do not have the medical diagnosis of rheumatoid arthritis may show mild increases in serum rheumatoid factor. Evidence of acute inflammation in clients with rheumatoid arthritis can be demonstrated by examination of the synovial fluid, which looks cloudy because of a high concentration of white blood cells. During early disease process, radiographs show soft tissue swelling and narrowing of articular space in the affected joints. As the disease process progresses over time (months to years), evidence is seen of articular erosion, which progresses most rapidly during the first 2 to 3 years (Luckmann, 1997; Sack, 1996).

The individual's level of ability is supported by history and physical findings. The client is observed for indications of pain, such as facial expressions, groaning on joint movement, and the manner in which joints are moved. The nurse should elicit subjective information related to pain when the joint is at rest as well as when activity is being performed. Functional ability is assessed to determine the client's capability to perform ADLs. The client is asked if the expected, usual (as described earlier) local symptoms are present and to what extent they are bothersome. The nurse should assess for presence of systemic symptoms and to what extent they interfere with the performance of ADLs. During the physical examination, ROM and muscle strength of the extremity are tested. The client's gait is observed to ascertain whether there is any joint edema and deformity. The involved joints are palpated to determine if warmth, swelling, and subcutaneous nodules are present.

Manifestations of rheumatoid arthritis, other than joint manifestations, may occur at any time during the course of the disease and may at times become more prominent and troublesome than the articular symptoms. These systemic manifestations need to be treated as soon as possible because they are major predictors of morbidity and, in some instances, mortality (Meyer, 1997).

CLINICAL FEATURES

Dermatological Presentation. Firm nontender subcutaneous nodules, ranging in diameter from 3 mm to 3 cm, may develop over pressure points. This is the best known of the rheumatoid extraarticular symptoms and is the most specific finding (Starkebaum, 1993). These nodules are rarely present early in the disease course but do occur in about 25% of those clients who have a positive serum rheumatoid factor. Rheumatoid vasculitis may lead to skin ulceration. Rheumatoid vasculitis is an inflammation of the small blood vessels outside the joints and, along with ulceration, may cause peripheral neuropathy. Biopsy may be done to determine the extent of the vasculitis. Symptomatic treatment—which includes smoking cessation, low doses of prednisone, antiplatelet agents, and ulcer care—is initiated (Meyer, 1997). Hemorrhage and purpura may occur as the result of rheumatoid vasculitis.

Respiratory Presentation. Pulmonary fibrosis is commonly seen in clients (approximately 28%) who have rheumatoid arthritis. Smoking contributes to this condition. Caplan's syndrome, pneumoconiosis, may develop in some who have rheumatoid arthritis. This condition consists of multiple large nodules throughout the lungs. It usually occurs in those with rheumatoid arthritis who have been occupationally exposed to silica. Varying treatment conditions are available (Meyer, 1997). Occasionally, dyspnea, stridor, and hoarseness develop if there is involvement of the cricoarytenoid joints.

Cardiac Presentation. For individuals who have rheumatoid arthritis, pericarditis is the most frequent cardiac manifestation, occurring in about 50% of those with the diagnosis. Glucocorticoid treatment yields a response. Disease of the mitral and aortic valves involves the development of nodules on the valves and thickening of the cusps (Meyer, 1997).

Ocular Presentation. Many of the ocular problems that are common to individuals who have rheumatoid arthritis are potentially blinding. Sjögren's syndrome, a chronic inflammatory condition, is the most commonly occurring ophthalmological condition in the client with rheumatoid arthritis. The eyes are dry, related to lymphocytic infiltration and destruction of the lacrimal glands by an autoimmune response. Scleritis and episcleritis, redness, and discomfort, may also be seen. Scleritis is the most harmful of the two conditions; it can cause severe eye pain and blindness. Hyperemic, painful nodules are present in the sclera secondary to vasculitis and can lead to ulcers of the cornea and glaucoma. This condition is treated with topical glucocorticoids and systemic antiinflammatory agents. If glaucoma does develop, then treatment for this is necessary as well (Meyer, 1997).

W e l l n e s s

❝*Many musculoskeletal conditions are more manageable today than they were in the past.***❞**

Neurological Presentation. Diffuse distal neuropathy secondary to peripheral nerve compression is usually associated with extensive synovitis. The client may complain of burning pain and paresthesias following the course of the nerve. Local injections of corticosteroids usually provide relief (Meyer, 1997).

Felty's Syndrome. Felty's syndrome, splenomegaly with concomitant leukopenia, may develop in clients who have severe rheumatoid arthritis (Akil and Amos, 1995). The client is at high risk for developing infections such as pneumonia and joint infections arising from the neutropenia. Felty's syndrome may be treated with the disease-modifying antirheumatic drugs for rheumatoid arthritis (e.g., gold salts) (Meyer, 1997).

Vasculitis. Vasculitis is composed of a group of disorders, including polyarteritis nodosa, systemic necrotizing vasculitis, and allergic agranulomatosis angiitis, that cause necrotizing inflammation of the blood vessels, leading to damaged large and small vessels with the consequence of end-stage organ damage. Symptoms manifested depend on the organ involved. Vasculitis is treated with corticosteroids (Meyer, 1997).

TREATMENT

The goals of treatment are to relieve the pain and discomfort, prevent joint destruction and deformity by arresting the inflammatory process, and maintain or improve joint and muscle function. A multidisciplinary approach is used that includes the following components: education, physical therapy, occupational therapy, psychosocial therapy, and nonpharmacological as well as a balance of pharmacological interventions.

Nonpharmacological modalities include using a variety of interventions in combination to accomplish the goals. It is important for the client with rheumatoid arthritis, especially an older adult, to attain a balance between *rest* and *activity*. *Exercising* helps to preserve joint mobility and muscle strength. Isometric exercises, a form of active exercise that does not alter the length of the muscle when performed againsta stable resistance, is a stabilizer of damaged joints, especially weight-bearing joints. Joint function is maintained or improved through the performance of gentle stretching exercises and ROM exercises.

Rest for the entire body aids in reducing joint inflammation. Fatigue is considered to be one measure of activity of the disease process. When inflammation is severe, the client tires earlier in the day than one whose inflammatory process is less severe. Clients should be encouraged to get more than 8 hours of sleep during the night and one or two restful naps during the day as well. When inflammation is severe, rest also includes inactivity for the inflamed joints. However, as inflammation begins to subside the client needs to begin to gradually increase activity so as to not lose joint mobility and function. Orthopedic splints and braces are used during periods of inflammation to ensure that the affected joints are rested and proper alignment is maintained. The occupational therapist instructs the client in the principles and strategies of joint protection—how to accomplish a task without pain.

Applications of *heat* or *cold* therapy are beneficial in pain relief. Wet or dry heat applications may be used depending on the preference of the client. Paraffin baths are sometimes used as a method of heat application. However, some clients believe that better pain relief is accomplished in an inflamed joint by the use of ice massage. The use of *assistive devices* for ambulation and *adaptive devices* are forms of support often used by a client with rheumatoid arthritis. See Box 16–7 for a list of uses of assistive devices.

Pharmacological management consists of administration of a variety of drugs: nonsteroidal antiinflammatory agents (NSAIDs), corticosteroids, remission-inducing agents, immunosuppressive drugs, experimental medications, and adjuvant medications. NSAIDs act rapidly, and a response is readily noticed, which makes them a good choice for initial treatment of the client who has rheumatoid arthritis. This class of drugs is used with the goal of inflammation reduction, but these medications are not capable of reversing the disease process. Thus, the bones continue with rough and weakened edges and the inflammation returns as the effects of the medication wear off (Meyer, 1997; Sack, 1996). *Aspirin* at one time was the first drug of choice of the NSAIDs with which to treat rheumatoid arthritis because of its analgesic, antiinflammatory, and antipyretic actions. Although still currently used, it is not prescribed as frequently as it once was because there are now a number of other drugs in this same class with less troubling side effects (Meyer, 1997). When aspirin is prescribed, a large quantity (10 to 20 tablets per day) must be taken to reach a therapeutic blood level, and thus compliance can be a problem (Sack, 1996). Such high doses place the client at risk for developing other troubling problems, such as gastrointestinal irritation and bleeding, impaired platelet function, and ototoxicity.

There is a growing number of other nonsteroidal antiinflammatory medications with simpler dosing schedules that are currently in

Box 16-7   ASSISTIVE DEVICES FOR AMBULATION

Crutches
- Must be the correct length.
- Never walk with crutches in stocking feet, slippers, or high heels.
- Teach the proper crutch walking gait.
- Teach how to be safe in the environment.
- The physical therapist usually measures for length and implements the appropriate teaching. The nurse usually reinforces what has been taught and assesses for correct use of the crutches.

Canes
- Must be long enough to allow for elbow extension and weight bearing on the hand holding the cane.
- Needs a rubber-tipped end for safety.
- Use on the side opposite the affected leg.
- Canes are used when only minimal support is necessary.

Walkers
- Supplies additional support for balance.
- The walker is advanced forward and the client then steps forward.

use, some of which can be purchased without a prescription. Those in common use include ibuprofen (Motrin, Advil), naproxen (Anaprox, Naprosyn), and sulindac (Clinoril) (Meyer, 1997). Because these medications can be so irritating to the gastrointestinal mucosa, a histamine receptor antagonist (e.g., ranitidine [Zantac]) is also prescribed for the client to reduce secretion of gastric acids (Deglin and Vallerand, 1997). Older adults seem to experience high incidences of severe gastrointestinal irritation and central nervous system toxicity related to the NSAIDs; thus, prescribing the lowest effective dose possible is a safety measure (Sack, 1996).

Low doses of oral *corticosteroids* tend to provide adequate symptomatic relief for some clients. As soon as symptomatic relief is achieved, the dose is gradually tapered to the lowest dose possible to control inflammation and pain, because these drugs are associated with serious side effects. This class of drugs is usually reserved for those clients who have had a poor response to the NSAIDs. Even in low doses these drugs inhibit absorption of calcium from the gastrointestinal tract, leading to bone loss as well as decreased bone re-formation (Sack, 1996). If the client enters a period of stress, however, the dose must be increased be-

cause the adrenal glands have been suppressed and will not be able to respond adequately.

Slow-acting agents, disease-modifying antirheumatic drugs, may be added to the treatment regimen when a rapidly acting antirheumatic drug has not completely eradicated the signs of inflammation. These medications slow progression of the disease process and provide short-term (maybe 5 years) benefit but do not alter the eventual outcome of the disease. Because these drugs act slowly, a perceptible effective response may require several months of administration of the drug. *Gold salts* have been used for the past 30 years to treat rheumatoid arthritis. There is a delay of 2 to 3 months before improvement is seen, and injections must be given frequently. The client must be monitored closely, with complete blood cell counts and urinalyses to monitor renal function (Meyer, 1997). Toxicity occurs readily but is reversible (Deglin and Vallerand, 1997). There is a form of gold that can be taken orally, but onset of effectiveness requires a longer period of time than the injectable form of gold and may not be quite as good (Sack, 1996). *Hydroxychloroquine (Plaquenil),* an antimalarial agent, has an unknown antiinflammatory action, is easily administered, and is relatively safe. About 6 months is necessary before improvement is seen, but the effectiveness of this drug is about the same as for the gold salts. Monitoring with frequent laboratory tests is not necessary, but it is important to schedule ophthalmological examinations before beginning the medication and every 3 to 6 months during therapy to evaluate for macular degeneration (Deglin and Vallerand, 1997). *Immunosuppressant agents* are also used to treat rheumatoid arthritis. They may be used when rheumatoid arthritis has not responded well to other agents. Examples of immunosuppressant drugs include azathioprine (Imuran), cyclophosphamide, and methotrexate.

Caring

"Encourage older adults to move slowly when changing positions so as to maintain balance."

Rheumatoid arthritis is also treated with experimental drugs such as biological response modifiers, immunomodifiers, antioxidants, and inhibitors of cartilage metabolism (Meyer, 1997). As with use of any experimental drug, clients are monitored closely so that medication dosage can be altered as needed. Examples of drugs included in this group are monoclonal antibodies and interferon (Luckmann, 1997).

Complications of rheumatoid arthritis are generally due to the disease process itself or the side effects of drug therapy or other treatment modality. Because the disease process affects body systems, complications can involve organs of the body as well. Organ involvement may be life threatening, as in pulmonary fibrosis and nodules and pericarditis. Inflammation in the tissues over the eyes (episcleritis) can develop when the disease process is advanced. Many clients experience severe symptoms and disabling deformities (Googe and Gerlach, 1992b). Depression may occur in the client who is trying to cope with the stress of living with a chronic condition such as rheumatoid arthritis. Pain and loss of independence can lead to low self-esteem, impacting depression. If the client views the disease process as one of continual loss, powerlessness, helplessness, and hopelessness will contribute to the state of depression.

The side effects of the different classes of medications used in the treatment of rheumatoid arthritis can lead to such problems as bleeding, gastrointestinal irritation and ulceration, and delayed healing, which are secondary to the NSAIDs. The hepatic and renal systems are at risk for becoming dysfunctional as the result of dosing with this group of medications. Those clients using aspirin, especially in high doses, are at risk for developing aspirin toxicity, hypersensitivity reactions, tinnitus, and hearing loss. Allergy, anemia, renal disorder, and bone marrow suppression are examples of other complications that can develop related to drug therapy for rheumatoid arthritis. Various drug-to-drug interactions are also a possibility (Meyer, 1997).

Surgical management is an approach to treating rheumatoid arthritis, in conjunction with medical management. Surgical techniques are currently being used early in the disease course as a prevention for deformity. Surgery is implemented to accomplish the same goals as the medical approaches, to relieve pain, to correct deformities, and to improve function. Such surgical approaches as tendon transfer and osteotomy, synovectomy, arthrodesis, and total joint arthroplasty may be used to accomplish the goals (see the section on osteoarthritis for further discussion of these procedures).

Older adult clients may have more difficulty with both medical and surgical management techniques than a younger person would have. Older adults may not wish to follow exercise regimens for fear of causing pain. This lack of compliance worsens the problem of pain. When one becomes sedentary, any movement is painful.

Older individuals fear appearing in public because of the possibility of embarrassment over slowness of ambulation and movement. They are more likely to participate in exercise programs if other older adults with similar problems are participants in the program. Water aerobics classes for arthritic clients are beneficial and enjoyable. The water seems to lessen the pain experienced on exercise. Older adults also are less likely than a younger person to choose surgery as a treatment method. The idea of surgery frightens most older adults because of dependency issues. Recovery time is generally longer for older adults than for younger people, which means a longer stay in a rehabilitation facility (Meyer, 1997).

Gouty Arthritis

Gout (or gouty arthritis) is a genetic defect of purine (protein) metabolism leading to an excess of uric acid that accumulates in joints. Men between 40 and 60 years of age are more commonly affected than women, in whom gout usually appears in the post-menopausal period. Gout develops either as an overproduction of uric acid or as an under-secretion of uric acid (Sack, 1996). An acute inflammatory reaction occurs in the joint spaces secondary to the deposition of uric acid crystals.

The typical presentation of an acute attack of gout is the sudden onset of pain and swelling, with limited movement in a distal joint—usually the feet, legs, or great toe—which is the target in 50% of first gouty attacks (Luckmann, 1997; Sack, 1996). The involved joint feels warm to touch, appears dusky red, and is extremely sensitive to touch. The serum uric acid level will be elevated (>7.0 mg/dL), and there is a family history of gout. Aspiration of synovial fluid from the infected joint reveals urate crystals, which provides a definitive diagnosis. After several episodes of acute gout, the gout becomes chronic. With the progression of the disease, degenerative arthritic changes occur, including cartilaginous destruction and joint space narrowing.

Management is considered in relation to the acute phase as well as long-term therapy (Lappe and Meyer, 1997). Dietary considerations are controversial but include a low-purine diet that eliminates many proteins. The individual is instructed to avoid red and organ meats, lunch meats, shellfish, sardines, anchovies, and meat gravies. Some physicians prescribe these dietary changes, others only eliminate red and organ meats, whereas still others prescribe no dietary changes.

Medication management of the acute phase includes the use of colchicine and the NSAIDs to decrease pain and relieve inflammation. Clients who are taking colchicine are monitored closely for signs of toxicity such as nausea, vomiting, and diarrhea because the therapeutic dose and the toxic dose are very close. When milder antiinflammatory drugs are not effective, corticosteroids may be initiated. Allopurinol, which suppresses uric acid production, or probenecid, which promotes resorption and excretion of uric acid, is prescribed for long-term therapy. Excessive alcohol intake and starvation diets should be avoided. The client with gouty arthritis should be placed on bed rest with the affected part immobilized during acute flareups. Ice packs or heat packs over the affected area may help relieve the pain.

C a r i n g

66*Heat application must be used cautiously because older adults may have impaired feeling in the area being treated and are thus at risk for a burn injury.*99

Fractures

A fracture occurs when there is a break in the continuity of a bone secondary to more stress being placed on the bone than the bone is able to absorb. Secondary injury to the surrounding structures—skin, subcutaneous tissues, muscles, blood vessels, nerves, ligaments, and tendons—may occur when the fracture occurs. The most immediate concern is with the possibility of hemorrhage and shock (Black, 1997; Luckmann, 1997). The highest incidence of fractures occurs in young males and in older adults, especially women who are 65 years and older. Older adults are likely to have problems with balance, gait, and/or mobility and to have chronic degenerative conditions placing them at a high risk for falls and resulting fractures (Marek et al., 1995). A younger person who falls is likely to fracture a wrist in an attempt to catch himself or herself, but an older individual who falls is more likely to fracture a hip (Ebersole and Hess, 1998). A fracture for an older adult can be devastating because it may interfere with a return to prefracture functional ability. The thought of becoming dependent is very frightening to older adults, so those who do sustain a fracture tend to work very hard at rehabilitation to restore their independence.

Fractures may be classified in many ways; some of the most common classifications (Luckmann, 1997) include

- By extent of damage: compound (open) or closed (simple)
- By fracture line: oblique or spiral
- By anatomical location: femoral head
- By a person's name: Pott's
- By appearance of the fracture: burst
- By the method that caused the fracture: bumper

Although fractures generally have a causative factor, in older adults a fracture may occur pathologically due to a disease process. For example, an older adult may stand up to leave the dinner table and suddenly fall. In these instances, it is difficult to determine if the fall caused the fracture or the fracture caused the fall. In the older adult population, fractures may occur and be asymptomatic. Sometimes the bony fragments of hip fractures are not displaced and there is no need to surgically repair the fracture. Nondisplaced fractures are treated with non–weight bearing or partial weight bearing on the affected side (Yang et al., 1996).

C a r i n g

Older adults may want to keep yogurt on hand to eat before taking calcium.

When a fracture occurs, the small blood vessels in the surrounding tissues rupture and bleed into the fracture site, forming a hematoma. Within 3 to 10 days after the fracture, the hematoma begins to break down and the *callus*, new tissue, begins to form. This provisional callus remodels and an ossified callus, rigid bone, forms. The length of time required for the permanent callus, bone healing, to occur depends on the location and extent of the

fracture and the individual's general condition at the time of fracture.

There is deformity of the extremity secondary to strong muscle spasms (involuntary contractions of the muscles surrounding the fracture site), which cause bony overriding changing the alignment of the bone. Swelling and bruising (ecchymosis) may develop rapidly because of local bleeding into surrounding tissues. Tenderness and pain, usually severe, occur due to overriding of bony fragments, muscle spasms, or injury to surrounding structures. Numbness and tingling or paralysis may occur related to nerve compression or damage. Normal functioning of the area is lost because of instability of bone, pain, and/or muscle spasm. Abnormal mobility in a body part that is normally not mobile may be seen. Grating sounds (crepitus) may occur from bony fragmented ends rubbing together when the injured part is moved. Hypovolemic shock may develop if there is a large amount of blood loss (Black, 1997; Luckmann, 1997; Marek et al., 1995).

Definitive diagnosis is based on radiography, fluoroscopy, and computed tomography to determine the exact location and the direction of the line of the fracture. Anteroposterior and lateral radiographs are taken before reduction of the fracture and include the joints above and below the fracture site. Radiographs of these same angles are taken after reduction is accomplished, as well as periodically during the course of the healing process. The possibility of joint injury may be determined by the use of arthroscopy. Other laboratory examinations that may be done to determine extent of concomitant injury include complete blood cell count, which gives an indication of the amount of blood loss; urinalysis, which shows presence of myoglobinuria; and serum studies of cardiac enzymes, which demonstrate evidence of cardiac contusion (Black, 1997; Luckmann, 1997). Careful history taking will provide information related to the mechanism of the injury. The client is observed for the need of initiation of acute care—the ABCs of airway, bleeding, circulation.

Treatment is geared toward the relief of pain, facilitating bone healing, and preserving function so that the client may return to preinjury status. Fractures are reduced either by closed reduction methods such as manipulation, casting, traction, or the use of an external fixator or by open reduction internal fixation methods. Open reduction internal fixation requires a surgical procedure with a fixating device implanted into the fracture site to maintain bony alignment. Immobilization is the other important aspect of fracture treatment. Open (compound) fractures are surgical emergencies and require antibiotic therapy, surgical debridement of dead tissue and foreign material from the wound, and closure of the wound as well as reduction of the fracture. If debridement needs to be repeated, it is done within 24 to 72 hours. Applications of cold are usually applied over the injury site for the first 24 to 48 hours after the injury occurs to decrease bleeding and swelling; then applications of heat may be used to improve circulation to the area, thereby promoting healing. For severe levels of pain, narcotic analgesics may be ordered. This class of drugs must be used very cautiously in the older adult population. As pain lessens, after the first couple of days, analgesia is achieved with nonnarcotic intervention. NSAIDs may also be prescribed for their analgesic, antipyretic, and antiinflammatory effects.

The client who has suffered a fractured bone is at risk for developing long-term complications. Prolonged immobilization leads to joint stiffness, which occurs more often in the upper extremities. Posttraumatic arthritis may develop because of the severity of the initial injury and may at a later date require a total joint arthroplasty. Avascular (aseptic) necrosis, the death of bone tissue, is related to the lack of blood supply to the tissues. Avascular necrosis is most often associated with fractures of the femoral head and carpal fractures. Delayed union, malunion, and nonunion are complications of fracture healing. *Delayed union* refers to slowing, but not complete stopping, of the healing process. Pain and tenderness may continue beyond a reasonable healing time because of distraction of the fracture fragments or infection. *Malunion* refers to healing of improperly aligned fracture fragments even with proper initial reduction. It is sometimes associated with weight bearing too soon. *Non-*

Caring

❝*Older adults may not be suited to use crutches because their upper extremities may not be strong enough to bear their weight on their hands. Use of crutches also requires good balance and coordination, which many older adults lack.***❞**

union refers to a situation in which fracture healing has not occurred within 4 to 6 months after the fracture was sustained. Nonunion may be due to poor blood supply to the fracture site or repetitive stress on the fracture site.

Although the prognosis for fracture healing is usually good depending on the age of the individual sustaining the injury, the location of the fracture (need a good blood supply), severity of the fracture, and method of treatment (fractures treated by open reduction internal fixation usually heal faster), older adults often are dealing with one or a number of chronic conditions other than the fracture. Those older adults who have osteoporosis, as well as the very frail, can expect a poorer prognosis.

Caring

❝*During the winter months, older adults may want to sleep under an electric blanket with a low heat to decrease pain and stiffness upon arising.***❞**

A fracture, as well as many other chronic musculoskeletal conditions, causes pain. Traditional methods of treatment are often effective in controlling the pain. However, when these interventions do not achieve effective pain management, complementary interventions may be implemented. See Box 16–8 for complementary *nonpharmacological pain* measures and techniques.

Self-care teaching related to prevention of the development of a musculoskeletal condition ideally is begun at a very early age. The fo-

Box 16-8   NONPHARMACOLOGICAL PAIN MEASURES AND TECHNIQUES

Behavioral Technique
- Meditation—Focuses attention away from pain
- Autogenic training—Uses relaxation and self-suggestion, which lead to self-control
- Progressive relaxation training—Uses alternating contracting and relaxing certain muscle groups leading to deep relaxation
- Guided imagery—Uses a combination of distraction and relaxation
- Rhythmic breathing—Combined relaxation and distraction
- Operant conditioning—Used for clients who have high levels of pain that impair functional ability
- Biofeedback—Assists the client in learning to control the physiological variables associated with pain

Therapeutic Touch
- Implemented by a nurse to realign the client's energy fields

Transcutaneous Electrical Nerve Stimulation
- Eliminates the pain possibly causing the body to secrete endorphins and enkephalin

Hypnosis
- Focuses attention away from the pain
- Uses distraction and relaxation

Acupressure
- Cutaneous stimulation over acupuncture points

cus of the self-care becomes one of health maintenance, and teaching is related to specific interventions that are designed to alleviate the problem and prevent complications. See Box 16–9 for teaching points for older adults with musculoskeletal disorders.

Summary

Musculoskeletal disorders are not uncommon among the older adult population. Many of these conditions are more manageable today then they were in the past. Newer medications and treatment modalities allow for greater manageability of the disorder. It is never too late to initiate self-care behavior. Many self-care behaviors if begun at an early age will prevent or lessen the impact of a disease process. Older adults need to be taught dietary considerations that will prevent further bone loss seen in osteomalacia, osteoporosis, and Paget's disease. Because pathological fractures are likely to occur when these conditions are present, extreme caution is used when helping a client to maneuver. Activity is encouraged to prevent demineralization from immobilization. For the older client with a rheumatoid condition, careful monitoring of the medication regimen is necessary. Polypharmacy among older adults makes this aspect of treatment a priority. Although the older adult is at risk for developing many chronic musculoskeletal conditions, there is self-care input that can be implemented to lessen the severity of these disorders.

Box 16-9 TEACHING POINTS FOR OLDER ADULTS WITH MUSCULOSKELETAL DISORDERS

The nurse should stress:

1. All aspects of the disease process that the older adult is experiencing.
2. The importance of complying to medication regimen.
3. Continuation of some type of weight-bearing exercise program.
4. The necessity of moving slowly and carefully.
5. Pharmacological and nonpharmacological interventions for pain control.
6. Appropriate use of pain relief methods to achieve maximum independence.
7. Appropriate use of heat/cold.
8. Measures that reduce strain on the lower back and allow appropriate body alignment without twisting.
9. The need to avoid sitting for long periods of time and to avoid sitting in chairs that are too low to the floor.
10. Sleeping on a firm mattress.
11. Balance rest and activity.
12. Correct use of assistive devices for ambulation as well as those used to accomplish ADLs.
13. Safety measures for injury prevention.
14. Appropriate use, application, and care of joint protective devices, splints, and braces.
15. The need to check with the physician before spending money on rheumatoid arthritis "cures" that may be unfounded and useless. Approximately $1 billion each year is spent on these types of treatments.
16. Importance of follow-up care such as doctor's appointments and laboratory appointments.

RESOURCES

Agency for Health Care Policy and Research Publications Clearinghouse
PO Box 8547
Silver Spring, MD 20907
(800) 358-9295

American Pain Society
5700 Old Orchard Road
Skokie, IL 60077
(708) 966-5595

Arthritis Foundation
2045 Peachtree Road NE
Atlanta, GA 30326
(404) 351-0454

Arthritis Information Clearinghouse
PO Box 34427
Bethesda, MD 20034
(301) 881-9411

National Arthritis and Musculoskeletal and Skin Diseases Information Clearinghouse
1 AMS Circle
Bethesda, MD 20892-3675
(301) 495-4484

National Chronic Pain Outreach Association
8222 Wycliff Court
Manassas, VA 22110
(703) 368-7357

National Institute on Aging Information Center
PO Box 8057
Gaithersburg, MD 20898-8057
(800) 222-2225

National Osteoporosis Foundation
1150 17th Street NW, Suite 500
Washington, DC 20004
(202) 347-8800

National Rehabilitation Information Center
8455 Colesville Road, Suite 935
Silver Spring, MD 20910-3319
(800) 346-2742

Paget's Foundation
200 Varick Street, Suite 1004
New York, NY 10014-4810
(212) 299-2588
(800) 23-PAGET

REFERENCES

Akil M, Amos R. (1995). ABC of rheumatology: Rheumatoid arthritis: Clinical features and diagnosis. BMJ 310:587–90.

Black JM. (1997). Nursing care of clients with musculoskeletal trauma or overuse. In Black JM, Matassarin-Jacobs E, eds. Medical-Surgical Nursing: Clinical Management for Continuity of Care. 5th ed. Philadelphia: WB Saunders.

Burke MM. (1997). Mobility. In Burke MM, Walsh MB, eds. Gerontologic Nursing: Wholistic Care of the Older Adult. 2nd ed. St. Louis: CV Mosby.

Carson P. (1997). Nursing care of clients with disorders of the spinal cord, peripheral nerves, and cranial nerves. In Black JM, Matassarin-Jacobs E, eds. Medical-Surgical Nursing: Clinical Management for Continuity of Care. 5th ed. Philadelphia: WB Saunders.

Clark JB, Queener SF, Kaib VB. (1993). Pharmacologic Basis of Nursing Practice. St. Louis: CV Mosby.

Deglin JH, Vallerand AH. (1997). Davis's Drug Guide for Nurses. 5th ed. Philadelphia: FA Davis.

Ebersole P, Hess P. (1998). Toward Healthy Aging, Human Needs, and Nursing Response. St. Louis: CV Mosby.

Fleming LA. (1992). Osteoporosis: Clinical features, prevention, and treatment. J Gen Intern Med 7:554–558.

Googe MC, Gerlach MJM. (1992a). Nursing management of adults experiencing musculoskeletal trauma and surgery. In Burrell LO, ed. Adult Nursing in Hospital and Community Settings. East Norwalk, CT: Appleton & Lange.

Googe MC, Gerlach MJM. (1992b). Nursing management of adults with disorders of the musculoskeletal system. In Burrell LO, ed. Adult Nursing in Hospital and Community Settings. East Norwalk, CT: Appleton & Lange.

Ignatavicius DD, Bayne MV. (1991). Medical-Surgical Nursing: A Nursing Process Approach. Philadelphia: WB Saunders.

Lappe J, Meyer CL. (1997). Nursing care of clients with musculoskeletal disorders. In Black JM, Matassarin-Jacobs E, eds. Medical-Surgical Nursing: Clinical Management for Continuity of Care. 5th ed. Philadelphia: WB Saunders.

Lonergan ET, Harris ST. (1996). Osteoporosis. In Lonergan ET, ed. Geriatrics: A Lange Clinical Manual. East Norwalk, CT Appleton & Lange.

Luckmann J. (1997). Manual of Nursing Care. Philadelphia: WB Saunders.

Marek JF. (1995). Assessment of the musculoskeletal system. In Phipps WJ, Cassmeyer VL, Lehman MK, eds. Medical-Surgical Nursing Concepts and Clinical Practice. 5th ed. St. Louis: CV Mosby.

Marek JF, Buergin PS, Paskert KM. (1995). Management of persons with inflammatory and degenerative disorders of the musculoskeletal system. In Phipps WJ, Cassmeyer VL, Lehman MK, eds. Medical-Surgical Nursing Concepts and Clinical Practice. 5th ed. St. Louis: CV Mosby.

Meyer CL. (1977). Nursing Care of Clients with Connective Tissue Disorders. In Black JM, Matassarin-Jacobs E, eds. Medical-Surgical Nursing: Clinical Management for Continuity of Care. 5th ed. Philadelphia: WB Saunders.

Miller CA. (1995). Nursing Care of Older Adults: Theory and Practice. Chicago: Scott, Foresman.

Parker KP, Clinton DRS. (1992). Nursing management of adults with disorders of the kidneys. In Burrell LO, ed. Adult Nursing in Hospital and Community Settings. East Norwalk, CT: Appleton & Lange.

Reimer M. (1997). Sleep and sensory disorders. In Black JM, Matassarin-Jacobs E, eds. Medical-Surgical Nursing: Clinical Management for Continuity of Care. 5th ed. Philadelphia: WB Saunders.

Sack KE. (1996). Musculoskeletal diseases. In Lonergan ET, ed. Geriatrics: A Lange Clinical Manual. East Norwalk, CT: Appleton & Lange.

Sagar SM. (1997). Gait instability and falls. In Lonergan ET, ed. Geriatrics: A Lange Clinical Manual. East Norwalk, CT: Appleton & Lange.

Sands JK. (1995). Human sexuality. In Phipps WJ, Cassmeyer VL, Lehman MK, eds. Medical-Surgical Nursing Concepts and Clinical Practice. 5th ed. St. Louis: CV Mosby.

Seidel HM, Ball JW, Dains JE, Benedict GW. (1995). Mosby's Guide to Physical Examination. 3rd ed. St. Louis: CV Mosby.

Sims LK, D'Amico D, Stiesmeyer J, Webster JA. (1995). Health Assessment in Nursing. Redwood City, CA: Benjamin/Cummings.

Starkebaum G. (1993). Review of rheumatoid arthritis: Recent developments. Immunol Allergy Clin North Am 13:273–289.

Townsend MC. (1996). Psychiatric Mental Health Nursing: Concepts of Care. 2nd ed. Philadelphia: FA Davis, 1996.

Yang KH, Shea KL, Demetropoulos CK, et al. (1996). The relationship between loading conditions and fracture patterns of the proximal femur. J Biomech Eng 118(11):575–578.

CRITICAL THINKING EXERCISES

Mrs. Emma Smith, a 78-year-old woman, visited her doctor for a routine check-up this morning. A bone density radiograph was taken, and she was told that she has osteoporo-

(continued on following page)

CRITICAL THINKING EXERCISES Continued

sis. Mrs. Smith told her physician that she is not a very active person but likes to sit and watch TV. She smokes two packs of cigarettes per day and usually drinks a liter of wine with dinner.

1. Compare Mrs. Smith's history with the known risk factors for osteoporosis.
2. Develop a care plan for Mrs. Smith, including possible nursing diagnoses for osteoporosis, dietary interventions, possible drug interventions, an exercise regimen, and teaching needs in relation to all factors of the disease process.
3. Discuss the pros and cons of estrogen replacement therapy for Mrs. Smith.

CHAPTER 17

Maintaining Wellness of the
Brain and Nerves

Paula Hudgins, MS, RNCS
Vergie M. Brannon, MSN RN-C

CHAPTER OUTLINE

OBJECTIVES

After completing this chapter, the reader will be able to:

1. Compare and contrast normal neurological functioning of the brain and nerves in adults and older adults.
2. Identify how memory, language/speech, visuospatial function, attention, concentration, executive function, and mood relate to the neuropsychological stability of a patient.
3. Write a teaching plan that incorporates modifications for the older adult learner.
4. Employ nursing strategies for the older adult experiencing a neurological disorder.

KEY TERMS

aphasia
bradykinesia
dysphagia
hemianesthesia
hemiparesis

The functions of the brain and nerves in humans are to (1) regulate internal body systems, (2) receive conscious and unconscious stimuli from both internal and external sources, (3) integrate and interpret stimuli, and (4) initiate or instigate responses that allow the individual to maintain a state of dynamic equilibrium and normal physiological functioning. The brain and spinal cord are part of the central nervous system, whereas the nerves outside the cranial cavity and the spinal column are part of the peripheral nervous system (Depace, 1994). Normal physiological function is dependent on the two systems integrating smoothly with each other, and changes in one invariably impact the function of the other.

The brain and nerves regulate, monitor, integrate, interpret, and influence all other body systems; therefore, during assessment of each body system, information is gathered about the overall neurological status of the client. Assessment of the nervous system, both peripheral and central, often begins unconsciously the moment the nurse meets the client(s). The following vignette can assist in conceptualizing a neurological assessment.

CASE STUDY

Mrs. A, age 88, has requested a complete physical examination. She is a small-framed, neatly dressed, clean woman. She is reading a magazine when called from the waiting room and asks if she can take the magazine with her to the examination room to complete an article. Her gait is stable and she quickly locates the examination room. When instructed to change into a gown, she asks where she is to put her clothing and begins the task. When you return to the room, Mrs. A is seated on the examination table.

Neurological examination of Mrs. A reveals an alert/oriented ×4 white female, with appropriate dress and behavior. Reasoning and arithmetic calculations are intact. Immediate, recent, and remote memory are intact. Her mood is pleasant and relaxed, and her affect is congruent with her mood. Her speech is clear and smoothly enunciated. Thought processes are well organized and logical. Thought content is negative for suicidal/homicidal thoughts. She denied hallucinations, delusions, and ideas of reference. Cranial nerves I to XII are intact. She wears a hearing aid and corrective lens. Proprioception and cerebellar function are intact. There is moderate loss of superficial touch and pain sensation bilaterally of the hands and feet. Deep tendon reflexes are 2+ bilateral in all extremities. Plantar reflex is negative bilaterally with no clonus.

Mrs. A clearly has an intact neurological system that is integrating internal and external stimuli smoothly and making appropriate responses to stimuli received. Mrs. A appears to be able to communicate well with others, and her physiological functions are all intact. She has adapted well to the aging process by having regular physical examinations and identifying changes within her neurological system that can be corrected to allow her to continue normal activities of daily living without distress.

HEALTH TEACHING

Weinrich and colleagues (1994) noted that despite their lack of knowledge regarding health topics, older adults were less likely to participate in health screening and assessment than younger adults. They noted that many sources have demonstrated that when older adults attend health education programs their adherence to specific health directions can be quite high. It was also noted that with the biophysical changes of aging, educational programs should be redesigned for the older learner and address issues relevant to decreased neurological functioning, including decreased cognitive response time and decreased sensory, visual, and auditory functions.

Older adults need to understand that changes in their neurological system do not lead to loss of vitality, general intellect, and ability to complete functions of daily life (Depace, 1994). The brain and nerves are a very complex system that works collaboratively, as well as independently, in assisting the individual to maintain normal body functions. While they will experience changes in their neuroanatomy, the changes focus on a decreased effectiveness in performing tasks rather than failure to perform the expected task.

Commonly occurring changes in the neurological system include a decrease in the sensory processes, short-term memory deficits, shortened attention span, difficulty with memory sequencing, and the ability to learn changes. All these factors are barriers to education and, without addressing the changes in the neurological system, teaching often is frustrating for the patient and the nurse. With these issues in mind, the nurse needs to focus teaching plans toward specific physical/neurological conditions and present the topic slowly, repetitively, and with multiple large-print aids that the client can take home to reinforce the learning.

Wellness and self-care teaching need to focus on normal changes older adults can expect to occur in their neurological system as they age and specific interventions they can pursue. Hand tremors when eating, drinking, or dressing can be very disturbing. Use of a straw to drink from a glass, eating utensils with broad surfaces, and clothing with no buttons to fasten can assist older adults in regaining a feeling of ability rather than continuing defeat.

Loss in short-term memory and slowing cognitive functions can be compensated for with use of notes and written daily schedules. Koch and Webb (1996) noted that memory problems were often related to being unable to retrieve information and that when given clues memory often improved. Having a large key-shaped holder by the door can be a reminder to store keys there as an individual enters the home and be a specific place to return to later when keys are needed. Lists of frequently called numbers and emergency numbers should be tied to the phone and done in large print so they are easy to read. Family members can also call older adults daily to inquire if they have taken medications, bathed, and eaten.

Caring

66The nurse needs to focus teaching plans toward specific physical/neurological conditions and present the topic slowly, repetitively, and with multiple large-print aids that the client can take home to reinforce the learning.99

Loss in sensory functions can be compensated for with the use of additional spices during cooking to improve the taste of foods. Homes should be brightly lit with overhead lighting rather than depending on eye level windows and lights. Special adapters are available for phones that increase the volume of both the ringer and the speaker. Temperature gauges are available to check the temperature of bath water before use to reduce the risk of burns. Glasses have long been accepted wear by individuals of all ages to correct visual acuity, and hearing aids should also be viewed as a way to correct a problem rather than a specific problem itself.

Wellness

66Wellness and self-care teaching need to focus on normal changes older adults can expect to occur in their neurological system as they age and specific interventions they can pursue.99

Loss of muscle tone and delays in nerve transmission can lead to falls or make rising from the sitting position difficult. Chairs and couches should have firm arms that can be used for support and assistance in standing. Rails can be installed in the bathroom next to the toilet and bathtub to reduce the risk of falls and provide assistance in rising. Storage in closets and kitchens can be rearranged so that items that are used frequently are at waist to shoulder height.

Older adults also need to be educated on how to minimize their risks through environmental changes. Area carpeting should be well maintained to reduce the risk of falls. Throw rugs should be eliminated wherever possible or anchored securely to the floor. Light bulbs should be bright and of high wattage and have protective covers that reduce glare. Fire and smoke detectors should be checked regularly by family members with the older adults in another room to ensure that they can still hear the alarms. Alarms are available that emit not only a sound but also a flashing light.

Because the aging process of the neurological system is slow and insidious, regular visits to a health care provider is necessary. Careful documentation of changes assist both the nurse and client in identifying "normal" from "unexpected" and allow for the development of a teaching plan and referrals. Sudden changes are never expected and are always a warning sign that medical attention is needed.

For the health care professional it is important to remember that a complete neurological assessment provides valuable information about not just the neurological system but other body systems as well. The neurological system works collaboratively with other systems, and alterations in one system (e.g., infection, malnutrition) can profoundly affect the neurological system. The health care provider must always be aware that normal aging changes can present consistent with other diagnoses.

■ AGE-RELATED CHANGES

As humans age there are certain predictable and expected changes in their central and peripheral nervous systems. However, Crigger and Forbes (1997) note that heredity, environment, and general health affect the timing, progression, and extent of age-related neurological changes in each individual. The brain and nerves all undergo specific structural, cellular, and neurotransmitter changes as individuals age (Depace, 1994).

Changes in the aging brain can include decreased cerebral blood flow, cerebral atrophy, and ventricular dilation; the development of neurofibrillary tangles and neuritic plaques; and alterations in the synthesis and metabolism of various neurotransmitters. Crigger and Forbes (1997) noted that after the age of 50, brain cells are believed to die at a rate of about 1% per year, resulting in a 6% to 11% loss in actual brain weight. Depace (1994) noted that, although these changes are not sufficient to alter the mental abilities of older patients, under times of stress, when metabolic requirements increase, the brain may be unable to accommodate the heightened demands. This may result in confusion and reduction in perception of pain (Depace, 1994).

Benuck and colleagues (1996) found that changes in enzymes and protein activity within the brain during aging reflect not only changes in enzyme properties but also changes in susceptibility to enzymes and proteins. Because neurons are the largest cells in the human body and have the largest amounts of distinct proteins per cell, these changes have profound effects (Dani et al., 1997). Dani and others also noted that the protein precipitation during neuronal aging might be responsible for the development of neuritic plaques and neurofibrillary tangles often found in the brains of individuals with Alzheimer's disease.

Conduction of nerve impulses in the spinal cord is diminished with age (Burke and Kamen, 1996). In addition, anterior horn cells decrease in the lumbosacral region and myelinated nerve fibers are decreased with age, especially in the posterior roots and peripheral nerves (Cruz-Sanchez et al., 1996). Vertebral body compression and intervertebral disk collapse lead to changes associated with osteoporosis related to demineralization of the bones (Depace, 1994). Although osteoporosis is currently a "normal expected change," with advances in pharmacological therapies, diet therapy, vitamin supplementation, exercise, and estrogen replacement therapy, this diagnosis may eradicate osteoporosis as an issue in the normal aging changes of the spinal column.

On the cellular level, RNA and mitochondria are both diminished in cytoplasm (Depace, 1994). Nuclei are decreased in size, dendrites atrophy, and axons degenerate with age. The older patient may experience some impairment of the peripheral nerve functions that is not attributable to any particular disorder. Evidence of segmental demyelination indicates Schwann cell damage, and wallerian degeneration has been demonstrated by some investigators (Bunge, 1993).

The sympathetic nervous system also slows with aging, which limits the smooth, effective boosting of the heart rate with response to stressors and physical activities (Depace, 1994). Depace also noted that hypothalamus responsiveness to temperature regulation slows, and therefore body temperature may not correlate with the severity of an infection. Also the body becomes less sensitive to changes in the external environment and may fail to activate the proper biofeedback mechanisms in a timely fashion.

Mild extrapyramidal dysfunction manifested as stooped, forward-flexed posture and slowed gait is also common in older adults. Slight tremors of the head or hands affect an estimated 4 million people. Essential tremors is among the most prevalent movement disorder in the United States. There is no known cure: however, propranolol (Inderal) and primidone

(Mysoline) are often prescribed. Essential tremors may gradually worsen and can affect the voice. Tremors occur when writing or eating or with hand movements. The individual is instructed that fatigue and extreme emotions aggravate the symptoms. The fear of Parkinson's disease is alleviated with the diagnosis of essential tremors. Information on controlling symptoms and drug therapy reassures the individual that essential tremor is not life threatening and is treatable. The use of a drinking straw and half-filled glass/cup and wearing of heavy bracelets may help eliminate problems with the tremors. The older adult client is often reassured when the differences between essential tremors and Parkinson's disease are pointed out.

The cranial nerves also experience predictable changes during the aging process (Ebersole and Hess, 1998). Because the cranial nerves interpret, integrate, and stimulate areas that include sensory functions, changes affect visual, auditory, taste, and kinesthetic functions. These physiological changes and the effect they have on function are outlined in Table 17–1. In many cases involving an older adult, a sensory impairment may be superimposed on an acute or preexisting illness, pain, or medication toxicity. In these situations, the client is at extended risk for adverse outcomes and a thorough examination and history are absolutely necessary to uncover underlying disorders.

TABLE 17–1. Common Age-Related Changes in Cranial Nerves, Effect on Older Adult, and Nursing Interventions

Cranial Nerve/Change	Effect on Older Adult	Nursing Interventions
Olfactory		
Decrease in number of sensory receptors	Decrease in sensitivity to smells	When testing, use familiar odors: coffee, oranges, lemons, alcohol.
Optic		
Lens yellow	Decrease in color discrimination	Use black lettering on white backgrounds.
Lens less pliable	Blurred images	Refer for corrective lens; use large print.
Lens develops opacities	Increased sensitivity to glare	Ensure bright overhead lighting, sit client with back to windows/mirrors; refer to ophthalmologist.
Retina has fewer cones	Impaired color discrimination	Use black lettering on white backgrounds. When colors are necessary focus on primary colors with good contrast.
Oculomotor		
Lens thickens and pupil diameter decreases	Less light enters eye	Ensure brightly lit room.
Pupillary accommodation slows	Decreased adaptation from light to shadow	Allow extra time for accommodation to occur.
Trochlear		
Decrease in number of motor nerves	Down and inner movement slower	Allow extra time for reading during examination.
Trigeminal		
Decrease in sensory nerves	Dry eyes; loss of blinking response	Administer isotonic eye drops to moisten eyes.
Decrease in motor nerves	Eyelids do not close completely; increase in lag time when opening eyes; difficulty chewing foods, and opening mouth for examination	Use isotonic eye drops to moisten eyes. Encourage cutting food into small pieces; soft foods. Use tongue blade to assist in visualizing back of oral cavity.
Abducens		
Decrease in number of motor nerves	Reduced side vision	Sit directly in front of client. Present material in front of client during examination.

TABLE 17–1. Common Age-Related Changes in Cranial Nerves, Effect on Older Adult, and Nursing Interventions (*Continued*)

Cranial Nerve/Change	Effect on Older Adult	Nursing Interventions
Facial Decrease in sensory and motor nerves	Loss of sensation to soft palate; decrease in facial expression; decrease in salivation and tearing	Cut foods into small pieces and chew slowly. Expect less expression on face. Encourage fluids with meal. Use isotonic eye drops to moisten eyes.
Acoustic Loss of neurons in cochlea; stiffening of basilar membranes	Impaired ability to hear high-pitched sounds and speech discrimination	Speak in louder voice tones, pronounce words carefully, ask client to repeat information heard to clarify understanding. Minimize masking noises during examination, such as radios.
Reduction in numbers of myelinated vestibular nerve fibers.	Decreased ability to maintain balance and correct imbalance	Encourage use of steadying devices when standing (arms, chairs, canes). Monitor for imbalance when client stands.
Glossopharyngeal Decrease in number of taste receptors.	Impaired ability to distinguish flavors Slowing of gag reflex	Use familiar tastes when testing (salt/sugar).
Increased threshold for stimulation of taste receptors	Decrease in ability to distinguish flavors	Use flavor enhancers during cooking. When testing, cover wider area of tongue.
Slowing of motor nerves.	Difficulty pronouncing words and swallowing	Encourage client to speak slowly and chew food slowly.
Vagus Slowing of sensory and motor nerves	Difficulty pronouncing words; slowing of feedback loops to control heart rate, respiratory rate, digestive tract, and enzyme excretion	Encourage client to speak slowly. Rates may not reflect current physiological status.
Spinal Accessory Slowing of motor nerves	Slower turning head, and swallowing	Allow extra time
Hypoglossal Decrease in motor nerves	Slower tongue movement during swallowing and pronouncing words	Allow extra time

GUIDELINES SPECIFIC TO ASSESSING NEUROLOGICAL PROBLEMS IN OLDER ADULTS

The neurological system of the aging adult can present with multiple challenges, even to the most experienced clinician. It is very important that improper assumptions are not made about the changes that occur to the brain and nerves. Many health care professionals and lay people believe that senility is a normal and expected part of the aging process. This is unfortunate because many mental status changes are directly related to an acute illness or other medical condition. The neurological system's complexity can lead to misinterpretation.

The aging adult requires a thorough baseline history and physical examination. This history should cover the areas of speech and communications, functional abilities, movement, personality, emotional state, and cognitive skills. It is noteworthy to mention that the clinician should schedule adequate time for history gathering from the aging adult. Often the history and physical examination are done on separate office visits.

Equally as important is the past medical history and medication history. The family history is often an overlooked and poorly explored area of the aging person's assessment. The assessor should try to elicit as much information as possible. Owing to decades of poor history recordings and poor communication, many neurological disorders will be omitted from subjective histories. If possible, the evaluator should solicit the help of other family members to provide a more reliable database.

The physical assessment of the aging adult's neurological system requires that the examiner have a thorough understanding of what is considered normal versus abnormal with this population. The examiner should be prepared to assess the patient's mental status, cranial nerves, communication ability, ability to move, responses to reflexes, functional status, and, if the client is hospitalized, rehabilitation potential.

Neurological assessment of mental status is generally completed using a test that combines verbal responses to orientation, memory, and attention functions and a component that requires the ability to write, draw, name objects, and follow oral and written instructions. Often the Folstein Mini Mental State Examination is utilized in clinical settings (see Figure 23–2). This instrument is scored with a maximum of 30 points; a score below 24 is considered abnormal, and further assessment is required (Depace, 1994). The primary value of the Mini Mental State Examination as an assessment tool is its ease of administration and the fact that it requires no equipment.

◼ COMMON DISORDERS

Parkinson's Disease

Parkinson's disease (PD) is characterized by tremors at rest, slowness and weakness of vol-

untary movement, and rigidity. It is second only to strokes as the most common geriatric neurological disorder (Caparros-Lefevre et al., 1995). Parkinsonism can be classified as idiopathic (primary) or symptomatic (secondary). There are other forms of this disease, which are classified as parkinsonism plus syndromes.

Primary, or idiopathic, PD has an unclear cause. There are many theories that support that PD may be genetic, viral, or environmental (McDermott et al., 1995). PD is more common in industrialized nations, which may help to support the theory that environmental toxins, along with the aging brain, may result in PD (Caparros-Lefevre et al., 1995). Secondary, or symptomatic, PD may be caused by certain drugs, infection, or illicit drug use. Drug-induced, dopamine-blocking parkinsonism may result from use of neuroleptics, antiemetics, and antihypertensive agents (Grandy, 1994).

The diagnosis of PD is based on a thorough history and physical assessment that includes a comprehensive neurological assessment. There is a clinical triad of PD (tremor, rigidity, and bradykinesia). The patient may present with one or more of the clinical triad of symptoms. Tremors are the most common reason patients seek medical evaluation (McDowell, 1994). The tremors result from the imbalance between dopamine and acetylcholine. The tremor is described as "pill rolling movements" for the fingers that occur at rest. The jaw, hands, and lower extremities are affected. The tremors stop when the patient is making purposeful movement or when the patient is asleep (McDowell, 1994). McDowell found that tremors worsen during times of high emotional stress or during periods of acute illness.

Rigidity may affect one side of the body or both sides. When muscles are rigid, this symptom is described as "lead pipe syndrome" because the bending mimics that maneuver. Cogwheel rigidity is a ratchet-like movement that appears when muscles cannot be flexed or extended easily but only with a sudden jerk (McDowell, 1994).

Bradykinesia affects movement and is often the major feature that renders the patient disabled. **Bradykinesia** refers to the inability to initiate movements or to change direction of the movement easily. Reaction time is very slow because the basal ganglia's ability to coordinate antagonistic muscle groups has decreased (Nichols, 1994). When they do not work together or when in opposition, the result is bradykinesia. The nurse should provide visual and auditory cues to initiate or to complete the movements. The nurse should expect slowness, hesitancy, and a shuffling gait caused by the rigidity. Patients hold their arms stiffly beside their bodies and do not swing them as they ambulate (McDowell, 1994).

Individuals with PD are at high risk for falls due to postural instability and the tendency to walk backward (retropulsion). Physical therapy can play an important role in working closely with the patient and the family on safety tips for ambulation. The patient with PD is additionally at risk for falls secondary to autonomic dysfunction, which causes hypotension and bladder dysfunction. Medications used to treat PD can also yield hypotension (McDowell, 1994). Disability for PD is rated according to five stages and included in Table 17–2.

The goal of nursing care is to assist the client and family to learn to manage the symptoms, identify risks to the client, identify risks in the environment for the client, teach the client

and family members coping skills, and provide referrals to resources available to them in the community. Nursing diagnoses used with clients with PD are included in Box 17–1.

The goal of medical care is to rectify the imbalance of two of the neurotransmitters—dopamine and acetylcholine. Drug therapy is the most important medical aspect of PD treatment. Drug therapy is initiated when impairment with ADLs begin. Drug therapy associated with PD is presented in Table 17–3.

Transient Ischemic Attacks

Transient ischemic attacks (TIAs) occur when there is any situation that reduces cerebral circulation. Reduced cerebral circulation may be caused by many factors such as physical positioning, medical illnesses, certain medications, and cigarette smoking. The classic feature of TIAs is the temporary nature of the CNS dysfunction, usually minutes to hours, that spontaneously resolves within 24 hours. Many elderly individuals ignore TIA signs and symptoms because they are short term and involve no permanent neurological disturbance. TIAs increase the patient's risk of cerebrovascular accidents (Bots et al., 1997) however, Bornstein et al. (1996) found no correlation between TIAs and the development of dementia.

Cerebral blood flow can be reduced by malpositioning of the head when sitting or lying. Older adults who fall asleep sitting in a chair may have impaired cerebral blood flow. The purchase of a new pillow or sleeping in a different bed can also change vascular alignment and affect blood flow to the brain. Postural hypotension, anithypertensive agents, and diuretics all lower blood pressure and decrease cerebral blood flow. Other factors to consider are carotid artery plaque formations and anemia.

Symptoms of TIAs include loss of short-term memory, hemiparesis, hemianesthesia, aphasia, unilateral loss of vision, diplopia, vertigo, nausea, vomiting, and dysphagia. These symptoms can appear singly or in a group depending on the area of the brain that has diminished cerebral blood flow. Alone, or as a group, these symptoms can be very frightening to the patient and family.

A complete examination documenting the foci of dysfunction and careful investigation of the etiology of the dysfunctional cerebral

TABLE 17–2. Five Stages of Parkinson's Disease		
Stage	**Involvement**	**Risk/Complications**
I	Unilateral	Low fall risk
II	Bilateral	Moderate fall risk
III	Bilateral	High fall risk
IV	Global	Severe fall risk Severe impairment
V	Global	Severe fall from chairs/bed High risk for infections

Box 17-1 NURSING DIAGNOSES FOR CLIENTS WITH PARKINSON'S DISEASE

Physical Mobility, Impaired, related to
Rigidity
Bradykinesia
Cogwheeling during movement
Unstable gait

Altered Thought Processes, related to
Confusion
Disorientation
Hallucinations
Medication effects
Decreased concentration
Decrease in short-term memory retention

Altered Nutrition, Body Requirements, related to
Difficulty chewing
Difficulty swallowing
Inability to feed self
Confusion regarding meal time

Altered Sleep Pattern, related to
Confusion
Disorientation to time
Decrease in need for sleep
Hallucinations

Altered Elimination, Constipation, related to
Loss of mobility
Side effect of medications
Low-fiber diet
Dehydration

Ineffective Coping, Family, related to
Reversal in role with parent
Overwhelming sense of loss
Need for placement/changes in lifestyle to care for parent

blood flow is very important. Ultrasound of cerebral blood flow is useful; however, results can vary. Baumgartner et al. (1997) noted that echo contrast sonography can provide conclusive examinations with greater reliability in many elderly patients.

Treatment, once the etiology is identified, focuses on correction. Education, counseling, anticoagulant therapy, and/or vascular reconstruction of the carotid artery are all options for treatment of TIAs. The nurse plays a key role during treatment by assisting the client and family in dealing with their fears, providing education, and problem solving (Mower, 1997).

Cerebrovascular Accident

A cerebrovascular accident (CVA), or stroke, is an acute disruption of the blood supply to the brain resulting in a cessation of blood flow to the affected portion(s) of the brain. Areas of the brain that are deprived of blood flow cease functioning related to lack of oxygen. Arteriosclerosis is one of the leading causes of CVA due to sclerotic plaque on the vessel walls promoting formation of thrombi. The thrombus is then transported through the vascular system until it lodges in an artery or capillary. Hypertension is another factor in CVA and may

TABLE 17–3. Medications for Parkinson's Disease

Drug	Usual Dosage	Indication for Use	Side Effects
Carbidopa/levodopa (Sinemet)	40/400 to 200/2000 (levodopa/ carbidopa) mg/d bid or tid	Tremor Rigidity	Orthostatic hypotension, nausea, confusion, visual hallucinations
Amantadine (Symmetrel)	100–300 mg/d qd or bid	Rigidity Bradykinesia	Leg edema, hallucinations
Bromocriptine (Parlodel)	4–6 mg tid or qid	Motor fluctuations (wearing off, dyskinesia, dystonia)	Hallucinations, mental cloudiness, orthostatic hypotension, confusion
Trihexyphenidyl (Artane)	6–10 mg/d bid	Drooling Tremor Rigidity	Dry mouth, urinary retention, constipation, blurred vision, tachycardia, exacerbation of glaucoma, behavioral changes
Benztropine (Cogentin)	0.5–8 mg/d bid	Drooling	Same as above plus nausea
Selegiline (Eldepryl)	10 mg qd	Rigidity Tremors Bradykinesia	Abdominal pain, dry mouth, nausea, dizziness, confusion, hallucinations, worsening dyskinesias

occur from either rupture of an aneurysm within the subarachnoid space or from bleeding into a localized area of the brain.

A CVA is generally defined by the area of the brain that is affected. A left CVA indicates there is a lesion on the left side of the brain causing right-sided weakness or paralysis. Conversely, a right CVA indicates a lesion on the right side of the brain and left-sided weakness. The signs and symptoms of neurological dysfunction help in identifying the location and extent of the CVA.

Kalra et al. (1998) noted factors that contribute to CVA, including hypertension, diabetes, obesity, cigarette smoking, alcohol intake, anticoagulant medications, elevated cholesterol levels, and a sedentary lifestyle. In one recent study regarding knowledge of risk factors for CVA, the researchers found that older adults are the least knowledgeable about stroke warning signs and risk factors (Pancioli et al., 1998). Public knowledge regarding risk factors and early symptom recognition are key issues in patient education.

Older adults have a higher mortality rate than younger individuals; however, those who do survive have an excellent chance of recovery (Gresham et al., 1998). Duncan et al. (1997) found that the consequences of a CVA affect all dimensions of health except pain. They maintain that assessment of functional ability must be evaluated across the entire continuum of health related functioning.

Complications of CVA may include: unstable blood pressure from loss of vasomotor control, fluid imbalances, malnutrition, infections, depression, contractures, and pulmonary emboli. Nursing considerations should include alteration in tissue perfusion due to impaired blood flow; impaired physical mobility due to decreased level of consciousness and damage to the motor pathway; impaired verbal communication due to impaired cognitive function or due to damage to speech centers in the dominant cerebral hemisphere; potential for injury due to sensory, motor, and cognitive impairments and psychosocial changes due to the illness's effects on family dynamics.

Nursing care during the acute phase focuses on maintaining physiological functioning at

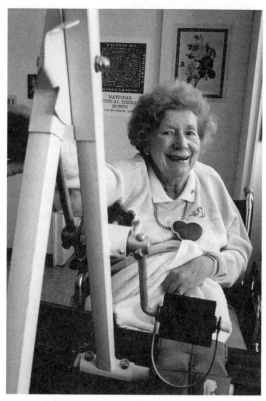

When physical impairment has occurred, it is necessary to reestablish neural pathways.

the highest level possible and preventing any further damage or deficits. Later, when the client enters the rehabilitation phase, the nurse assists the client and family in learning how to compensate for the deficits to regain as much independence as possible.

Caring

"Nurses play an important role in providing education in the older adult patients and families before and during decline in physical functions."

Summary

The neurological system controls, regulates, integrates, and initiates changes in the aging adult. Many of the neurological health problems observed by nurses are directly related to dysfunction and degenerative changes in the brain and nerves. An understanding of the normal and abnormal changes that occur will assist the nurse in providing quality nursing care.

In the July 1996 issue of the *Journal of Gerontological Nursing,* nurses were asked to respond with the four most important wellness concepts every nurse should teach the elderly. Generally, the nurses' responses included remaining socially and physically active; remaining involved in family, community, and world issues; eating a balanced diet; and being involved in routine preventive care activities. Hudson and Sexton (1996) compared older adults' and nurses' priorities of care and found that they were ranked differently. Older adults focused more on relief of specific problems they were currently experiencing and less on concepts of wellness and maintaining well-being.

How, then, can nurses ensure that older adults maintain a healthy functional neurological system? It begins with the professional nurse acknowledging the indispensability of assessing the clients' needs before developing a plan of care. The nurse should have a good understanding of the changes that occur with normal aging. The nurse should also ensure that the physical environment is supportive to completing a comprehensive neurological evaluation and that extra time be allowed. The nurse must include documentation of each finding of the neurological examination so that tracking of dysfunction and diminished responses can be monitored over time.

Many of the changes that are consistent with aging place older adults at high risk for stereotyped behaviors. This often results in discrimination and the assumption that they will have memory impairment, inability to perform ADLs, and difficulty managing and maintaining personal affairs. Older adults also stereotype themselves and do not seek the medical attention they need when dysfunction is noted, often owing to fears that they will be told it is normal.

The aging adult is also at high risk for injury and accidents related to the normal changes in gait, visual acuity, sensory decline, and neurological changes. Accidents are one of the leading causes of death among older adults. Many accidents could be prevented if older adults had pursued health care that would help identify the degree of dysfunction and had adapted to the use of corrective aids and supportive equipment. Aging is a normal process that can be completed successfully through learning to cope effectively with changes.

Nurses play an important role in providing education to the patients and families before and during decline in physical functions. The education that a client and family receive can reduce or eliminate dysfunction. The nursing care and education that a client receives is equally as important as any medical treatment.

RESOURCES

American Parkinson Disease Association
1250 Hylan Blvd
Staten Island, NY 10305
(800) 223-2732

Amyotrophic Lateral Sclerosis Association
(800) 782-4747

Brain Tumor Foundation
(800) 934-CURE

Head Injury Foundation
(800) 444-6443

Headache Foundation
428 West Street
James Place
Chicago, IL 60614
(800) 843-2256

Medicare-Medicaid Complaint Line
(800) 597-0724

National Parkinson Foundation, Inc.
Bob Hope Road
1501 NW 9th Ave
Miami, FL 33136
(800) 327-4545

Parkinson's Educational Program
(800) 334-7872

REFERENCES

Baumgartner RW, Arnold M, Gonner F, et al. (1997). Contrast-enhanced transcranial color coded duplex sonography in ischemic cerebrovascular disease. Stroke 28:2473–2478.

Benuck M, Banay-Schwartz M, DeGuzman T, Lajtha A. (1996). Changes in brain protease activity in aging. J Neurochem 67(5):2019–2029.

Bornstein NM, Gur AY, Treves TA, Reider-Groswasser E, et al. (1996). Do silent brain infarctions predict the development of dementia after first ischemic stroke? Stroke 27:904–905.

Bots ML, van der Wilk EC, Koudstaal PJ, et al. (1997). Transient neurological attacks in the general population. Prevalence, risk factors, and clinical relevance. Stroke 28:768–773.

Bunge R. (1993). Expanding roles for the Schwann cell: Ensheathment, myelination, trophism, and regeneration. Curr Opin Neurobiol 3:805–809.

Burke J, Kamen G. (1996). Changes in spinal reflexes preceding a voluntary movement in young and old adults. J Gerontol 51A(1):M17–M22.

Caparros-Lefevre D, Pecheux N, Petit V, et al. (1995). Which factors predict cognitive decline in Parkinson's disease? J Neurol Neurosurg Psychiatry 58:51–55.

Crigger N, Forbes W. (1997). Assessing neurologic function in older patients. Am J Nurs 97(3):37–40.

Cruz-Sanchez F, Moral A, Rossi L, et al. Synaptophysin in spinal anterior horn in aging and ALS: An immunohistological study. J Neural Transm 103:1317–1329.

Dani S, Pittella J, Bodhme A, et al. (1997). Progressive formation of neuritic plaques and neurofibrillary tangles is exponentially related to age and neuronal size. Dementia Geriatr Cogn Disord 8:217–27.

Depace D. (1994). In Barker E, ed. Neuroscience Nursing. St. Louis: CV Mosby.

Dippel DW, Koudstaal PJ. (1997). We need stronger predictors of major vascular events in patients with a recent transient ischemic attack or nondisabling stroke. Stroke 28:774–776.

Duncan PW, Samsa GP, Weinberger M, et al. (1997). Health status of individuals with mild stroke. Stroke 28:740–745.

Ebersole P, Hess P. (1998). Toward Healthy Aging: Human Needs and Nursing Response. 4th edition St. Louis, Mo. CV Mosby.

Grandy S. (1994). Other degenerative disorders of the nervous system. In Hazzard W, Bierman E, Blass J, et al., eds. Principles of Geriatric Medicine and Gerontology. 3rd ed. New York: McGraw-Hill.

Gresham GE, Kelly-Hayes M, Wolf RA, et al. (1998). Survival and functional status 20 or more years after first stroke: The Farmingham Study. Stroke 29:793–797.

Hudson K, Sexton D. (December 1996). Perceptions about nursing care: Comparing elders' and nurses' priorities. J Gerontol Nurs 22(12):41–53.

Kalra L, Perez I, Melbourn A. (1998). Stroke risk management: Changes in mainstream practice. Stroke 29:53–57.

Koch T, Webb C. (1996). The biomedical construction of aging: Implications for nursing care of older people. J Adv Nurs 23:954–959.

McDermott, M, Jankovic J, Carter J, et al., and the Parkinson Study Group. (1995). Factors predictive of the need for levodopa therapy in early, untreated Parkinson's disease. Arch Neurol 52:565–570.

McDowell F. (1994). Parkinson's disease and related disorders. In Hazzard W, Bierman E, Blass J, et al., eds. Principles of Geriatric Medicine and Gerontology. 3rd ed. New York: McGraw-Hill.

Mower DM. (1997). Brain attack. Treating acute ischemic CVA. Nursing 27:34–39.

Nichols M, Meador K, Lorin D, et al. (1994). Age-related changes in the neurologic examination of healthy sexagenarians, octogenarians, and centenarians. J Geriatr Psychiatry Neurology 7(1):1–7.

Pancioli AM, Broderick J, Kothari R, et al. (1998). Public perception of stroke warning signs and knowledge of potential risk factors. JAMA 279:1288–1292.

Your Turn (editorial). (1996). J Gerontol Nurs 22(7):50–52.

Weinrich S, Weinrich M, Boyd M, et al. (1994). Teaching older adults by adapting for aging changes. Cancer Nursing 17:494–500.

CRITICAL THINKING EXERCISES

Assess your community for available resources to assist patients who are diagnosed with Parkinson's disease, post CVA, and other neurological disorders and report back to your class.

Mrs. Worth, age 97, was found unconscious in her home by her daughter and brought to the emergency department by ambulance. Her daughter states that when she visited the previous day her mother was alert and orientated. Vital signs are stable and normal. The physician orders a urinanalysis in addition to multiple other laboratory tests. When Mrs. Worth regains consciousness she reports she thinks she fell and hit her head.

1. What are two possible causes for Mrs. Worth to be unconscious?
2. What are two possible consequences of her falling related to her neurological system?
3. What are discharge planning considerations that need to be addressed with her daughter?

CHAPTER 18

Maintaining Wellness of the
Skin

Carol Dennis, DSN, RN

CHAPTER OUTLINE

OBJECTIVES

After completing this chapter, the reader should be able to:

1. Differentiate age-related changes of the skin from abnormal findings.
2. Describe preventive measures for skin disorders.
3. Compare and contrast the various skin lesions experienced by older adults.
4. Formulate a plan to lessen the psychological impact of skin conditions.
5. Describe nursing management for integumentary disorders.
6. Teach a classmate how to recognize and manage malignant skin tumors.
7. Apply preventive interventions for pressure ulcers.

KEY TERMS

erythema
Koebner's phenomenon
lichenification
papule
plaque
pruritus
pustule
vesicle
tinea
tissue load
xerosis

The largest and most visible organ in the body is the integument, or the skin, which weighs about 9 pounds. The surface of the skin measures 15 to 20 square feet. One square inch of skin contains large quantities of other structures, such as blood vessels and nerves (15 to 20 feet), sweat and oil glands (hundreds), and cells (more than 3 million), which undergo the continuous process of death and replacement. The skin is the body's first line of defense because it acts as a protective barrier between the body and the environment. Assessment of an individual's integumentary system provides valuable data about the person's interaction with the internal and external environment (Weaver and Long, 1995). The skin is important to an individual's physical and mental health.

▅▅ HEALTH TEACHING

The skin should be examined daily for any changes, especially changes in moles or other skin lesions. Skin changes or lesions that do not heal should be reported to a physician. Scratching dry skin should be avoided because scratching leads to itching, which becomes cyclical. With aging, bathing should be changed from a daily routine to three or four times per week and hot water should not be used. A daily sponge bath is acceptable. Harsh skin cleansers should be avoided, and only superfatted, nondeodorant soaps should be used. Emollients or lotions should be applied generously after bathing. Rubbing alcohol is very drying and should not be used on aging skin. If bath oils or mineral oils are used in the tub, caution is essential to avoid a fall. Unless contraindicated, the older adult needs to drink several glasses of water each day. Humidifiers are good for dry skin during the winter months. People should avoid overexposure to sunlight, especially from 10 AM until 3 PM, and use sunscreens with an SPF of at least 15 and protective clothing (e.g., hats, long sleeves) when possible. It is important to avoid getting burned by the sun; a "healthy" tan really does not exist. Box 18–1 presents risk factors for the development of skin problems.

An intact skin provides the body's first line of defense against invasion by bacteria and other foreign substances (Sparks, 1997). The skin also provides protection from damage by

---

Box 18-1   RISK FACTORS FOR THE DEVELOPMENT OF SKIN PROBLEMS

- Poor personal hygiene
- Immunodeficiency
- Hot, dry climate
- Poor nutrition
- Obesity
- Increasing age
- Emotional distress
- Family history of certain disorders
- Overexposure to sunlight
- Fair skin, blue or green eyes, and blond or red hair

mechanical, chemical, thermal, and solar means. It protects the body against the loss of water and electrolytes (Sims, D'Amico, Stiesmeyer, and Webster, 1995). It also provides sensory perception through special senses that respond to a variety of stimulation. The skin allows individuals to perceive touch, pressure, temperature, and pain. It is responsible for keratin synthesis. Keratinocytes originate in the basement membrane, develop, and then migrate to the surface of the skin. Blood vessels in the skin regulate body temperature by vasodilation and vasoconstriction. Also, the skin uses the mechanisms of radiation, conduction, convection, and evaporation in body temperature regulation. The excretion of waste products such as sweat, sodium chloride, urea, and lactic acid occurs via the skin. Blood pressure regulation is impacted by the blood vessels found in the skin because of their ability to constrict, increasing cardiac output and blood pressure. Surface wounds can be repaired by the skin-replacing cells. The skin allows for vitamin D synthesis.

Wellness

"The care of the skin is essential to maintaining health and should always be a part of any plan of management for older adults."

AGE-RELATED CHANGES

Photo aging (environmental effects) and intrinsic aging (physiological effects), two closely related but distinct entities, are responsible for the predictable age-related changes that occur in the integumentary system (Ghadially, 1996; Sparks, 1997). As part of the aging process, the epidermis and dermis become thinner secondary to a decreased number of fibroblasts and fibers. Less collagen, elastin, and other proteins are produced, and cells are replaced more slowly, resulting in decreased elasticity and wrinkling, with wound healing requiring a longer period of time (Ghadially, 1996; Murray et al., 1997). Decreased elasticity is promoted by cigarette smoking. In a 70-year-old individual, skin cells are viable for an average of 46 days, whereas in a 30-year-old person the average

age is 100 days. The loss of fat cells, especially in the face and extremities, contributes to wrinkling and sagging. The tissue over bony prominences decreases, predisposing the individual to the development of pressure ulcers. Older adults are susceptible to chilling because of their decreased cutaneous blood flow and the decrease in fat cells. There is less ability to retain fluids, leading to drier, less flexible skin. The number of sweat glands decreases, as does the output of sebaceous glands, leading to dry flaky skin. Hair growth declines and hair becomes thin and loses its color (because of decreased melanin), becoming gray to white (Ghadially, 1996). Women experience an increase in facial hair, especially on the upper lip and chin, related to decreased estrogen levels. Nails grow more slowly, and the calcium deposition is greater, leading to thicker nails with ridges. There is a decreased response to pain sensation and temperature changes, which places older adults at greater risk for injury (Lueckenotte, 1994). Table 18–1 summarizes these age-related changes.

GUIDELINES SPECIFIC TO ASSESSING THE INTEGUMENTARY SYSTEM IN OLDER ADULTS

Assessment of the integumentary system is usually incorporated throughout the physical examination (Lueckenotte, 1994). This type of assessment requires inspection, palpation, olfaction, and measurement and the use of a transparent pocket ruler and a penlight. Data pertinent to describing a skin lesion include size, color, distribution (area of body affected and comparison to similar other body areas), and configuration (grouping of lesions in respect to each other). The major symptoms experienced by individuals with dermatological problems are **erythema** (redness), **pruritus** (itching), and **xerosis** (dry skin). Thus, it is important to determine the significance of these symptoms by questioning the client as to length of time the symptoms have been present. Has the client experienced similar symptoms in the past? If yes, under what circumstance?

Overall skin color is noted, remembering that areas with less pigmentation demonstrate

TABLE 18–1. Summary of Age-Related Changes to the Skin	
Change	**Assessment Findings**
Increased number of fibroblasts and fibers	Thinner epidermis and dermis
Decreased collagen, elastin, and proteins	Decreased elasticity with wrinkling and increased wound healing time
Cells replaced more slowly	
Cells have shortened life span (46 days)	
Decreased fat cells	Wrinkling and sagging
Decreased tissue over bony prominences	Increased risk of pressure ulcers
Decreased cutaneous blood flow and fat cells	Increased susceptibility to chilling
Dry, less flexible skin	Increased loss of fluids
Decreased number of sweat glands	Decreased perspiration and dry, flaky skin
Decreased sebaceous gland output	
Decreased melanin	Gray-to-white, thin hair with decreased growth
Decreased estrogen levels in females	Increased facial hair, especially on upper lip
Increased calcium deposits in nails	Thick, rigid nails
Decreased response to pain or temperature change	Increased potential for injury

abnormal findings more readily than do heavily pigmented regions. Moisture in the skin is noted to determine hydration. Skin temperature is felt with the dorsum of the hand; the skin should feel uniformly warm. Integumentary assessment should provide information related to skin texture, turgor, edema, tenderness, odor, and lesions, including location, distribution, and size, arrangement, color, and configuration (shape). Inspection of the hair and nails is included as part of the integumentary assessment (Luckmann, 1997; Nicol, 1997a).

The normal age-related changes taking place in the integumentary system may have a negative effect on the self-esteem of an older adult. This becomes a more serious problem when there is an abnormal integumentary condition. So, in addition to the basic integumentary assessment, there should be some assessment of the individual's social relationships, roles, and sexuality. Also, the client should be questioned about the level of stress, because stress may trigger or exacerbate certain skin conditions. The nurse should ask the older adult about any skin changes that have been noted over the past several years. Is there itching anywhere on the skin? Is there any difficulty encountered when caring for the skin, hair, and nails?

COMMON DISORDERS

Senile Pruritus

Older adults commonly complain of pruritus, the sensation of itching. The etiology of pruritus is multifactorial. Nonidiopathic pruritus may be due to xerosis, a natural consequence of the aging process experienced by older adults, which may be related to decreased moisture content in the skin and aggravated by excessive bathing or the use of harsh skin cleansers (Sims et al., 1995). Environmental factors, such as exposure to temperature changes, low humidity (air conditioning), extensive bathing in water that is too hot, certain types (woolen) of clothing or tight-fitting clothing, harsh skin cleansers, and natural drying of the skin also contribute to pruritus.

CLINICAL FEATURES

Pruritus, which is a symptom and not a disorder itself, is the most common symptom noted in many dermatological disorders (Luckmann, 1997). Idiopathic pruritus is an underlying symptom of a systemic disease; it may be related to hepatic, renal, or thyroid problems and to drug reactions.

The pruritic itching sensation is frequently

described as a tingling or crawling, unpleasant sensation yielding a strong desire to scratch (Luckmann, 1997; Nicol, 1997a). The more one scratches, the more one itches, until a vicious itch/scratch cycle is created. Skin damage is likely to develop as a complication of scratching in a client who has pruritus. The client's fingernails should be cut short to minimize skin trauma. This symptom may be a continuous sensation or intermittent but often worsens at bedtime. Pruritus most frequently affects three areas of the body—the anus (pruritus ani), vulva (pruritus vulvae), and the ear (otitis externa) (Dains, 1997).

C a r i n g

❝When caring for an older adult who has a pressure ulcer, keep the ulcer moist and the rest of the skin dry.❞

A thorough history is taken and a careful physical examination is completed on the older adult with the complaint of pruritus, to determine if the problem is drug related or if a disease process is present (Dains, 1997; Ghadially, 1996). Specimens are screened with a complete blood cell count with differential and to look for thyroid, liver, and kidney disease; and a chest radiograph is taken, searching for an underlying pathophysiological problem.

MANAGEMENT

If an underlying problem is identified, it needs to be treated and corrected; if no cause is found, measures to treat the itching are used. When environmental factors are the cause of the itching sensation, they need to be corrected. For example, the temperature of bath water can be reduced so that it is not too hot, bathing can be done with nondetergent cleansers, an emollient can be added to the bath water (a controversial issue for an older adult, safe only if a nonskid rubber bath mat is also used), and humidification can be added to the ambient air. Clients may use emollients with or without a mild antipruritic agent added on the area of the body that is bothersome (e.g., camphor, 1% to 3%, or menthol, 0.25% to 0.5%). A systemic antihistaminic medication

such as hydroxyzine may be administered—cautiously to older adults, owing to the side effect of drowsiness—every 4 to 6 hours. When the pruritus is associated with a disease process, other specific interventions may be applied, such as adding lidocaine to dialysis fluids for the treatment of uremic pruritus (Ghadially, 1996; Luckmann, 1997; Nicol, 1997b).

Nursing assessment is directed toward gathering data related to the pruritus, lesion involvement, and environmental factors pertinent to the condition. The client is questioned about the severity of the pruritus. The nurse can present a continuum of 1 to 5, with 5 being the worst in severity, and ask the client which number best describes the itching being experienced. Where on the body is the itching located? Is there a seasonal or diurnal pattern associated with the problem? Are the lesions erythematous, scaling, excoriated, or fissured? How are the lesions distributed over the body? Are there aggravating factors in the environment? Is the client stressed or experiencing tension? The nurse should ask the client "Do you feel depressed?" If the answer is yes, relevant information related to depression needs to be explored (Dains, 1997).

Pruritus Ani

Pruritus ani is a condition involving perianal itching, irritation, or superficial burning (Norris, 1996) that occurs mainly in males (Dains, 1997). Many factors contribute to the cause of pruritus ani, which may be associated with a variety of disease conditions. Cleansing the perianal area using harsh soaps or vigorous rubbing with a washcloth or with toilet paper can be a contributing factor. Poor perianal hygiene can, likewise, cause the problem. Straining to defecate may lead to local, minor trauma, contributing to the cause of the condition. Other contributing factors include hypersensitivity to certain environmental factors: perfumed or colored toilet tissue; spicy foods; some medications; excessive sweating related to manual labor; high levels of stress, irritability, or depression; tight-fitting clothing; long periods of sitting; and anal skin tags. Pruritus ani is sometimes associated with systemic disease, especially diabetes. Other skin lesions, such as the skin carcinomas, as well as fungal or parasitic infections and local anorectal disease (hemor-

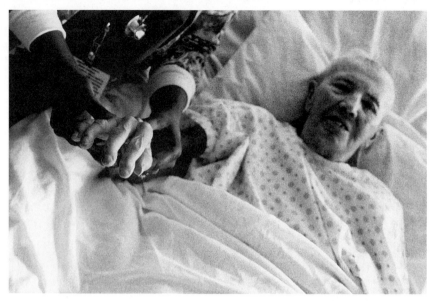

Massage is one way of supporting healthy skin in patients who are bedridden.

rhoids), may lead to the development of pruritus ani (Norris, 1996).

CLINICAL FEATURES

The clinical manifestations associated with pruritus ani are perianal erythema and scratches, or gross excoriation in acute cases, in the area that may involve all of the gluteal fold. In long-standing chronic conditions, **lichenification** (cutaneous thickening and hardening from continued irritation) or fissures develop (Dains, 1997). The chief complaint of the client is perianal itching or burning after defecation, during times of stress, or at night.

The diagnosis of pruritus ani is made only after a very careful and detailed client history is taken. A rectal examination is done to determine the presence of fissures and fistulas. A biopsy may be taken to rule out the possibility of cancer. To determine if the problem is allergy related, allergy testing may be indicated (Norris, 1996).

MANAGEMENT

Management is symptomatic after the underlying cause is eliminated. The condition and causes of the condition are explained to the client, ensuring that the client understands, which is especially important for the older client. The teaching should include the necessity for the client to avoid use of all items that could contribute to the condition. The older adult is instructed in appropriate methods of maintaining a clean and dry perianal area. The area can be cleansed with witch hazel pads, and cotton balls may be kept in the gluteal fold to absorb moisture (Dains, 1996).

Pruritus Vulvae

Many factors provide cause for the development of pruritus vulvae, and this condition is associated with various disease processes. In the early stages, the episodes of pruritus vulvae are intermittent, but they may progress to full-blown pruritus. The labia majora become erythematous, progressing to the development of lichenification when long-standing disease is present. This condition may also affect the perianal region. The situation is aggravated by tightly fitting clothing (e.g., jeans), heat, perspiration, motion, sitting, and lying down. This condition is commonly caused by an allergic reaction to such items as hygiene sprays, douches, detergents, clothing, toilet paper, and poor personal hygiene. In older adult women, pruritus vulvae may be attributed to atrophy of the vaginal mucosa because of decreasing levels of estrogen, predisposing the individual to bacterial invasion. Treatment is the same as that described for other pruritic conditions (Dains, 1997; Norris, 1996).

Eczematous Dermatitis (Eczema)

Eczematous dermatitis is a term that may be used interchangeably with *dermatitis* to describe a group of dermatological conditions; it is not a disease process itself. Eczema is a superficial inflammation of the skin that erupts in lesions. Eczematous dermatitis can be described as a reaction pattern of the skin (Dains, 1997). Dermatitis may be classified based on specific features, such as cause, pattern, age, or method of treatment necessary. Although used synonymously with dermatitis, the term *eczema* usually refers to chronic dermatitis. Some of the common forms of eczematous dermatitis include contact dermatitis, atopic dermatitis, seborrheic dermatitis, and stasis dermatitis. No matter what the cause, the lesions of any type of dermatitis adhere to a characteristic pattern. The initial appearance of the eczema is one of erythema with local edema, which is followed by the formation of oozing vesicles that then crust and scale. Scratching and rubbing the affected area leads to excoriation and eventually thickened brownish skin. Dermatitis is a common skin disorder in older adults (Nicol, 1997a; Weaver, 1995). Eczematous dermatitis is the prototype for understanding the other forms of dermatitis. Clinical management and nursing care are basically the same for all types of dermatitis (Dains, 1997).

Eczematous dermatitis can be categorized as acute, subacute, or chronic. The skin reacts to noxious stimuli with an inflammatory response in which there is vasodilation and edema of the dermis and inflammatory cell infiltration of the dermis and epidermis with breakdown of the epidermal cells leading to the formation of vesicles. The skin surface appears erythematous, edematous, and eroded or crusted from vesicle formation and accumulated exudate and/or infection. Acute dermatitis becomes subacute due to natural healing processes or treatment. Subacute dermatitis may heal or be-

come chronic with continued exposure to the noxious stimuli. All three states of dermatitis may occur simultaneously (Dains, 1997).

W e l l n e s s

"Careful examination of the skin in an overall assessment can prove invaluable to older adult patients who may be unaware of early cancers."

CLINICAL FEATURES

Clinical features include reddened, swollen pruritic skin with exudate and crusting from weeping **vesicles,** which are small sacs containing fluid. As the acute phase subsides and the condition becomes subacute, the erythema lessens and the vesicles become more dry. There is some excoriation with scaling, and pruritus continues. The chronic phase is dry but scaling continues, as does the pruritus. Lichenification (cutaneous thickening and hardening) develops because of the continued irritation (Dains, 1997).

MANAGEMENT

Management and nursing care include the administration of a variety of medications. Antihistamines (e.g., cyproheptadine [Periactin] 12 to 16 mg/d by mouth) in divided doses are administered to combat the pruritus. Systemic or topical corticosteroids are administered (e.g., prednisone [Deltasone] 40 to 80 mg/d by mouth, depending on the severity of the dermatitis, in divided doses [systemic], or hydrocortisone [Cortef] 1% applied three or four times per day topically). Systemic antiinfective agents are prescribed when a secondary infection is present, with the drug of choice depending on the infecting organism. Topical antiinfective agents include bacitracin or neomycin (often combined with polymyxin B [Neosporin]) applied three or four times per day. Topical antifungal medications such as nystatin applied twice per day may be used as well. Keratolytic agents added to corticosteroids (e.g., salicylic acid 3% to 5% in a topical corticosteroid) are used once or twice weekly. During the acute phase, dressings wet with Burow's solution, saline, or tap water help provide relief and promote healing. When the eczematous dermatitis enters the subacute phase, oil-in-water compresses are applied and emollient creams are used. When the condition becomes chronic, oil soaks or water compresses may be applied and hydration of the skin is important (Dains, 1997).

Nursing assessment is based on observation of manifestations. Is there secondary infection? The nurse needs to observe for drainage that is purulent and check the client's temperature. Is tenderness noted? Are the regional lymph nodes enlarged?

Stasis dermatitis is a common skin condition of the lower extremities in older adults. It is usually preceded by venous insufficiency and varicose veins. The condition includes the development of very dry areas of skin on the lower extremities that may degenerate to shallow ulcers. Because of an inadequate blood supply to bring oxygen and nutrients to the tissues and to take away waste products, tissues become hypoxic and irritated. With the pooling of the blood, hemoglobin is released from the red blood cells into the tissues, causing necrosis. The development of leg ulcers is a major source of morbidity for older adults. Varicose veins are more common in women than in men. Pregnancy, obesity, pelvic tumors, traumatic interruption of the venous system, and occupations requiring long periods of sitting or standing worsen the situation by leading to relaxation of the venous musculature and interrupting capillary blood flow by placing backpressure on the venules.

Clinical manifestations include reddened, edematous skin with pruritus that is often severe, visibly enlarged cutaneous veins in the lower extremities, a feeling of heaviness in the legs, and pigmentation (brown-stained scaly skin), with open eroded lesions. A secondary infection may occur if scratching is severe, introducing bacteria via the hands, clothing, and other sources. These lesions heal very slowly because of the lack of circulating oxygenated blood. The ulcer typically develops above the medial malleolus.

Clinical management for the problem of stasis ulcer depends on the clinical picture, which may dictate the use of several approaches simultaneously. The goal of treatment is to improve venous return. This can be accomplished by applying fitted support hose or elastic wraps daily (which also reduces edema), elevating the legs to relieve the legs from a dependent position, and avoiding prolonged sitting or standing. The client should be taught not to cross the legs and not to sit in a chair in which the edge of the chair presses on the backs of the legs, thereby impeding circulation. Sometimes it is beneficial for the older adult client to elevate the foot of the bed with 2 × 4 blocks or books. For a client who is ambulatory, walking is encouraged (rather than standing) so that circulation is enhanced.

Mild-to-moderate potency topical corticosteroids may be used in the treatment of stasis dermatitis. The ulcers may be treated with moisture-retentive dressings or gradient pressure wraps. When infection is present, ulcers may be placed in antibacterial soaks followed by an application of an antibacterial cream (e.g., silver sulfadiazine). Surgical removal of varicosities is an option for younger people but may not be a viable option for an older adult (Ghadially, 1996; Nicol, 1997b; Weaver, 1995).

Seborrheic Dermatitis

Seborrheic dermatitis is a disorder that is localized to areas of the body having a concentration of sebaceous glands. However, there is no abnormality of the composition, production, or flow of sebum with this disorder; its cause is unknown, but it seems to have a genetic predisposition.

CLINICAL FEATURES

Seborrheic dermatitis is a chronic, noninfectious, eczematous (inflammatory) condition with typical traits of erythema and scaling. This condition has a significant prevalence and is a major source of pruritus among the older adult population. In older adults, seborrheic dermatitis often accompanies neurological abnormalities, such as Parkinson's disease, facial paralysis, and hemiplegia. Emotional stress may be a precipitating factor. The condition is exacerbated by stress, infection, hormonal fluctuations, and poor nutrition. There is an inverse association between the frequency of shampooing and the incidence and severity of seborrheic dermatitis.

Clinical manifestations include lesions that may be mild to severe and are pruritic, erythematous, greasy, scaly, or crusting and occur on areas of the body that have an abundance of sebaceous glands (scalp, face, and trunk). The eruptions tend to be symmetrical, typically appearing in the eyebrows, in the nasolabial folds, in the postauricular folds, on the scalp, and in intertriginous areas where bacterial counts are high and secondary infections are likely to develop. Periods of remission and exacerbation are common to this condition, with flareups commonly experienced during cold weather. The diagnosis is made based on client history and physical findings, and is especially evident when lesions are distributed in areas of the body where sebaceous gland concentration is high. Psoriasis is ruled out before a definitive diagnosis is made (Dains, 1997; Ghadially, 1996; Norris, 1996).

MANAGEMENT

Clinical management is straightforward, aimed at controlling the condition and relieving any underlying stress. Mild, nonfluorinated corticosteroid creams (e.g., hydrocortisone 1%) may be used on the face and intertriginous areas. Betamethasone, a midpotency corticosteroid, can be used on general body areas. Keratolytic and keratoplastic shampoos, containing tar, sulfur, selenium, or salicylic acid, alone or in combination, are used daily or twice a week to remove the scales. Topical antifungal creams (ketoconazole) or systemic antibiotic therapy may be indicated in resistant cases (Ghadially, 1996; Luckmann, 1997).

Nursing assessment includes observation of the lesions for redness, scaling, excoriation, fissures, and inflammation. The patient is asked to describe the associated pruritus. The nurse needs to be alert to the potential for the development of secondary infection, observing for purulent discharge, tenderness, fever, and enlarged lymph nodes in the area. Does the client have concerns about body image?

Intertrigo

Intertrigo, a superficial inflammatory dermatitis, develops where two skin surfaces rub, preventing adequate ventilation to the area. In the older adult population, predisposing factors include obesity, incontinence (one of the most common causes), poor hygiene, and diabetes, all of which are prevalent conditions among this age group. Areas of the body where intertrigo is commonly found include neck creases, axillae, antecubital fossae, perineum, finger and toe webs, abdominal skin folds, and beneath the breasts. Intertrigo occurs more commonly when the weather is hot and humid.

CLINICAL FEATURES

Clinical manifestations include a glazed, bright erythema, maceration, itching, and burning that arise from the friction caused by movement, heat, and moisture. Before treatment begins, other skin conditions, such as psoriasis, seborrheic dermatitis, and contact dermatitis, must be ruled out.

MANAGEMENT

The goal of clinical management is to reduce moisture, eliminate maceration, and decrease friction by promoting drying and aeration between the skin folds. The client should be instructed to wear loose-fitting cotton clothing, especially underwear, avoiding clothes that fit tightly (e.g., jeans) and to avoid activity that promotes sweating. Clothing may need to be removed at intervals to allow for drying of affected areas. Care to the involved area depends on the condition of the skin. When the skin is still intact, the area should be bathed gently twice daily with tap water and dried thoroughly and a generous amount of dusting powder applied that contains talc or cellulose (Zeasorb) to reduce friction and for extra absorption. Use of cornstarch must be avoided because it promotes the growth of *Candida albicans*. If incontinence is the predisposing factor, zinc oxide paste may be applied to create a barrier. Low-potency topical corticosteroids (hydrocortisone 1% to 2.5%, cream or lotion) are used when inflammation is present or a corticosteroid-antibiotic-antifungal (e.g., Vytone 1%) combination may be applied to the area on a short-term basis. When secondary infection or eroded areas are present, moist compresses of tap water or Burow's solution 1:20 are applied several times daily to remove exudate and promote comfort. Castaderm, an antifungal-astringent-antiseptic drying preparation, may be applied once a day, but it is messy and stings on application. Folded gauze squares or cotton handkerchiefs placed between skin folds enhance healing by keeping skin surfaces apart. The major complication occurring with this disorder is from secondary infections such as **tinea** (fungal infection of plantlike organisms that consume organic matter), candidiasis (fungal infection), or erythrasma (bacterial).

Caring

"*For the older adult, who may already be taking several medications for chronic illnesses, medication management for herpes zoster must be very closely monitored. Start low and go slow.***"**

Neurodermatitis (Lichen Simplex Chronicus, Essential Pruritus)

Neurodermatitis is a superficial chronic inflammation of the skin that occurs as a result of repeated scratching. This condition is common among the older adult population. Psychotropic factors are hypothesized to be an underlying cause. The disorder is more common in women and Asians but may occur in both genders and in all races.

CLINICAL FEATURES

Itching initiates the condition of lichen simplex chronicus in normal skin, and in the early phase the disorder is characterized by papular eruptions that are more commonly found in the occipital region of the scalp, hands, perineum, and legs. If the scratching were to stop, these lesions would disappear. When the itch/scratch cycle, which is often more pronounced at night, is begun, scratching becomes a habit. Continual scratching or rubbing of the **papules** (reddened, elevated circumscribed areas on the skin) produces excoriated skin that results in lichenified **plaques** (patches on the skin) that are thick and well circumscribed. This condition may progress to a worsened state called prurigo nodularis, which includes picking at the skin, mainly on the extremities (Ghadially, 1996; Norris, 1996; Weaver, 1995). The diagnosis is established by physical findings.

MANAGEMENT

Management consists of stopping the scratching so that the lesions will disappear, which occurs within about 2 weeks of cessation. Application of potent corticosteroid creams covered by occlusive dressings to protect the area from scratching is often successful. Corticosteroid injections of triamcinolone acetonide, 5 to 10 mg/mL, directly into the lesions may be necessary to effect improvement. A corticosteroid tape may be used on nonhairy areas to cover the lesion and prevent scratching. Client education about the underlying cause is necessary.

Neoplastic Disorders

Actinic keratoses (e.g., solar, senile), the most frequently occurring precancerous skin lesions in older adults, are caused by exposure to the sun, and these lesions become progressively more obvious with age, occurring most frequently in white-skinned people and affecting almost 100% of the older adult white population (Ghadially, 1996; Nicol, 1997a; Sparks, 1997).

CLINICAL FEATURES

The lesions are composed of keratinocytes and melanocytes, are light pink to reddish-brown, and occur mostly on the face, scalp, trunk, and arms, the sun-exposed areas of the body. The lesion begins as a small irregularly shaped macule or papule with indistinct borders. It gradually becomes rough and warty and erythematous, with a hard overlying keratotic scale that is periodically shed or peeled off only to regrow. The size of the lesion can vary from pinhead to several centimeters; it is often more easily palpated than seen. A single lesion may be noted, but more often there is a group of lesions on a background of sun-damaged skin (Ghadially, 1996; Nicol, 1997a; Sparks, 1997). The risk of these lesions turning into malignancies is small but definite.

MANAGEMENT

Actinic keratoses are treated topically with 5-fluorouracil (Efudex), a topical antimetabolite, 1% to 2% lotion applied twice a day for 2 to 3 weeks. This medication removes premalignant and superficial malignant lesions and at the same time destroys those lesions that have gone clinically undetected. This treatment offers the advantage that large areas of disease can be treated at the same time but carries the disadvantage of a therapeutic inflammatory response associated with successful treatment. This inflammatory response is seen as a sequence of the following events: erythema, usually followed by vesiculation, erosion, ulcerations, necrosis, and epithelialization. A glove should be worn during application of the medication, and the eyes, nose, mouth, and scrotum should be meticulously avoided. A porous dressing may be applied over the medication for cosmetic reasons, but occlusive dressings must not be used because of increased inflammatory response. When the inflammatory response reaches the stage of erosion, necrosis, and ulceration, the use of the medication is discontinued. Toward the end of therapy, 2 to 4 weeks, the client may require administration of an analgesic medication to relieve discomfort. When 5-fluorouracil is discontinued, a corticosteroid cream may be applied to reduce inflammation and provide further comfort. Other forms of treatment consist of liquid nitrogen cryotherapy, local destruction using curettage, and electrodesiccation (Ghadially, 1996; Nicol, 1997b; Sparks, 1997). Clients who have senile keratoses should be taught to avoid exposure to sunlight as much as possible and to use sunscreens.

Epitheliomas (Cancers of the Skin)

Skin cancer is the most common form of human malignancy in the United States (Dains, 1997; Nicol, 1997a), with approximately 800,000 cases diagnosed each year. Basal cell and squamous cell carcinomas, both curable, comprise the majority of skin cancers; however, deaths due to skin cancer are increasing at a rapid rate. Skin cancers are specific to a layer of skin and are distinguished by the types of cells involved, with basal cell carcinoma, squamous cell carcinoma, and malignant melanoma being the three most common types of skin cancer. Ninety percent or more of the skin cancers are either basal cell or squamous cell carcinomas. Basal cell and squamous cell carcinomas are slow-growing tumors that have a cure rate of 95% or higher when diagnosed and treated early. The increasing incidence of all skin cancers is thought to be related to a change in lifestyle, with increasing numbers of successive generations having greater exposure to sunlight.

Wellness

"Prevention is the key to healthy skin in old age, with regular checking of the skin status as part of daily care."

Both basal cell and squamous cell carcinomas are noted more frequently in light-skinned individuals who live closer to the equator. Both types of cancers are more commonly found in males, with basal cell carcinoma being more prevalent in persons older than age 40 and squamous cell carcinoma being more prevalent in individuals older than age 60. Prolonged exposure to ultraviolet rays from the sun is the cause of all skin cancers, especially if sunburn and blistering occur. Most skin cancers occur in individuals who have had excessive exposure to sunlight and arise on areas of the body unprotected by clothing. Although all persons are at risk for the development of skin cancer, some are at greater risk than others. Those who are most susceptible are individuals with red, blond, or light brown hair and light complexions or freckles. Individuals who experience occupational or recreational exposure (e.g., farmers, construction workers, sailors, swimmers, surfers, sunbathers) to the sun are at greater risk. Other risk factors include occupational exposure to coal, tar, pitch, creosote, arsenic compounds, and radium.

CLINICAL FEATURES

Basal cell carcinoma, the most common malignant epithelial tumor of the skin, arises from the basal cells of the epidermis. This type of skin cancer is usually painless and slow growing. The vast majority of these tumors are related to excessive exposure to ultraviolet rays of the sun. The tumor usually presents as a small, firm, nodular, dome-shaped papule that is flesh-colored with raised edges and pearly (shiny) white borders related to the fact that it does not keratinize. Telangiectatic vessels, overlying the tumor, may be seen through the epidermis. With enlargement, the center of the lesion may become flat, ulcerated, and bleed. Basal cell carcinomas rarely metastasize, but if left untreated they can be locally destructive by invasion through vital structures such as blood vessels, lymph nodes, nerve sheaths, cartilage, bones, lungs, and the dura mater. When diagnosed and treated early, surgical destruction or destruction by radiation therapy is curative in 90% to 95% of the cases. The potential for recurrence of a tumor, indicating incomplete destruction initially, is seen within the first 2 years. A client who has had one basal cell carcinoma is at greater risk for developing another (Dains, 1997; Nicol, 1997; Sparks, 1997).

Squamous cell carcinoma, the second most common type of skin cancer, is a tumor of the epidermal keratinocytes and is noted on areas of the body exposed to the sun, the rim of the ear, the face, the lips and mouth, and the dorsa of the hands. The lesion is scaly and slightly elevated and may or may not have a cutaneous horn. There is usually a history of actinic keratoses. These lesions are poorly marginated and are more difficult to differentiate from the surrounding sun-damaged skin than are basal cell carcinomas. The presentation of a squamous cell carcinoma can be varied and may resemble an ulcer, a flattened red area, a cutaneous horn, an indurated plaque, or a hyperkeratotic papule or nodule. Although these tumors grow more rapidly than basal cell tumors, with early intervention and complete tumor destruction the prognosis is good, but without early treatment squamous cell carcinomas can metastasize. Cure rates for squamous cell lesions are 75% to 80% with surgical or radiation therapy treatment. Precancerous lesions should receive prompt attention and removal (Dains, 1997; Nicol, 1997a; Sparks, 1997).

A biopsy, incisional or total excisional, is performed to confirm the diagnosis of basal cell or squamous cell carcinoma. The surgery performed for removal of the tumor is tumor excision with a wide margin of normal-appearing skin and subcutaneous tissue. Chemosurgery or Mohs' procedure (a lengthy technique based on a series of incisions to remove one layer of cells at a time) may be used, especially in areas where normal skin preservation is a consideration, such as eyelids, pinnae, and nasolabial folds. Cryosurgery and electrodesiccation and curettage are also surgical options for both basal cell and squamous cell carcinoma. The antineoplastic medication fluorouracil can be a treatment option, as is radiation therapy. Prevention is the best treatment for both types of skin cancers. Exposure to the sun should be avoided and all individuals should use sun-blocking agents generously (Ghadially, 1996).

Malignant melanoma, a cancer of the melanocytes, is the deadliest form of skin cancer, with the incidence and death rate rising worldwide by 7% to 15% per year in countries populated by fair-skinned individuals. Individuals who develop malignant melanoma tend to have histories of blistering sunburns, a family history of melanoma, or an atypical mole. Approximately 5500 (75%) deaths per year from skin cancer are the result of malignant melanoma. The incidence for white populations is 10 times greater than for black populations and is equal between males and females. The most frequent age range for occurrence is between the ages of 30 to 60, but it is also found in people 65 years of age and older. In older adults, target areas include the back and lower extremities. Intensity of sunlight exposure, not duration, continues to be one of the most important causes of melanoma. Other theories considered as possible causes of melanoma are hereditary factors, hormonal factors, and an autoimmune effect. These lesions are easily identifiable in the initial stages and should be suspected in a client who had an already existing nevus that demonstrated change in appearance.

The following are characteristics of malignant melanomas:

- Various shades of brown and black with red, white, or blue and pink or gray within one lesion
- An irregular periphery with notching or indentation and pigment extending from the edge
- An irregular and raised surface that may appear eroded, ulcerated, or crusted
- A skin lesion that is bleeding or that has changed size, thickness, or color over a pe-

riod of several months. (These changes include doubling in size over 3 to 8 months, change in diameter, enlarging diameter, bleeding, itching, erosion, change of color, and the occurrence of a palpable lymph node.)

When metastasis occurs it is usually to the brain, lungs, bone, liver, and skin and is fatal. A lesion that is not metastatic at the time of diagnosis and excision carries a better prognosis when its depth is superficial. The more superficial and thin the lesion, the better the prognosis.

CASE STUDY

Paul Sims, a 70-year-old man, had been doing construction work all of his working life. He enjoyed the work and loved being outside for most of the day. During the warm months, Mr. Sims did not even wear his shirt while he worked. He mostly clothed himself in shorts, socks, and boots and never applied sunscreens. At the age of 70, Mr. Sims noticed a small "place" on his anterior neck with an irregular, raised, eroded surface. The color of the "place" was black with red areas. The periphery of the "place" showed indentations. Mr. Sims was not alarmed by this "place" but maintained a watchful attitude toward it. In about 4 months, Mr. Sims felt that this "place" had doubled in size and he became alarmed. He was seen by his physician, who diagnosed the "place" to be malignant melanoma and performed a wide excision of the lesion. The lesion was found to be superficial, improving Mr. Sims' prognosis.

There are four common classifications of melanoma and one relatively rare form. It is of much greater importance to recognize early melanoma before it invades the dermis and metastasizes than to recognize its type.

Superficial spreading melanoma (SSM), the most common form of melanoma, is a lesion that changes slowly, with the most rapid change developing just before diagnosis. Initially, this disorder appears as a small, irregularly shaped brown lesion containing shades of red, white, and blue. Superficial spreading melanoma accounts for approximately 70% of the melanomas and tends to develop anywhere on the surface of the body. This type of lesion may be present for 1 to 5 years before invasion of deeper layers of the skin, as evidenced by the development of papules and nodules. The average age of occurrence is 50 years old.

Caring

"Although there are many preventive interventions for pressure ulcers, pressure relief is crucial, especially in the older adult who is at greater risk of developing a pressure ulcer owing to the normal age-related changes in the integumentary system."

Nodular melanoma (NM), the second most common form of melanoma (15% of the cases), is a rapidly growing and aggressive tumor with a shorter clinical onset time than superficial spreading melanomas. These lesions occur on a variety of body areas, especially the trunk, head, and neck. The tumor appears as a 1- to 2-cm lesion with a smooth, scaly, or ulcerated surface. These lesions are usually brown or black and more uniform in color. Nodular melanoma metastasizes by invasion of the dermis and then the lymph nodes.

Acral lentiginous melanoma, accounting for approximately 10% of the melanomas, is more common in dark-skinned, older (60 years) individuals and occurs most frequently on the light pigmented areas of the body such as the palms, soles, nail beds, and mucous membranes. Acral lentiginous melanoma lesions are large (about 3 cm in diameter), flat brown spots requiring a few months to years to become nodular and pigmented, which indicates vertical invasion. These lesions may be misdiagnosed as corns, and metastasis is likely.

Lentigo maligna melanoma (Hutchinson's freckle) accounts for about 5% of melanomas and is found in older adults. This lesion grows slowly and is usually located on areas of the body exposed to sunlight, such as the face and hands. Typically, this type of melanoma affects white women and may have been present for 5 to 15 years when diagnosed. It appears as a large, flat lesion resembling a brown (may contain various shades of brown) stain on the skin. Metastasis from lentigo maligna melanoma is less common than from other types of melanoma.

TABLE 18–2. Skin Cancers

Type	Clinical Manifestations	Treatment
Basal cell carcinoma	Arises from epidermal basal cells Slow growing and usually painless Usually occurs in individuals older than 40 Presents as small, firm, nodular, dome-shaped papules Flesh-colored, with raised edges and pearly white borders Telangiectatic vessels overlie tumor Rarely metastasizes, but may invade locally Cure rate of 90% to 95%	Excision of tumor Chemotherapy, 5-fluorouracil Mohs' procedure Cryosurgery Electrodesiccation Curettage Radiation therapy
Squamous cell carcinoma	Arises from epidermic keratinocytes Lesion is scaly and slightly elevated Usually a history of actinic keratoses Difficult to differentiate from surrounding sun-damaged skin May metastasize Grows more rapidly than basal cell carcinoma Cure rate of 75% to 80% Occurs in those 60 years and older	Excision of tumor Chemotherapy, 5-fluorouracil Mohs' procedure Cryosurgery Electrodesiccation Curettage Radiation therapy
Malignant melanoma	Arises in the melanocytes Deadliest form of skin cancer History of blistering sun burns Family history of malignant melanoma History of atypical mole Occurs in those 30 to 60 years, or 65 and older Nevus with change Various colors: brown, black, red, white, blue, pink, or gray Irregular, raised, eroded, ulcerated, or crusted surface Bleeding, change in size, thickness or color Can metastasize	Surgical excision of tumor Dissect regional lymph nodes when advanced tumor Chemotherapy Immunotherapy Radiation therapy

Desmoplastic melanoma is a rare melanoma. In its neurotrophic form it may invade neural tissue (Table 18–2) (Dains, 1997; Ghadially, 1996; Nicol, 1997a; Sparks, 1997; Norris, 1996).

DIAGNOSIS

A deep margin skin biopsy including subcutaneous fat with histological examination confirms the diagnosis of malignant melanoma, including the type of melanoma and stage of disease, and distinguishes this lesion from those of a benign nevus, seborrheic keratosis, and pigmented basal cell epithelioma. Tumor thickness is also established by these techniques. During the physical examination, particular attention is paid to lymph nodes to determine metastatic involvement. Laboratory studies include a complete blood cell count with differential, an erythrocyte sedimentation rate, a platelet count, liver function chemistries, and urinalysis. Other diagnostic studies—radiography, computed tomography of the chest and abdomen, bone scan, and computed tomography of the brain—may be needed, depending on the depth of tumor invasion and metastasis.

MANAGEMENT

Clinical management consists initially of high suspicion for any type of skin cancer, especially melanoma. As with all suspected cancers, the necessity for early diagnosis and intervention cannot be overemphasized with suspected malignant melanoma. Any and all warning signs should initiate immediate attention to the situation.

Surgical excision of the tumor, with resection of a wide, deep margin of normal-appearing skin, with skin grafting when excision is extensive, is the mainstay of treatment for malignant melanoma. Regional lymph nodes should also be dissected when the lesion is advanced. The surgical excision may be performed after a frozen section examination while the patient is still on the operating table; other surgeons prefer to wait for the results of permanent section pathological diagnosis and perform the surgery usually within 1 week of biopsy. There is no evidence to indicate that this 1 week's wait for surgery is harmful to the patient. During this wait, the patient is allowed time to prepare, physically and psychologically, for undergoing the surgery.

When the tumor has metastasized, most clients do not live beyond 1 year. Metastatic melanoma cannot be cured, but there are treatment options that may offer an improved quality of life. Chemotherapy and immunotherapy are implemented to eliminate or re-

duce the number of tumor cells. Whereas radiation therapy, usually administered when metastasis has occurred, does not extend the life expectancy with metastatic melanoma, it does tend to reduce the tumor size and provide relief from pain. Follow-up supervision is an intense, close, long-term approach aimed at detecting metastasis and recurrences of the melanoma (which occur in about 13% of the cases 5 years after the primary surgery was completed).

There are scales to help determine the individual prognosis of survival. The Clark scale looks at invasion of the tumor into different skin layers. Breslow's microstaging relies on tumor thickness to indicate prognosis (Dains, 1997; Ghadially, 1996; Luckmann, 1997: Nicol, 1997b; Norris, 1996).

Caring

66*Early detection and intervention provide the best prognosis, so teach older adults how to do skin inspection and what to look for when doing the inspection.*99

Herpes Zoster

Herpes zoster, commonly known as "shingles," occurs most frequently in the age group older than 50. This infectious skin disorder is an acute vesicular, often painful inflammation of the dorsal root ganglia with the herpesvirus varicella-zoster, which is also the cause of chickenpox. Herpes zoster occurs as a reactivation of the varicella-zoster virus, a previous episode of chickenpox being the primary infection. This disorder occurs in 5 to 10 individuals per 1000. Most of these indi-viduals experience only one episode of herpes zoster, but there is a 4% chance that the disorder will recur. Individuals who have not had chickenpox may develop it after being exposed to someone with herpes zoster. An increased incidence of herpes zoster has been noted in individuals who have lymphoma, leukemia, and acquired immunodeficiency syndrome (AIDS), theoretically due to their decreased immunological response. Risk factors predisposing an individual to the development of herpes zoster include increasing age, physical trauma, debilitated or immunosuppressed states, systemic illness, emotional stress, and fatigue.

CLINICAL FEATURES

Herpes zoster typically runs a course of classic symptomatology, but serious complications do occasionally occur. The typical onset is one of fever and malaise, with the primary vesicular lesions presenting in a group on an erythematous base along a dermatome, 1 to 4 days after pain (which may be severe), itching, and burning initiate along that area. In older adults, the acute neuritic pain is a major factor of rash eruption. Initially, the pain may be misdiagnosed as pleuritic pain, myocardial infarction, or appendicitis until the characteristic eruptions form. These lesions are typically unilateral because they follow nerve pathways. The lesions progress from purulent fluid-filled vesicles into **pustules** (small elevations of the skin filled with pus) that rupture and dry, forming scabs; they heal within 7 to 14 days and may leave residual scarring. When the vesicles rupture, the client is at risk for developing a secondary infection. After the lesions have gone, the individual may experience postherpetic neuralgia, residual pain, and itching. The pain experienced in postherpetic neuralgia can remain with the client for weeks to months to years. In older adult clients, postherpetic neuralgia tends to remain for months to years.

◼ CASE STUDY

Mary Jones, aged 74 years, felt tired and irritable, with a fever for the past few days before the development of skin lesions on one side of her lower chest area. The lesions appeared as vesicles on an erythematous base. She described the pain she began to experience about 3 days before lesion development as intolerable. Mary went for an appointment with her physician and was diagnosed with herpes zoster. After about 10 days the skin lesions were mostly gone, but severe pain in the area remained for the next year, at which time Mary was diagnosed with leukemia and died within a few months.

Zoster ophthalmicus, a complication of herpes zoster, is infection in the ophthalmic branch of the trigeminal nerve or the oculomotor nerve. Trigeminal ganglion involvement is a serious condition that leads to associated eye pain and potential corneal and scleral damage, with impaired vision or total loss of vision. Oculomotor involvement, occurring rarely, leads to conjunctivitis, extraocular weakness, ptosis, and paralytic mydriasis. Both conditions necessitate immediate ophthalmic examination and intervention. Another complication of herpes zoster is Ramsay Hunt syndrome, which is an uncommon condition resulting from infection of the geniculate ganglia, causing pain and vesicle formation in the external auditory ear canal. The client may also present with ipsilateral facial palsy, hearing loss, dizziness, and loss of taste in the anterior two thirds of the tongue.

DIAGNOSIS

A positive diagnosis of herpes zoster is made only when the skin lesions appear. Before this time, the pain is suggestive of other conditions. Physical findings include the observation of characteristic clustered vesicles distributed along a nerve dermatome, generally associated with pain and itching. A Tzanck test is done to examine vesicular fluid and infected tissue for multinucleated giant cells, and a viral culture is helpful in identifying the varicella virus to make a definitive diagnosis. Staining of the vesicular fluid isolates antibodies that can be differentiated under fluorescent light from those of herpes simplex.

MANAGEMENT

Analgesia for the pain may be accomplished with the use of aspirin 300 mg orally every 4 hours or acetaminophen 250 mg orally every 4 hours for mild pain. More severe pain may be controlled with codeine orally in doses that provide relief, especially during the eruptive phase or for postherpetic neuralgia. A tranquilizing agent, chlorpromazine (Thorazine), 25 mg orally four times a day, may be indicated for severe postherpetic pain. Acyclovir, an antiviral agent, may be administered orally in doses of 800 mg every 4 hours for 7 to 10 days during the eruptive phase or intravenously 10 mg/kg every 8 hours in immunocompro-

TABLE 18–3. Clinical Management of Herpes Zoster

Agent	Dose and Route	Frequency
Analgesic Agents		
Aspirin	300 mg PO	q4–6h prn, for mild pain
Acetaminophen (Tylenol)	250 mg PO	q4h prn, for mild pain
Codeine	PO; dose to provide relief	During eruptive phase or for postherpetic neuralgia
Tranquilizing Agent		
Chlorpromazine (Thorazine)	25 mg PO	For severe postherpetic pain qid
Antiviral Agent		
Acyclovir	800 mg PO, or 10 mg/kg IV	q4h × 7–10 days in eruptive phase or q8h if client is immunocompromised
Famciclovir	500 mg PO	tid × 7 days
Corticosteroid		
Prednisone	20 mg PO	tid × 7 days, followed by 20 mg PO bid × 7 days; then 20 mg PO qd × 7 days
Postherpetic Phase		
Capsaicin (Zostrix)	0.075%	Apply topically tid to qid
Amitriptyline (Elavil) (tranquilizer) with	75–100 mg PO	qd, for months
Perphenazine (Trilafon)	4 mg PO	tid to qid, for months

mised patients. Acyclovir is beneficial in reducing pain and accelerating healing only when administration is begun within the first 72 hours after the rash is apparent. Another antiviral agent also used is famciclovir, 500 mg orally three times a day for 7 days. A controversial treatment is the administration of systemic corticosteroids during the eruptive phase for the purpose of preventing postherpetic neuralgia. Prednisone, 20 mg orally three times a day for 7 days, followed by 20 mg orally twice a day for 7 days and then reducing the dose to 20 mg by mouth each morning for another 7 days, is usually the regimen of choice when systemic corticosteroids are used. After the acute phase, when the client is actually experiencing post-herpetic neuralgia, a combination of medications may be prescribed. Capsaicin (Zostrix) 0.075% may be applied topically. A combination of tranquilizing agents, such as amitriptyline (Elavil), 75 to 100 mg orally daily, with perphenazine (Trilafon), 4 mg orally three to four times a day, may be necessary for months. Table 18–3 presents clinical management for herpes zoster.

General management consists of cryosurgery for the management of postherpetic pain. Transcutaneous electric nerve stimulation may be helpful in relieving the pain of postherpetic neuralgia. Topical therapy for symptom relief includes cool compresses to the affected areas, applications of cooling antipruritic agents (e.g., Estar gel), and implementation of methods to prevent secondary infection.

Nursing assessment focuses on location and characteristics of the lesions. Pain assessment and effectiveness and side effects of analgesics are necessary components of the nursing assessment. The nurse should assess for signs and symptoms of secondary infection. During the postherpetic phase, discomfort may continue to be a problem requiring further assessment (Dains, 1997; Nicol, 1997b; Warner, 1996; Norris, 1996).

Psoriasis

Psoriasis, a chronic, recurrent, erythematous, inflammatory disorder, is a noninfectious disease of keratin synthesis, marked by epidermal proliferation. The characteristic lesions are dry papules and plaques that are commonly covered by silvery-white scales and varied in severity and distribution. The onset of the disease is slow, and the course is long and unpredictable, with periods of exacerbation and partial remission. The recurrences tend to last for increasingly longer periods of time. There is no known cause for psoriasis, but there may be a hereditary defect underlying the overproduction of keratin as well as other immunological and cellular abnormalities. Psoriasis affects both sexes equally, with 3% to 5% of the U.S. population being affected, with a higher incidence among whites. In about 40% of the cases there is a family history. Although psoriasis can occur at any age, it tends to occur between the ages of 10 and 40 years. Individuals are at risk of developing psoriasis when there is a family history of the disorder, with exacerbations of the condition being related to emotional stress, trauma, systemic illness, cold weather, and hormonal changes.

The normal length of time required for cellular division in the basal layer to the cellular shedding from the stratum corneum is about 28 days; however, when psoriasis is present, this process requires only 3 to 4 days, so the cells are immature and the stratum corneum becomes thick and flaky. These rapidly proliferating cells form lesions of various sizes. Pruritus can be severe from this condition.

CLINICAL FEATURES

Psoriatic lesions are usually symmetrical, affecting mainly the scalp, elbows, knees, extensor surfaces of the extremities, lower back, sacrum, intergluteal fold, and the genitalia. In some clients, psoriasis spreads to the fingernails, causing thickening, pitting, and yellow or brown discoloration. The lesions cause disturbances in self-esteem, and the individual may be emotionally distressed related to the lesions themselves. In 5% to 20% of clients who have psoriasis, there is also an associated arthritis, with symptoms that may affect one or more joints of the fingers or toes or the sacroiliac joints. These individuals may complain of morning stiffness, with the joints demonstrating periods of remission and exacerbation similar to that of rheumatoid arthritis. A newly traumatized area of skin may develop psoriatic lesions; this is known as **Koebner's phenomenon**.

MANAGEMENT

The diagnosis is based on client history and the appearance of the lesions. A skin biopsy may be done to provide a definitive diagnosis. An elevated uric acid blood level is due to the rapid nucleic acid degradation; however, signs and symptoms of gout are not evident. There is no cure for psoriasis, so treatment depends on the extent of the disease process, the patient's response to therapy, and the effect of the disease process on the patient's lifestyle. The goal of treatment is to bring about and maintain remission and relieve symptoms. The treatment for psoriasis is varied and may include careful exposure to sunlight (without burning), applications of topical agents, intralesional corticosteroids, and stress reduction techniques.

Topical nonfluorinated corticosteroids, hydrocortisone 2% to 3% used sparingly twice to three times a day, may be applied to lesions on the face and intertriginous areas; and for lesions on the scalp, body, and extremities, fluocinolone 0.025% to 0.01% may be used sparingly two, three, or four times a day. If low-potency agents are not effective, then high-potency agents are tried. The use of systemic corticosteroids is controversial. Keratolytic agents, such as coal tar preparations (Alphosyl), may be used as shampoo or bath oil or applied directly to the lesion. Photosensitizing agents and oral retinoids may be used as part of combination therapy for severe, recalcitrant forms. Antineoplastic agents, such as methotrexate, an antimetabolite, 5 to 7.5 mg, may be administered weekly orally, intramuscularly, or intravenously, with the dose being increased by 2.5 to 5 mg weekly up to 30 mg and then placed on a tapering schedule. Antiinfective agents are utilized when secondary infection is present. Penicillin, 250 mg orally four times per day for 10 days, may be given. With widespread disease, whole-body irradiation with ultraviolet light may be accomplished to retard rapid cell production. Various combinations of these treatment methods may be employed.

NURSING ASSESSMENT

Observation of the lesions will aid in identifying the characteristics. The client is asked questions relating to symptoms of arthritis to determine if this associated condition is present. The nurse should identify if there are conditions in the environment, emotional stress, or items that could cause skin injury that might lead to exacerbation of the condition when it is in remission (Dains, 1997; Luckmann, 1997; Nicol, 1997a; Norris, 1996; Weaver, 1995).

Pressure Ulcer

Pressure ulcers, formerly known as "decubitus" ulcers, bedsores, or pressure sores, occur in 3% to 8.5% of hospitalized clients per year; while they are in long-term care facilities, the prevalence is higher, at about 23%. Debilitated individuals are likely to develop pressure ulcers, which are areas of necrotic tissue. Older adults are therefore good candidates for the development of pressure ulcers, especially when they are immobile, dependent, malnourished, and bedridden—thus experiencing friction and shearing force. In very debilitated individuals, permanent tissue damage can occur in less than 2 hours and a pressure ulcer may develop in as short a time as 24 hours. Seventy percent of pressure ulcers in hospitalized clients develop within the first 1 or 2 weeks of hospitalization. These ulcers occur when the external pressure on the skin, usually over bony prominences, is greater than capillary hydrostatic pressure, which compromises local tissue perfusion and oxygenation. This problem can be avoided with adequate preventive care. During the early stages of development, pressure ulcers usually respond well to treatment and may entirely clear; however, in later stages of development these ulcers are very difficult to treat. An individual is at greater risk for the development of a pressure ulcer when certain factors are involved: moisture, nutritional deficits, shear stress, alterations in mobility and perception, and abnormal albumin and hemoglobin levels. It is estimated that the development of a pressure ulcer adds 1 to 6 weeks to a hospital stay and will potentially increase the cost of that individual's care by $10,000 to $20,000. It has been further estimated that the annual cost for treatment of all pressure ulcers is as high as $11.5 billion. Another estimate indicates that approximately 60,000 individuals die each year of complications secondary to pressure ulcers.

CLINICAL FEATURES

Identifying individuals who are at risk for the development of pressure ulcers is the first step toward prevention (Box 18–2). The Braden scale and the Norton scale are assessment tools used to evaluate an individual for the risk of developing pressure ulcers. In the initial development of a pressure ulcer, a blister may form when the damage has only occurred in the superficial tissues. A necrotic area of tissue may be noted when damage has occurred in underlying tissues. As the body tries to get rid of this necrotic area and prepare the tissue for healing, it undergoes inflammation. Areas of the body where pressure ulcers most often develop include the greater trochanter, heel, sacrum, and ischial tuberosities. Pressure ulcers may display tissues that are yellow, white, brown, or black. When a pressure ulcer is covered by

---

Box 18-2 RISK FACTORS FOR THE DEVELOPMENT OF A PRESSURE ULCER

- Malnutrition
- Incontinence
- Immobility
- Skin shearing
- Decreased sensory perception
- Decreased activity
- Increased skin friction

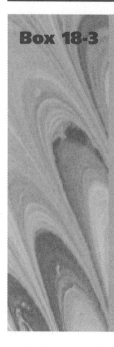

Box 18-3   PREVENTION OF PRESSURE SORES

- Perform daily (or every shift) skin inspection.
- Maintain clean skin (routine, and at time of soiling). Use warm, not hot, water and mild cleanser, with a minimum of force and friction.
- Use skin moisturizers (cream is best).
- Do not massage bony prominences.
- Avoid skin exposure to moisture and use absorbent products that provide a quick-drying surface to the skin.
- Utilize appropriate positioning, transferring, and turning techniques, using pillows to keep bony prominences from rubbing together, and develop a written schedule for turning and repositioning.
- Maintain adequate intake of protein and calories through self-feeding or enteral or parenteral feedings.
- Maintain activity, mobility, and range of joint motion.
- Lift clients who need to be moved; do not drag them.
- Utilize pressure-reducing devices (foam or gel pads, foam mattresses, alternating air mattresses) for clients at risk for developing pressure ulcers.

Adapted from Black JM, Matassarin-Jacobs E, eds. (1997). Medical-Surgical Nursing, 5th ed., p. 2217. Philadelphia: WB Saunders.

necrotic tissue, the necrotic tissue must be removed to properly stage the ulcer. Pressure ulcers are described in four stages. Stage I involves soft tissue swelling or ulceration lasting 24 hours or longer; a nonblanchable erythema of the intact skin heralds the lesion of a pressure ulcer. Stage II is a partial thickness ulcer penetrating the dermis. Clinically, pressure ulcers in this stage appear to be superficial and look like abrasions, blisters, or shallow craters. Stage III pressure ulcers display full-thickness skin loss with necrosis of the subcutaneous tissue extending to, but not through, the fascia. An ulcer in this stage looks like a deep crater with or without undermining of adjoining tissue. Stage IV includes a full-thickness loss of skin and demonstrates extensive destruction, tissue necrosis, or involvement of muscle, bone, or supporting structures and possibly exposure of the underlying bone (Luckmann, 1997; Nicol, 1997a).

MANAGEMENT

A thorough history is taken, with the goal of identifying factors that potentially contributed to the development of a pressure ulcer. A complete physical examination is also necessary. Prevention of the development of a pressure ulcer is the best treatment and can be accom-

plished by identifying risk factors for each client on an individual basis (Box 18-3). Skin assessment is an ongoing intervention and must be completed at least daily, but it is best if this can be done on every shift. For those clients who are incontinent, the skin must be cleansed thoroughly after each episode of incontinence is noted. Absorbent products that control moisture and skin exposure should be used for clients who are incontinent of urine and/or feces. Nutritional supplementation must be considered when malnutrition is suspected and/or evidenced by an albumin level less than 3.5 g/dL, a total lymphocyte count less than 1800 mm^3, the client is not eating, or the body weight is less than 80% of the ideal weight. If there are no gastrointestinal disorders, the client may take oral nutritional supplements or supplements per tube. If gastrointestinal disorders are a problem, then total parenteral nutrition may be an option. The client is assessed for signs of dehydration, including thirst, skin turgor, and dry mucous membranes. Nutritional status should be followed closely and assessed every 3 months.

Tissue load (distribution of pressure, friction, and shear on the tissues) is another management issue. Interventions for distributing pressure include the use of special beds (e.g., air-fluidized bed, Roho mattress), establishing a turning schedule for the client, and increasing the client's activity when possible (e.g., by ambulation and range of motion exercises) (Luckmann, 1997; Nicol, 1997b; Sparks, 1997).

When alterations in mobility and activity are risk factors, the client must be repositioned every 2 hours. Heels should be elevated off the bed by using supportive pillows, and heel protectors should be worn to decrease friction. Clients who sit in wheelchairs for long periods of time need to be taught to shift weight frequently.

For an established pressure ulcer, debridement is necessary to remove the moist, devitalized tissue that supports bacterial growth. Several methods of debridement may be used. Sharp debridement requires the use of a scalpel to cut away devitalized tissue (**eschar**). This method demonstrates best results when the eschar is thick and adherent. The use of wet-to-dry dressings, hydrotherapy, wound irrigation, and dextranomers (e.g., Debrisan) are forms of mechanical debridement. Topical debriding agents (e.g., collagenase) may be applied to achieve enzymatic debridement. Autolytic debridement is accomplished by covering the ulcer with a synthetic dressing and permitting enzymes in the ulcer bed to digest the devitalized tissue (Table 18–4). This type of debridement is slow and is generally used when the client cannot tolerate the other forms of debridement. Ulcers located on the heels are not debrided unless they are definitely infected. Analgesics should be administered before debriding a pressure ulcer wound because all forms of debridement, except autolytic, are painful.

■ NURSING DIAGNOSES

Most clients experiencing disorders of the skin are at risk for developing a number of nursing diagnoses, such as impaired (potential) skin integrity, which may be related to a number of factors, such as skin dryness or itching. Other diagnoses that apply to clients with skin disorders include

- Potential for Infection, related to scratching or pressure ulcer
- Impaired Tissue Integrity, related to stasis ulcer
- Knowledge Deficit of skin care
- Body Image Disturbance
- Low Self-Esteem, related to cosmetic effect of skin disorders
- Alteration in Comfort, Pain, related to skin disorder

TABLE 18–4. Products Useful for Clients with Pressure Ulcers

Product	Example
Absorption	
Dextranomer beads	Debrisan, HydraGran, Bard absorption dressing
Copolymer starch dressings	Duoderm granules
Calcium algenates	Sorbsan
Debridement	
Enzymatic wet-to-dry dressings	Elase ointment, Travase, Granulex; 4 × 4-inch gauze pads and Rirlex (usually with normal saline)
Wound Protection, Insulation, and Mild Absorption	
Hydrocolloids	Duoderm, Confeel, Tegasorb
Transparent dressings	Tegaderm
Polyurethane foam	Allevyn
Hydrogel dressings	Elasto-gel

Data from Weaver V, Long BC. (1995). Assessment of the skin. In Phipps WJ, ed. Medical-Surgical Nursing Concepts and Clinical Practice. 5th ed. St. Louis: CV Mosby; and Ebersole P, Hess P. (1998). Toward Healthy Aging: Human Needs and Nursing Response. 4th ed. St. Louis: CV Mosby.

Caring

"Because the normal age-related changes can be stressful for an older adult, it is especially important to have an empathetic approach, use appropriate communication techniques, and be thorough in data gathering."

Interventions are determined by the specific disorder and have been discussed with each condition.

Summary

The care of the skin is essential to maintaining health and should always be a part of any plan of management for older adults. The older adult is at greater risk for various disorders of the integumentary system simply due to the aging of the skin and the insults to which it has been exposed, particularly through excessive exposure to the sun. Prevention is the key to healthy skin in old age, and health teaching for clients of all ages needs to underscore the hazards of sun exposure at every age from infancy onward.

For patients who are bedridden in either acute or long-term care facilities, the potential for development of pressure ulcers is always present. Again, prevention is the most effective response, with regular checking of the skin status a part of daily care. Gentle transferring and repositioning, regular cleansing, and use of special mattresses or other devices can prevent ulcers from forming and contribute to their healing if they already exist.

Skin cancers need to be identified and addressed as early as possible, so an alert nurse who includes careful examination of the skin in an overall assessment can prove invaluable to patients who may be unaware of early cancers.

RESOURCES

Administration on Aging
330 Independence Avenue S.W.
Washington, DC 20201
(202) 619-0556

Age and Aging
Bailliere Tindall
7-8 Henrietta Street
Covent Garden
London, England WCZE 8QE

American Association of Retired Persons (AARP)
601 E Street N.W.
Washington, DC 20049
(202) 434-2277

American Cancer Society
777 Third Avenue
New York, NY 10017
(212) 371-2900

American Federation for Aging Research (AFAR)
1414 Avenue of the Americas, 18th Floor
New York, NY 10019
(212) 752-AFAR; fax (212) 832-2298

American Geriatrics Society
770 Lexington Avenue, Suite 300
New York, NY 10021
(212) 308-1414

American Health Care Association
1201 L Street N.W.
Washington, DC 20005-4014
(202) 842-4444

American Pain Society
5700 Old Orchard Road
Skokie, IL 60077
(708) 966-5595

American Society on Aging
833 Market Street, Suite 512
San Francisco, CA 94103-1824
(415) 882-2910

Center for Social Gerontology
2307 Shelby Avenue
Ann Arbor, MI 48103-3895
(313) 665-1126

Federal Council on Aging
330 Independence Avenue S.W.
Room 4280 HHS-N
Washington, DC 20201

Gerontological Nutritionists
4103 44th Street
Sacramento, CA 95820
(916) 451-7149

Help for Incontinent People
Box 544
Union, SC 29389
(803) 585-8789

National Cancer Institute
Office of Cancer Communications
Building 31, Room 10A18
Bethesda, MD 20205
(800) 492-6600

REFERENCES

Dains JE. (1997). Integumentary system. In Thompson JM, et al., eds. Mosby's Clinical Nursing. 4th ed. St. Louis: CV Mosby.

Ebersole P, Hess P. (1998). Toward Healthy Aging: Human Needs and Nursing Response. 4th ed. St. Louis: CV Mosby.

Ghadially R. (1996). Skin. In Lonergan ET, ed. Geriatrics: A Lange Clinical Manual. Stamford, CT: Appleton & Lange.

Lonergan ET, Stone JT. (1996). Pressure sores. In Lonergan ET, ed. Geriatrics: A Lange Clinical Manual. Stamford, CT: Appleton & Lange.

Lueckenotte AG. (1994). Pocket Guide to Gerontologic Assessment. 2nd ed. St. Louis: CV Mosby.

Murray RB, Zentner JP, Pinnell NN, Boland MH. (1997). Assessment and health promotion for the person in later maturity. In Murray RB, Zentner JP, eds. Health Assessment Promotion Strategies Through the Life Span. 6th ed. Stamford, CT: Appleton & Lange.

Nicol NH. (1997a). Assessment of clients with integumentary disorders. In Black JM, Matassarin-Jacobs E, eds. Medical-Surgical Nursing: Clinical Management for Continuity of Care. 5th ed. Philadelphia: WB Saunders.

Nicol NH. (1997b). Nursing care of clients with integumentary disorders. In Black JM, Matassarin-Jacobs E, eds. Medical-Surgical Nursing: Clinical Management for Continuity of Care. 5th ed. Philadelphia: WB Saunders.

Norris J, ed. (1996). Handbook of Diseases. Springhouse, PA: Springhouse Corporation.

Saunders Manual of Nursing Care (1997). Philadelphia: WB Saunders.

Sims LK, D'Amico D, Stiesmeyer JK, Webster JA. (1995). Health Assessment in Nursing. Redwood City, CA: Addison-Wesley.

Sparks SM. (1997). Integument. In Burke MM, Walsh MB, eds. Gerontologic Nursing: Wholistic Care of the Older Adult. 2nd ed. St. Louis: CV Mosby.

Warner L. (1996). Infectious disease. In Lonergan ET, ed. Geriatrics: A Lange Clinical Manual. Stamford, CT: Appleton & Lange.

Weaver V. (1995). Management of persons with problems of the skin. In Phipps WJ, et al., eds. Medical-Surgical Nursing Concepts and Clinical Practice. 5th ed. St. Louis: CV Mosby.

Weaver V, Long BC. (1995). Assessment of the skin. In Phipps WJ, et al., eds. Medical-Surgical Nursing Concepts and Clinical Practice. 5th ed. St. Louis: CV Mosby.

CRITICAL THINKING EXERCISES

Mrs. Nora Smith, an 89-year-old white woman who lives alone, has had chronic pruritus for the past 30 years. She has not been diagnosed with a specific condition but has periods of extreme itching, especially when she is emotionally stressed. Sometimes the itching is so annoying that she scratches the area until bleeding occurs. In a couple of places on her shoulders, she has developed hard, thickened skin because of the years of continual itching and scratching.

1. What predisposing factors might play a role in Nora's chronic skin condition?
2. Develop a plan of care for Nora and other clients with chronic skin conditions. Give thought to altered comfort, risk for infection, sleep pattern disturbance, anxiety, altered self-esteem, knowledge deficit of appropriate skin care.
3. One area of Nora's pruritus has become an open, oozing wound. What methods of debridement are available for treatment of this area?
4. Formulate a self-care health-promotion maintenance teaching plan for Nora.
5. Nora has isolated herself socially because of the continual scratching. What approach could be implemented to increase Nora's socialization?

CHAPTER 19

Maintaining Wellness of the
Metabolic System

Vanessa Jones Briscoe, RN, MSN

CHAPTER OUTLINE

OBJECTIVES

After completing this chapter, the reader should be able to:

1. Teach a classmate the age-related changes of the endocrine system and how these changes potentially affect homeostasis in older adults.
2. Compare and contrast type 1 and type 2 diabetes, including symptoms and incidence.
3. Create a teaching plan for an older adult patient with type 2 diabetes.
4. Specify three acute complications of diabetes and present interventions for each.
5. Differentiate between hypothyroidism and hyperthyroidism, including symptoms and complications.
6. Create a teaching plan for older adults with the following endocrine disorders: diabetes, hypothyroidism, parathyroid adenoma.

KEY TERMS

hormones
myxedema
thyroid storm

The combined functions of the endocrine and neurological systems enable our bodies to maintain metabolic control. The endocrine glands aid this regulatory process by secreting **hormones,** chemical transmitters, in response to metabolic depletion or overproduction; thus, they constitute a biochemical feedback system. These hormones are transported by the bloodstream to the target organs on which they have a specific regulatory effect. This chapter addresses age-related changes that occur within the endocrine system and how metabolic function is affected in older adults. Common disease processes that are associated with age-related endocrine changes are discussed along with their nursing assessment and treatment.

◼ HEALTH TEACHING

Most of the diseases discussed in this chapter are preventable with appropriate lifestyle modifications and early detection through regular screening. One of the essential elements in prevention of metabolic problems is a healthy, balanced diet. Often, older adults need information about dietary modification. For example, reducing dietary fat to less than 30% of total caloric intake will increase life expectancy and decrease deaths associated with heart attacks (Fishman, 1996). Other dietary modifications that lead to reductions in incidence of chronic diseases and disabilities associated with endocrine dysfunctions include restricting sodium intake; encouraging consumption of more vegetables, fruits, and dietary fiber; and, for postmenopausal women, increasing calcium intake (via supplement or dairy products). Clients who are less likely to meet these dietary goals include individuals living alone and alcoholics (Patterson and Chambers, 1995).

According to Patterson and Chambers (1995), regular aerobic exercise is a cornerstone of primary prevention of disease. Exercise is considered a primary mode of intervention for individuals with diabetes. The nurse should discuss with clients the benefits of a regular exercise program: increased sense of well-being, increased cardiovascular and respiratory function, and increased bone mass and muscle strength.

If clients use tobacco products, they should be encouraged to stop. Smoking increases the risk of many chronic diseases (cardiac and respiratory) and disabilities. The nurse should also emphasize the importance of the (one-time) Pneumovax and (annual) influenza inoculations. Immunization reduces the incidence of, and mortality rate associated with, influenza and pneumonia.

Health teaching also needs to include screening for and treatment of already existing conditions. For the endocrine system, these would include teaching regarding the importance of controlling hypertension. The use of screening programs for early detection of breast, colon, and prostate cancers should be encouraged.

◼ AGE-RELATED CHANGES

Older adults constitute a heterogeneous population. Current research is investigating factors that may regulate the rate and progression of the aging process. Many of the age-related endocrine changes exhibit little to no effect on the body's ability to maintain metabolic control. The pituitary gland continues to produce substantial levels of crucial hormones throughout life, although many studies have confirmed decreased production of growth hormone (GH). This GH deficiency state can be associated with symptoms of fatigue, insomnia, decreased muscle and bone mass, increased body fat, and a decreased sense of well-being (Kowal and Hornick, 1997). However, the overall effect of decreased GH production does not profoundly modify metabolism control.

Altered thyroid function causes older adults to be more susceptible to states of hyperthyroidism or hypothyroidism. Studies indicate that, with aging, there is a decreased production of thyroxine (T_4) and possibly triiodothyronine (T_3) (Felicetta, 1996). The basal metabolic rate begins its decline during young adulthood and continues progressively throughout life. Older adults likewise experience decreases in oxygen consumption and, as noted earlier, decreases in lean body mass, making the effects of this decreased metabolic rate less noticeable.

Pancreatic function also appears to decrease with aging. Studies have shown that with age comes decreased glucose tolerance; hence, pe-ripheral organs are less sensitive to the effects of insulin.

Adrenal function does not alter appreciably with advancing age, and adequate levels of hormones are produced to meet bodily needs. Table 19–1 summarizes the actions of the hor-

TABLE 19–1. Endocrine Hormones and Age-Related Changes

Hormone	Target Organ	Action	Change with Age
Pituitary Gland (Posterior Lobe)			
Antidiuretic hormone (ADH)	Kidney	Water balance	Increased secretion
	Asterioles	Blood pressure control	
Oxytocin	Uterus	Contraction	*
Pituitary Gland (Anterior Lobe)			
Growth hormone (GH)	General	Cell and tissue growth	Decreased secretion during sleep
Adrenocorticotropic hormone (ACTH)	Adrenal gland		*
Thyroid-stimulating hormone (TSH)	Thyroid gland		*
Prolactin	Mammary glands	Secretion of milk	*
Follicle-stimulating hormone (FSH)	Ovaries		Increased levels
	Testes		
Luteinizing hormone (LH)	Ovaries		Increased levels
	Testes		
Thyroid Gland			
Thyroxine (T_4)	General	Increases rate of metabolism	*
Triiodothyronine (T_3)	General	Increases rate of metabolism	Decreased levels
Calcitonin	Bones	Promotes calcium absorption in bones	Decreased levels
Islet Cells of the Pancreas			
Insulin	General	Promotes entry of glucose to cells	Decreased peripheral sensitivity
Glucagon	Liver	Increases release of stored glucose	Unknown
Sex Glands (Male)			
Testosterone	Testes	Growth of male sex organ and secondary sex characteristics	Decreased levels
Sex Glands (Female)			
Estrogen			
	Ovaries	Growth of male sex organ and secondary sex characteristics	
	Mammary glands		
Progesterone	Mammary glands	Maintenance of pregnancy and lactation	
	Uterus		

*No sufficient changes with aging.

mones and their age-related secretional changes.

GUIDELINES SPECIFIC TO ASSESSING THE METABOLIC SYSTEM IN OLDER ADULTS

The endocrine system is regulated by feedback mechanisms that involve hormonal interactions between the brain and the endocrine glands (pituitary, thyroid, parathyroid, adrenals, ovaries, and testes). Its function supports and maintains homeostasis, which involves growth and development, energy production, fluid and electrolyte balance, and reproduction.

Many of the early clinical findings associated with endocrine disorders are vague and may be attributed to "getting old" by the patient. The astute nurse realizes that the abnormal secretion of any of these hormones can produce physical symptoms and alter the function of the entire system. The ovaries, testes, and thyroid gland are the only endocrine glands that can be assessed directly by physical examination; assessment of other endocrine function must be observed indirectly via the body systems. For example, bradycardia or tachycardia observed during examination of the cardiovascular system may be due to hyposecretion or hypersecretion of thyroid hormones. Altered levels of consciousness experienced by the older adult may be due to increased levels of parathyroid hormone, insulin, or thyroid hormone. While inspecting the patient's skin, the nurse may find changes in hair texture, altered facial appearance (moon facies), or increased bruising, which indicate the need to assess cortisol level or even thyroid hormone.

Confirmation of endocrine dysfunction will be with laboratory values for the specific hormones. When making assessment of endocrine function, the nurse should keep in mind that, although this system may show some age-related alteration in function, function is usually normal unless the organ is stressed. As the reader proceeds to read about specific disorders of the endocrine system, the following will become obvious in the assessment of the older adult patient:

- Older individuals are prone to certain endocrine diseases.

- Other than laboratory findings, most of the clinical manifestations associated with these diseases of the endocrine are nonspecific.

COMMON DISORDERS

Diabetes

Diabetes mellitus (DM) is a major health concern for older Americans, affecting 10% of the population older than age 65 years and 20% to 23% of the population older than age 80 years (Byrd, 1994; Miller, 1996). The prevalence of type 2 diabetes in persons older than 65 is expected to be as high as 44% in the next 20 years (Byrd, 1994). It is the sixth leading cause of death in older adults, with high morbidity rates having an enormous negative impact on quality of life, as well as on the health care system (Byrd, 1994). There is an explosion of diabetes in the elderly minority population. In particular, African Americans, Hispanics, and Native Americans are more susceptible to diabetes and its devastating complications.

Caring

"*The nurse emphasizes healthy lifestyle modifications, especially a prudent diet and regular physical activity, in maintaining an adequately functioning endocrine system.***"**

CLINICAL FEATURES

Diabetes is a chronic disorder in which there is an inadequate amount of insulin and/or diminished function of insulin. This insulin deficiency causes deteriorating glucose tolerance that results in the abnormal metabolism of carbohydrates, fats, and proteins. Over time, this chronic disorder leads to numerous complications affecting the heart, eyes, kidneys, and peripheral nerves and vasculature. Studies indicate that some of the deteriorating glucose tolerance may be due to normal aging process. With aging comes some decrease in peripheral glucose uptake and slightly higher postprandial blood glucose levels. Additionally, other factors such as lack of exercise, obesity, chronic illness, and polypharmacy contribute to dwindling glucose tolerance (Miller, 1996; Le and Tuck, 1994).

There are several classifications of diabetes. The two major groups are *type 1,* also called insulin-dependent diabetes mellitus, and *type 2,* or non–insulin-dependent diabetes mellitus (Table 19–2). The probability of acquiring type 2 diabetes increases with each decade of life after age 30 (Le and Tuck, 1994).

The etiology of type 1 diabetes involves pancreatic beta cell destruction that often leads to absolute insulin deficiency. It is believed multifaceted, with genetic and environmental factors triggering an autoimmune process in individuals susceptible to diabetes. The autoimmune process causes destruction of the "islet" cells of the pancreas. People with type 1 diabetes make no endogenous insulin and require daily insulin injections to stay alive. This scenario most often occurs in children and young adults.

Type 2 diabetes, on the other hand, is a metabolic disorder whose etiology ranges from varying degrees of insulin resistance with relative insulin deficiency to a secretory defect that causes insulin resistance. It is the most common form of the disease and is nearing epidemic proportions in some of our minority populations.

The diagnosis of DM is based on a fasting plasma glucose level of 126 mg/dL or greater on at least two occasions (Report of the expert committee, 1997). Another diagnostic test for diabetes used for older adults is the oral glucose tolerance test; however, this test has many adverse reactions in older adults. Additionally, the oral glucose tolerance test results can be influenced adversely by acute illness, stress, alterations in diet, and polypharmacy, which can result in false-positive results (Reed and Mooradian, 1992). These situations often occur in the lives of older clients. The diagnostic test of choice is the fasting plasma glucose.

MANAGEMENT

The Diabetes Control and Complications Trial (DCCT) was a 10-year study undertaken to determine how best to control the complications of type 1 diabetes. The study concluded the best way to decrease the risk of developing long-term complications associated with DM (e.g., retinopathy, neuropathy, nephropathy)

TABLE 19–2. Comparison of Type 1 and Type 2 Diabetes Mellitus

Type 1*	Type 2†
• It usually occurs before age 30 but can occur at any age.	• It usually occurs after age 40.
• Abrupt onset of signs and symptoms occurs with insulinopenia.	• Obesity is present in 80%–90% of cases.
• There may be multiple causative factors: genetics, immunologic response, and/or environmental trigger (i.e., virus).	• Relative insulin deficiency is due to islet cell defect; reduced insulin receptor sites and/or peripheral resistance to insulin.
• Patient is ketoacidosis prone and dependent on insulin therapy to sustain life.	• Patient is usually not ketoacidosis prone nor dependent on exogenous insulin for survival.
• Treatment comprises nutrition therapy, exercise, and insulin.	• Treatment includes nutrition therapy and exercise. If blood glucose level is not controlled, individual may be treated with medication (oral hypoglycemics or insulin).
• Acute complications include ketoacidosis and hypoglycemia.	• Acute complications include hyperglycemic hyperosmolar nonketotic coma and hypoglycemia (if on medication that causes this side effect).
• Chronic complications include heart disease, neuropathy, retinopathy, and nephropathy.	• Chronic complications include heart disease, neuropathy, retinopathy, and nephropathy.

*Affects 5%–10% of individuals with diabetes.
†Affects about 90% of individuals with diabetes.
 Adapted from classification developed by the Report of the Expert Committee on the Diagnosis and Classification of Diabetes Mellitus, 1997. Diabetes Care 20:1183–1197.

or of suffering further progression of these conditions was to achieve and maintain tight blood glucose control (Diabetes Control and Complications Trial Research Group, 1993). Diabetes-related complications were cut by 50% or more in those clients on an intensive regimen aimed at keeping their blood glucose as close as possible to normal physiological levels. Even though the study was conducted using only individuals with type 1 diabetes, the results are believed by some sources to be generalizable to individuals with type 2 diabetes.

Treatment of diabetes in older adults is very important because the effects of hyperglycemia cause increased morbidity. Blood glucose levels of 200 mg/dL or greater may produce symptoms of urinary frequency, visual impairment, memory retention deficits, increased complaints of pain, and enhanced platelet adhesiveness (Reed and Mooradian, 1992). Hence, treatment is mandated to not only improve quality of life but also to reduce long-term complications associated with this catastrophic disease. There are a wide variety of treatments for DM in older adults. These include nutrition therapy, exercise, and pharmacological agents.

W e l l n e s s

"Most of the diseases discussed in this chapter are preventable with appropriate lifestyle modifications and early detection through regular screening."

Nutrition therapy is recognized as the cornerstone for management of DM. However, the primary reason individuals fail to respond adequately to diet alone is because of poor compliance (Briscoe, 1998; Williams, 1994). Dietary regimens are often complex, requiring multiple behavioral changes on the part of the client. The diet, in the case of diabetes, is employed as a means to control, rather than a cure. Hence, the diet regimen and associated behavioral changes must be a lifelong commitment. Both of these characteristics of a dietary regimen adversely affect client adherence.

A common goal of diet therapy when treating diabetes is to enhance metabolic control. In older adults, weight reduction is often recommended. Calories may also be restricted

for the client with normal weight, to compensate for the decreases in activity level and the decline in lean muscle mass. These factors decrease the amount of calories needed to maintain weight. There are a variety of dietary regimens aimed at assisting the client with DM in maintaining glucose control. The type of diet therapy used must be tailored to the individual's lifestyle (e.g., cultural, ethnic, and socioeconomic status) to increase the likelihood of compliance with the prescribed regimen. If the client has difficulty in learning the diet, and food choices are very restricted and differ greatly from present dietary habits, nonadherence to the prescribed meal plan will be the likely outcome.

Controversy still exists regarding the composition of a diet that best facilitates glucose control in adults with diabetes. However, the most recent American Diabetes Association (ADA) recommendations emphasize that the nutrient therapy achieve and maintain a reasonable body weight, lower blood glucose levels, and lower cholesterol levels (ADA, 1994).

Exercise is the second component of treatment for diabetes. Studies have shown that exercise benefits older individuals in many ways in spite of potential risks from some exercise programs (e.g., musculoskeletal injuries, hypoglycemic episodes) (Graham, 1994). Some benefits related to DM are improvement of glucose tolerance and improvement of insulin action. The exercise program should be carried out on a regular basis, tailored to address the individual's preexisting health conditions. The older client may only be capable of engaging in a "stretcherize" program or some type of chair exercises. Any regularly occurring activity will benefit the client. Exercise should be of a creative nature to encourage continued participation.

Medication is the third component of the DM treatment regimen and is not always necessary if diet and exercise adequately control blood glucose. The medication regimen can comprise oral agents to lower blood glucose levels or insulin. In some cases, medications may be used in combination.

Until recently, only two types of medications were available in the United States to aid in the control of hyperglycemia in persons with diabetes: oral sulfonylureas and insulin. Recently, however, the Food and Drug Administration

TABLE 19–3. Oral Hypoglycemic Agents

Generic Name	Brand Name
Sulfonylurea Drugs (First Generation)	
Tolbutamide	Orinase
Chlorpropamide	Diabinese, Glucamide
Tolazamide	Tolinase
Acetohexamide	Dymelor
Sulfonylurea Drugs (Second Generation)	
Glipizide	Glucotrol
	Glucotrol XL
Glyburide	DiaBeta, Micronase
	Glynase
Glimepiride	Amaryl
Biguanide	
Metformin	Glucophage
Alpha-Glucosidase Inhibitor	
Acarbose	Precose
Thiazolidinedione	
Troglitazone	Rezulin

has approved several new types of oral medications and a new type of insulin (Tables 19–3 and 19–4). Research is continuing to introduce new oral agents and new insulin preparations. Because the options for pharmacological therapy are expanding in the quest to control the hyperglycemia associated with diabetes, it is essential for the nurse to keep up to date. When oral medications are used to control hyperglycemia, the nurse should remember that the individual usually has to have some remaining endogenous insulin secretion; therefore, oral preparations will most likely be prescribed for individuals with type 2 diabetes.

Chlorpropamide (Diabinese) is not the drug of choice for the older adult client with diabetes because of its long duration of action and side effects (e.g., inappropriate antidiuretic hormone syndrome, hyponatremia). Also, renal insufficiency prolongs the activity of this drug.

The use of insulin (see Table 19–4) is reserved for those individuals in whom oral agents, dietary modification, and exercise fail to result in a satisfactory blood glucose level. Visual deficits and poor coordination may make insulin administration problematic in some older clients. However, there are many devices on the market to aid in insulin administration. Individuals are often started on insulin as outpatients; hence, an intensive education program needs to be in place. Intermediate-acting preparations are often used; however, the newer brands of "mixed" type of insulins are gaining popularity of usage in this age group. Once-a-day dosing is often adequate in this age group because insulin secretory capacity remains in most clients with type 2 diabetes. Human insulins should be used when insulin therapy is short term (e.g., during surgery or acute illness when blood glucose levels are out of control).

MONITORING BLOOD GLUCOSE CONTROL

Monitoring blood glucose control has become an important part of diabetes care now that home glucose monitoring is readily available.

TABLE 19–4. Insulin Preparations

Insulin	Onset of Action	Peak Action	Duration of Action
Lispro	10–15 minutes	30–90 minutes	<5 hours
Regular	30 minutes	2–5 hours	5–8 hours
NPH/Lente	1–3 hours	6–12 hours	16–24 hours
70/30, 50/50	30 minutes	7–12 hours	16–24 hours
Ultralente	4–6 hours	8–20 hours	24–36 hours

Note: Times will vary in different insulin preparations and among individuals.

Adapted from American Diabetes Association, 1994. Medical Management of Non-Insulin Dependent (Type II) Diabetes. 3rd ed. Alexandria, VA.

Data from Anderson JH (jr), Brunelle RL, Kiovisto DA, et al. and the multicenter insulin Lispro study group (1998). Reduction of post prandial hyperglycemia and frequency of hypoglycemia in IDDM patients on insulin—analog treatment. Diabetes 46(16):265–270.

Before home glucose monitoring, the only way to monitor blood glucose levels at home was indirectly by urine testing. The information solicited from urine testing was limited. The test informed the client that blood glucose was *negative,* meaning the blood glucose was 180 mg/dL (the renal threshold for glucose) or lower, or that blood glucose was *positive,* meaning the blood glucose level was greater than 180 mg/dL. Additionally, these values were only accurate if the individual had normal kidney function. With aging, there is a normal decline in kidney function. One result is an increased renal threshold for glucose; hence, in this population the glucose urine test results are unreliable. Urine testing for ketones is still to be used when the client is sick or has a blood glucose level that is over a certain range (usually 250–300 mg/dL or greater).

W e l l n e s s

"The astute nurse realizes that the abnormal secretion of any hormone can produce physical symptoms and alter the function of the entire body."

Home glucose monitoring is a valuable tool. It lets the individual know if the blood glucose level is high, low, or within normal range. It is useful to tell the client what is an acceptable range. For instance, one client may have a blood glucose target range of 100 to 180 mg/dL because he or she does not experience early symptoms of hypoglycemia. Another client may have a blood glucose range of 80 to 140 mg/dL. There are many blood glucose monitoring products available for sale on the market today. A consideration for older adults, when prescribing a particular glucometer, is whether the individual can operate the machine easily. If only visual monitoring is prescribed, the individual should be able to distinguish greens and blues, because these are the colors frequently used to identify glycemic states. The yellowing of the lens that occurs with aging affects the ability to discriminate these low-tone colors.

Two other tests used to elicit blood glucose control are the glycosylated hemoglobin and fructosamine tests. The glycosylated hemoglo-

bin test provides the clinician with a measure of the average blood glucose concentrations over the preceding 10 to 12 weeks before the drawing of the blood sample. Results are affected, however, by renal impairment and use of certain medications (e.g., acetylsalicylic acid) (Reed and Mooradian, 1992). The fructosamine test provides the clinician with an approximation of blood glucose control over the previous 2 to 3 weeks. The fructosamine test is recommended by some clinicians over the glycosylated hemoglobin because results are not affected by age and the cost of the test is lower (Reed and Mooradian, 1992).

ACUTE COMPLICATIONS

Hypoglycemia is the most common complication of insulin treatment in clients with diabetes. The lower the mean blood glucose level, the more likely the client will experience hypoglycemia. The risk of severe or fatal hypoglycemia increases in the older adult client because of altered counterregulatory hormone response to low blood glucose, altered sensorium, and decreased awareness of the symptoms of hypoglycemia (Meneilly et al., 1994). Precipitating factors of hypoglycemia are overdose of insulin or sulfonylurea, missed or delayed meal, and excessive exercise without carbohydrate compensation. The client may experience a combination of the following symptoms: headache, weakness, diaphoresis, tachycardia, confusion, visual disturbances, or seizure activity. Treatment for hypoglycemia, if the client is alert and can ingest items by mouth, consists of 15 to 20 g of quick-acting carbohydrates (e.g., orange juice, candy, glucose paste, or tablets), repeating every 15 minutes until the blood glucose level is within normal range. If the client is unconscious, glucagon intramuscularly or 50% dextrose given by intravenous push can be dispensed. Another acute complication of diabetes experienced by some older adults is *hyperglycemic hyperosmolar coma (HHC).* Characteristic symptoms and signs help the physician distinguish this syndrome from *diabetic ketoacidosis (DKA).* DKA is a serious complication of diabetes and is seen most frequently in individuals with type 1 diabetes. It results from an absolute or relative deficiency of insulin and is characterized by hyperglycemia, hyperketonemia, and severe

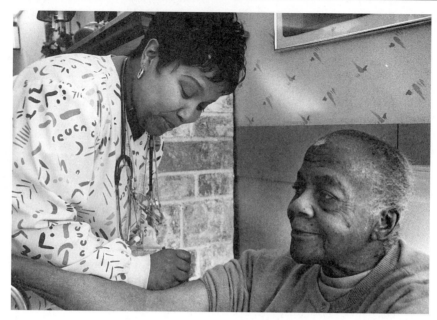

A diabetic patient receives an injection of insulin.

electrolyte and fluid imbalance. Client assessment may reveal a history of polyuria, polydipsia, fatigue, signs of dehydration, Kussmaul's respiration, acetone breath odor, and hypotension. Treatment consists of fluid replacement, insulin, potassium, and sodium bicarbonate (if acidosis is severe) (Genuth, 1997).

HHC presents most often in individuals with type 2 diabetes. Most of the patients are older adults and have had a rather benign history of diabetes. However, some stressors (i.e., myocardial infarction, sepsis, dehydration, initiation of steroid therapy) increase insulin requirements above the limit and trigger this syndrome. The major pathological processes associated with HHC are severe hyperglycemia and hyperosmolarity without meaningful ketosis. The absence or minimal nature of ketosis is what differentiates HHC from DKA. It is not completely understood why ketosis does not develop in HHC, but it is believed to be related to the fact that there is some circulating plasma insulin. This insulin production, along with the hyperosmolarity, is believed to inhibit the formation of significant ketosis (Genuth, 1997). Treatment consists of fluid and electrolyte replacement, supplemental potassium after es-

tablishing adequate urinary output, and insulin.

CHRONIC COMPLICATIONS

Preventing the chronic complications that develop 10 to 15 years after the onset of diabetes is one of the ultimate goals of therapy. The three most common complications of diabetes mellitus are: macrovascular diseases, microvascular diseases, and neuropathies. As indicated in the DCCTRG (1993) study cited earlier, there are positive correlations among the incidence and severity of chronic complications and the degree of metabolic control.

The primary characteristic of microvascular disease in the client with diabetes is capillary basement membrane thickening. The retina and kidney are primarily affected. With normal aging, there is a decline in glomerular function, and the renal problems that develop with nephropathy only compound the problem. In nephropathy, the client with diabetes often experiences frequent, recurrent infections, and these assaults contribute to the pathology by affecting the permeability of the capillary walls.

Retinopathy is seen in about half of all individuals with diabetes who are older than age 50 years. Diabetes is the leading cause of new blindness among adults (ADA, 1994). In older adults, retinopathy often occurs in addition to the other eye changes, including macular degeneration, cataracts, and glaucoma.

Neuropathy is a common complication of diabetes. The symptoms depend on which body systems are affected. Peripheral nerve degeneration is the type that usually affects the lower extremities. There are losses of vibratory sense. The client experiences episodes of pain, hyperesthesia, and "burning" sensations in legs or feet, which become more nagging and constant at night. Finally, the client experiences a painless neuropathy and does not perceive pain in the affected extremities. It is important to teach foot care to the individual with diabetes because delay in the treatment of a foot problem can result in an amputation.

Another type of neuropathy involves damage to the autonomic nerves. Symptoms experienced from this type of neuropathy include impotence in males, orthostatic hypotension, and bladder and gastrointestinal system atony.

Macrovascular complications seen in diabetes result from atherosclerosis. In diabetes there is an abnormal metabolism of fats, in addition to the abnormal metabolism of carbohydrates and proteins. Individuals with diabetes are at higher risk for high blood pressure, heart disease, and cerebrovascular accidents. It is often difficult to get the client to understand the relationship between atherosclerosis and diabetes because diabetes is seen only in terms of an abnormal carbohydrate metabolism dysfunction. Also, atherosclerosis causes decreased blood supply to the feet, affecting healing abilities of any type of foot lesions.

W e l l n e s s

"*Exercise is considered a primary mode of intervention for individuals with diabetes.***"**

Hypothyroidism

Alterations in immune function, mismanaged hyperthyroidism, and certain medications all contribute to the high incidence of hypothy-

roidism in older adults. Additionally, its presentation may differ dramatically from those symptoms commonly seen in younger adults (e.g., weight gain, cold intolerance, dry skin, thinning of body hair, constipation, lack of energy). The nurse's index of suspicion should increase if the older adult patient presents with the following problems: unexplained elevation in serum cholesterol or triglyceride levels, congestive heart failure, fecal impaction, anemia, vague arthritic complaints, and depression (Felicetta, 1996). Other symptoms that suggest the need for further evaluation include syncope, seizure activity, and impaired cerebellar function (Felicetta, 1996). Additional examination findings that may heighten suspicion of decreased thyroid function include goiter, family history of thyroid disease, thyroidectomy scar, and past treatment with radiolabeled iodine. Diagnosis is usually made by a low free T_4 index, which assesses total T_4 and thyroid-binding proteins, and an elevated thyroid-stimulating hormone level (Barzel, 1997). The older adult client may experience few or no symptoms until the dysfunction is critical. In clients with hypothyroidism, the effects of analgesics, sedatives, and anesthetic agents are augmented. Discretion is necessary when considering these medications for use in older clients. Additionally, older adults may respond more acutely because of age-related changes in liver and renal function.

Treatment of hypothyroidism is thyroid hormone replacement. When treating the elderly, the drug of choice is usually levothyroxine. Precaution should be taken to start with low doses and increase gradually to prevent cardiovascular (angina, rhythm disturbances, or myocardial infarction) and neurological side effects. Response to treatment will demonstrate a regression in symptoms, increased metabolism, diuresis, and improved mental and motor functions. Thyroid function should be monitored while the client's dose is being titrated to therapeutic levels, and thereafter. Observation for signs of thyrotoxicosis and heart dysfunction should be a routine part of the client's follow-up assessment.

Myxedema Coma

Myxedema coma is the result of prolonged, untreated hypothyroidism; it is a life-threatening situation. The coma is often precipitated by a stressful event: exposure to cold, infection, trauma, or surgery. Most of the patients seen with this condition are elderly. Clinical presentation often includes the presence of hypothermia, bradycardia, hypotension, electrolyte abnormalities, hypoglycemia, altered consciousness, convulsive states, and coma. Timely and aggressive treatment is paramount to save the life of the patient. Therapy includes giving intravenous thyroid hormone, correcting electrolyte imbalances, and conserving body heat.

Caring

❝Nurses will find that individuals living alone, and alcoholics, need special attention in meeting their dietary goals.❞

Hyperthyroidism

The signs and symptoms of hyperthyroidism (e.g., weight loss, palpitations, heat intolerance, smooth moist skin, exophthalmos) presented in the young adult are often stifled in older adults (Barzel, 1997). The accelerated thyroid state overloads the heart of the older adult in such a manner that the presenting diagnosis is often congestive heart failure, masking the underlying diagnosis of hyperthyroidism (Felicetta, 1996). Other clinical features of thyrotoxicosis in older adults may be apathy, constipation, and weight loss (Kowal and Hornick, 1997).

Diagnosis of hyperthyroidism rests heavily on laboratory findings. Elevated T_4, elevated free T_4 or free–T_4 index and/or T_3, and fully suppressed thyroid-stimulating hormone are the cardinal findings of this disease (Barzel, 1997). In examining test results, however, one must take into account that certain medications may influence the results. For example, estrogen preparations and propranolol (medications commonly prescribed for this population) will affect thyroid function tests.

Treatment is always administered if the diagnosis of hyperthyroidism is confirmed (with or without the presence of symptoms). These actions are mandated because the client is at risk of developing the life-threatening medical

emergency associated with hyperthyroidism called *thyroid storm* (Barzel, 1997). Major forms of therapy consist of the administration of radioactive iodine (^{131}I) and/or antithyroid medications and surgery. Radioactive iodine is principally prescribed for older adult clients. This treatment modality is performed on an outpatient basis. Advantages include simple administration (^{131}I is given orally in water) and economy. Disadvantages include the possibility that the ^{131}I destroys too many thyroid cells, resulting in myxedema. **Myxedema** is the medical emergency of hypothyroidism. Therefore, the nurse should always monitor the client for symptoms of hypothyroidism after ^{131}I therapy. When hyperthyroidism is treated with antithyroid medications, thioamides (propylthiouracil or methimazole) are used. Propylthiouracil corrects hyperthyroidism by impairing thyroid hormone synthesis. Methimazole (Tapazole) acts by blocking the action of the thyroid hormone in the body. The clinical effects of these drugs take 2 to 4 weeks to develop. Adrenergic blocking agents such as propranolol (Inderal) may be given as adjunctive therapy to control systemic manifestations of the disease (e.g., tachycardia, tremors).

Inorganic iodine preparations, such as Lugol's solution or saturated solution potassium iodide (SSKI), are used to interfere with the release and utilization of the thyroid hormone. Iodine therapy is often initiated to reduce the vascularity of the thyroid gland before thyroid surgery or to treat thyroid storm. Iodine preparations temporarily act to prevent release of thyroid hormone into the circulation by increasing the amount of thyroid hormone stored within the gland. However, the stored thyroid hormone will eventually be released into the circulation, producing symptoms of hyperthyroidism. For this reason, treatment with iodine preparations is usually given only before surgery.

Thyroid Storm (Thyrotoxic Crisis)

Thyroid storm is an emergency situation that results from untreated or undiagnosed hyperthyroidism. With this condition the patient's metabolic rate climbs dramatically without regard for any body system. Clinical presentation includes high temperature (102°F–106°F), severe tachycardia (resulting in arrhythmias and congestive heart failure), restlessness, psychotic behavior (usually mania), diaphoresis, vomiting, and diarrhea. Treatment includes medications to block thyroid hormone action, synthesis, and secretion; intravenous fluid replacement; and measures to reduce the fever.

Thyroid Cancer

Differentiated thyroid carcinoma includes papillary and follicular thyroid carcinoma and variants of these condition. Papillary carcinoma is the most common type of thyroid cancer and constitutes about three fourths of all thyroid cancers (Hershman and Gordon, 1997). Most thyroid adenomas are well encapsulated and do not spread to other tissues. Higher mortality rates are associated with thyroid cancer in the older adult.

Thyroid carcinoma occurs more frequently among clients who have received large doses of radiation to the head and neck; hence, if a client is to receive radiation to these areas, the thyroid area is shielded when possible. Additionally, follow-up assessment is necessary for these clients. The major manifestation of thyroid cancer is the appearance of a hard, painless nodule in the thyroid gland. Thyroid cancer is diagnosed by fine-needle aspiration and biopsy.

Medical treatment may consist of chemotherapy, ^{131}I radiotherapy, or external radiation for metastasis. Surgical treatment usually includes removal of all or part of the thyroid. If the client has a total thyroidectomy, replacement of thyroid hormone is necessary. The client should be checked at regular intervals for recurrence and also should have thyroid function monitored.

Parathyroid Adenoma

Hyperparathyroidism is estimated to occur in 1 per 1000 men and 2 per 1000 women older than age 60; however, this disease is often overlooked in older adults (Black and Matassarin-Jacobs, 1993). Hyperparathyroidism is classified as primary, secondary, or tertiary. Primary hyperparathyroidism is a metabolic disorder in which there is hypersecretion of parathyroid hormone (PTH) from one or more adenomatous or hyperplastic parathyroid glands. Excessive amounts of PTH lead to bone damage, hypercalcemia, and kidney damage. Normally, PTH functions to increase bone resorption of calcium, thereby maintaining the proper calcium:phosphorus ratio in the blood. The finding of elevated serum PTH levels in the presence of elevated serum calcium levels confirms the diagnosis (Attie, 1997). Hence, screening of serum calcium level is important in at-risk individuals. Primary hyperparathyroidism is a disease that may be asymptomatic. However, on careful questioning, one or more mild symptoms may be revealed (e.g., weakness, fatigue, headache, depression, bone pain, polydipsia, polyuria, pruritus, anorexia, nausea, vomiting, or constipation (Attie, 1997). Or it may present with a myriad of symptoms arising from bone diseases and/or kidney impairment or gastrointestinal and neurological abnormalities. Medical management may include lowering elevated calcium levels by hydration and calciuresis.

Wellness

"Immunization reduces the incidence of, and mortality rate associated with, influenza and pneumonia."

Calciuresis is achieved by using diuretics to increase urinary calcium excretion. Another medical therapy may involve the use of drugs such as mithramycin (Mithracin), gallium nitrate (Ganite), phosphate, or calcitonin to increase bone reabsorption of calcium and lower serum calcium level. Dietary restriction may also be prescribed, including diets low in calcium and vitamin D.

Surgery is the treatment of choice for hyperparathyroidism and involves removing the gland(s) causing the hypersecretion of the PTH (Attie, 1997).

Summary

There is no general effect of aging on endocrine function. Typically, function is adequate unless the organ is stressed. It is important to emphasize healthy lifestyle modifications, especially a prudent diet and regular physical activity, in maintaining an adequately functioning endocrine system.

When assessing older adults, the nurse should remember that they are prone to certain endocrine diseases (e.g., type 2 diabetes and hypothyroidism). The presentation of endocrine disorders is often subtle. Symptoms are frequently attributed to the aging process by the patient and family members. When abnormal endocrine states are diagnosed, education is key to preventing complications and misunderstanding regarding any treatment that may be initiated. This will especially hold true for older adults with conditions that dictate lifelong therapy. Continual reassessment of knowledge level, skills, and physical limitation will be necessary to avoid serious complications that can result from the patient's inability to effectively carry out the treatment plan.

RESOURCES

American Association of Diabetes Educators
444 N. Michigan Avenue
Suite 12340
Chicago, IL 60611
(312) 644-2233 or (800) 338-3633

American Diabetes Association
1660 Duke Street
P.O. Box 25757
Alexandria, VA 22314
(800) 232-3472

American Dietetic Association
430 North Michigan Avenue
Chicago, IL 60611
(312) 822-0330

American Heart Association
7320 Greenville Avenue
Dallas, TX 75231
(800) 242-1793

National Diabetes Information Clearinghouse
Box NDIC
Bethesda, MD 20892
(301) 468-2162

REFERENCES

American Diabetes Association. (1994). Medical Management of Non-Insulin-Dependent (Type II) Diabetes. 3rd ed. Alexandria, VA: American Diabetes Association.

Attie JN. (1997). Primary hyperparathyroidism. In Bardin WC, ed. Current Therapy in Endocrinology and Metabolism. 6th ed. St. Louis: Mosby–Year Book.

Barzel US. (1997). Thyroid disease after the sixth decade. In Bardin WC, ed. Current Therapy in Endocrinology and Metabolism. 6th ed. St. Louis: Mosby–Year Book.

Black JM, Matassarin-Jacobs E. (1993). Nursing care of clients with thyroid and parathyroid disorders. In Black JM, Matassarin-Jacobs E, eds. Luckmann and Sorensen's Medical-Surgical Nursing. 4th ed. Philadelphia: WB Saunders.

Briscoe VJ. (1998). Management of the client with type 2 diabetes mellitus. Contin Ed Med Ed Resource, Course #12 pp 1–22.

Byrd JH. (1994). Managing and monitoring diabetes in the elderly patient. Drug Topics 138(11):124.

Diabetes Control and Complications Trial Research Group. (1993). The effect of intensive treatment of diabetes on the development and progression of long-term complications in insulin-dependent diabetes mellitus. N Engl J Med 329:977–985.

Felicetta JV. (1996). The aging thyroid: Its effects—and how it affects diagnosis and therapy. Consultant 36(4):837.

Fishman P. (1996). Healthy people 2000: What progress toward better nutrition? Geriatrics 51(4):38.

Genuth SM. (1997). Diabetic ketoacidosis and hyperglycemic hyperosmolar coma. In Bardin WC, ed. Current Therapy in Endocrinology and Metabolism. 6th ed. St. Louis: Mosby–Year Book.

Graham, C. (1994). Exercise and aging: Implications for persons with diabetes. Diabetes Ed 17(3):189–195.

Hershman JM, Gordon HE. (1997). Differentiated thyroid carcinoma. In Bardin WC, ed. Current Therapy in Endocrinology and Metabolism. 6th ed. St. Louis: Mosby–Year Book.

Kowal J, Hornick TR. (1997). General principles of endocrine function after the sixth decade. In Bardin WC, ed. Current Therapy in Endocrinology and Metabolism. 6th ed. St. Louis: Mosby–Year Book.

Le CM, Tuck ML. (1994). How it differs in the elderly: Diabetes mellitus. Consultant 34(7):1008.

Meneilly GS, Cheung E, Tuokko H. (1994). Counterregulatory hormone responses to hypoglycemia in the elderly with diabetes. Diabetes 43(3):403–408.

Miller M. (1996). Type II diabetes: A treatment approach for the older patient. Geriatrics 51(8):43–50.

Patterson C, Chambers L. (1995). Preventive health care. Lancet 345:1611–1615.

Reed RL, Mooradian AD. (1992). Diabetes. In Ham RJ, Sloane PD, eds. Primary Care Geriatrics: A Case-Based Approach. 2nd ed. St. Louis: Mosby–Year Book.

Report of the Expert Committee on the Diagnosis and Classification of Diabetes Mellitus, 1997. Diabetes Care 20:1183–1197.

Williams G. (1994). Management of non-insulin-dependent diabetes mellitus. Lancet 343:95–100.

CRITICAL THINKING EXERCISES

Mrs. Brown, an African American, age 68, lives alone. She enjoys a very active social life revolving around religious and civic volunteer activities. She says these activities help give meaning and purpose to her life. They keep her mind active and allow her to maintain contact with former co-workers at the college where she worked before she retired. Many of these activities require some walking. Mrs. Brown comes to her physician's office for a routine follow-up visit for mild hypertension. On this visit she is diagnosed with type 2 diabetes. Because a fasting plasma glucose level is 210 mg/dL on one occasion and 250 mg/dL on another, the physician prescribes the following treatment regimen: 1200 calorie ADA diet; 30 minutes of moderate activity daily; daily whole blood glucose monitoring (before breakfast); and metformin, 500 mg bid. She is being seen by a home health nurse to continue her diabetes education and assist with home blood glucose monitoring. Two weeks later, Mrs. Brown has an acute episode of bronchitis. The physician orders prednisone, 60 mg/d, in addition to a bronchodilator. During the next home visit, the nurse notes that Mrs. Brown appears lethargic and has problems concentrating. The nurse attributes these symptoms to advancing age. Two days later, a family member visits Mrs. Brown. She is complaining of going to the bathroom more frequently, increasing thirst, weakness, and tiredness. The family member takes Mrs. Brown to a nearby ambulatory clinic.

Mrs. Brown is 5'5" tall and weighs 200 pounds. She appears very dehydrated, tachycardic, and confused. The family member reports that Mrs. Brown stopped taking her diabetes medication several days earlier because it was making her nauseated and unable to eat.

On admission, her laboratory values are
Plasma glucose: 1000 mg/dL
Serum osmolality: 360 mOsm/dL
Potassium: 5.2 mEq/L
Serum acetone: negative
Glycosylated hemoglobin: 13.5%
Urinalysis: 2% glucose, negative ketones

She is admitted to the hospital.

1. What is the etiology of type 2 diabetes? What are the risk factors for acquiring this type of diabetes?
2. What acute complication of diabetes is Mrs. Brown experiencing? What most likely precipitated this acute problem?

Mrs. Brown survives her initial hospitalization after being treated with intravenously administered fluids (for dehydration), insulin (for the hyperglycemia), and potassium (for her electrolyte imbalance). She is discharged on 25 units of intermediate insulin, SQ each morning; with a target blood glucose range of 100 to 150 mg/dL. Her home monitoring records reveal blood glucose levels that vary between 180 and 250 mg/dL. She is subsequently switched to a twice-daily dose of sliding scale Regular Insulin. The home health nurse who continues to assist Mrs. Brown with her blood glucose monitoring and insulin regimen notes that Mrs. Brown is now experiencing frequent episodes of hypoglycemia.

3. What is hypoglycemia? What are the symptoms? What is the treatment?
4. Why is it important for Mrs. Brown to perform whole blood glucose monitoring and keep records of the values?
5. There are many chronic complications of diabetes. Name the type that causes blindness?
6. Why is it important for the person with diabetes to have regular evaluation of kidney function?

CHAPTER 20

Maintaining Wellness of the
Immune System

Carol Sue Holtz, RN, PhD

CHAPTER OUTLINE

Health Teaching
Age-Related Changes
Guidelines Specific to Assessing the Immune System
    in Older Adults
Common Disorders
Infections
  Pneumonia
  Tuberculosis
  Acquired Immunodeficiency Syndrome (AIDS)

Urinary Tract Infection
Skin Infections
  Management
Occupational Health Risks
Infection Control
Summary
Resources
References
Critical Thinking Exercises

OBJECTIVES

After completing this chapter, the reader should be able to:

1. Teach a classmate the physiological changes in the immune system that are due to normal aging.
2. Differentiate between the immune response and autoimmune response and the physiological changes in them that affect older adults.
3. Compare and contrast the susceptibility to infection and the ability to combat infection between middle-aged and older adults.
4. Formulate a care plan for a 78-year-old man who is hospitalized with pneumonia.
5. Teach a client with tuberculosis why TB is a challenging issue for the older adult.
6. Specify the reasons that AIDS in older adults is a growing health issue.

KEY TERMS

acquired immunity
antibody
antigen
autoantibody
autoimmune reaction
B cell
immune response
immunity
innate immunity
leukocytes
phagocytosis
T cell

The immune system protects the body by seeking out and destroying foreign agents such as viruses, bacteria, fungi, and sometimes the person's own cells (if the individual is going through neoplastic changes). The cells and molecules of the immune system are distributed throughout the body, circulating within the blood and lymph. Major lymphoid organs include the thymus, spleen, lymph nodes, and bone marrow. Other structures that contain lymphatic tissues include the tonsils, skin, and linings of the respiratory system and gastrointestinal tract. Immune system cells include macrophages, Langerhans cells of the skin, and lymphocytes. Immune responses depend on the number of different cells and tissues and their interactions (Bennett and Plum, 1996; Digiovanna, 1994; Rhoades and Tanner, 1995; Wingate and Wright, 1995).

An **antigen** (immunogen) is any substance that can cause an immune response. An antigen must be recognized as foreign, or non-self. When an antigen such as a bacterium enters the body, the antigen may cause the formation of lymphocytes. Some of these lymphocytes stimulate the production of antibodies and others neutralize and destroy the bacterial cells or their toxins. In addition, the antigen may stimulate the lymphocytes to produce cell-mediated reactions, such as delayed hypersensitivity or destruction of foreign tissue grafts and tumors. An **antibody** (immunoglobulin) is a protein molecule produced by the immune system plasma cells that adheres to an antigen and assists in combating antigens. The binding of the antigen to the antibody benefits the

body by detoxifying toxins, inactivating viruses, or causing direct lysis of cells. A nonspecific defense mechanism, such as **phagocytosis** (which is the intake of extracellular material, including cellular debris, foreign material, and bacteria), is often initiated (Bennett and Plum, 1996; Digiovanna, 1994; Moffett et al., 1993; Rhoades and Tanner, 1995; Wingate and Wright, 1995).

Major antibodies (immunoglobulins) are mainly classified as IgG, IgM, or IgA. IgG makes up 75% to 80% of the immunoglobulins and is mainly responsible for the following functions: (1) providing the newborn with a temporary natural passive immunity, (2) toxin neutralization, (3) viral and bacterial inactivation, and (4) certain types of hypersensitivity. IgM constitutes 7% of the immunoglobulins in the blood and acts as a protector against (1) viral and bacterial invasions of the blood, (2) certain types of hypersensitivities, and (3) autoimmune diseases such as rheumatoid arthritis. IgA constitutes 10% of the immunoglobulins. It is found in body secretions and protects the mucosal surfaces of the respiratory, digestive, and genital tracts (Bennett and Plum, 1996; Rhoades and Tanner, 1995; Wingate and Wright, 1995).

The primary cells of the immune system are derived from the stem cells of the bone marrow. These cells of the immune system are types of lymphocytes. The **T cell** is a type of lymphocytic cell that undergoes differentiation under the influence of the thymus gland. T cells are responsible for assisting with cell-mediated immunity. A **B cell** is a type of lymphocyte that matures independent of the thymus. These cells are responsible for the production of immunoglobulins and the humoral immune response (Bennett and Plum, 1996; Rhoades and Tanner, 1995; Wingate and Wright, 1995).

The immune system has two major divisions: the humorally mediated system and the cell-mediated system. The humorally mediated system provides **immunity** against (1) bacteria that produce acute infections; (2) bacterial exotoxins, such as diphtheria, botulinus, and tetanus toxins; (3) viruses; and (4) organisms entering from the mucosal tissue. The cell-mediated system provides immunity from (1) chronic bacterial infections (tuberculosis or syphilis); (2) viral infections (measles, herpesvirus, chickenpox); (3) fungal infections;

(4) parasitic infections; and (5) transplanted or transformed cells (tissue transplants). One or both systems may be dysfunctional, causing vulnerability to infection (Bennett and Plum, 1996; Rhoades and Tanner, 1995; Wingate and Wright, 1995).

The immune system is unique because it is capable of self-recognition, which means that it can distinguish between those substances that are a normal part of the body and those that are foreign to it. Recognition of the self is also known as self-tolerance. If this system identifies a foreign substance, it can elicit an **immune response** against it. Any foreign substance that causes an immune response is an antigen. The immune response operates against only one specific antigen, so a different immune response must occur with each different foreign substance (antigen). Once the immune system has responded to an antigen, later encounters with that antigen will produce a stronger and faster response (Wingate and Wright, 1995). In addition, the phagocytic cells act nonspecifically to kill foreign cells and cancer cells. Memory cells, which are a residual set of lymphocytes and long-lasting antibodies, are developed each time a person is exposed to a particular antigen (Bennett and Plum, 1996; Digiovanna, 1994; Rhoades and Tanner, 1995). An autoimmune reaction causes the immune system to produce antibodies against normal parts of the body to the extent of causing tissue injury.

HEALTH TEACHING

Nurses are in excellent positions to influence other people's behavior positively through example as well as through teaching. We can motivate clients to maintain health by avoiding actions that are harmful and forming habits that are beneficial. Each client has a unique personality, set of cultural values, and array of environmental influences that must be identified before teaching strategies are developed. Teaching is an integral part of nursing care of the older adult with an immunological disorder. Within the lymphatic system there is a decrease with age in number and size of nodes, which causes a decreased ability of the body to resist infection. Nurses can teach older clients how to maintain optimal health and prevent

certain illnesses. Health teaching for the immune system is incorporated into the chapters that deal with other body systems specifically (see Chapters 14 through 19, 21, and 22).

AGE-RELATED CHANGES

The involution of the thymus and decreased T-cell activity cause a decline in the function of the immune system. This decline results in increased rates of infections, autoimmunity, and sometimes cancer. Many elderly persons have chronic conditions such as nutritional deficiencies that decrease host defenses. *Acquired immunity* is immunity resulting from development of active or passive immunity as opposed to natural or innate immunity. *Innate immunity* is natural immunity.

Changes in the immune system cause infections to be more severe and individuals to have a slower recovery time and less chance of developing immunity after the infection. There is also an increase in tumors and autoimmune disorders because of the decreased ability to recognize foreign material (Fletcher, 1995). Decreases occur in

- Immune system function
- Chemical barriers within many organs
- Mechanical functioning of body organs with ciliary action, as well as gastric emptying
- Skin thickness, vascular flow, and collagen
- Mucosal barriers

Nutritional problems and chronic illnesses also can cause older adults to be more vulnerable to infection (Fletcher, 1995).

After mid life, the thymus and T-cell activity declines. Normal antibody levels also decline with age, starting shortly after the involution of the thymus. Changes in the immune system are found among older people as a result of thymic involution, with a progressive decline in serum thymic hormonal activity. The thymus gland plays a role in the production of mature peripheral lymphoid cells. As the thymus gets smaller, there is an increase in immature T lymphocytes in the thymus and in the peripheral blood. The aging process significantly impairs specific antibody responses to foreign antigens. Normal immune response requires a proliferation of lymphocytes. Thus, with age, specific antibody responses to foreign antigens are greatly impaired (Bennett and Plum, 1996;

Rhoades and Tanner, 1995; Saxon and Etten, 1994; Stanley and Beare, 1995).

Autoimmune disorders may increase in older adults, concomitant with the decrease in immunological function. The body becomes less able to recognize or tolerate "self" antigens, causing antibodies to act against self tissues. Older adults have increased levels of autoantibodies, lymphocytes, and plasma cells. Older individuals frequently lose some of the immune tolerance to their own tissues. This loss occurs after the destruction of the body tissues, which releases large quantities of antigens that circulate in the body. Some of these antigens combine with bacteria or viruses to form a new type of antigen that can then cause immune reactions. The result is that activated T cells and antibodies attack the body's own tissues (Bennett and Plum, 1996; Rhoades and Tanner, 1995; Saxon and Etten, 1994).

Aging also affects the T cells that regulate antibody response. T cells are responsible for protecting the body against viruses, fungi, and some types of bacteria. T cells also prevent the growth of some neoplasms and regulate the antibody production to a large number of antigens. This decreased immune response can lead to a variety of problems related to infections. Older people, when stressed with an infection, may not be able to maintain homeostasis by increasing cellular production to compensate for cellular destruction. Also, responses to influenza, pneumonia, and tetanus vaccines are less effective. Inflammatory defenses decrease, and inflammation may be atypically present in older adults with low-grade fever and minimal pain (Saxon and Etten, 1994).

Wellness

66Activities that protect the immune system include stress reduction, getting adequate rest, avoiding hot baths and showers, staying indoors in unusually hot or cold weather, and avoiding crowds and people with known infections.99

The later the age at which an antigen is first encountered, the greater the amount of injury caused by a second encounter with the antigen.

The primary immune responses diminish with aging, resulting in fewer memory cells and therefore less residual antibody for subsequent exposures. As the immune memory declines, the initial secondary immune response against an antigen also declines in speed and strength. The antigen also may cause more frequent injury because additional secondary responses may be needed before acquired active immunity develops. In spite of the decline, there may be only slight alterations in the total amount of antibody formed after antigenic stimulation. Because memory decreases with age, vaccines are best received before age 60, but they can be beneficial at any age (Digiovanna, 1994; Saxon and Etten, 1994).

The thymus shrinks until age 50, becoming 5% of its original size; and thymic hormone production reaches zero by age 60. This ends the development of the immune response capabilities against additional antigens. Other immunoglobulins, such as **autoantibodies,** are thought to be produced by older adults along with the decrease in specific antibody production (Digiovanna, 1994; Saxon and Etten, 1994). See Box 20–1 for physiological changes that affect the immune response in older adults.

Infection can become widespread among older adults and have potentially devastating consequences (Stanley and Beare, 1995; Saxon and Etten, 1994). Ciliary action and coughing, both primary defenses against respiratory infection, are decreased with advancing age. In addition, IgA, a secretory immunoglobulin found in the respiratory tree that helps neutralize viruses, is reduced. Macrophages in the alveolar area of the lungs also have decreased function. These changes can lead to increased rates of pneumonia, tuberculosis, and other respiratory diseases in older adults. The integumentary system is affected by the aging process, and skin diseases are more prominent in older adults. The skin is drier, has less elasticity, and has a decreased vascular supply. When the skin is broken, the body's first line of defense is gone, making the older person more prone to skin diseases. In addition, the number of epidermal cells that can recognize foreign antigens is reduced by 50% between early and late adulthood, which may also be a factor in decreased immune functioning in older adults (Janeway and Travers, 1994; Saxon and Etten, 1994; Stanley and Beare, 1995).

Risks increase with the age at which the antigens or carcinogens are first encountered.

Box 20-1   PHYSIOLOGICAL CHANGES THAT AFFECT THE IMMUNE RESPONSE IN OLDER ADULTS

Skin—decreases in thickness and elasticity, tensile strength, and neurosensory function cause the skin to be more vulnerable to trauma, invasion of organisms, and decreased awareness of injury.

Respiratory system—decreases in ciliary action, reduced respiratory muscle strength, and impaired gag or cough reflexes cause decreased removal of inhaled organisms.

Cardiovascular system—decreases in cardiac output and increases in peripheral resistance cause decreased circulation to tissues, possible delayed inflammatory response, and increased risk of ischemic injury.

Gastrointestinal system—decreases in ciliary action, gastric emptying, secretion of hydrochloric acid and some digestive enzymes cause decreased organism removal, decreased digestion, and decreased production of serum proteins.

Genitourinary system—decreases in glomerular filtration rate, relaxed muscles, decreased mucosal barrier, and decreased estrogen cause increased urinary tract and vaginal infections.

Lymphatic system—decreases in number and size of lymph nodes cause decreased ability to resist infection.

Adapted from Fletcher K. (1995). Assessment of the immune system. In Phipps WJ, Cassmeyer VL, Sands JK, Lehman MK, eds. Medical-Surgical Nursing. St. Louis: CV Mosby.

There is an increased incidence of infection from the bacteria causing tuberculosis and the virus causing herpesvirus varicella (chickenpox). The immune memory against these diseases decreases, and the weakened immune system allows a reactivation of the infectious agents causing tuberculosis. The chickenpox virus can be transported down sensory neurons to skin areas, causing herpes zoster (shingles). Shingles is characterized by localized skin eruptions and pain, and the incidence increases with age. It is also dependent on a previous chickenpox infection. In older adults, antibodies decrease with time and the virus can reactivate. This virus is harbored within the spinal nerve fibers and is reactivated when the older adult's immunological system function has decreased (Janeway and Travers, 1994; Saxon and Etten, 1994; Stanley and Beare, 1995).

Many autoimmune diseases resulting from childhood or young adulthood continue to cause progressive damage. Some autoimmune diseases affecting older adults include atrophic gastritis, rheumatoid arthritis, rheumatic heart disease, multiple sclerosis, and myasthenia gravis (Digiovanna, 1994). The immune system protects the older adult from diseases such as cancer, atherosclerosis, and (possibly) Alzheimer's disease. The damaging agent in Alzheimer's disease may be potentiated by a subsequent autoimmune attack on the brain cells by the immune system. It is also possible that diabetes mellitus, biliary cirrhosis, and multiple sclerosis may be caused by an autoimmune response (Janeway and Travers, 1994; Saxon and Etten, 1994; Stanley and Beare, 1995).

The difference in the immunity between the young and older adults is not in the total number of T cells but in the percentage of T cells that can be activated and reproduce in sufficient quantities to give protection against disease. In older adults, T lymphocytes do not function well because they cannot reproduce as they did when the person was younger. Older adults have 50% to 80% functional T lymphocytes, as compared with young people. At present, research using growth factors such as interleukin-2 is designed to stimulate older adults' T cells to reproduce. In addition, research is being conducted to see whether it would be possible to convert some of the nonresponsive lymphocytes to responsive lymphocytes by replacing some of the activities of the thymus gland. Older adults who are given thymic proteins are reported to have an improved response to influenza (Janeway and Travers, 1994; Saxon and Etten, 1994; Stanley and Beare, 1995).

The Langerhans cells of the epidermis play a role in activating an immune response in the skin. Older adults have a 50% decrease in these cells, and the number could be further reduced by sun damage in the skin. The decreased numbers of Langerhans cells in the skin may partly explain the decreased immune responsiveness of older skin and its increased potential for sensitization to allergic substances and may also be implicated in the increased production of skin tumors (Janeway and Travers, 1994; Morton, 1993b; Saxon and Etten, 1994).

GUIDELINES SPECIFIC TO ASSESSING THE IMMUNE SYSTEM IN OLDER ADULTS

Assessment of the immune system in older adults should begin with a thorough history of the client, focusing on the chief complaint, present and past history of allergies, family history of allergies, present medications, and a psychosocial history including environmental stressors. The nurse needs to report the symptoms and assist in identifying the allergens. Allergens include the following (Bennett and Plum, 1996; Black and Matassarin-Jacobs, 1993; Morton, 1993a; Phipps et al., 1995):

- Inhalants (pollens, molds, dust, spores)
- Contact agents (dyes in clothing, metals in jewelry, plant oils, topical drugs)
- Ingested agents (foods, food additives, and drugs)
- Injectable agents (drugs, vaccines, insect venom)

The client must be asked about past episodes of drug and food allergies and reactions, whether they are seasonal, and how they were treated.

The client can minimize disease exacerbations by identifying and avoiding conditions that trigger them. Typical triggers include stress, fatigue, temperature extremes, infection, and trauma. Activities should include stress reduction, getting adequate rest, avoiding hot baths and showers, staying indoors in unusually hot or cold weather, and avoiding crowds and people with known infections. Clients should be taught to seek treatment for all fevers and infections. The physical assessment of the immune system in older adults consists of an overall evaluation of the client's general health and appearance while looking for evidence of acute or chronic illness.

The older adult client with a disorder of the immune system may have signs and symptoms that are nonspecific. Signs of acute illness include grimacing and profuse perspiration. Chronic illness may be evidenced by emaciation, listlessness, and nonagreement of age and appearance (chronic diseases and nutritional deficiencies make clients look older than their chronological ages). The nurse should ask the client about general fatigue, chills, fever, sweating, pruritus, malaise, and reactions to foods, medications, or drugs.

C a r i n g

"*Nurses can teach older clients how to maintain optimal health and prevent certain illnesses.***"**

The immune system is interconnected to many other body systems, some of which must also be assessed to complete the evaluation. A particular area of concern is the lymphatic system. The lymph nodes should not be visible or palpable in the normal healthy client. Generally, the number and size of the nodules decrease with age. Box 20–2 presents the regions of the head and neck that should be inspected. Abnormal findings of lymph nodes include the following (Morton, 1993a; Saxon and Etten, 1994):

- *Enlargement.* This can be due to increased lymphocytes and reticuloendothelial cells. The clinical significance increases with age; therefore, it is an important and serious finding in older adults.
- *Red streaks on skin with palpable nodes.* This indicates a lymphatic disorder.
- *Tenderness.* This indicates an infection.
- *Generalized lymph adenopathy* (three or more in a group). This indicates an autoimmune disease such as lupus, an infection, or a neoplastic disorder.

Box 20-2   REGIONS OF THE HEAD AND NECK TO INSPECT FOR LYMPHATIC HEALTH

- Parotid
- Preauricular
- Postauricular (mastoid)
- Occipital
- Submandibular
- Submental
- Superficial anterior cervical
- Supraclavicular

Axillary and epitrochlear nodes include

- Subclavian
- Subscapular
- Epitrochlear

Inguinal and popliteal nodes include

- Superior superficial inguinal
- Inferior superficial inguinal
- Popliteal

- *Spleen.* Normally the spleen is unpalpable. It must be three times its normal size to be palpated. Tenderness and enlargement indicate infection or injury. The client should be asked about recent infections such as measles, mononucleosis, influenza, and viral infections; neoplasms; injuries; and date of last tetanus toxoid injection.

COMMON DISORDERS

Infections

Infections are a leading cause of morbidity and mortality in older individuals. The aged have altered defenses, a deteriorating immune system, chronic illnesses, and many environmental factors that cause a greater vulnerability to infections. Infections can present in atypical ways (e.g., no fever, "normal" white blood cell counts), which may cause delays in diagnosis and treatment. In addition, older adults have slower rates of antibiotic absorption, metabolism, and excretion, which necessitate more effort in selection of antibiotics and their correct dosages (Morton, 1993b; Saxon and Etten, 1994).

Pneumonia and influenza are the leading infections causing death in older adults and the fourth most common cause of death in the overall population; delays in diagnosing older adults contribute to their high death rate from these diseases. The usual symptoms of fever, chills, and sputum production found in a younger population are often absent in older adults. Chest radiographs are not specific and frequently show incomplete lung consolidation. Therefore, diagnosis is more difficult to make in the older adult. The many immunological defenses of the lungs include the alveolar lining fluid, alveolar macrophages, T lymphocytes, and polymorphonuclear neutrophils (Janeway and Travers, 1994; Noble, 1996).

Older adults have many physiological changes in their bodies that increase the risk for infection. Changes in the immune system cause infections to be more severe and require a slower recovery time. These changes may cause older adults to have a decreased chance of developing immunity after the infection. There are also increases in tumors and autoimmune diseases because of the older body's decreased ability to recognize foreign material (Fletcher, 1995).

T cells that respond to new antigens decline as thymic involution occurs and as the production of thymic hormones diminishes. Most T cells in an older person have already had antigenic exposure. This explains why older adults respond to antigens that they have encountered previously but not to new antigens. However, the response is slow in an older adult, increasing the risk of reactivation infection with pathogens such as *Mycobacterium tuberculosis* and varicella-zoster virus.

Wellness

"We can motivate clients to maintain health by avoiding actions that are harmful and forming habits that are beneficial."

Health care environments (e.g., hospitals, long-term care facilities) provide special risks for nosocomial infection. Factors such as group activities, common washing and dining facilities, and crowding provide many opportunities for direct contact between clients and health care personnel. In addition, patients are frequently transferred to and from hospitals, providing greater opportunities for exchange of pathogens. Extensive and inappropriate use of antibiotics further contributes to the increasingly drug-resistant pathogens sometimes found in nursing homes (Saxon and Etten, 1994).

Pneumonia, urinary tract infections, skin infections, and soft tissue infections are the most common infections in older adults. Because many of these infections respond to antimicrobial therapy, life spans may be increased by treating infections. Defects in the immune system and malnutrition are major factors that affect the aged person's ability to fight infection. Older people often eat poorly because of their living circumstances, and they may also have difficulties absorbing some nutrients (e.g., folate). Nutrient supplements can modify the delayed immune mechanism and help to minimize some infections in older adults. Vitamin supplements, particularly the antioxidants E, C, and beta-carotene, may be useful in helping the immune system fight infections (Butler et al., 1994; Saxon and Etten, 1994).

The older adult is predisposed to various infections because of an aging immune system; yet there are risk factors that can be reduced.

Patients can be taught to take meticulous care of their skin to reduce the risk of soft tissue infection. Good oral hygiene can be helpful. Correction of urinary tract obstructions and relying on indwelling urinary catheters only when necessary can help reduce the risks of urinary tract infections. Medications that may cause impairment of cognitive function should be monitored carefully because they could cause an individual to aspirate, leading to pneumonia. In addition, correction of malnutrition may improve cell immunity and skin integrity, leading to a reduced risk of infection. Inflammatory periodontal diseases in older adults are increased by dental plaque and a decreased functioning of the immune system (Saxon and Etten, 1994).

Pneumonia

Pneumonia is a common infection in older adults and one of the leading causes of death. Many older adults have chronic obstructive pulmonary disease, nutritional deficiencies, or changes in mental status, which are some predisposing factors. Many bacterial pneumonias seen in the community are caused by *Streptococcus pneumoniae*, *Haemophilus influenzae*, and *Mycoplasma pneumoniae*. Nosocomial pneumonias are often caused by *Staphylococcus aureus*, *Klebsiella pneumoniae*, *Pseudomonas aeruginosa*, and *Escherichia coli*. Aspiration pneumonia is also common in older adults because of colonization of gram-negative bacteria in the posterior pharynges, chronic disease, debility, abnormal swallowing reflexes, or a history of strokes.

Pneumonia in older adults often has atypical signs and symptoms as compared with younger adults. Fever is frequently delayed because of decreases in the immune response and decreases in the inflammatory response. Crackles, wheezing, and pleuritic chest pain may be absent in older adults who have pneumonia. Instead, the older adult with pneumonia may appear with anorexia, changed mental status, changed activity patterns, confusion, and weight loss (Fraser, 1993). A respiratory rate of greater than 26 breaths per minute is often a reliable indicator of a lower respiratory tract infection. In the presence of emphysema, the signs of pneumonia may be quite subtle. Pulmonary consolidation may be absent and rales and pleural effusions could be easily con-

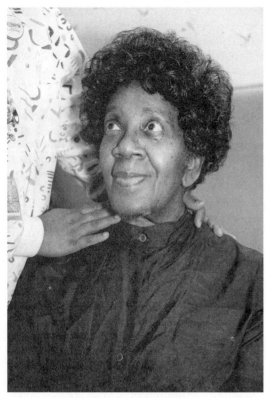

A compromised immune system is sometimes signaled by swollen lymph nodes.

fused with congestive heart failure (Brown, 1993).

In older people with community-acquired pneumonia, the white blood cell count is usually slightly increased, and about 25% of all blood cultures will be positive, depending on the pathogen. Gram stain of the sputum is very important for diagnosis and should be obtained in all patients suspected of having community-acquired pneumonia. Chest radiographs are also necessary to document the extent of the pneumonia and to provide a baseline to gauge therapeutic response (Brown, 1993; Saxon and Etten, 1994).

Some older adults may be aspirating chronically and may not have a swallow reflex. These pneumonias could be caused by *Legionella* or *Chlamydia.* In the hospital, aspiration pneumonia may occur in patients who are in postoperative or critical care units and in patients who are constantly in a supine position; simply ele-

vating the head of the bed can reduce the incidence of aspiration pneumonia significantly.

A low blood pH of some critically ill older adults may contribute to nosocomial pneumonia by not suppressing microorganisms. Older adults with no fever may have nonspecific signs and symptoms such as falling, confusion, and failure to thrive. Others may have a cough and low-grade fever (Butler et al., 1994).

TREATMENT

Community-Acquired Pneumonia. This is caused by *Haemophilus influenzae, Staphylococcus aureus,* or bacteria such as *Chlamydia, Legionella,* and *Mycoplasma;* it could be caused by aspiration. It is treated by broad-spectrum antimicrobial agents.

Hospital-Acquired Pneumonia. This arises from anaerobes and gram-negative organisms. It is treated by aminoglycosides, plus aminopenicillin or cephalosporin, plus additional agents such as vancomycin if *Staphylococcus* is suspected; the head of the bed is elevated to prevent aspiration pneumonia, and hygiene of endotracheal tubes is monitored.

Long-Term Care Facility–Acquired Pneumonia. This is caused by colonization with gram-negative organisms. It is treated by aminoglycosides plus aminopenicillin or by clindamycin if aspiration is suspected. The nurse should monitor the patient for aspiration pneumonia, inadequate oral hygiene, and/or impaired sensory perception (Butler et al., 1994).

Immunization. Only 14% of adults older than 65 years of age have been immunized against pneumococcus, and only 30% have received influenza vaccinations. The pneumococcal vaccinations have been estimated to produce immunity in about 60% of all people, although protection rates are only about 46% in people age 85 and older. These vaccinations do not always establish immunity but can be very helpful (Butler et al., 1994). Pneumococcal vaccine is usually given once and is safe and inexpensive. For very old patients, a repeat vaccine in 7 years is recommended. The viral influenza vaccine must be given annually, typically in late autumn. It is safe and approximately 75% effective in older adults (Brown, 1993; Saxon and Etten, 1994).

Tuberculosis

Tuberculosis (TB) in older adults has increased in incidence since the mid-1980s. It crosses all levels of society but is not proportionally distributed by region or ethnicity. Within the United States, the highest incidences of TB are among the following groups (Lancaster, 1993):

- Hispanics, African Americans, Asians and Pacific Islanders, Native Americans, and Alaskans
- Residents of correctional institutions, mental institutions, nursing homes, and other long-term care facilities
- Alcohol and drug users
- People who have immunosuppression (from chemotherapy or acquired immunodeficiency syndrome)
- Foreign-born people who come from an area with a high prevalence of TB

The risk of TB in older adults living in the community is twice that of the general population (Hopkins and Schoener, 1996).

People who are merely infected with TB will have a positive tuberculin skin test, a normal chest radiograph, and *negative* sputum smears or cultures for TB, and they are not infectious to others.

People who have active pulmonary TB will have a positive TB skin test, a positive sputum or bronchoscopy for acid-fast bacillus smear, symptoms of a cough, sputum production, and occasional hemoptysis or chest pain. They may also have fever, night sweats, and weight loss, and they are infectious to others (Lancaster, 1993). Among older adults, the majority of clients have a recurrence of previous TB infections because of the decrease in immune function, many chronic diseases, or poor nutritional status. The classic signs and symptoms (e.g., night sweats, chest pain, hemoptysis) are not often seen in older individuals; instead, more vague findings such as coughing, weight loss, and weakness are present (Fraser, 1993).

Hopkins and Schoener (1996) recommend various activities for the prevention and control of TB in long-term care facilities providing care for older adults. They include

- *Surveillance,* which is the routine screening for TB for all residents and employees using the Mantoux test (intradermal test)
- *Case finding*
- *Containment or isolation* of all people until they have become noninfectious
- *Treatment,* including drugs such as isoniazid, rifampin, pyrazinamide, ethambutol, or streptomycin
- *Preventive therapy,* including education about the signs and symptoms of TB

When the immune system is compromised, as in aging, there is a potential for dormant bacilli to become active. The reactivation is called secondary TB, which is found in 80% of older adults with TB (Hopkins and Schoener, 1996).

> ### C a r i n g
>
> **66**Nurses are in excellent positions to influence other people's behavior positively through example as well as through teaching.**99**

Acquired Immunodeficiency Syndrome (AIDS)

The diagnosis of AIDS in older adults is a major problem because it often presents in the form of other illnesses that can mislead the diagnostician. For example, AIDS may present as a form of dementia and is sometimes confused with Alzheimer's disease.

Perhaps an even greater problem is that AIDS is often completely undiagnosed in older adults. Many people continue to believe that AIDS is one disease unlikely to be found in older adults (Letvak and Schoder, 1996; Schuerman, 1994). Homosexual or bisexual behavior remains the predominant risk factor for human immunodeficiency virus (HIV) infection in individuals up to 70 years of age.

According to Wallace, Paaiw, and Spach (1993, p. 61):

The number of AIDS patients over 60 years of age has risen steadily in the past decade, with more than 1400 cases reported in 1991. In the coming decade, the proportion of AIDS patients who are 60 or older is expected to rise from 3 to approximately 10%. In the United States, it is estimated that there are 1 million homosexual men over 65 years of age. Given the long incubation period between HIV acquisition and AIDS (average, 8 to 10 years), even if the last sexual exposure was years ago, these patients may remain at high risk for developing AIDS well into their seventies.

Dementia, malnutrition, and pneumonia, commonly seen in many hospitalized elderly patients, are also characteristics of AIDS. Although older patients with AIDS are treated in the same manner as younger patients, older adults have unique problems. They may require more functional assistance sooner and may not have a family support system at home (Schuerman, 1994). Disease progression is more rapid in older adults, but the shorter survival time may be partly due to delays in diagnosis. Symptoms in older adults are often nonspecific: weight loss, fatigue, anorexia, and decreased physical and cognitive function (Fan, Conner, and Villareal, 1996; Letvak and Schoder, 1996; Wallace et al., 1993).

Spouses of those with HIV infection and those who participate in unprotected anal or vaginal intercourse outside a monogamous relationship are also at risk. Elderly women may be at a higher risk for acquiring HIV than elderly men, because the changes in the vaginal tissue that occur with aging allow a greater possibility for disruption of the vaginal mucosa. In addition, rare use of condoms by partners also places elderly women at greater risk (Fan, Conner, and Villareal, 1996; Letvak and Schoder, 1996; Schuerman, 1994).

A study at Grady Memorial Hospital between 1985 and 1992 of 32 elderly persons with HIV infection (27 men and 5 women) revealed that the majority of patients at this hospital acquired the HIV virus from sexual intercourse or intravenous drug use. Gordon and Thompson (1995) state that the diagnosis of HIV infection in older adults is usually not considered until the disease has progressed to its later stages. They recommend that those who care for older adults who have a history of recent sexually transmitted diseases or high-risk behaviors should include a complete sexual history and offer sexual education, HIV testing, and counseling (Gordon and Thompson, 1995).

Urinary Tract Infection

Urinary tract infections are often found in older adults. At least 10% of men and 20% of women older than age 65 years have bacteriuria. *Escherichia coli* is the most frequent causative organism, but urinary tract infections can also be caused by staphylococci, enterococci, anaerobes, or yeast. Asymptomatic is more common than symptomatic bacteriuria. These infections can be caused by

- Incomplete emptying of the bladder
- Benign prostatic hypertrophy
- Presence of a Foley catheter
- Bladder obstructions
- Neurogenic bladder

Seventy thousand to 140,000 men and even more women in long-term health care settings have indwelling Foley catheters. Each person with an ongoing Foley catheter insertion averages about one urinary tract infection per year that requires hospitalization (Butler et al., 1994; Saxon and Etten, 1994).

Because frequency, urgency, and stress incontinence are associated with the normal aging process, a urinary tract infection with similar symptoms may be difficult to differentiate; yet in older adults a new episode of incontinence is a classic sign of a urinary tract infection. Fever may be delayed, but the older adult may also have confusion, disorientation, nausea and vomiting, and abdominal pain (Butler et al., 1994; Fraser, 1993; Saxon and Etten, 1994).

Skin Infections

Skin chronically exposed to sunlight exhibits a decrease in the production of Langerhans cells, which leads to a decrease in the processing and presentation of antigens in the skin, thus increasing the risks of skin infection and cancer. In addition, there is a delayed hypersensitivity reaction, which may cause decreased signs and symptoms such as swelling, itching, and rash that could warn of the presence of harmful substances (Fraser, 1993; Saxon and Etten, 1994).

Skin infections are a great problem for older adults. Changes in the skin arising from the normal aging process (e.g., thinning, decreases in vascular supply, drying) may cause the older person to be more susceptible to infections. These infections are mainly due to *Staphylococcus aureus, Staphylococcus epidermidis*, and *Streptococcus A* and *B*. In addition, fungal infections of the skin are found more frequently in older adults. Candidiasis occurs most often in areas of the body that may remain moist, such as under the breast, the perineum, and in the mouth. Herpes zoster also is more common in the older adult. It is a reactivation of a latent varicella virus, and the infection is an open weeping lesion. This reactivation occurs in older adults because of the loss of normal epidermal protective coverings, a decreased immune system function, high stress levels, and nutritional deficiencies. Nurses need to check all areas of the body for ulceration, especially bony prominences and areas with decreased peripheral circulation (Fraser, 1993; Saxon and Etten, 1994).

Caring

"Nurses should be well educated about nursing care of the client with an altered immune system and the nursing care needed for prevention and treatment of pathological conditions.**"**

Debridement of pressure ulcers that cover a large area (greater than 10 cm) may be enough to decrease the need for further surgical intervention and the incidence of sepsis. Pressure ulcers, especially in the sacral area (where fecal material may cause further contamination), may contain *Streptococcus* and *Staphylococcus* and are often treated with a broad-spectrum antibiotic. Prevention of skin infections is of utmost importance. The older adult with decreased mobility, obesity, incontinence, impaired consciousness, and decreased pain perception must be carefully monitored. Frequent turning, dry bedding, cushions, mattress pads, or special mattresses to decrease pressure points are needed for both prevention and treatment. In addition, patients should be monitored for dehydration or overhydration, which can lead to tearing of fragile skin (Butler et al., 1994; Saxon and Etten, 1994; Stanley and Beare, 1995).

MANAGEMENT

Assessment for skin infection in older adults includes monitoring the integrity, temperature, odor, and color of the skin. For respiratory tract infections, respiratory rate and rhythm, gag reflex, auscultations of lung sounds, and possible presence of a cough are essential to assess and analyze. For urinary tract infections, the urine color and appearance and the presence of a distended bladder are also important factors to evaluate. Laboratory data that may indicate an infection include leukocytosis and elevated numbers of polymorphonuclear **leukocytes.** Many older people may have normal or even low white blood cell counts. Bacterial counts on cultures may not show urinary tract infections, because bacteriuria is always present in clients having Foley catheters. Positive blood cultures may indicate upper respiratory tract infections. A decreased serum albumin level may indicate a poor diet, which can lead to greater infection risk. Arterial blood gases need to be monitored in assessing for pneumonia. Measures to prevent infections are essential in older adults. Adults older than 65 should have influenza immunizations if they are not allergic to eggs. Nutritional education to prevent infections is also important (Saxon and Etten, 1994; Stanley and Beare, 1995).

OCCUPATIONAL HEALTH RISKS

The Bloodborne Pathogen Standard of December 1991 states that all workers with the potential exposure to human blood and body fluids to which universal precautions apply are eligible to receive a free hepatitis B vaccine. This is given intramuscularly in the deltoid in three doses over a 6-month period, and more than 90% of healthy adults produce an adequate antibody response to it. About 50% of the vaccinated people lose antibody response within 7 years, yet they are still protected against infection (Spechko, 1993).

Wellness

"Older adults within a long-term care facility need an infection control program.**"**

Health care workers exposed to a bloodborne pathogen need a postexposure management program that includes a mechanism for assessment of the source of the patient's risk factors (Saxon and Etten, 1994; Spechko, 1993; Stanley and Beare, 1995), including

- Hepatitis B virus and HIV serological status of the patient
- Testing that is periodically and confidentially done (usually a baseline 6 weeks and 3, 6, and 12 months after exposure)
- Assessment for the need for zidovudine prophylaxis

> ## Wellness
>
> **"Basic infection control principles include good handwashing by staff, universal precautions, and barrier precautions such as enteric, respiratory, and contact isolation."**

INFECTION CONTROL

Older adults within a long-term care facility need an infection control program. Some basic elements of this program should include systematic data collection to identify nosocomial infections in residents; a system for the detection, investigation, and control of infections; an isolation system; infection control policies and procedures; in-service education for prevention and control; a resident health program; an employee health program; a system for antibiotic review and control; a process for disease reporting that is sent to the public health department to complete compliance with all federal, state, and local regulations; and an infection control person who is responsible for the directing of infection control activities (Prichard, 1993).

> ## Wellness
>
> **"Clients should be taught to seek treatment for all fevers and infections."**

Basic infection control principles include good handwashing by staff; universal precautions, designed to prevent the transmission of the HIV and bloodborne organisms; and barrier precautions such as enteric, respiratory, and contact isolation, which are still indicated in some conditions such as TB. Antibiotic use should be limited to those who have positive cultures, and treatment of asymptomatic bacteriuria should be avoided, especially when patients have an indwelling catheter (Saxon and Etten, 1994; Stanley and Beare, 1995).

Summary

Involution of the thymus and decreased T-cell activity cause a decline in the function of the immune system with age. This decline results in increased rates of infections, autoimmunity, and sometimes cancer. Infections in older adults are problematic because they are a leading cause of morbidity and mortality. Many unrecognized signs and symptoms cause a delay in diagnosing an infection, which often delays treatment. Many older adults also have chronic conditions, such as nutritional deficiencies, that decrease host defenses. Pneumonia, TB, urinary tract infections, and skin infections are commonly found in the older adult population, and AIDS in older adults has recently become a new health concern. Nurses must be well educated about nursing care of the client with an altered immune system and the nursing care needed for prevention and treatment of related pathological conditions.

RESOURCES

Growing Younger
Healthwise Inc.
P.O. Box 1989
Boise, ID 83702

National Clearinghouse on Aging
SCAN Social Gerontology Resource Center
P.O. Box 231
Silver Spring, MD 20907

Children of Aging Parents
2761 Trenton Rd.
Levittown, PA 19056

SAGE (Senior Actualization and Growth Exploration)
1713 Grove Street
Berkeley, CA 94709

Department of Health and Human Services (DHHS)
Publications Clearinghouse
P.O. Box 8547
Silver Spring, MD 20907
(800) 358-9295

National Institute on Aging
NIA Information Center
2209 Distribution Circle
Silver Spring, MD 20910
(301) 495-3455

Centers for Disease Control and Prevention (CDC)
1600 Clifton Road NE
Atlanta, GA 30333
(404) 639-3534 for public inquiries
PHS Aids Information Hotline (800) 342-AIDS; in Spanish (800) 344-SIDA

REFERENCES

Bennett J, Plum F. (1996). Cecil Textbook of Medicine. Philadelphia: WB Saunders.

Black J, Matassarin-Jacobs E. (1993). Luckmann and Sorenson's Medical-Surgical Nursing. Philadelphia: WB Saunders.

Brown R. (1993). Community-acquired pneumonia: Diagnosis and therapy of older adults. Geriatrics 48(2): 43–50.

Butler R, Cali T, Louria D, et al. (1994). Rational use of broad-spectrum antibiotics in the elderly. Geriatrics 49(Suppl 1):s-2–s-16.

Digiovanna A. (1994). Human Aging. St. Louis: CV Mosby.

Fan H, Conner R, Villareal L. (1996). AIDS: Science and Society. Boston: Jones & Bartlett.

Fletcher K. (1995). Assessment of the immune system. In Phipps WJ, Cassmeyer VL, Sands JK, Lehman MK, eds. Medical-Surgical Nursing. St. Louis: CV Mosby.

Fraser D. (1993). Patient Assessment: Infection in the Elderly. J Gerontol Nurs 19(7):5–11.

Gordon S, Thompson S. (1995). The changing epidemiology of human immunodeficiency virus infection in older persons. J Am Geriatr Soc 43(1):7–9.

Hopkins M, Schoener L. (1996). Tuberculosis and the elderly: Living in long-term care facilities. Geriatr Nurs 17(1):27–32.

Janeway C, Travers P. (1994). Immunobiology: The Immune System in Health and Disease. New York: Garland.

Lancaster E. (1993). Tuberculosis comeback: Impact on long-term care facilities. J Gerontol Nurs 19(7):16–21.

Letvak S, Schoder L. (1996). Sexually transmitted diseases in the elderly: What you need to know. Geriatrics 17(4):156–160.

Moffett D, Moffett F, Shauf C. (1993). Human Physiology. St. Louis: CV Mosby.

Morton P. (1993a). Health Assessment in Nursing. Philadelphia: FA Davis.

Morton P. (1993b). Physical Assessment. Philadelphia: FA Davis.

Noble J. (1996). Textbook of Primary Care Medicine. St. Louis: CV Mosby.

Phipps W, Cassmeyer V, Sands J, Lehman M. (1995). Medical-Surgical Nursing. St. Louis: CV Mosby.

Prichard V. (1993). Infection control: Programs for long-term care. J Gerontol Nurs 19(7):29–32.

Rhoades R, Tanner G. (1995). Medical Physiology. Boston: Little, Brown.

Saxon S, Etten M. (1994). Physical Change and Aging. New York: Tiresias Press.

Schuerman D. (1994). Clinical concerns: AIDS in the elderly. J Gerontol Nurs 20(7):11–17.

Spechko P. (1993). Bloodborne pathogens: Can you become infected from your older adult? J Gerontol Nurs 19(7):12–15.

Stanley M, Beare P. (1995). Gerontological Nursing. Philadelphia: FA Davis.

Wallace J, Paaiw D, Spach D. (1993). HIV infection in older patients: When to suspect the unexpected. Geriatrics 48(2):61–70.

Wingate A, Wright ER. (1995). Inflammatory and immune responses. In Phipps WJ, Cassmeyer VL, Sands JK, Lehman MK, eds. Medical-Surgical Nursing. St. Louis: CV Mosby.

CRITICAL THINKING EXERCISES

Mr. Richard Jones, age 75, is HIV positive and also has active TB. He remains sexually active. His family's response is shock and disbelief.

1. Explain to Mr. Jones and his family the relationship of the aging immune system and the increased vulnerability to AIDS and TB.
2. Why do you think the family is so shocked? Prepare a plan to dispel the myths about older adults and sexual activity that you could share with the family.
3. Formulate a care plan for Mr. Jones. Why would his diseases be even more difficult to treat than those of a younger individual?

Ms. Sally Brown, age 92, lives in a nursing home and has recently acquired pneumonia. Her diagnosis was made late and medical care was not initiated at an early stage. Ms. Brown's roommate had already been diagnosed with the same bacterial pneumonia.

1. Prepare an in-service teaching plan for the nursing home where Ms. Brown lives. Include prevention and control measures for communicable diseases that could be easily used in this long-term care facility. What are the most important goals and how could they be measured?

(*continued on following page*)

CRITICAL THINKING EXERCISES Continued

2. Teach a classmate how to assess the respiratory system of an older adult client in a long-term care facility. What changes in the immune system of an older client would affect the findings of the assessment?
3. Would treatment for Ms. Brown's pneumonia differ from that for a younger client living at home? Explain why Ms. Brown would be more vulnerable to a respiratory tract infection.

Mr. Mohammed Farouk is a 77-year-old hypertensive retired farmer who lives by himself and enjoys daily work in his small vegetable garden. He lives on a fixed income, adheres to a strict Islamic diet, and prepares all his meals for himself. Other than his medication-controlled hypertension, he has been in good health and remains active. Recently he had a physical examination that revealed a squamous cell carcinoma lesion on his nose and the right side of his face.

1. Explain why Mr. Farouk is vulnerable to skin cancer. How could he modify his lifestyle to decrease his vulnerability?
2. Mr. Farouk told his nurse that many of his friends the same age are constantly having colds and flu. He is very interested in maintaining his health by eating a healthy diet. Plan a diet for Mr. Farouk that would help him maintain his health and reduce his chances for infection while addressing his hypertension and his strict Islamic diet.
3. When assessing the integumentary system in an older adult such as Mr. Farouk, what are important areas to include? If the integumentary system is compromised, what might be some expected findings?

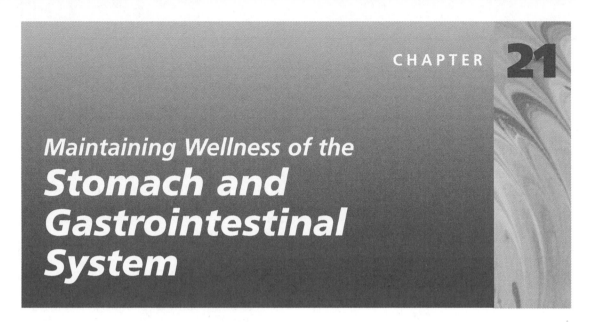

CHAPTER **21**

Maintaining Wellness of the
Stomach and Gastrointestinal System

Joyce Lusan, RN, MA

CHAPTER OUTLINE

OBJECTIVES

After completing this chapter, the reader should be able to:

1. Describe the impact of the aging process on the structure and function of digestive and gastrointestinal organs.
2. Discuss the pathophysiology, clinical manifestations, diagnoses, and interventions for a number of pathological conditions of the digestive and gastrointestinal system.
3. Assess the older adult with alterations in the digestive and gastrointestinal system.
4. Describe management and care of the older adult experiencing alterations in digestive and gastrointestinal functions.
5. Employ nursing strategies for the older adult experiencing alterations in digestive and gastrointestinal functions.

KEY TERMS

achalasia
chyme
diverticula
dyspepsia
dysphagia
motility
odynophagia
volvulus

The aging process may have only minimal adverse effects on the normal functioning of the body, and most older adults are able to cope by making changes in their activities of daily living. However, for others, organ anatomy and function undergo many adverse changes that place them at high risk for morbidity and mortality from a number of diseases and conditions.

■ CASE STUDY

> Ms. LG, a 92-year-old client in a local home care program, has a short-term memory so stunning that she elicits curiosity regarding her formative years. Although physically ill, she participates in all facets of decision-making regarding her care. This older adult was experiencing swallowing difficulties and abdominal cramps, and she stated that she had experienced these cramps all of her adult life but the swallowing difficulties were new. She also said that she had always been able to fight off her illnesses, but this time she was finding it difficult to do so. "Anyway," she stated philosophically, "At my age, what do I expect?"

The digestive and gastrointestinal system, with its rapid turnover of cells, high motility or ability to move substances precisely, and secretive, absorptive, and protective functions, is vulnerable to an unusual share of these disorders. And, although many of the problems may begin in the younger adult years, their incidence and prevalence increase significantly in older adulthood. For example, certain benign conditions with the potential for malignancy may evolve in that direction with time. The needs of older adults are challenging, and gerontological nurses must be prepared for the challenge presented by digestive and gastrointestinal disorders. For example, it takes time, patience, and fortitude to feed someone who is experiencing dysphagia and does not want to eat or to assist in keeping the elimination process intact for a patient who is bedridden. It is difficult to utilize the usual parameters for assessing poor nutrition and dehydration because normal aging changes such as sunken eyeballs and dry skin are not unusual for the old-old client (Bennett and Greenough, 1993). Research has, however, made available new diagnostic techniques and management strategies to assist in meeting these challenges.

■ HEALTH TEACHING

The role of a healthy diet to the well-being of the individual cannot be overstated. Many strides have been made in the quantity and quality of nutritional supplements produced with the expressed intention of keeping us healthy; there are numerous protein, vitamin, and mineral preparations available for nutritional supplementation. Although our nutritional needs change as we age, there is little change seen in the basic elements necessary for cellular activity.

Older adults, as with all age groups, need adequate nutrition to maintain health and extend longevity, and the nurse can play a significant role in assisting them to meet this need. The client can be educated regarding the importance of maintaining a well-balanced diet while restricting fats and cholesterol to decrease the incidence of heart disease, high blood pressure, stroke, and cancer. Limiting the intake of excess carbohydrates and sweets also helps to decrease adult onset of diabetes mellitus. Spicy foods, and foods cured in concentrated salt and nitrites, should be taken in limited quantities because of their irritating effects on the gastrointestinal mucosa.

Some factors that influence nutritional intake in older adults include changes in social status and economic resources, poor dentition, depression, and other adverse health conditions. To ensure nutritional intake for older adults of limited means, the nurse can make a referral to a food stamp program. If there is a problem with shopping and preparation of food, a referral can be made to the "Meals on Wheels" program, in which a meal is delivered daily to the homebound client.

Caffeine and alcohol are substances that are irritating to the gastrointestinal mucosa, and they are often implicated as predisposing factors in conditions such as gastritis, ulcer disease, and malignancies of the gastrointestinal tract. Overindulgence in alcohol delivers empty calories to the body, which leads to poor nutrition and often results in damage to vital organs such as the brain and the liver. The nurse can give information concerning the deleterious effects of these substances and encourage older adults to give up these habits. For cigarette smokers there are many aids available (e.g., nicotine patch or gum) that reduce the intense craving for nicotine and decrease the addictive behavior. Older adults who are experiencing problems with alcohol may be referred to support groups such as Alcoholics Anonymous (AA) to assist them in the fight to overcome the habit.

Older adults need information pertaining to disease-causing organisms found in food and their potential for causing serious illnesses. They should be taught correct handling and preparation of foods, such as storing meat in the freezer compartment of the refrigerator until ready for cooking and refraining from consuming meats that are not thoroughly cooked. In this situation, the nurse may meet resistance because many older adults are not inclined to change their eating habits, either because of habit or of confidence in the food supply in this country.

W e l l n e s s

"Most older adults live at home and are well. Home health care professionals can provide an alternative to lengthy hospitalization or institutionalization for those with impaired health."

The benefits of dental care should also be emphasized to older adults, because, in spite of current information on the benefits of tooth retention, many individuals do not make themselves available for dental care and tend to accept tooth loss as part of the normal aging process. According to the American Dental Association (ADA, 1997), regularly scheduled dental care can assist the older adult in fighting tooth decay, diseased gums, and dry mouth; when necessary, older adults can be provided with well-fitted dentures. If cost of care is a problem, the ADA can provide information related to the offsetting of expenses. Many older clients with chronic illnesses and contractures may find it difficult to sit or recline in a dental chair for any period of time, so procedures need to be done with the client in an upright chair and in short intervals. Most dentists recommend that older adults seek dental care every 6 months, or more often if necessary.

The nurse should reinforce the need for regular exercise during the later years to keep muscles toned and bones strong. Exercise also influences the release of endorphins that are beneficial as a mood elevator. Finally, the nurse should teach all clients to wash their hands often, especially before and after self-care, to decrease the likelihood of coming into contact with microorganisms or germs that cause diseases.

◼ AGE-RELATED CHANGES

All body cells need nutrition, and this need is continuous throughout the life span. Our bodies receive nutrients from the food we eat, which, through the process of digestion, releases the energy necessary for cellular function. This process is accomplished by the organs of the gastrointestinal system. Good nutritional status is also ensured by the central nervous system through the feeding and satiety centers that regulate the consumption of food. Changes in structure and function of the digestive system and/or changes in the central nervous system place an individual at risk for poor nutrition if the process of digestion is altered. Many adults, as they age, present with significant changes in the gastrointestinal system that not only affect the nutritional status but also cause pain and discomfort, and may even result in morbidity and mortality. It is sometimes difficult, however, to identify these changes as age related or as effects of diseases and the medications used for therapy. For example, it is questionable whether dry mouth, noted as a physiological change in an older adult, is related to altered hydration or to the side effects of polypharmacy. In previous years, many studies that described changes in the gas-

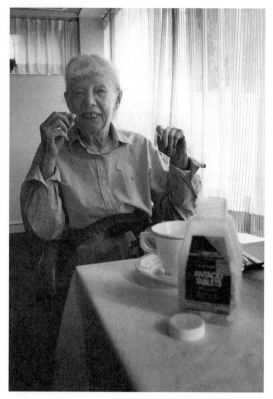

Although many older adults frequently feel the need for antacids, it is essential that serious sources of gastrointestinal discomfort be ruled out.

trointestinal system as being age related were conducted on sick, institutionalized individuals, and results are now been disputed by more recent studies conducted on healthy older adults. However, some of the findings of these recent studies are controversial and must be applied judiciously. Nevertheless, although surveys show that 20% of people older than 65 claim to have some type of chronic digestive disease (Hampton, 1991), it is evident that, for the majority, gastrointestinal function remains intact even when some changes are present.

Digestion begins in the mouth, where the teeth, tongue, and saliva play a very important role in the primary preparation of food for its passage through the system. Common changes that are evident in the oral cavity of older adults include tooth loss related to dental or periodontal problems, malocclusion of the teeth related to temporomandibular joint syndrome, alteration in the integrity of the mucosal lining, and decrease in the quality and

quantity of saliva. Although still controversial, many studies point to the fact that taste thresholds rise related to a decrease in the number of taste buds on the tongue (Bartoshuk and Weiffenbach, 1990). All these changes can have adverse effects on the nutritional health of the elderly.

Motility in the esophagus, which is important for the propulsion of food and fluids into the stomach, is accomplished through esophageal peristalsis. Peristaltic waves are of two types: *primary*, which occur just after swallowing, and *secondary*, which occur when the upper end of the esophagus is distended locally. In certain circumstances a series of spontaneous, nonperistaltic contractions termed *tertiary* occur after swallowing and seem to increase with age. Therefore, they are seen more often in the esophagus of older adults and are accompanied by a decrease in normal peristaltic waves, delayed relaxation of the lower esophageal sphincter (LES), and delayed esophageal emptying. This syndrome is referred to as *presbyesophagus* (old esophagus). However, newer studies by Hollis and Castell, (1974) on healthy aged men conclude that "in normal healthy individuals, the physiological function of the esophagus is well-preserved with increasing age, save for, perhaps, in very old age." Therefore, "presbyesophagus" may be related to entities other than aging.

In the area of gastric motility and secretory function, studies seem to indicate that solid food emptying appears to be unaffected by age whereas liquid emptying may be somewhat delayed. The significance of this information is the time variance in which drugs may pass from the stomach into the intestines. Some studies also identify thinning with loss in volume of the gastric mucosa and the muscularis (atrophic gastritis) as occurring more frequently in older adults. However, the correlation between age and atrophic changes is still in question, because other studies suggest that gastric infection with *Helicobacter pylori* may be pathogenically responsible for the development of atrophic gastritis in both the young and older adult (Peterson, 1993). In this case, there is also reduced production of hydrochloric acid and delayed gastric emptying. There is less controversy, however, over the decline in the production of gastric acid secretion, which seems to occur more often in older adult men (Altmann, 1990).

The main function of the small intestine is the absorption of nutrients from the **chyme** (material produced by the digestion of food). Through sequential movements called *segmentation*, the chyme is moved back and forth so that it can be mixed with and be acted on by the gastric juices. It is then propelled by peristaltic movements into the large intestine, small amounts at a time. No change with aging has been found for the small intestine in terms of the transit time of chyme or the degree of absorption of most nutrients as they pass through. This means that there is no decrease in the absorption of fats, carbohydrates, vitamins, iron, or proteins with aging.

The process of digestion is completed in the large intestine as the chyme is moved along by churning and peristalsis. Water is absorbed, and bacterial action on the solids produces vital substances needed by the body. The process of defecation is reflexive but is under voluntary control in the adult, and any alteration in nervous stimulation may put one at risk for constipation and incontinence.

Caring

" *The nurse assists the patient with therapeutic measures that are being used for palliation when a cure is not expected.* "

A significant change seen in the large intestine is weakness in the musculature that results in decreased forcefulness of contractions and a slowing down of peristaltic activity. These changes may be more related to a general decrease in physical activity, alteration in the diet related to chewing difficulties, and the effects of medications, rather than to aging alone. There is also a tendency for the formation of **diverticula** or herniation of the mucosa into the weakened musculature.

Pancreatic activity is in response to chyme in the small intestines, whose mucosa produces secretin, which stimulates the production of pancreatic juice, and cholecystokinin, which stimulates the secretion of digestive enzymes. There seems to be little change in the function of the pancreas with age, except for a slight reduction in the number of cells, which may be reflected in the quantities of pancreatic lipase produced.

In general, liver/biliary functions remain intact with aging except for some decrease in liver storage capacity and in the production of some enzymes essential for metabolism and clearance of certain substances from the body. This may have an effect on drug metabolism in older adults, making it necessary to adjust the choices of medication and the dosages prescribed for them. Older adults should also be carefully monitored for drug absorption and side effects of medications. The gallbladder continues to contract in response to chyme in the small intestines; however, there seems to be an increase in the incidence of gallstones that may be related to a change in the ratio of cholesterol/phospholipid in the bile with age.

GUIDELINES SPECIFIC TO ASSESSING GASTROINTESTINAL PROBLEMS IN OLDER ADULTS

Pain

Pain and discomfort in the gastrointestinal system may signify local irritation of the mucosa, ulcer disease, malignancy, increased motility, or an obstruction. The nurse should assess for the location of the pain; ask the client to describe the pain in terms of intensity, type, time of onset; and determine if it is accompanied by any other symptoms such as nausea, vomiting, and/or diarrhea.

Periodontal disorders and irritation of the mucosa are problems of the oral cavity that often result in pain for the individual. The nurse should assess for the presence of broken or rocking teeth, malocclusion of the teeth, or poorly fitting dentures, which may be causing the problem. The assessment should also include an examination of the soft tissue for any irritation or ulceration that may suggest the presence of an infection or malignancy.

If the client complains of painful swallowing, the nurse can make a referral to the speech pathologist for further evaluation. Pain related to problems in the esophagus may mimic that of angina, and the client may fear a heart attack. Therefore, the nurse must explore the quality and extent of the discomfort, and the factors that aggravate its onset and duration, in an effort to differentiate the symptoms and assist the client with appropriate therapeutic measures. For example, the nurse may gain information that the client consumed spicy food that is irritating to the mucosal lining or drank fluids that were too hot or cold and initiated or exacerbated the esophageal spasms.

The location of abdominal pain can give information regarding the organ or organs affected. For example, pain in the right upper quadrant may signify liver, gallbladder, or duodenal pathology; pain in the left upper quadrant may be associated with the stomach and pancreas, and pain in the left and right lower quadrant may indicate intestinal involvement. The nurse utilizes the four techniques (i.e., inspection, palpation, auscultation, percussion) to assess the client's complaints. Inspection may be used to check for abdominal distention, ascites, or visible peristaltic movements. Visible peristalsis may indicate intestinal obstruction and, if observed, should be reported to the physician promptly. The nurse may also assess for the presence or absence of bowel sounds by auscultation, percussion (to assess the size of solid organs), and gentle palpation (to ascertain the presence of a mass).

Nausea and Vomiting

Nausea and vomiting most commonly are manifestations of gastrointestinal disturbances, but they may also be presenting signs of conditions affecting other body systems. Although nausea may occur independent of vomiting, nausea and vomiting often occur together and are treated as one problem. The nurse may assess vomiting in an older adult as related to difficulty in swallowing, esophageal problems, or a simple response to mucosal irritation. The irritant may be chemical or bacterial and related to an infectious process, food poisoning, intestinal obstruction, or a metabolic condition. Nausea and vomiting are also side effects of many medications that are prescribed for the elderly.

The nurse questions the client regarding occasions when vomiting occurs and the precipitating factors. An assessment is also made of the amount of vomitus, its color, and a description of its contents. Vomiting of partially digested food at least 5 hours after a meal is suggestive of gastric outlet obstruction or delay in

gastric emptying. The color of the vomitus may yield important information regarding the patency of the gastrointestinal tract and integrity of its lining. For example, vomitus that is bile stained or has a fecal odor indicates intestinal obstruction beyond the pylorus. A "coffee ground" appearance suggests blood remaining in the stomach and being acted on by the gastric secretions, whereas bright red blood indicates active bleeding from tears in the mucosal lining, a gastric or duodenal ulcer, a neoplasm, or bleeding esophageal varices.

Diarrhea and Constipation

When an elderly person complains of diarrhea or constipation, a careful history of usual bowel habits should be obtained. Our concepts of normal bowel activity vary, and an individual may actually be expressing a slight difference between his or her concept of a normal bowel movement and what is actually the norm. Whatever the situation, the client's complaints should be taken seriously and investigated fully, because slight changes in bowel habits can signify the presence of devastating conditions such as a severe infection or a malignancy. Normal bowel activity ranges from three bowel movements per day to one bowel movement every 3 days, although having more than three per day does not mean that diarrhea is present if the stool is formed (just as not having a bowel movement every day does not signify constipation if the stool is soft and defecation takes place at regular intervals). Diet, fluid intake, and activity have great influence on bowel activity.

■ COMMON DISORDERS

Disorders of the Oral Cavity

Normal functioning in the oral cavity may be compromised because of changes in the integrity of the mucosal lining, which may become thin, smooth, and dry; salivary gland disorders that alter the quality and quantity of saliva can result in dryness of the mouth (xerostomia) and the presence of lesions such as leukoplakia. These changes may lead to an inability to moisten food for chewing and swallowing and some difficulty speaking. Experience has shown that these changes may not be entirely related to aging but are systemic responses to certain types of medications that stimulate or depress sympathetic and parasympathetic activity.

A mild decrease in taste sensation (and sense of smell) may also be a problem for the older adult, because these sensations have a major impact not only on the consumption of food but also on alerting the person to substances that may be poisonous or spoiled. Because many medications and disease states seem to affect chemosensory function, it is difficult at this time to attribute a reduction in the acuity of the senses of taste and smell to the aging process alone. However, as new information becomes available, differentiating chemosensory dysfunction from loss through the aging process or other causes will become easier (Bartoshuk and Weiffenbach, 1990). What is important for caregivers to remember is that many older adults do verbalize a difference in the taste of food as they get older, and this can have an impact on their nutritional intake.

Dental and periodontal problems also impact on the nutritional health of the older adult. In the past, tooth loss and gum disease were accepted as normal processes of aging. However, with early dental education on the benefits of tooth retention, more individuals are availing themselves of dental care. This education was not available for the present older adult population. Even though dental and oral problems increase with age, older adults are poor utilizers of dental services, perhaps in part because of the cost of dental care.

A thorough assessment of the oral cavity is needed to determine what interventions may be needed. Radiographs are useful for diagnosis of structural deformities, and inspection and palpation are important for identification of soft tissue problems.

The management and care of oral problems in older adults depend on the presenting problems. For those who can participate and benefit from education, good oral hygiene is taught. A diet that can be chewed comfortably with plenty of fluids (if not contraindicated) and regular dental follow-up are encouraged. For those who are unable, an oral care plan with input from dentistry, physiotherapy, and nursing must be developed and executed. Assistive devices for handling the toothbrush may be provided for those who can manage. The nurse provides daily (and as often as needed) mouth care for removal of food and debris from the teeth and tongue and to moisten the mucous membrane.

Teeth that cannot be salvaged by fillings and sealings may have to be extracted. Although tooth extraction is a simple procedure, many older adults with chronic illnesses and contractures may find it difficult to sit or recline in a dental chair for any period of time. Therefore, the procedure may be done with the patient in an upright chair and in short intervals. The wearing of dentures should be encouraged and problems with fitting referred to the dentist. Antibiotics are used to treat any infections that may be present; lesions and tumors are treated appropriately.

The nurse must be aware that dental problems and dental care involve an element of discomfort, and what may appear to be noncompliance by the patient may actually be a reflection of fear of this discomfort. Therefore, emotional support should be offered and strategies to decrease anxiety discussed. Explanation of new techniques available to decrease painful stimuli in dentistry may also be helpful.

Disorders of the Esophagus

Swallowing difficulties include **dysphagia,** which may be expressed as a sensation of or actual difficulty swallowing, **odynophagia,** or painful swallowing, and **pseudodysphagia,** which is experienced after a meal and expressed as a sensation of "fullness" or a "lump" in the throat. This sensation does not interfere with swallowing and may even disappear with swallowing. Older adults may also experience *small swallow,* in which case the individual can swallow saliva and fluids but cannot swallow food. Small swallow may be the result of dryness of the mouth or a pharyngoesophageal pathological process.

DYSPHAGIA

Based on presenting signs and symptoms, dysphagia may be divided into two distinct syndromes: oropharyngeal dysphagia and esophageal dysphagia. Oropharyngeal dysphagia may be associated with many conditions. They include neurological deficits after a cerebrovascular accident or major stroke; alterations in the neuromuscular mechanisms that control movements of the tongue, pharynx, and the upper esophageal sphincter (UES); neck tumors; or outpouching in the pharyngeal wall (Zenker's diverticulum) immediately above the UES. Abnormalities of the UES include hypotensive and hypertensive functions that may result in its incomplete or delayed relaxation.

The clinical manifestations of oropharyngeal dysphagia depend on the underlying cause. Generally, the patient presents with the holding of fluid, semisolids, or solids in the mouth and expresses a feeling of difficulty or painful swallowing. If Zenker's diverticulum is present, food may be retained in the sac, which can become large enough to produce a visible mass in the neck. This results in coughing, a feeling of fullness in the neck, and regurgitation after eating. The patient is at high risk for aspiration of food and fluid into the lungs.

The history and finding on physical examination along with diagnostic tests are important in the diagnosis of oropharyngeal dysphagia. The patient is referred to the speech pathologist, who evaluates the swallowing reflex. The tongue is held in place with a tongue depressor while the throat is examined. Then the patient is asked to move the tongue from side to side and up to the roof of the mouth. Water is given to drink while the throat is palpated to see how strong the swallowing reflex is, or if it is present at all. Then food is offered, with the consistency increasing from applesauce to a dry cracker while the pathologist again evaluates the swallowing reflex and checks to see if any food has been left in the mouth.

Other studies include examination of the pharynx and upper esophagus under barium radiography with videofluoroscopy. The patient is required to swallow barium sulfate under direct fluoroscopy, and the examiner is able to identify any alterations in the anatomy or any lesions that are present. Manometric studies are used to detect any alteration in the peristaltic activity of the esophagus (Society of Gastroenterology Nurses and Associates, 1993).

Treatment depends on the underlying cause. Neuromuscular diseases are treated appropriately, and physiotherapy is given for restoration of function if the problem is related to a cerebrovascular accident. The speech therapist works with the patient to see which therapeutic intervention is most helpful (e.g., which position of the head enables the patient to swallow more efficiently). The nurse works very closely with the dietitian to determine the appropriate diet, and every consistency of food is tried to assist the patient to maintain oral feeding. For patients who are experiencing difficulty swallowing fluids, a thickening substance is added to the fluid that makes it heavy and easier to swallow.

Because the main goal is to maintain adequate nutrition, tube feeding may have to be an alternative until the swallowing reflex is adequate. The nurse teaches, clarifies, and encourages the patient to meet the goals of therapy.

ACHALASIA

Achalasia is the result of defective innervation to the lower end of the esophagus and the LES. There is absence of peristaltic motility in this area, accompanied by narrowing of the tube and failure of the LES to relax in response to swallowing. The esophagus above the affected area becomes dilated as it fills with air, fluid, food, and saliva. This condition may be idiopathic or the sequelae of malignant lesions in the esophagus.

The patient complains of difficulty in swallowing fluids and food, a sensation of oppressive fullness in the lower chest, and regurgitation of undigested food, which may lead to nocturnal coughing and aspiration pneumonia. Chest pains or a burning sensation in the chest may also be experienced.

Radiography of the chest, barium swallow, and endoscopy are useful for diagnosis. However, manometry gives a definitive diagnosis by showing the lower end of the esophagus to be dilated and aperistaltic, with low pressure and incomplete relaxation of the LES.

Achalasia can be treated medically or surgically; and for the older adult, who may have other debilitating conditions, medical intervention may be more suitable. This involves introducing a pneumonic dilator into the esophagus, then inflating the bag at the end of the tube under fluoroscopy to dilate the affected area. About 75% of patients are helped by this procedure, but there is a 3% incidence of perforation of the esophagus (Brunner and Suddarth, 1992), which is a serious complication. Surgical intervention involves the separation of muscle fibers (myotomy) in the constricted area. Complications of this procedure include gastroesophageal reflux. Smooth muscle relaxants such as isosorbide or nifedipine may be effective in enhancing relaxation of the LES and improve dysphagia during meals. Sitting upright for at least two hours after ingestion of a meal will also prevent regurgitation and possible aspiration.

W e l l n e s s

"Older adults, as in all age groups, need adequate nutrition to maintain health and extend longevity; the nurse can play a significant role in assisting them to meet this need."

GASTROESOPHAGEAL REFLUX DISEASE

The integrity of the esophagus is maintained by the UES and LES, which are zones of high pressure under muscular, neural, and hormonal control. The UES guards the opening between the pharynx and esophagus, and the LES guards the opening between the esophagus and the stomach. The angle at which the esophagus enters the stomach and the area of high pressure around the orifice help to maintain sphincter closure, which prevents the reflux of gastric contents into the esophagus (Kahrilas, 1997). The mechanism that alters LES sphincter control is still unknown, but its inappropriate relaxation with subsequent reflux of gastric contents into the esophagus is a quite common occurrence in the general population, and its incidence seems to increase with aging.

The clinical manifestations of gastroesophageal reflux disease vary with the degree of gastric reflux. The client complains of heartburn (pyrosis), which is a burning sensation in the substernal or retrosternal area. If reflux is severe, the pain may radiate to the neck or jaw and may migrate to the back. It tends to worsen when the individual bends over, strains, or is in a recumbent position. Other symptoms the nurse may assess include regurgitation without belching or nausea, and water brash, which is a reflex salivary hypersecretion in response to the reflux. Also, the client may report a sensation of fluid in the throat that does not have a sour or bitter taste. Gastroesophageal reflux disease, if uncontrolled, can progress to dysphagia or difficulty swallowing.

Management of the client with gastroesophageal reflux disease involves a collaborative effort of physician, dietitian, and nurse in providing a regimen of diet therapy, medications, and lifestyle changes. The nurse utilizes an interactive approach of educating the client about the disease process and the therapeutic measures necessary for control or recovery, keeping in mind that many older adults may not benefit from this approach because of physical or mental impairment. Many of the interventions may have to be accomplished for them.

Therapeutic measures for gastroesophageal reflux disease begin with the elimination of those entities that are related to its cause. The nurse assists the client and significant others with choosing a diet that is low in fat and to eliminate substances such as tea, coffee, cola, chocolate, and alcohol. Spicy foods and acidic foods such as orange juice should also be avoided until irritated tissues heal in order to decrease heartburn. To decrease gastric pressure, the client should be encouraged to consume four to six small meals daily, instead of the usual three large ones, avoid evening snacks, and eat no food for at least 3 hours before bedtime. The client should also be assisted with proper positioning, such as elevating the head of the bed or placing foam wedges under the head and shoulders. The client is also encouraged to loose weight, if obese, to stop smoking, if indicated, and to avoid restrictive clothing and bent-over stooped positions. The nurse emphasizes that these adaptations are essential for control of this condition.

If antacids are not effective, systemic drugs such as histamine-2-receptor blocking agents ranitidine (Zantac), famotidine (Pepcid), or nizatidine (Axid) may be ordered. Surgery to anchor the LES below the diaphragm and reinforce the high-pressure area is indicated for clients who do not respond to aggressive antireflux therapy. However, they are encouraged to continue antireflux therapy after surgery, which decreases the rate of relapse.

HIATAL HERNIA

The area at which the esophagus passes through the diaphragm has a physiological tightness that keeps the stomach securely in the abdomen. A hiatal hernia occurs when the opening becomes enlarged enough to allow the upper end of (or the entire) stomach to move into the lower thorax. The hernias are of two types depending on the extent of the defect. Type 1, which occurs in 90% of patients (Brunner and Suddath, 1992), is known as a sliding hiatal hernia, in which the gastroesophageal junction and the upper end of the stomach slide in and out of the thorax. There may or may not be gastric reflux; therefore, the patient may be asymptomatic or complain of heartburn, belching, regurgitation, and dysphagia. Type 2 is a rolling hernia, in which all or part of the stomach pushes through the diaphragm. Symptoms of gastric reflux may not be present because the gastroesophageal sphincter remains closed. However, the patient may complain of a sense of fullness in the chest, breathlessness or suffocation after eating. Hiatal hernias are confirmed by radiographic studies and fluoroscopy.

The patient is encouraged to consume small frequent feedings and to remain in a sitting position for at least 1 hour after eating to prevent reflux or movement of the hernia. The head of the bed is also kept elevated to prevent movement of the hernia by gravity. If these measures are unsuccessful, surgery is performed to anchor the stomach to the abdominal wall and prevent complications such as strangulation, obstruction, and peptic stricture.

TUMORS

Tumors of the esophagus may be benign or malignant, with squamous cell carcinoma occurring most frequently. Predisposing factors include chronic irritation of the esophageal mucosa from chronic or persistent reflux, drinking excessively hot fluids, heavy smoking and alcohol consumption, and lack of roughage in the diet. The patient usually presents with dysphagia and odynophagia to solid food and eventually to liquid. Other signs and symptoms include hoarseness, cough, and pain, which may be substernal and radiating to the back. The condition may progress with weight loss and anemia, which are consequences of poor nutrition and slow bleeding.

The signs and symptoms may be indicative of many conditions occurring in the esophagus. However, a definitive diagnosis is obtained by endoscopy, from which a cytological examination can be made and tissue samples obtained for biopsy. The mediastinum is also visualized to determine if the disease has spread to those areas. The mode of treatment depends on the stage of the disease. The goal is to effect a cure if possible, which may not be realized because in most cases the disease is caught in the late stages.

The condition of the patient and the attending physician determine the interventions that will be most beneficial. Surgery, radiation therapy, laser treatment, and chemotherapy may be used individually or in any combination. Surgical intervention involves excision of the tumor and utilizing a portion of the colon for reconstruction. In situations in which surgery would not be helpful, a gastrostomy tube is placed for feeding and the patient is managed symptomatically. The prognosis for the patient experiencing cancer of the esophagus is poor, with a survival rate of less than 3% (Nelson and Castell, 1991).

Initially, the patient and significant others are assisted in coping with the news of a devastating disease. After finding out what they have been told by the physician, the nurse offers explanations and clarification as needed. Emotional support is offered, giving them the opportunity to ventilate feelings of sadness and loss. The nurse must also be aware that not all patients are willing or emotionally able to deal with a fatal disease and they should not be forced to do so until they are ready. Nurses, however, should remain supportive of the patient and family regardless of the behavior, constantly giving reassurance and care.

The goal of therapy is to enhance and maintain nutritional status and to prevent aspiration pneumonia, obstruction, and infection. The caloric and protein contents of the diet are increased, and the patient is fed orally as tolerated. If hardship is being experienced with oral feedings, then enteral or parenteral feedings are started. Preoperatively, the patient and family are educated as to what to expect with the different types of therapeutic interventions. Postoperatively, the nurse caring for this client is challenged to work closely with the physician in terms of correct positioning, management of nasogastric suctioning, and the handling of prostheses.

Disorders of the Stomach

GASTRITIS

Inflammation of the stomach mucosa may result from the consumption of foods that are too spicy or that contain infective bacteria, alcoholic beverages, or caustic substances such as nonsteroidal antiinflammatory medications (NSAIDs); systemic conditions such as kidney and liver disease or pernicious anemia; and radiation therapy. Especially for the elderly, the use of NSAIDs to treat arthritis places them at high risk for injury to the gastric mucosa. Because prostaglandin is important in maintaining the mucosal integrity of the gastrointestinal tract, the injury is believed to be produced by the inhibitory effect on prostaglandin synthesis by NSAIDs.

Older adults may also be afflicted with chronic atrophic gastritis, which affects the glandular portion of the mucosa, resulting in a decrease in mucus production and the infiltration of inflammatory cells, mainly of lymphocytes, into the area. This may be a premalignant lesion.

Another form of gastritis seen more often in males is Ménétrier's disease, where the mucosal cells proliferate into giant folds or convolutions. The cause of this condition is unknown, and the patient is usually asymptomatic unless the area becomes ulcerated with loss of protein and immunoglobulins from the folds. Then edema and signs of compromised immune defenses may be evident. The patient may complain of nausea and vomiting, abdominal pain, hiccups, anorexia, diarrhea, malaise, and headache.

Endoscopic examination may reveal edema, ulceration, bleeding, and changes in the mucosal lining of the stomach. Tissue samples may be removed for histological studies and the presence of other pathology. Where the symptoms are related to dietary indiscretion, they may be self limiting and resolve in about 3 days. For the patient on NSAIDs, enteric-coated agents are helpful in protecting the mucosa from injury. These agents should never be crushed for administration because they would lose their protective effect.

ULCERS

Any condition that disrupts the integrity of the mucosa may lead to ulcer formation. Included are those conditions mentioned earlier as being responsible for an irritating effect, as well as hypersecretion of hydrochloric acid and pepsin accompanied by a decrease in the production of mucus; reflux of duodenal contents containing acid and bile salts onto the stomach mucosa related to an inefficient pyloric sphincter; and infection with bacteria (e.g., *Helicobacter pylori*). Autoimmune responses in the development of ulcer disease are under investigation and remain controversial. Gastric ulcers occur more often in older adults, although duodenal ulcers are not uncommon.

The usual symptom of ulcers is epigastric pain, dull and radiating to the back which may be temporarily relieved by food. The patient may lose weight, or there may be weight gain as food is often consumed for the relief of pain. Nausea, vomiting, and constipation are other signs and symptoms that may be present. If erosion is deep enough to involve blood vessels, bleeding will be evident in vomitus, which is either bright red or resembles coffee grounds. Bleeding may also be evident as melenic stools.

Ulcers in some older adults assume unusual characteristics. The "giant gastric ulcer" usually associated with lesions larger than 3 cm in diameter is an example. These may not give typical ulcer symptoms; instead, the patient may be pain free or have an unusual pattern of pain that radiates to the chest, periumbilical region, or lower abdomen. An interesting variation of gastric ulcer in older adults is the "geriatric ulcer," located high in the gastric fundus, along the lesser curvature. This may present as a form of chest pain (Nelson and Castell, 1991). Diagnostic measures include a physical examination, an upper gastrointestinal tract series, endoscopy, gastric secretion studies, stool for occult blood, a breath test for *Helicobacter pylori,* and cytological studies to rule out the presence of malignancies.

The therapy that is chosen depends on the type and extent of the lesion. Diet is modified to decrease intake of substances that would increase acid production and motility. Foods that contain caffeine, alcohol, and preserved meat products should be avoided; however, the patient may have three regular meals as tolerated. Milk, which coats the stomach mucosa and was previously thought to be protective, has been found to increase gastric acid secretion; therefore, milk is no longer recommended for ulcer therapy. For most patients, drug therapy is very effective. Commonly used drugs for older adults are cimetidine (Tagamet), famotidine (Pepcid AC), and nizatidine (Axid). These drugs are convenient because of the single dosage at bedtime and because they are available in liquid form.

CARCINOMA

Carcinoma of the stomach is most often noted in individuals older than age 40 years, and its incidence increases with age. It is twice as common in men as in women. The etiology is related to factors involved in gastric mucosal irritation and injury. Factors implicated in the risk of stomach cancer are the overconsumption of highly salted, nitrate-cured fish and meat, a diet low in fruits and vegetables, previous gastric surgery, adenomatous polyps, gastric ulcers, pernicious anemia, type A blood, and situations that lower the production of hydrochloric acid. Although the incidence has been decreasing in the United States, incidence of gastric cancer still remains high in other countries such as Japan, Chile, Iceland, and Finland. However, the survival rate is highest in Japan, where routine screening is done on well individuals. This means an early diagnosis, or catching the lesion while it is still limited to the submucosal layer and may be cured by surgery.

Malignant tumors are most often seen in the antrum or along the lesser curvature of the stomach, with the majority of lesions being adenocarcinomas and lymphomas. Initial lesions spread very easily, either locally through the submucosal layer causing the stomach to become rigid and nondistensible "leather bottle stomach" or to other organs in the area, such as the liver, lungs, and lymph nodes.

The signs and symptoms of gastric cancer mimic those of other conditions in the stomach: pain that is relieved by eating, weight loss, **dyspepsia** (indigestion after meals), and anemia. By the time the lesion, especially the carcinoma, is identified, it is too late to effect a cure. Therefore, the mortality rate is high. Late symptoms include abdominal mass, ascites, infected lymph nodes (especially those of the supraclavicular fossa [Virchow's sign]), hypoalbuminemia, and dysphagia for solid foods. Any patient with dyspepsia for more than 4 weeks should be evaluated for stomach cancer.

Double-contrast barium swallow, endoscopy for biopsy, and cytological washings are the usual diagnostic studies. Computed tomography and magnetic resonance imaging are also used to differentiate the lesion from the surrounding tissues.

Early diagnosis and surgical excision is the only hope for a cure; however, because most stomach cancers are discovered too late to effect a cure, treatment is usually palliative to relieve symptoms of complications such as obstruction, dysphagia, and chronic bleeding. Cytotoxic substances such as 5-fluorouracil may be used, but most tumors do not respond and the drugs have their own toxic side effects.

When a cure is not expected, the nurse assists the patient with therapeutic measures that are being utilized for palliation. The issues of death and dying must also be addressed and worked through with the patient and family, although they may be in a state of denial. Especially for the old-old patient, the nurse may rationalize that death is expected and therefore its coming should be easier to bear, but for some patients this may not be true, because developmentally the tasks of old age have not been resolved; therefore, conflicts in this area should be expected and planned for. The nurse should also include the spiritual leader, family, and significant others in the plan of care so that the patient has support from all sources.

VOLVULUS

Volvulus is torsion or complete twisting of an organ on itself, and in the gastrointestinal tract this may happen to the stomach or to a loop of intestine. The condition is rare but does occur in older adults and may be related to relaxation of supportive structures, especially the ligments that support the stomach. Complete torsion can result in interruption of circulation and obstruction. The patient with volvulus of the stomach presents with severe epigastric pain, initial vomiting, then retching without vomiting, and absence of belching. It may also be impossible to pass a nasogastric tube. The condition is diagnosed by abdominal radiography and may require emergency surgery. Care of the patient is the same as for a patient in shock and pain with circulatory compromise and increased anxiety.

Disorders of the Small Intestine

The main function of the small intestine is the absorption of nutrients from the food that we eat. Therefore, the conditions that affect this area of the tract are reflected in signs and symptoms of malabsorption syndrome and deficiency anemias. Adult celiac disease, also known as celiac sprue, idiopathic or gluten-induced enteropathy, is a condition in which the individual shows intolerance to gluten made from barley, wheat, rye, and oats. The gluten influences changes in the epithelium, which result in partial or complete atrophy of the villi of the jejunum, leading to malabsorption of all nutrients such as fats, protein, carbohydrates, vitamins, minerals, and water. The actual cause of this disease is unknown, but it may be related to an immunological response to the gluten.

The main symptoms are diarrhea, steatorrhea, weight loss, signs of multiple vitamin deficiencies, abdominal distention, and excessive flatulence. When taking the history the nurse may obtain information that connects the bout of diarrhea with the intake of substances containing gluten. The nurse also assesses for allergies to other foods, or if the client can remember eating a particular food that did not taste right. The nurse also asks the client to describe the color and consistency of the stool, because steatorrhea indicates that there is some form of malabsorption of fat in the small intestines. The stool from the client with sprue is fatty and foul smelling. If for some

reason the disease escaped an earlier diagnosis, the older adult may present with anemia and fractures related to metabolic bone disease. The osteomalacia is related to calcium and vitamin D malabsorption, and the anemia, to vitamin B_{12}, iron, and folate malabsorption. Other problems the client may present with include water and electrolyte imbalance from loss of sodium and potassium, hypotension and edema from protein loss, bleeding diathesis from vitamin K deficiency, and abdominal distention. Malabsorption syndrome should also be suspected in clients who exhibit neurological symptoms, such as peripheral neuropathy and depression, that do not improve with treatment.

Caring

"The nurse should include the spiritual leader, family, and significant others in the plan of care so that the older adult patient has support from all sources."

The client is placed on a strict gluten-free diet, high in protein, calories, vitamins, and minerals. The nurse collaborates with the dietitian in assisting the client to identify foods from which to abstain and foods that may be consumed. The client is taught to read labels carefully and, when eating in restaurants, to make inquiries regarding ingredients utilized in recipes, such as flour added to soups and gravies. Caregivers must also be aware that medications that are absorbed in the jejunum will not be available to the client with celiac sprue, and adjustments may need to be made in the prescription. The physician may prescribe codeine sulfate for the relief of diarrhea and abdominal pain. Complications of celiac disease include no response to the gluten-free diet, a high incidence of cancer, bleeding, and perforation that is often fatal.

Disorders of the Colon, Rectum, and Anus

The incidence of disorders of the colon, rectum, and anus seem to increase with age. Mutation and damage of cells occurring earlier in the life cycle become manifested in later years, showing up as serious disease entities that disturb adequate functioning in the elderly population. For example, alteration in motility may result in muscle spasms, diarrhea, constipation, and fecal incontinence. Lesions can cause pressure or narrowing of the lumen, resulting in changes in bowel habits and obstruction. Erosion of the lining (epithelium) with exposure of blood vessels may result in bleeding, and infections may readily occur because of weakening and decrease in surveillance of the immune system.

CANCER OF THE COLON

Cancer of the colon is the most commonly occurring cause of death except for lung cancer (Parker et al., 1996). Adenocarcinoma (epithelial neoplasm) is the most common type, and the incidence increases in individuals older than 70 with a death rate of almost 50% of those affected (Levine, 1992). Factors that place the individual at high risk include a diet low in fiber and high in red meats, a family history of colonic cancer, metastasis from other areas of the body, and a history of inflammatory bowel disease. There is also conflicting evidence of alcohol, cigarette smoking, and viral involvement.

The client may be asymptomatic or complain of new onset of constipation, diarrhea, mucous discharge, rectal bleeding, and symptoms of abdominal obstruction. The nursing assessment may reveal abdominal blotting and distention, the presence of an abdominal mass, and an enlarged liver. The nurse encourages and assists the client to comply with scheduled procedures arranged by the physician and explains and clarifies information as needed. Screening procedures for early detection is very essential in preventing the high rate of morbidity and mortality from this disease (Bond, 1997). The nurse must teach the elderly client that age-related changes in the intestine increase the risk of malignancies; therefore, participation in screening procedures is very important. A tumor that is detected early can be eradicated completely, thus prolonging the life of the individual.

Surgical intervention is successful in the treatment of these lesions, but the exact procedure used depends on the location and the extent of the lesion present. A colonoscopic polypectomy may be sufficient for the removal of polyps and other free-hanging lesions. However, surgical resection is required for large lesions to effect a cure or prevent obstruction. There are also new treatment modalities that have been successful in the treatment of colorectal cancer. Therapy such as cryosurgery, which is a destruction of malignant tissue by freezing and thawing, has been used successfully. Laser and new chemotherapeutic agents are also available for treatment. For example, 5-fluorouracil was not absorbed and utilized well when administered orally. However, prodrugs of this substance, which are well absorbed from the gastrointestinal tract and enzymatically converted to 5-fluorouracil in the liver or within the tumor itself, have solved this problem (Waters et al., 1997).

The nursing care of the client with colorectal cancer is directed toward assessments and interventions for the relief of pain, hemorrhage, respiratory complications, altered nutrition, and other effects of immobility. Care is also directed toward giving the client and family the emotional support needed to deal with fear of a life-threatening illness. Complications of advanced disease include metastasis to other organ systems, hemorrhage that leads to anemia, hepatomegaly, hypotension, and kidney failure. The goal of therapy is to effect a cure without an altered body image.

DIVERTICULAR DISEASE

This disease is very common in the elderly; approximately 40% of individuals are affected (Levine, 1992). The development of diverticulosis may be a sequela of a low-residue diet (because it is more prevalent in developed countries), constipation, and forceful evacuation. Stress and obesity are also implicated as predisposing factors.

Changes in the muscular wall of the intestine allow the mucosal layers to herniate through sites where it is normally perforated by blood vessels. Diverticulosis occurs in any area of the intestines; however, the most common sites are in the sigmoid and descending colons. The patient may not have any symptoms of its presence until complications such as bleeding and inflammation with abscess formation (diverticulitis) set in. Scarring and spasms after bouts of diverticulitis result in narrowing of the lumen with symptoms of obstruction.

The client may complain of nausea and vomiting, rectal bleeding, abdominal pain, constipation, urinary problems, diarrhea or alternating constipation and diarrhea, and abdominal distention. Fever, rigors, and leukocytosis are evidence that sepsis is present.

Physical examination would reveal abdominal mass, signs of obstruction, and sepsis if present. A more definitive diagnosis can be obtained through radiographic examination to identify diverticular disease and narrowing of the lumen; angiography will identify abscess and bleeding complications.

For the majority of patients, increasing the dietary fiber is helpful. Avoiding consumption of small seeds or hard particles also prevents irritation, pain, and infection in some individuals. For others, treatment is symptomatic and includes nothing by mouth, bed rest, and fluid and electrolyte therapy. Nasogastric suctioning is used to treat vomiting and other signs of obstruction, and antibiotic therapy is administered to treat infections caused by anaerobic bacteria that are natural inhabitants of the colon. These antibiotics may be used alone or in combination for maximum effect. Ampicillin and gentamicin, or gentamicin and cefoxitin sodium (Mefoxin), may be given.

Surgical resection of the affected bowel is indicated if more conservative therapy is not effective. Postoperatively, the patient may be placed on nasogastric suctioning for decompression and given intravenous feeding in order to rest the bowel for the first few days.

The nurse collaborates with the dietitian in teaching and assisting the patient to identify and combine foods for a high-fiber diet. If the patient is unable to chew high-fiber foods, a teaspoon of bran may be sprinkled over food to supply extra fiber. Bran is added slowly to the diet, because too much of it at a time may cause nausea. Irritants such as alcohol and hot spices are also eliminated from the diet.

Mouth care is given when the patient is taking nothing by mouth. The nares are assessed for pressure from the nasogastric tube, strict intake and output is maintained to prevent fluid overload, and drainage is replaced as ordered by the physician. If pain is present, the patient is managed with an analgesic that would not increase gastric irritation.

DIARRHEA, CONSTIPATION, AND FECAL IMPACTION

Diarrhea is defined as the passage of frequent loose or watery stools that may be self-induced or the result of a variety of problems in the tract. It may be related to the overuse of cathartics, malabsorption syndrome, inflammation and ulceration of the mucosa, malignancies, bacterial and parasitic diseases (e.g., infection with *Clostridium difficile*). Motility disorders related to diabetic or drug-induced neuropathy, impaction, and medications such as antibiotics, the xanthines, antacids, and digoxin are also implicated in diarrhea.

The main issues for the patient are altered nutrition, fluid and electrolyte imbalance, abdominal discomfort, and irritation of the perianal tissues. The goal of therapy is to treat the underlying cause or causes. Diagnostic measures are used to identify disease conditions of the gastrointestinal tract, fluid and electrolyte imbalances are corrected, and drug therapy is evaluated for possible changes in medications.

Constipation occurs when fecal material in the bowel is too dry and hard to be passed comfortably or when bowel movements are so infrequent that they interfere with the sense of well-being. As with diarrhea, constipation may be secondary to a number of conditions, such as aganglionic megacolon (a congenital defect), which if not corrected early in life will cause problems in older adults; dietary changes, because loss of dentition makes it difficult to chew high-fiber foods; systemic changes related to hypothyroidism or diabetic neuropathy; neuromuscular damage related to stroke; myasthenia gravis or parkinsonism; injudicious use of laxatives through the years; and immobility.

The goal of treatment includes diagnosis and management of underlying diseases and increasing dietary fiber and fluids in the diet. The nurse should assist the client in choosing appropriate foods such as prune juice, bran (either sprinkled on food or made into muffins), stewed or preserved cooked fruits, and vegetables. Stool softeners, laxatives, and enemas are also helpful. Fluids should be encouraged as tolerated, but caution should be used in older adults with heart disease to avoid problems with fluid overload.

Fecal impaction occurs when there is alteration in the mechanism of defecation. Poor peristalsis, or lack of response to the defecation reflex, causes stool to pool in the rectum and become dry and compacted. Liquid stool may seep around the mass, or the patient may vomit dark-colored fluid that may be mistaken for digested blood from a stomach ulcer.

Fecal impaction includes management of constipation. Protocol may include use of a stool softener, laxatives, or enemas administered on a schedule, either standing facility orders or individual physician orders. Adequate fluid intake and regular exercise are also encouraged. A rectal examination should be performed if stool is not passed within 3 days, and appropriate treatment is administered.

INCONTINENCE

Fecal incontinence is loss of normal elimination function in an individual who was previously toilet trained, and it not only affects the patient's life but also impacts on the lives of family members. About 20 million older Americans suffer from some form of incontinence, and the impact on financial status, social life, and sexual function cannot be overstated. It is one of the many conditions that make it necessary for older adults to leave home, family, and community to enter a long-term care facility. Many older adults are admitted in a continent state, but a number of psychological and environmental factors may influence their becoming incontinent, such as lack of privacy, dependence on others for transfer to the bedpan or toilet, and being in unfamiliar surroundings. Incontinence is also secondary to age-related changes and disease processes that influence diarrhea, constipation, and fecal impaction. Conditions such as anorectal sphincter dysfunction, motility disorders that lead to impaction, and neurological and cognitive impairment related to stroke or diabetic neuropathy are also causes. As this discussion shows, age-related changes alone do not predispose to incontinence. A thorough investigation should always be done to identify the cause or causes.

A bowel history should be obtained by the nurse on admission of the patient, and a plan put in place for maintenance. If incontinence is present, and the patient is cognitively aware and psychologically able, a bowel rehabilitation program should be included in the plan of care. The patient should never be given the impression that incontinence is normal. Treatment requires a multidisciplinary team effort: gastroenterologist, nurse, certified nursing assistant, dietitian, and social worker.

Liver Disease

Physiologically, the liver ages in conjunction with aging in other parts of the body. There is a slight decrease in weight. Standard liver tests do not show significant decrease in production of enzymes, serum albumin, and bilirubin levels. However, heart disease may decrease blood flow to the organ and poor nutrition may result in decreased albumin levels (Vistal et al., 1990). Problems that affect the liver in older adults include drug-induced hepatitis, viral hepatitis, cirrhosis, and cancer.

One of the prime organs that metabolizes and detoxifies substances in the body, the liver is heavily impacted by the increased consumption of drugs in older adults. They may suffer from drug-induced hepatocellular jaundice or drug-induced hepatitis because of the many substances given to them, and also many caregivers have difficulty determining the correct dosage of a drug for the older adult.

Previously, acute viral hepatitis was seen less frequently in older adults. However, this has changed with the advent of more invasive diagnostic and surgical procedures with blood and blood products replacement therapy. Infections with hepatic viruses such as cytomegalovirus, hepatitis A virus, and hepatitis B virus are quite common, with type B hepatitis occurring more frequently and having greater morbidity and mortality. If left untreated, hepatitis B may progress to a chronic type, hepatitis C, resulting in liver cirrhosis and cancer (Blum, 1997).

Cirrhosis is damage of liver cells, which are replaced with fibrotic tissues that alter the normal anatomy of the organ. Damage may be the result of ischemia from low circulating blood volume, a pyrogenic abscess, or long-standing alcohol abuse. Cirrhosis in older adults, however, is often of unknown etiology and clinically silent.

Most cancerous tumors of the liver develop as a result of metastasis from other sites in the body, especially the gastrointestinal tract, the breast, and the lungs. The clinical manifestations of liver disease depend on the causative agent. They include fever, malaise, anorexia, nausea and vomiting, pain in the right upper quadrant, jaundice, dark urine, and clay-colored stool if there is intrahepatic obstruction. If portal hypertension is present, this may lead to esophageal varices, hemorrhoids, and ascites. The nurse should assess for activity intolerance, alteration in nutrition, and, if isolation measures are utilized, separation anxiety. Testing may reveal the presence of hepatic viruses and evidence of damage such as elevated liver enzymes and abnormal cells. Management includes physical and psychological rest; small frequent feedings with enough protein, calories, and vitamins to promote healing; and drug therapy to help with the nausea, vomiting, infection, and pain. The nurse should instruct the patient in the transmission of hepatitis and safety measures to be employed.

Gallbladder Disease

The incidence of cholelithiasis increases with age. Severe complications may result if the stones are not removed either by surgery or dissolution. Most gallstones are silent unless they enter the common bile duct, causing acute pain and biliary tract infection. Many are unable to pass down the physiologically narrow ampulla of Vater, causing obstructive jaundice and infection from refluxed bile filled with intestinal flora. The presence of stones in the gallbladder may lead to complications such as carcinoma, which occurs more often in women older than 70 years; pressure ulceration; and perforation of the wall of the gallbladder, which is found more often in men. The stones can also find their way into the small intestines, causing gallstone ileus or obstruction. Perforation may also result in peritonitis from bile draining into the abdominal cavity.

Symptoms are usually nonspecific in the older adult: who may complain of fatigue, nausea, vomiting, and anorexia. The nurse should assess the presence of fever of unknown origin, jaundice, and sepsis. Diagnosis is made by biliary contrast radiology, computed tomography, or biliary ultrasonongraphy. Initially, the patient is treated medically unless complications are present. A low-fat diet, antispasmodics, and antibiotics are given for up to 6 months; then surgery is performed to remove the stones and drain the bile duct. Bile acid therapy is also ef-

fective in dissolving certain types of bile stones and may be utilized for older adults who are poor surgical risks.

Pancreatitis

Acute pancreatitis is related to gallbladder disease, endocrine metabolic disorders, medication, obstruction from tumors, hypothermia, and surgery with closed loop obstruction. There are two types: if the microcirculation of the organ remains intact, it is known as interstitial pancreatitis. If it is disrupted, there is necrosis of pancreatic cells and hemorrhage. This may result in multisystem failure and a very high death rate in the elderly (Banks, 1993).

Females are affected more often than males. The nurse should assess the presence of upper abdominal pain that radiates to the back, abdominal tenderness, decrease in bowel sounds, nausea, vomiting, fever, agitation, and hypovolemia. The patient often leans forward in a guarding manner.

Laboratory evaluation reveals elevated amylase levels, elevated white blood cell count, and blood urea nitrogen levels that suggest an infectious process and hypovolemia. Electrocardiographic changes simulating a myocardial infarction and blood-stained pleural effusion suggesting respiratory involvement may be evident. However, their relationship to the disease is unclear and may be related to an imbalance in circulating pancreatic hormones.

During the acute phase, the nurse assists with nonsurgical management of placing the patient on NPO, starting nasogastric drainage for stomach decompression, and IV therapy for nutritional replacement. The replacement of each nutrient is dependent on the extent of damage to the organ. The patient's energy and nitrogen balance should be maintained (McClave et al., 1997). Bedrest and pain management with meperidine (Demerol) are also instituted. The prognosis depends on the causative factors; however, the condition can become chronic, necessitating pancreatic enzyme replacement and oral hypoglycemics to combat lack of pancreatic stimulation.

Summary

Nutrition and elimination are processes essential to the existence of the human organism, and the digestive and gastrointestinal system does an excellent job meeting these needs. The fact that it functions so well through the life cycle into old age deserves extra recognition, considering the assaults heaped on it by various diets, eating habits, and lifestyles. The aging process impacts in various ways on the system mainly by slowing down its motility, secretory, and absorptive abilities. However, these age-related changes, although they put the older adult at risk for disorders that impact on the system, are not supposed to result in death. Many diseases that affect older adults are not unique to them but are seen in earlier periods of life.

Nevertheless, older adults do succumb to conditions that severely impact on nutrition, hydration, elimination, and even life itself, because they are influenced not by the aging process only but by disease entities that become worse in old age. Dysphagia, neoplasms, malabsorption syndrome, hemorrhage, and incontinence all play a significant role in increasing morbidity and mortality in the later years.

The health care team, especially the nursing staff, is constantly challenged to tailor strategies and interventions to meet the needs of both the well and the sick older adult client. Good nursing care begins with primary intervention through health teaching, health screening, and appropriate interventions for other problems and needs as they arise. As research is done, and new sources of information become available, the gerontological nurse is challenged to find creative ways in which to apply interventions in the care of the older adult client.

REFERENCES

Altman FA. (1990). Changes in gastrointestinal, pancreatic, biliary, and hepatic function with aging. Gastroenterol Clin North Am 19:227–232.

American Dental Association. (1997). Preventative care for the older adult: The 12 most often asked questions (draft). Chicago: American Dental Association.

Banks PA. (1993). Acute pancreatitis: Identification of high risk patients and aggressive treatment. Gastrointest Dis Today 2(1):2–9.

Bartoshuk M, Weiffenbach M. (1990). Chemical senses and aging. In Schneider EL, Rowe JW, eds. Handbook of the Biology of Aging, 3rd ed. New York: Academic Press.

Bennett RG, Greenough WB. (1993). Approach to acute diarrhea in the elderly. Gastroenterol Clin North Am 22:517–533.

Blum HE. (1997). Update hepatitis A-G. Digestion 58(1):33–36.

Bond JH. (1997). Fecal occult blood testing for colorectal cancer: Can we afford not to do this? Gastroenterol Clin North Am 26:57–69.

Bond JH. (January 1997). Screening for colorectal cancer. Hosp Pract 59–61. January 15th 1997.

Brunner LS, Suddarth DS. (1992). Digestive and gastrointestinal function. In Brunner LS, Suddarth DS, eds. Textbook of Medical-Surgical Nursing. 7th ed. Philadelphia: JB Lippincott.

Hampton JK Jr. (1991). The Biology of Human Aging. San Luis Obispo, CA: WC Brown.

Hollis JB, Castell DO. (1974). Esophageal function in old men: New look at "presbyesophagus." Ann Internal Med 80:371–374

Kahrilas PJ. (1997). Anatomy and physiology of the gastroesophageal junction. Gastroenterol Clin North Am 26:467–471.

Levine DS. (1992). Colonic and anorectal disorders: Diagnosis and treatment. Geriatrics 47(10):22–23.

McClave SA, Snider H, Owens N, Sexton LK. (1997). Clinical nutrition in pancreatitis. Digestion 42:10:2035–2040.

Nelson JB, Castell DO. (1991). Gastroenterology. In Cassel CK, et al., eds. Geriatric Medicine. 2nd ed. New York: Springer-Verlag.

Parker SL, Tong T, Bolden S, et al. (1996). Cancer statistics. Cancer 46(5):3.

Peterson WL. (1993). Recurrent ulcers revisited: When to eradicate *Helicobacter pylori?* Gastrointest Dis Today 2(5):7–15.

Society of Gastroenterology Nurses and Associates Core Curriculum Committee. (1993). Gastroenterology Nursing: A Core Curriculum. Philadelphia: Mosby–Year Book.

Vistal ER, Cusak BJ. (1990). Pharmacology and aging. In Schneider EL, Rowe JW, eds. Handbook of the Biology of Aging. 3rd ed. New York: Academic Press.

Waters JS, Ross PJ, Popescu RA, Cunningham D. (1997). New approaches to the treatment of gastrointestinal cancer. Digestion 58:508–510.

CRITICAL THINKING EXERCISES

1. Discuss with a group of older adults at the community senior center specific guidelines for identifying gastrointestinal problems in their age group.
2. In what ways do age-related changes impact dental health and dental care pertaining to the digestive and gastrointestinal system?
3. Describe factors that should be identified in obtaining a bowel history from an older client.
4. Design a bowel rehabilitation plan that would involve a multidisciplinary team effort and suggest the role of each team member.

CHAPTER 22

Maintaining Wellness of the
Genitourinary System

Ellen Shipes, RN, MN, CETN

CHAPTER OUTLINE

OBJECTIVES

After completing this chapter, the reader should be able to:

1. Describe alterations in genitourinary function related to aging.
2. Create a teaching plan to address the psychosocial consequences of urinary incontinence for frail older adults and their families.
3. Differentiate among the common genitourinary tests and correlate them with presenting symptoms.
4. Isolate the critical components of a comprehensive genitourinary assessment.
5. Formulate a care plan for an older adult client in your own teaching facility.

azotemia
dyspareunia
oliguria
phimosis
rugae
trabeculae

Many older adults maintain genitourinary health throughout their life span. Older adults are expressing their sexuality into their 80s and beyond, with modification of their practices to suit the slower responsiveness of an aging body. Urinary disorders are not uncommon in older adults, particularly men, but many maintain adequate function throughout life. Genitourinary disorders can affect all age groups, but they are more problematic as people age. Resources (e.g., finances, transportation, access to health care) may be scarce, and the ability to deal with the condition may be lessened by physical or mental infirmities and psychosocial concerns.

HEALTH TEACHING

Health teaching to prevent or minimize genitourinary problems is centered on reducing risk factors, pursuing screening services and immunizations, maintaining and promoting sexual activity, suggesting environmental modifications, and enhancing a healthy lifestyle (including smoking cessation and weight control).

Teaching specific to the genitourinary system includes emphasis on a variety of factors that impact the system directly and indirectly. Adequate fluid intake decreases bacterial counts in urine and reduces the irritative voiding symptoms of concentrated urine. A high-fiber diet that includes vitamin C and foods such as cranberries, prunes, plums, grains, eggs, and fish acidifies urine to help prevent infection and avoid constipation, which can increase incontinence or retention. Maintenance of good hygiene, especially of the genital area, discourages bacterial invasion of the genitourinary system and maintains healthy skin. Regular toileting, bowel management, and exercise of the pelvic floor muscles help prevent urinary stasis and retention (McConnell, 1997; Burggraf, 1996).

It is also beneficial to control medical conditions that affect genitourinary function (e.g., cardiovascular disease, diabetes, Parkinson's disease, multiple sclerosis), so as to lessen the impact of the disease on genitourinary health. Nurses engaged in health teaching should also provide individuals with a list of medicines that impact voiding. These include diuretics, sedatives, antihistamines, antidepressants, anticholinergics, prolonged use of calcium-based antacids, and some antibiotics (Finkbeiner and Bissada, 1994; McIntosh and Richardson, 1994). Another important component of genitourinary teaching is participation in regular screening for cervical, bladder, testicular, and prostate conditions (Lowdermilk, 1995).

AGE-RELATED CHANGES

All cells and tissues are altered anatomically by the aging process. These changes result in altered function of the organs. A fundamental understanding of genitourinary changes associated with aging provides a basis for helping older adults maintain optimal genitourinary function and for early intervention to prevent deterioration of the upper tract.

There are both structural and functional changes in the *kidneys*. Because of the ability of the kidney to adapt, most older adults are able to maintain homeostasis despite these changes. Structural changes include a decrease in kidney size related to a reduction in the cortical mass that occurs as a result of loss of nephrons and a decrease in the number of glomeruli. Thickening of tubular membranes and sclerotic changes in blood vessels also occur. Cysts and diverticula may occur in the tubules as well. These changes mean that there is less filtering area, with an associated lessened ability to concentrate urine, impaired ability to maintain blood flow, loss of diurnal urine production, decreased response to salt intake, and decreased renin and aldosterone levels (Brundage and Linton, 1997; Chambers, 1995). These changes can be summarized as follows:

- The aging kidney is more susceptible to trauma or disease.

- Creatinine clearance is a more accurate test for renal function when administering potentially nephrotoxic drugs.
- Anemia may occur with a decrease in erythropoietin.
- Excretion of drugs is altered, leading to risk of toxicity.
- There may be hyperglycemia without glucosuria.
- Nocturia may be common. Limited water intake, increased water loss, and use of high-osmolarity agents (intravenous contrast media) may lead to renal failure.
- Slow response to salt intake and loss of salt with illness may result in cardiac, renal, and mental alterations.
- Dehydration can cause mental confusion.
- Increased salt intake by means of diet, intravenous fluids, or medicines may result in dehydration and hyperosmolarity.

Health teaching includes signs and symptoms of sodium and potassium loss or excess, the need to monitor fluid intake, the importance of learning actions and side effects of medicines, the use of a night light, and removal of loose rugs between the bedroom and bathroom.

As the *bladder* ages, the detrusor muscle becomes less elastic and weakens. There is a diminished ability to empty completely. **Trabeculae,** fibrous cords of connective tissue, and diverticula may form as smooth muscle is replaced with connective tissue. In addition, there is a general weakening of all supporting pelvic floor structures and atrophy of pelvic organs (Brundage and Linton, 1997; Chambers, 1995; Ganabath et al., 1994). Implications include

- Incomplete emptying and urinary stasis results in an increased incidence of urinary tract infections.
- Decreased capacity leads to increased frequency of voiding.
- Urine retention occurs if the bladder wall is overstretched.
- Decreased ability to postpone voiding results in urge incontinence.
- Dribbling indicates retention and overflow.
- Shortened urethra in women due to weak pelvic floor muscles results in stress incontinence.
- There is increased incidence of urinary tract infections related to incomplete emptying.

- There is an increased risk of reflux and upper tract damage.
- Skin irritation and the potential for bacterial infection and candidiasis result from maceration from the urine leak.

Health teaching includes the importance of adequate fluid intake to avoid concentrated urine, which increases irritative voiding symptoms and supports bacterial growth; the need to decrease fluid intake 2 to 4 hours before bedtime; scheduled toileting and double voiding to facilitate emptying; a night light and removal of loose rugs for safety; perineal hygiene to prevent skin breakdown; and education as to the signs and symptoms of urinary tract infection and retention (Pierson, 1995).

W e l l n e s s

"Urinary disorders are not uncommon in older adults, particularly men, but many maintain adequate function throughout life.**"**

The major change in the aging *prostate* is that of hyperplasia. It usually begins after the age of 40. As the condition develops, symptoms of retention appear (Jones, 1995; Lindeman, 1994):

- Obstructive voiding symptoms (hesitancy, frequency, feeling of incomplete emptying) develop. Symptom severity depends on the degree of obstruction.
- Decreased force of stream with poor control develops as the bladder muscle weakens from efforts to overcome the obstruction.
- Dribbling is related to retention and residual urine.
- Bleeding occurs as the bladder strains to empty and microvessels rupture.
- There is a potential for damage to the upper tract if the obstruction is severe.
- Increased urinary tract infections are related to incomplete bladder emptying.
- Bladder wall hypertrophy occurs as the bladder exerts itself to overcome the narrowed outlet.
- Bladder diverticula are possible because of increased voiding pressures.
- Acute retention can develop suddenly and is a urological emergency.

Health teaching includes signs and symptoms of urinary tract infection and retention; double voiding to enhance emptying; avoiding medicines that relax the bladder muscle or cause sphincter spasm; and the importance of regular prostate examinations.

Women experience a generalized atrophy of *genitalia* related to hormonal changes. These include decreased fat, external hair loss, and labial flattening. The vagina becomes smooth and shiny, drier, narrower, and shorter. Tissues lose elasticity and **rugae,** or folds, become thinner, and have an increased pH (Brundage and Linton, 1997; Gallo et al., 1995; Lowdermilk, 1995). The following may occur:

- There is an increased risk of vaginal trauma with tissue damage and bleeding.
- An increased risk of pruritus and infection, especially with *Candida,* may be noted because of higher pH.
- Altered sexual responses, such as delayed lubrication, **dyspareunia** (painful coitus), and uterine cramps with orgasm, may occur.
- The emotional impact of sexual dysfunction may be hidden.

Health teaching includes normal sexual response with aging; measures to aid in lubrication; importance of good hygiene; signs and symptoms of infection along with topical treatments; pros and cons of estrogen replacement therapy; and sexual positions to decrease discomfort.

As men age they develop lesser degrees of atrophy. The penis and scrotal structures appear smaller as fat is lost. In some men the scrotum may appear larger because of loss of elasticity of supporting tissues. Although men can be sexually active into their 90s, there may be varying degrees of erectile and ejaculatory dysfunction. These are seldom related to hormone depletion and are often associated with decreased blood flow to the penis; comorbid conditions such as cardiovascular, peripheral vascular, or pulmonary disease; arthritis; diabetes; or medicines that affect penile nerve, vascular, or muscle function; and surgical procedures that interrupt nervous innervation of the penis (Gallo et al., 1995; Lowdermilk, 1995). Implications include the following:

- Medical conditions need to be controlled to reduce their impact on sexual function.
- Surgical procedures may restore blood flow in some conditions.

- There are some nerve-sparing operations that preserve erectile function.
- Medicines may need to be changed or doses altered.
- Emotional impact of sexual dysfunction may be hidden.

Health teaching includes normal sexual function with aging; need to question physician and pharmacist regarding the impact of medicines on sexual function; need for regular examination of genitalia; if uncircumcised, good hygiene to prevent phimosis; and importance of maintaining good general health state.

■ GUIDELINES SPECIFIC TO ASSESSING THE GENITOURINARY SYSTEM IN OLDER ADULTS

Components of a genitourinary assessment encompass a medical history with a focus on urinary symptoms; a list of current medications; an appraisal of functional, mental, and emotional status; a psychosocial history; an estimate of existing support systems; and the physical examination (McIntosh and Richardson, 1994).

The medical history focuses on previous or current medical conditions that cause or contribute to genitourinary problems. Some of the most prominent are cerebrovascular accident, diabetes, cardiovascular disorders, pulmonary disorders, parity for women, prostate disorders for men, and gynecological or genitourinary operations. If there are urinary symptoms or symptoms of voiding difficulty, it is important to determine the type and degree of problems. Questions should address hesitancy, straining, dribbling, dysuria, difficulty starting stream, poor stream, or hematuria. Other considerations are onset of symptoms; factors that worsen or improve the condition; location, onset, duration, and severity of pain; frequency of incontinence; leaking of urine, with estimated amount and frequency; amount and type of fluid intake; past and current treatments and outcomes; and incontinence aids used (Norton, 1991; Pierson, 1995). There are more than 20 medications that cause or contribute to urinary incontinence (Finkbeiner and Bissada, 1994; Karch, 1998).

Assessment of functional status examines mobility and activity, use of mobility aids such as walkers, difficulty transferring onto toilet, difficulty with clothing, sensory changes, dietary habits, elimination patterns, sleep-rest patterns, sexual activity, and ability to perform activities of daily living. Exploration of mental status includes cognition, depression, anxiety, or recent mood changes. Evaluation of emotional state involves reactions to aging and consequent alterations in activities and lifestyle, response to illness, and coping strategies. Environmental assessment includes toileting facilities, number of people using the toilet, obstacles to toileting, and bathing and laundry facilities (Lekan-Rutledge, 1997; Norton, 1990).

Physical assessment includes observation, palpation, percussion, and auscultation and examination of the skin, genitalia, bladder, prostate, kidneys, and urine, with a determination as to whether incontinence is present. Table 22–1 presents symptoms and related tests, and Table 22–2 sets forth the diagnostic tests and their results and implications.

In assessing the individual's *skin,* the nurse should look for overall signs of poor hygiene, dehydration, and edema. The perineal skin is checked for irritation, redness, lesions, and *Candida.* The external *genitalia* is observed for lesions, atrophic changes, irritation, vaginal or urethral discharge, and the condition of surrounding tissues. The color and distribution of pubic hair is noted. The examiner should also check for lice and scabies. The labia and scrotum should be palpated for masses, lesions, pain, or edema. Any unusual odor is noted. The nurse should note the location of the meatus as well as any purulent or bloody discharge. The client should be referred for a thorough gynecological or genitourinary examination if one has not been done in a year (Chambers, 1995; Lowdermilk, 1995).

In assessing the *bladder,* the examiner should inspect the abdomen for asymmetry, ecchymoses, redness, or swelling. Percussion is done of the abdomen over the suprapubic area; dullness indicates bladder fullness. The abdomen is palpated for bladder height and fullness, pelvic masses, and pain. If necessary, a catheter is placed for postvoid residual (Chambers, 1995; Ganabath et al., 1994; Albertson, 1997).

During assessment of the prostate, the individual is asked to void first, then lie supine. The abdomen is percussed and palpated for blad-

TABLE 22–1. Tests Related to Genitourinary Signs and Symptoms

Sign or Symptom	Test
Frequency	Urinalysis
Burning	Culture and sensitivity
Odor	
Fever	
Flank/abdominal pain	
Hematuria	
Leaking	Urinalysis
Dribbling	Urodynamics
Urgency	Culture and sensitivity
Pain	Urinalysis
Frequency	Culture and sensitivity
Hematuria	Kidney-ureter-bladder radiography
Painless hematuria	Kidney-ureter-bladder radiography
	Cystoscopy
	Blood urea nitrogen/creatinine/creatinine clearance/computed tomography/ultrasonography
Incomplete emptying	Digital rectal examination
Dribbling	Cystoscopy
Suprapubic discomfort	Blood urea nitrogen/creatinine/creatinine clearance
	Urinalysis
	Culture and sensitivity

der distention. The bladder requires 150 mL to be palpated. Then the individual is placed in the knee-chest position or bent over the examination table. A digital rectal examination is done to detect masses, size, consistency, and sphincter tone. The prostate should be smooth, of a uniform consistency, nontender, and about the size of a walnut. An increase in size usually indicates cancer or benign prostatic hypertrophy. The prostate is assessed for signs and symptoms of obstruction: hesitancy, irritative voiding symptoms, decreased force and caliber of the stream, and postvoid dribble. A postvoid residual catheterization is done if there is a concern about residual urine. The client is referred for a thorough urological examination if any abnormalities are detected

TABLE 22–2. Diagnostic Tests, Results, and Implications

Test	Results	Implications
Urinalysis	Color change	Medicines/blood/bile
	pH > 7.0	Urinary tract infection/high-alkali diet/ use of antacids/systemic alkalosis
	pH < 5.0	High-protein diet/fever/metabolic or respiratory acidosis
	< Specific gravity	Diabetes insipidus/renal problems/ hypercalcemia/hypokalemia
	> Specific gravity	Congestive heart failure/dehydration
	Red blood cells	Inflammation/stones/necrosis
	White blood cells	Infection/renal disease
	Bacteria	Infection
Blood urea nitrogen	Decreased	Liver damage/malnutrition
	Increased	Renal disease
Creatinine	Increased	Renal damage
Creatinine clearance	Decreased	Reduced renal blood flow/renal disease
Kidney-ureter-bladder radiography	Shows kidney size, position, structure; may show stones, other lesions	
Excretory urography	Allows visualization of structure of kidneys, ureters, bladder, urethra; may show stones, lesions	
Retrograde cystography	Helps diagnose bladder trauma, urinary tract infection, neurogenic bladder, fistulas, reflux	
Voiding cystourethrography	Helps identify reflux, chronic urinary tract infection, incontinence, genitourinary abnormalities	
Ultrasonography	Shows internal structures, lesions, fluid accumulation, anomalies	
Urodynamics	Identifies voiding problems	
Uroflow		
Cystometrography		
Urethral pressure profile		
Electromyography		

(Ganabath et al., 1994; Jones, 1995; Albertson, 1997).

When assessing the *kidneys,* the abdomen is inspected for swelling, ecchymoses, redness, or asymmetry. The examiner should auscultate over the midclavicular line for bruits, which indicate renal artery stenosis or obstruction. With the individual lying supine, all four quadrants of the abdomen are palpated for masses or tenderness. One hand is placed under the kidney, and the other is on the abdomen below the rib cage. Each kidney is palpated in turn, looking for change in size, nodules, or pain. The costovertebral angle is percussed to detect pain. The same area is palpated for dullness (Chambers, 1995).

Urine characteristics such as clarity, odor, blood, and sediment are checked. Dark urine signifies concentration, whereas very light urine indicates dilution. A red/brown color signifies blood or the presence of some medications. A foul odor usually denotes infection. Cloudiness is significant for infection or increased amount of sediment. An increased pH may indicate infection by urea-splitting organisms, dietary changes, or renal disease (or that the specimen is old) (Chambers, 1995).

A female client is tested for *stress incontinence* by having her drink a glass of water. Once a sense of bladder fullness is reached, she is asked to stand, hold gauze or a pad over the perineum, and then cough actively. The pad is checked for the amount of urine lost. Another test is to wait for sensation of bladder fullness, have the woman in the lithotomy position, and ask her to cough and observe for urine leak. Urge incontinence can be tested by observing time from sensation of need to void to actual voiding. Clients are asked to keep a bladder record for at least 1 week. They record the amount, time, and type of fluid intake, the time and estimate of leakage, and the number of pads used per day. Some records also note activity occurring at the time of leak.

COMMON DISORDERS

Acute Renal Failure

Acute renal failure occurs when there is an abrupt drop in the glomerular filtration rate. Causes may be (1) intrinsic: thromboembolic incidents, acute tubular necrosis due to nephrotoxic substances, damage to the cortex, or acute glomerulonephritis; (2) prerenal: shock, sepsis, congestive heart failure, volume depletion; and (3) postrenal: obstruction related to tumor, stones, strictures, clots, and benign prostatic hypertrophy (Brundage and Linton, 1997). The most common signs and symptoms include altered mental status, acidosis, azotemia, oliguria, hyperkalemia, and increased blood urea nitrogen and creatinine levels (Brundage and Linton, 1997).

Caring

"Nurses must be sensitive to the fact that older people may believe that urinary incontinence is a normal part of aging or be too embarrassed to introduce the subject."

Treatment options include removal of the obstruction, if possible; initiation of hemodialysis or peritoneal dialysis for hyperkalemia, fluid overload, and/or **azotemia** (presence of nitrogenous bodies, especially urea in the blood); administration of antibiotics for infection; placement of a nephrostomy tube to provide drainage until the kidney recovers; correction of any acidosis; and dietary and medicine modifications (Brundage and Linton, 1997). Dietary alterations are focused on the prevention or reduction of uremic symptoms, on hypotension/hypertension, on slowing the progression of the disease, on control of hy-

pertension, and on maintenance of an optimal nutritional state. Medication changes include avoiding nephrotoxic elements such as aminoglycosides, contrast media, analgesics, phenacetin, acetylsalicylic acid, and nonsteroidal antiinflammatory drugs (American Dietetic Association, 1996).

Chronic Renal Failure

Chronic renal failure is irreversible loss of kidney function. Causes include diabetic neuropathy, obstructive uropathy, nephrotoxic agents, hypertensive neuropathy, and multiple myeloma. Signs and symptoms are **oliguria** (diminished amount of urine formation); azotemia; edema; itchy, dry skin; fatigue; nausea and vomiting; malaise; weakness; mental status changes; anemia; increased blood urea nitrogen and phosphate levels; and decreased creatinine and creatinine clearance (Chambers, 1995; Jones, 1997). Dietary planning and drug modification are the same as for acute renal failure.

Treatment consists of controlling hypertension and diabetes; managing anemia with iron supplements or erythropoietin; electrolyte adjustment; regulating medicine dosage to avoid toxicity related to impaired renal excretion; restriction of protein, potassium, and sodium; control of infection, if present; dialysis; and transplantation. Dialysis is used to maintain homeostasis. Caution is needed when hemodialyzing older adults because the stress of the procedure, anticoagulation, and fluid changes may increase risk for those with cardiac disease (Brundage and Linton, 1997). In these instances, peritoneal dialysis may be used. Transplantation for those older than 60 has been successful.

Renal Stones

The etiology of renal (kidney) stones is multifactorial and includes infection, increased urinary pH, chronic diarrhea, decreased mobility and urinary stasis, dehydration, increased elimination of uric acid, and hypercalcemia. Symptoms are pain, hematuria, and the irritative voiding symptoms of frequency, urgency, and the feeling of incomplete emptying.

Treatment of stones is directed at removing the etiology and relieving the symptoms. Elec-

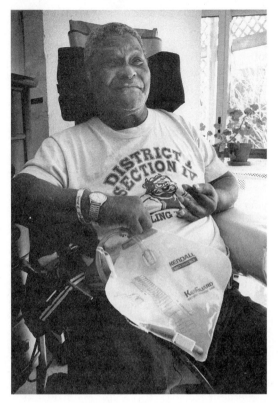

Utmost care must be taken to maintain adequate cleanliness and to prevent irritation in patients with indwelling catheters.

trocorporal shock wave lithotripsy (ESWL) or percutaneous nephrolithotomy are the most common interventions for stone removal. ESWL lithotripsy is usually reserved for stones less than 1.5 cm and ureteral stones. Percutaneous nephrolithotomy is used for stones greater than 2.5 cm, when there is obstruction distal to the stone or renal anomalies, when it is not possible to position the person for ESWL, or for an impacted stone (Fuchs et al., 1994). Some physicians advocate dietary intervention to prevent stone recurrence. Dietary changes are directed at prevention of saturation of the urine with salts and minerals that form the nidus of stones and at decreasing intake of substances that might contribute to increased urinary excretion of these products. Increased fluid intake is the most important factor, because it decreases urinary saturation levels. Because most stones are calcium oxalate stones, the individual may need to decrease in-

take of dairy foods and foods high in oxalate. These include beer, chocolate, instant tea and coffee, grits, wheat bran, nuts, berries, beets, beans, and dark leafy vegetables (American Dietetic Association, 1996). It is important to control the intake of medicines that contribute to stone formation. These include salicylates, thiazides, probenecid, nonsteroidal antiinflammatory drugs (especially phenylbutazone [Butazolidin]), chronic corticosteroid use, carbonic anhydrase inhibitors, and vitamin D intoxication.

Glomerulonephritis

Chronic glomerulonephritis is not uncommon in older adults. Symptoms may be vague and may be attributed to other medical conditions. They include fatigue, nausea, vomiting, anemia, edema, arthralgias, anorexia, pain, hypertension, and an increased sedimentation rate. There may be headache, followed by altered mental status and coma due to cerebral edema as the disease progresses. Antibiotics, protein and sodium restriction, and close monitoring of intake and output are basic management strategies. Drug toxicity is a concern, so regulation of medicines is vital.

Pyelonephritis

Chronic pyelonephritis is often associated with habitual overuse of phenacetin-containing drugs. Fever, frequency, urgency, hematuria, burning, and bacteriuria are common and may be mistaken for cystitis. Costovertebral angle pain of varying severity and pyuria confirm the diagnosis of pyelonephritis. Treatment consists of antibiotics specific to the causative organism and careful monitoring of fluid intake. If left untreated, the chronic form of the disease can lead to progressive kidney damage.

Bladder Cancer

Bladder cancer is the second most common urological cancer (Skinner and Skinner, 1994; American Cancer Society, 1994). Smoking is the primary risk factor for bladder cancer. Environmental factors such as industrial exposure to dyes, rubber, leather, paint, organic chemicals, and aluminum products are also associated with the development of bladder cancer. The presenting sign of bladder cancer is usually gross, painless hematuria, although individuals may present with symptoms of infection. Retention may develop if bleeding results in clot formation. Diagnosis is made with a biopsy, usually through cystourethroscopy.

The stage of the cancer dictates treatment parameters. Superficial cancers may be treated with fulguration and/or intravesical instillation of chemotherapeutic agents. Invasive cancers without metastasis usually result in partial or radical cystectomy. A radical cystectomy is most often accompanied by bilateral pelvic lymph node dissection. Radical cystectomy requires diversion of the urinary tract, and individuals may have the option of a standard ileal conduit, colon conduit, continent diversion, or orthotopic neobladder. Bone or lymph node metastasis is usually treated with chemotherapy and/or radiation therapies (Skinner and Skinner, 1994).

W e l l n e s s

❝*Health teaching includes the importance of adequate fluid intake to avoid concentrated urine, which increases irritative voiding symptoms and supports bacterial growth.***❞**

Urinary Tract Infection

There is an increasing prevalence of urinary tract infection in older adults. The most common of these conditions are urethritis and cystitis (Nicolle, 1994). Risk factors include poor fluid intake, which results in urinary stasis and concentration; increased pH; catheterization; sexual activity; and urinary tract abnormalities. Causes are decreased estrogen in women, the use of external urinary collection devices such as condom catheters and bedside drainage bags, indwelling catheters, and systemic diseases. The most common are neurogenic bladder related to diabetes and Alzheimer's disease, benign prostatic hypertrophy, and retention. Cystitis can be noninfectious and infectious. Noninfectious cystitis is caused by chemotherapy and radiation therapy and interstitial cystitis. Infectious cystitis is caused by bacteria, fungi, viruses, and parasites. The causative organisms are usually *Escherichia coli, Proteus, En-* *terobacter, Klebsiella, Staphylococcus aureus,* and *Candida.* Organisms ascend the tract from external sources. Symptoms include irritative voiding symptoms, hematuria, and foul odor (Nicolle, 1994; Pierson, 1995). Diagnosis is made from symptoms and culture or biopsy. Because older adults are at great risk for sepsis, early intervention is imperative.

Appropriate antibiotics are given based on the identified organism. Common antibiotics are quinolones, nitrofurantoin, trimethoprim-sulfamethoxazole, amoxicillin, and cephalosporins. Urinary acidification with vitamin C, cranberry juice, or methenamine (Mandelamine) may be recommended, although there is controversy related to the effectiveness of this treatment. Bladder spasms are treated with antispasmodics or suppositories. Fluid intake is increased to flush the system and dilute the urine. It is important to teach risk factors and methods for preventing reinfection, such as voiding immediately after sex, adequate fluid intake, good perineal hygiene, and a regular voiding schedule with double voiding, if needed, to completely empty the bladder (Brundage and Linton, 1997; Nicolle, 1994; Pierson, 1995).

Urinary Retention

Urinary retention may be acute or chronic. Acute retention is a urological emergency and demands immediate intervention. Chronic retention develops slowly over time. Retention is the result of obstruction. Causes include stones, bladder or prostate cancer, benign prostatic hypertrophy, **phimosis** (inability to retract the foreskin), stricture or trauma, stenosis, uterine prolapse, neurological problems, fecal impaction, and medications. Symptoms are inability to void, overflow dribbling, a palpable suprapubic mass, and pain. Protracted retention may result in azotemia and upper tract damage. Assessment reveals a distended bladder, dribbling with overflow, and varying degrees of discomfort (Brundage and Linton, 1997).

Bladder drainage is essential. If trauma or stricture prevents urethral catheterization, then a suprapubic approach is used. Other treatments are directed at removing or reducing the cause. Obstructive pathology is removed surgically, if possible. If surgery is not a choice, intermittent catheterization is the preferred method of emptying the bladder on a regular basis (Brundage and Linton, 1997).

Vaginitis

Atrophic, or senile, vaginitis is common in estrogen-deprived older women. As tissues thin and become dry, the women are more vulnerable to trauma and infection. Symptoms are pruritus, burning, dyspareunia, and bleeding. The main line treatment is estrogen replacement therapy or topical estrogen. Health teaching includes methods of lubrication, avoidance of trauma by reducing or discontinuing douching, use of coital positions that limit deep penetration or damage, and the importance of good perineal hygiene. Other management options are vitamin therapy with vitamins A, B-complex, C, and E, increased ingestion of foods rich in beta-carotene, and the addition of cultured yogurt to the diet.

Benign Prostatic Hypertrophy

As men age, the prostate develops an increased number of cells (hyperplasia), which leads to enlargement of the gland (hypertrophy) (Jones, 1995). Benign prostatic hypertrophy occurs in 80% of men older than age 60. The incidence increases with each decade. By age 50 years, 50% of men have the disorder. Of these, 50% have some degree of voiding difficulties. Ten percent of these men need surgery to relieve their symptoms. Benign prostatic hypertrophy is thought to be hormonal, although investigators are examining the role of chronic inflammation and nutrition in its development. The process is asymptomatic until the growth impinges on the bladder outlet. Presenting symptoms are urinary tract infections, difficulty starting the stream, postvoid dribbling, a feeling of incomplete emptying, decreased size and force of the stream, irritative voiding symptoms, and nocturia. As the obstruction progresses, the bladder muscle decompensates and retention occurs. Overflow incontinence, reflux, and hydronephrosis develop (Jones, 1995). Assessment includes history and symptoms, percussion and palpation of the bladder for residual urine, digital rectal examination, and cystoscopy (Jones, 1995).

Treatment options are surgical or pharmacological. Surgical interventions include transurethral resection of the prostate, suprapubic prostatectomy, retropubic prostatectomy, and perineal prostatectomy. Balloon dilation of the prostatic urethra, placement of stems, cryosurgery, and microwave hyperthermia are options for poor surgical candidates. Pharmacological therapy with alpha-adrenergic blocking agents is used to decrease sympathetic stimulation of the prostate and bladder neck. Antiandrogens decrease prostate size and improve urinary flow (Jones, 1995; National Association for Continence, 1995).

Prostate Cancer

Prostate cancer is the most common cancer in men (American Cancer Society, 1994). By 2000 there will be a 90% increase in the total number of cases (Dreicer and Williams, 1994). The etiology is uncertain, although dietary fat might be implicated to some degree. Prostate cancer is the slowest growing of all cancers. Although over 50% of men older than age 70 will have prostate cancer, less than 3% will die of the disease (Abrams et al., 1995). Metastasis is usually to lymph nodes and bone. Gross, painless hematuria is usually the presenting symptom, although the signs and symptoms of outflow obstruction may also be present (Jones, 1995). Diagnosis is made by digital rectal examination, transrectal ultrasonography, and biopsy. Measuring levels of prostate-specific antigen is a good screening tool for early detection and determination of response to therapy but is not a reliable predictor of the stage of the disease (Dreicer and Williams, 1994). Treatment is based on stage and the ability of the individual to withstand therapy. It includes surgery, radiation, and hormone therapy. Health teaching focuses on management strategies for the side effects of therapies, diet and fluids, pain management, and resumption of activities of daily living to the optimum permitted by the person's health status.

Urinary Incontinence

Urinary incontinence is defined as the involuntary loss of urine that is demonstrable and is a social and/or hygienic problem (Brundage and Linton, 1997; Kincaid, 1993). Urinary incontinence affects approximately 10 million people in the United States, mostly older adults. It affects 15% to 30% of noninstitutionalized people older than age 60 and 50% or more of those in institutional facilities (U.S. Department of Health and Human Services, 1992). Nurses must be sensitive to the fact that older adults may believe that urinary incontinence is a normal part of aging or be too embarrassed to introduce the subject. The initial interview should be set to elicit responses that will initiate a discussion of the particular incontinence problem. It is important to understand that urinary incontinence is a symptom of an underlying problem not a disease. A thorough assessment is necessary to determine the underlying cause so that appropriate treatment(s) may be initiated as soon as possible. Urinary incontinence may be transient or established. Transient incontinence is treated by eliminating the underlying etiology. An acronym for the causes of transient urinary incontinence is DIAPERS:

D = delirium
I = infection
A = atrophic vaginitis or urethritis
P = pharmacological, psychological
E = endocrine, excessive urine production
R = restricted mobility
S = stool impaction

The Agency for Health Care Policy and Research (U.S. Department of Health and Human Services, 1992) has defined three primary categories of established urinary incontinence: stress, urge, and overflow. Two other frequently addressed classifications are mixed and functional.

STRESS INCONTINENCE

Stress incontinence is the involuntary loss of urine during coughing, sneezing, laughing, or other physical activity that increases abdominal pressure (Gray, 1992; U.S. Department of Health and Human Services, 1992). The cause is most often hypermobility and displacement of the urethra and bladder neck junction during activity. Another cause of stress incontinence is internal urethral sphincter deficiency (Gray, 1992; U.S. Department of Health and Human Services, 1992). The weakness may be the sequelae of multiple pregnancies, prosta-

tectomy, radiation therapy, trauma, or sacral cord pathology. A complete evaluation includes the interview and components of the physical examination as previously described. Specific information needed to diagnose stress urinary incontinence follows. The history includes

- Symptoms, duration, and precipitating factors
- Parity with difficult deliveries; gynecological or genitourinary surgeries
- Previous treatments and outcomes
- Use of pads or other urine collectors

Caring

❝Nurses can position themselves to coordinate care across the spectrum of health maintenance, prevention, interventions, and treatment, thus enhancing quality while ensuring cost-effectiveness.❞

The physical examination focuses on provocative stress testing—asking the individual to cough vigorously with full bladder to determine the amount of leak and urodynamic testing by a qualified specialist if necessary.

Basic interventions include treatment of chronic cough and constipation, weight loss (if needed), and modification of activities that exacerbate the problem. A variety of treatments are effective for stress urinary incontinence. They include pelvic-floor exercises, pharmacological intervention, pessaries, and surgery. Tables 22–3 through 22–6 present interventions for incontinence of various causes.

Pelvic floor muscle exercises (sometimes called Kegel exercises) strengthen the muscles of the pelvic floor, including those of the sphincters. They are most effective for mild to moderate degrees of stress urinary incontinence. Consistency and adherence to the regimen is necessary for success. Evaluation of the effectiveness of the program is through subjective reports of fewer incontinent episodes by the individual, perineometry to measure muscle strength, a urethral pressure profile to assess sphincter competence, or documentation of increased muscle strength when inserting a finger into the vagina (Gray, 1991a).

Pessaries are ring-, donut-, oblong-, or

TABLE 22–3. Behavioral Interventions for Incontinence

Intervention	Method	Uses
Bladder training	Resist/inhibit urge Postpone voiding Void on timetable	Stress Urge
Habit training	Timed voiding Scheduled toileting	Intractable Cognitively impaired
Prompted voiding	Teach to know when incontinent—ask for help	Dependent people Cognitively impaired
Pelvic muscle exercises	Contraction of pubococcygeal and pelvic muscles	Stress Urge After prostate and gynecological operations
Vaginal cones	Contract muscles with cone in place to strengthen pubococcygeal and pelvic muscles	Stress
Biofeedback	Electronic display to relay information about ability to change physiological response	Stress

Data from U.S. Department of Health and Human Services, Agency for Health Care Policy and Research. (1992). Clinical Practice Guidelines: Urinary Incontinence in Adults, pp 27–34. Washington, DC: U.S. Government Printing Office.

TABLE 22–4. Pharmacologic Interventions for Urge Incontinence

Medication	Actions
Propantheline	Anticholinergic—blocks bladder contractions
Oxybutynin	Anticholinergic and smooth muscle relaxer
Calcium channel blockers	Block calcium influx; inhibit bladder contractions
Terodiline	Anticholinergic Calcium channel blocker
Tricyclic antidepressants	Anticholinergic Alpha agonist—improves urethral resistance
Flavoxate	Smooth muscle relaxant
Dicyclomine	Anticholinergic Smooth muscle relaxer

Data from U.S. Department of Health and Human Services, Agency for Health Care Policy and Research. (1992). Clinical Practice Guidelines: Urinary Incontinence in Adults, pp 38–42. Washington, DC: U.S. Government Printing Office.

TABLE 22–5. Pharmacological Interventions for Stress Incontinence

Medication	Actions
Phenylpropanolamine	Alpha-adrenergic agonist—improves urethral resistance
Estrogen	May restore urethral coaptation, increase tone
Combination of alpha-adrenergic agonist and estrogen therapy	Improves urethral resistance and tone
Imipramine	May improve urethral resistance
Propranolol	Beta-adrenergic blocker; may improve urethral resistance

Data from U.S. Department of Health and Human Services, Agency for Health Care Policy and Research. (1992). Clinical Practice Guidelines: Urinary Incontinence in Adults, pp 43–47. Washington, DC: U.S. Government Printing Office.

TABLE 22–6. Surgical Interventions for Incontinence		
Type of Incontinence	**Surgery**	**Action**
Stress bladder	Urethral suspensions	Anatomic repositioning of neck and urethra
	Teflon/collagen injections	Compress urethra
	Artificial sphincter	Compress urethra
Overflow due to obstruction	Prostatectomy	Removes etiology of obstruction
	Removal of other obstruction	
Bladder dysfunction	Urinary diversion	Provides continent (internal) or incontinent (external) mechanism for urine drainage

sphere-shaped devices that are inserted into the vagina. They work by mechanically restoring the sphincter to a more anatomically correct position. Pessaries can be used for severe stress urinary incontinence or for women who are not surgical candidates. Teaching is important. It involves correct pessary placement and hygiene. Follow-up is vital to monitor for effectiveness and for potential problems such as vaginal wall erosion (Gray, 1991a,b).

Estrogen deficiency responds to topical or systemic estrogen therapy. The pharmacological interventions of alpha-adrenergic drugs (ephedrine, pseudoephedrine, phenylpropanolamine/chlorpheniramine [Ornade]) work by increasing urethral resistance. Health teaching includes drug side effects, the need to avoid drugs and foods that contain caffeine, good hygiene, and reportable signs and symptoms (Gray, 1991a,b).

Surgical procedures are designed to suspend the urethra in the correct anatomical position. Periurethral Teflon and collagen injections can achieve the same outcome. A urologist should discuss pros and cons of each procedure before a choice is made (Gray, 1991b; National Association for Continence, 1995).

W e l l n e s s

"Older adults are expressing their sexuality into their 80s and beyond, with modification of their practices to suit the slower responsiveness of an aging body.**"**

URGE INCONTINENCE

Urge incontinence is loss of urine with a sudden urge to void (U.S. Department of Health and Human Services, 1992). Involuntary bladder contractions may or may not be present. Evaluation includes

- The usual assessment parameters
- Symptoms: a report of an urge to void with an almost immediate leak of urine. The woman will report that she cannot get to the toilet in time.
- Check of the postvoid residual to be certain the bladder is emptying properly
- Urinalysis to assess for infection, which can cause incontinence
- Use of a voiding record for 2 weeks to determine amount and frequency of voiding
- Cystometry: a voiding cystometrogram measures detrusor contractility. Simple cystometry involves filling the bladder using a catheter and saline. Bladder capacity can be determined when an involuntary contraction occurs.

Treatment usually involves fluid and dietary management, bladder training, electrical stimulation, biofeedback, and drug therapy (Gray, 1991b; National Association for Continence, 1995).

Fluid management includes intake of fluids on a regular schedule until about 2 L has been consumed. Excessive fluid intake (over 2000 mL) should be avoided. Leaking can occur when the bladder is overwhelmed with large amounts of urine. Dietary changes consist of eliminating or reducing foods or drinks containing caffeine, alcohol, and hot seasoning because these are all bladder irritants (Gray, 1991a,b; National Association for Continence, 1995).

Bladder control is often restored with prompted voiding (scheduled toileting) or bladder drill (Gray, 1991b). Both use a regular schedule of voiding, approximately every 2 hours. Bladder drill differs in that it requires a gradual increase in the interval between voidings until an acceptable level of 3 to 4 hours is reached (Gray, 1991b).

Electrostimulation uses a probe placed in the rectum or vagina. Stimulation inhibits bladder contractions. Treatments last for 20 minutes and are done daily or as prescribed by the physician. Treatments can be done in the office or at home (Gray 1991b; National Association for Continence, 1995). Biofeedback is used to confirm the person's physical ability to inhibit unstable contractions after pelvic floor muscle exercises or electrostimulation. Electrodes are placed in the anal area. The number and strength of the contractions are shown on a screen. A printout is available (Gray, 1991b; O'Donnell, 1994; National Association for Continence, 1995). Antispasmodic and anticholinergic medicines increase bladder capacity by decreasing bladder contractility. Health teaching includes correct dose and schedule and side effects (Gray, 1991b).

OVERFLOW INCONTINENCE

Overflow incontinence is caused by a hypoactive bladder or bladder outlet obstruction (e.g., stones, tumors, strictures) (Gray, 1991b; National Association for Continence, 1995). The presenting symptom is usually dribbling and a complaint that the bladder does not feel empty after voiding. There may also be frequency and hesitancy. Urodynamic studies confirm the cause. The goal of treatment is to remove or reduce the obstruction. Healthy bowel habits will prevent fecal impaction. Surgical removal of obstruction is optimal.

If surgery is not an option, an indwelling catheter may be the treatment of choice. Because the indwelling catheter is a foreign object, complications are frequent. They include infection, meatal trauma, and bladder neck trauma. If long-term use is anticipated, specific

guidelines need to be followed. Silicone or hydrogel catheters cause less irritation or mucosal trauma than latex. An increase in latex allergies makes these catheters even more appealing. For most adults, a French size of 16 or 18 is sufficient. It is helpful to develop a procedure for routine catheter maintenance. Information to include is listed below:

1. Adequate daily fluid intake to enhance flow and prevent obstruction related to increased sediment
2. Provision of a drainage system—leg bag for daytime use and bedside bag for night use
3. Proper taping of the catheter—on the abdomen or lateral thigh for men and on the lateral thigh for women
4. Procedure for meatal care and routine cleaning of drainage bag. Half vinegar and half water or a light bleach/water mix is recommended.
5. Provision for routine change and reevaluation (Gray, 1991a,b). Infection is treated with appropriate antibiotics.

If the cause of the obstruction is a hypoactive bladder, intermittent self-catheterization is the treatment of choice. If the obstruction is mild, double voiding will facilitate bladder emptying. The person is taught to void once, remain on the toilet for a few minutes, then void again. Fluid intake is managed by scheduling fluids on a regular basis throughout the day. Fluids can be restricted 2 hours before bedtime. This is helpful in controlling frequency and nocturia (Gray, 1991a,b; U.S. Department of Health and Human Services, 1992). Health teaching includes medication side effects and schedule, hygiene, CIC (clean intermittent catheterization) or catheter care, fluid and dietary requirements, and reportable symptoms.

FUNCTIONAL INCONTINENCE

Functional incontinence is related to impaired physical or cognitive functioning. A comprehensive workup is needed to ensure that there is no physiological basis for the incontinence. Management goals include measures to improve mobility (walker, cane, braces, proper footwear, attention to visual needs, improved access to the toilet, bedside commode, urinal, environmental safety) and dexterity (Velcro

TABLE 22–7. Other Management Options for Incontinence

Option	Uses
Self intermittent catheterization	Inoperable overflow
	Inoperable detrusor/sphincter dyssynergia
	Acute/chronic retention
	Neurogenic bladder
	Large residual volumes
External collection products	Total incontinence
	Cognitive impairment
Penile clamps	Total incontinence
Pessaries	Inoperable urethral problems
Containment products	Total incontinence
	Inoperable conditions
Skin care	Cleansers—nonirritating, no rinse, emollients, surfactants
	Protective barriers (creams, sprays, ointments)—provide protective barrier
	Moisturizers (creams, lotions, salves)—keep skin supple
	Medicated powders, creams, gels (antibacterial and antifungal)—treat specific skin problems

Data from U.S. Department of Health and Human Services, Agency for Health Care Policy and Research. (1992). Clinical Practice Guidelines: Urinary Incontinence in Adults, pp 59–65. Washington, DC: U.S. Government Printing Office.

tabs instead of buttons or zippers, avoidance of layers of clothing, avoidance of underwear) and methods for enhancing cognition and motivation (scheduled toileting, behavioral therapy) (Gray, 1991a,b).

MIXED INCONTINENCE

Mixed incontinence is relatively common in older people. It is a combination of stress and urge incontinence. Treatment is focused on managing the causes and symptoms (U.S. Department of Health and Human Services, 1992). Table 22–7 presents further intervention options for incontinence.

▌ CARE PLANNING

Developing a plan of care is a multidisciplinary process that begins with the first contact and proceeds across the health care continuum. The plan of care includes a care plan or collaborative path, home care instructions for procedures, medicine instructions, and a discharge plan. The discharge plan usually in-

cludes the person's health goals, the treatment goals and expected outcomes, health teaching, support system, discharge needs (education, diet, supplies, equipment, medicines, and referrals (clinic, home health, extended care, physical therapy, occupational therapy). The multidisciplinary team documents all findings and treatments in the plan of care to facilitate communication among all team members and record progress toward goal achievement.

C a r i n g

"Nurses engaged in health teaching should provide older adults with a list of medicines that affect voiding."

Summary

Most aging individuals adjust to changes in the genitourinary system and are able to maintain homeostasis. Working with an older population requires a basic knowledge of these changes, assessment parameters, signs and symptoms of disease, treatments, and expected outcomes.

Health teaching is one of the nurse's most important functions, and for the healthy aged it has multiple objectives: maintaining health, preventing or reducing complications, and adjusting to health problems and treatments.

Changes in the health care environment have mandated an increase in preventive management and early intervention. Nurses can position themselves to coordinate care across the spectrum and enhance quality while ensuring cost-effectiveness.

RESOURCES

Agency for Health Care Policy and Research
Urinary Incontinence Update Panel
PO Box 8547
Silver Spring, MD 20907
(800) 358-9295
website: http://www.ahcpr.gov

Alliance for Aging Research
2021 K Street, NW
Suite 305
Washington, DC 20006
(202) 293-2856; fax: (202) 785-8574

American Cancer Society
National Home Office
1599 Clifton Road, NE
Atlanta, GA 30329-4251
(800) 227-2345; fax: (404) 325-2217
website: http://www.cancer.org

American Foundation for Urologic Disease
300 West Pratt Street
Suite 401
Baltimore, MD 21201
(800) 242-2383; fax: (410) 528-0550
e-mail: admin@afud.org

American Kidney Fund
6110 Executive Blvd.
Suite 1010
Rockville, MD 20852
(301) 881-3052; fax: 301-881-0898
website: http://www.arbo.kidney/com

Bladder Health Council American Foundation for Urological Disease
300 West Pratt Street
Suite 401
Baltimore, MD 21201
(800) 242-2383
e-mail: admin@afud.org

Continence Restored, Inc.
407 Strawberry Hill Avenue
Stamford, CT 06902
(914) 285-1170

Enu-Care Foundation, Inc.
100 Main-Sumner
Coos Bay, OR 97420
(541) 269-0746; fax: (541) 296-6900

Incontinence Information Center
PO Box 9
Minneapolis, MN 55440
(800) 543-9632

The Mathews Foundation for Prostate Cancer Research
817 Commons Drive
Sacramento, CA 95825-6655
(916) 567-1400; (800) 234-6284;
fax: (916) 927-5218
e-mail: mathews@sna.com

National Association for Continence
PO Box 8310
Spartanburg, SC 29305
(854) 579-7900; (800) BLADDER;
fax: (854) 579-7902
website: http://www.nafc.org

The Simon Foundation for Continence
PO Box 835
Wilmette, IL 60091
(847) 864-3913; (800) 23-SIMON;
fax: (847) 864-9758

United Ostomy Association
36 Executive Park
Suite 120
Irvine, CA 92714
(714) 660-8624; (800) 826-0826;
fax: 714-660-9262
website: http://www.gulf.net/civic/uoa/org

REFERENCES

Abrams W, Beers M, Berkow R, et al., eds. (1995). Merck Manual of Geriatrics. 2nd ed. Whitehouse Station, NJ: Merck Research Laboratories.

Albertson P. (1997). Urologic "nuisances": How to work up and relieve men's symptoms. Geriatrics 52(February):46–54.

American Cancer Society. (1994). Cancer Facts and Figures. Atlanta: American Cancer Society.

American Dietetic Association. (1996). Manual of Clinical Dietetics. Chicago: American Dietetic Association.

Brundage D, Linton A. (1997). Age-related change in the GU system. In Matteson MA, et al., eds. Gerontological Nursing: Concepts and Practices. 2nd ed. Philadelphia: WB Saunders.

Burggraf V, Barry R. (1996). Health Teaching in Geronto-logical Nursing: Current Practices and Research. 2nd ed. Thorofare, NJ: Slack.

Chambers J. (1995). Interventions for clients with renal/urinary problems. In Ignatavicius D, et al., eds. Medical-Surgical Nursing: A Nursing Process Approach. 2nd ed. Philadelphia: WB Saunders.

Dreicer R, Williams R. (1994). Management of prostate cancer. In O'Donnell P, ed. Geriatric Urology. Boston: Little, Brown.

Finkbeiner A, Bissada N (1994). Urologic effects of current medical therapy. In O'Donnell P, ed. Geriatric Urology. Boston: Little, Brown.

Fuchs G, Kang Pang K. (1994). Electroshock wave lithotripsy. In O'Donnell P, ed. Geriatric Urology. Boston: Little, Brown.

Gallo J, Reichel W, Anderson L. (1995). Handbook of Geriatric Assessment. Gaithersburg, MD: Aspen.

Ganabath K, Zimmern P, Leach P. (1994). Evaluation of voiding dysfunction. In O'Donnell P, ed. Geriatric Urology. Boston: Little, Brown.

Gray M. (1991a). Assessment and investigation of urinary incontinence. In Jeter K, et al., eds. Nursing for Continence. Philadelphia: WB Saunders.

Gray M. (1991b). Management of urinary incontinence. In Doughty D, ed. Urinary and Fecal Incontinence: Nursing Management. St. Louis: CV Mosby.

Gray M. (1992). Genitourinary Disorders. St. Louis: CV Mosby.

Jones K. (1995). Interventions for clients with problems of the reproductive organs. In Ignatavicius D, et al., eds. Medical-Surgical Nursing: A Nursing Process Approach. 2nd ed. Philadelphia: WB Saunders.

Karch M. (ed). (1998). Nursing Drug Guide. Philadelphia: Lippincott-Raven.

Kincaid E. (1993). Urinary retention. In Loftis R, Glover T, eds. Decision Making in Gerontological Nursing. St. Louis: CV Mosby.

Lekan-Rutledge D. (1997). Functional assessment. In Matteson MA, et al., eds. Gerontological Nursing: Concepts and Practices. 2nd ed. Philadelphia: WB Saunders.

Lindeman R. (1994). Specific urologic problems in the elderly. In O'Donnell P, ed. Geriatric Urology. Boston: Little, Brown.

Lowdermilk D. (1995). Assessment of the reproductive system. In Ignatavicius D, et al., eds. Medical-Surgical Nursing: A Nursing Process Approach. 2nd ed. Philadelphia: WB Saunders.

McConnell E. (1997). Conceptual basis for gerontological nursing practice: Model, trends, issues. In Matteson MA, et al., eds. Gerontological Nursing: Concepts and Practices. 2nd ed. Philadelphia: WB Saunders.

McIntosh L, Richardson D. (1994). Thirty-minute evaluation of incontinence in the older woman. Geriatrics 49(2):35–37.

National Association for Continence. (1995). Clinical Guide to Incontinence. Spartanburg, SC: NAC.

Nicolle L. (1994). Urinary tract infections. In O'Donnell P, ed. Geriatric Urology. Boston: Little, Brown.

Norton C. (1991). Assessment and investigation of urinary incontinence In Jeter K, et al., eds. Nursing for Continence. Philadelphia: WB Saunders.

O'Donnell P. (1994). Behavioral treatment for incontinence. In O'Donnell P, ed. Geriatric Urology. Boston: Little, Brown.

Pierson C. (1995). Interventions for clients with urinary problems. In Ignatavicius D, et al., eds. Medical-Surgical Nursing: A Nursing Process Approach. 2nd ed. Philadelphia: WB Saunders.

Skinner E, Skinner D. (1994). Management of bladder cancer. In O'Donnell P, ed. Geriatric Urology. Boston: Little, Brown.

U.S. Department of Health and Human Services, Agency for Health Care Policy and Research. (1992). Clinical Practice Guidelines: Urinary Incontinence in Adults. Washington, DC: U.S. Government Printing Office.

CRITICAL THINKING EXERCISES

1. Susan Jones, a 38-year-old woman, presents with complaints of urinary frequency, burning, pain, and occasional spots of blood. What questions would you ask to determine the etiology of her symptoms? What health teaching would you do?

2. Sam Smith is a 68-year-old man who reports the following symptoms: difficulty starting the urinary stream, postvoid dribbling, a feeling of incomplete emptying after voiding, and some irritative symptoms. What assessment would you do? What treatments are appropriate for this condition?

3. Ellen Black is a 42-year-old woman with six children who has a long history of urinary leak when she coughs, sneezes, or does strenuous work. She has been using peripads, but the problem has become worse and interferes with her life. What evaluation parameters would you include in your examination? What treatment options would you discuss?

4. Elsie Johnson is 62 years of age. She and her husband have had a loving relationship but she is having dyspareunia on a regular basis and also has occasional pruritus. She would like to continue her sexual relationship, but the discomfort is interfering. What assessment would you do? What interventions and health teaching are appropriate?

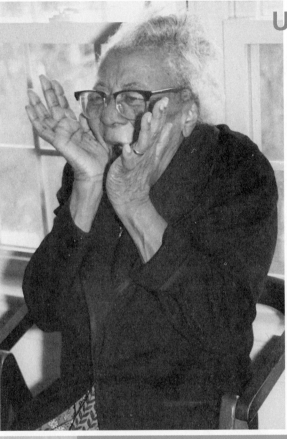

UNIT **VI**

Cognitive Challenges of Aging

CHAPTER 23

Addressing Cognitive Issues

Vimala Philipose, RN, PhD

CHAPTER OUTLINE

OBJECTIVES

After completing this chapter, the reader should be able to:

1. Teach a classmate the three essential components of cognitive function.
2. Differentiate between intelligence and wisdom and give five examples of each.
3. Compare and contrast the major types of reversible and irreversible dementia.
4. Specify the five assessments that are utilized to rule out reversible causes of dementia.
5. Write a teaching plan outlining practical interventions in the daily care of an Alzheimer's disease patient living in a health care facility who is in the second phase of the disease.
6. Write a teaching plan for a presentation to a group of family caregivers of patients with Alzheimer's disease.

Even older adults who are maintaining good health and vigor into their later years are inclined to ask themselves the following questions: Is my memory still good? Can I think clearly? Can I learn as quickly and as well as I did in earlier years? Can I solve problems like I used to? These are not idle questions. They are directly connected to the individual's ability to remain an integral part of society and to maintain control over daily activities, living arrangements, and lifestyle. All of these components are interrelated and are integral aspects of cognition.

▪ COGNITION

Cognition includes intelligence, learning, and memory. Hooyman and Kiyak (1991) identified each of these three components. Deficits in any one, or in all, of these will either interfere with or influence a person's performance in almost every aspect of life, including relationships with family and friends and with the community at large.

Intelligence

Intelligence is difficult to define, because it cannot be measured directly. Huyck and Hoyer (1982) described intelligence as a range of abilities in a person that includes the ability to deal with symbols and abstractions, comprehend and acquire new information, appreciate or create new ideas, and adapt to new situations. Horn was one of the pioneers who described two types of intelligence—fluid and crystallized. *Fluid intelligence* (also called "native intelligence") consists of skills that are biologically determined (innate) in a person; it is independent of experience or learning. *Crystallized intelligence* refers to the knowledge and abilities that a person acquires through lifelong experiences and education.

Various tests are used to elicit the two types of intelligence, which demonstrate different patterns as a person grows older (Horn and Donaldson, 1980). Performance on these tests by older adults may be influenced by a variety of factors, including anxiety when taking tests, changes in sensory and perceptual abilities, and slowed psychomotor skills. Older adults generally exhibit a slower reaction time, owing to delay in receiving and processing information due to the altered physiology in their sense organs. As a result, they do not score well on time-limited tests. Verbal skills are stable and vocabulary improves as people get older, although performance skills may decline (Horn and Donaldson, 1980). Educational level generally correlates with occupational level and has an impact on intelligence test scores. Older adults who continue to use their cognitive abilities in occupations that require thinking and problem solving show less decline in cognitive tests than those who do not continue to work or otherwise remain mentally active.

Also, people who use verbal skills in their jobs (e.g., lawyers, teachers) continue to perform well in intelligence tests pertaining to verbal skills. Deteriorating intelligence is not so much related to education and occupation, however, as it is to a decline in physical health, disability, or sensory and other losses. There is rapid decline in cognitive functioning and test scores in older individuals whose physical health deteriorates (Katz, 1991).

Learning and Memory

The other two components of cognition are learning and memory, and these should be considered together. *Learning* is the process by which new information, both verbal and nonverbal, or skills are placed in memory. *Memory* is the process of recalling, as needed, information that has been stored in the brain. Memory is the function of the brain that retains what is learned throughout a person's lifetime (Jarvik and Falek, 1963).

Older adults usually become concerned when they cannot retrieve information from memory. If the problem persists and increases, the anxiety this creates can lead to a decreased self-image and may contribute to poor performance of tasks. It is not unusual for worry over loss of one's memory to cause depression. Nurses who care for cognitively impaired adults can help to enhance their patients' mental state and ability by offering them positive feedback and also by providing them with familiar and relevant information frequently.

C a r i n g

"Nurses who care for cognitively impaired adults can help to enhance their mental state and ability by offering them positive feedback and also by providing them with familiar and relevant information frequently."

Another way of improving memory in those who are experiencing increased problems with daily cognitive functioning (e.g., recalling names, words, phone numbers, performing independent activities of daily living [IADLs]) is to encourage them to make use of cognitive aids (e.g., imagery, word association) or memory joggers (e.g., lists, notes). Many older adults have acquired a large array of techniques for remembering as a part of formal education and subsequent life experiences. However, an older person with minimal education and limited experiences may not have this advantage.

Eighty to 90% of older adults eventually have small amounts of memory loss known as *benign senescence forgetfulness.* However, these individuals are able to recall, a little later, what they have previously forgotten. But in patients with Alzheimer's disease, large segments of life events are forgotten and there is no later recall. This is known as *malignant intellectual failure.*

Wisdom and Creativity

Wisdom and creativity are closely related to cognitive development. Wisdom, like intelligence, is difficult to quantify or define. It encompasses both cognitive development and mastery over the emotions and is a skill that comes with age. According to Butler and Gleason (1985), **wisdom** is a combination of experience, introspection, reflection, intuition, and empathy, all of which are integrated into a person's interaction with the environment. Wisdom also implies that the individual does not act on impulse but attempts to review all aspects of a life situation objectively. Not all older adults have matured into wisdom. It is dependent on the quality and quantity of each individual's cumulative life experiences. As Butler and Gleason suggested, a person with wisdom has the ability to aspire beyond the limitations of basic needs such as health, income, and housing. The individual should also have continuous opportunities for growth and creativity (Butler and Gleason, 1985). Unfortunately, not all people have such opportunities.

Creativity is the ability to apply unique and practical solutions to new situations and to come up with original ideas. Creativity in a person is generally inferred from the individual's productivity. Many older adults, both after retirement and in very advanced age, have discovered hidden talents in themselves, such as writing poetry or short stories, painting or sculpting, and other creative activities. Many older people would like to leave something of their life experiences behind for the edification of posterity, if they have had personal fulfillment in their own life experiences (Butler and Gleason, 1985).

COGNITIVE IMPAIRMENT: THE DEMENTIAS

Dementia is an *acquired* neuropsychiatric illness that is a global organic mental disorder of the brain (cortex). It is characterized by a general gradual loss of intellectual abilities involving memory, reasoning, judgment, and abstract thinking in persons who previously engaged in normal social and occupational activities (Katz, 1991). Current demographic projections seem to indicate that the dementias, especially *dementia of the Alzheimer's type,* will be a predominant health problem in the 21st century. Although dementia and aging are not synonymous, the **incidence** (number of new cases in a particular period of time) of dementia does increase with an individual's age. Many of the dementias might have similar symptoms and treatment modalities, but their etiologies may vary.

Some probable causes for the **prevalence**

Box 23-1   ETIOLOGIES OF DEMENTIA

Primary Diseases (usually affect the brain globally as the disease progresses)

- Senile dementia of the Alzheimer's type (SDAT), which occurs in individuals older than 65
- Dementia of the Alzheimer's type, which occurs in individuals younger than 65
- Pick's disease—frontal lobe disease with personality changes in the individual
- Huntington's disease—a genetic disease that usually manifests in the 40s and 50s

Secondary Causes: Vascular (focal)

- Multi-infarct dementia (includes stroke)
- Multiple transient ischemic attacks (TIAs)

Secondary Causes: Intracranial

- Subdural hematoma
- Brain tumor (primary or metastasis)
- Normal-pressure hydrocephalus

Secondary Causes: Metabolic (treatable with early diagnosis and treatment)

- Hypothyroidism
- Deficiencies of vitamin B_{12} or folate
- Other metabolic disorders

Secondary Causes: Viral Infections

- Syphilis (rare)
- Acquired immunodeficiency syndrome (becoming more common)
- Creutzfeldt-Jakob disease

Exogenous

- Polypharmacy
- Substance abuse

Psychological

- Pseudodementia (treatable)
- Psychosis (untreatable)

(number of all new and old cases of a disease or occurrences of an event during a particular period of time) of dementing illnesses are reversible (Box 23–1). The more common of these include:

- Nutritional deficiencies, including vitamin B_{12}, and excessive fat intake
- Long-term therapeutic polypharmacy
- Excessive and chronic alcohol intake, with associated Wernicke-Korsakoff illness
- Brain tumors

- Endocrine problems (e.g., hypothyroidism, hyperthyroidism)
- Neurosyphilis
- Normal-pressure hydrocephalus (early stage)
- Metabolic imbalances and abnormalities
- Autoimmune deficiencies (e.g., dementia of acquired immunodeficiency syndrome)
- Depression (pseudodementia)

Many of these conditions may be reversible with early diagnosis and treatment (Morris, 1994).

There are other diseases that contribute to dementias that are not reversible. Of these, Alzheimer's disease accounts for more than 75%. Alzheimer's disease can frequently coexist with vascular disease, alcoholism, or Parkinson's disease. Some of the other irreversible dementias include Creutzfeldt-Jakob disease, Pick's disease, Huntington's chorea, and normal-pressure hydrocephalus (later stage). Some may result from head trauma (with loss of consciousness) such as "boxer's dementia" (dementia pugilistica).

Evidence has surfaced of causal links between Down syndrome and Alzheimer's disease. In the past decade, researchers have found that there is a higher incidence of Down syndrome in families with a history of Alzheimer's disease. Additionally, the brain pathology in Down syndrome (if the individuals live into their 40s, or age prematurely) is typical of that in patients with Alzheimer's disease (Heston, 1982).

A very small number of individuals suffer from *idiopathic dementia;* brain autopsy in these patients shows none of the typical pathological changes present in the dementias, but the individuals present with observable behavioral problems typical of patients with dementias (Heston, 1982). Box 23–2 is a guide to assessment of dementia. The best indicator and predictor of the dementias is deterioration of the functional capabilities of the individual. Because Alzheimer's disease is the most common of all dementias, it is the focus of this chapter.

W e l l n e s s

"The philosophy of treatment for the patient with Alzheimer's disease can be summarized as the highest degree of humaneness; it encompasses the components of empathy, compassion, therapeutic touch, gentleness, tolerance, and patience."

Alzheimer's Disease

Alzheimer's disease (AD) is a progressive, degenerative disease that affects the cortex of the brain and results in impaired memory, thinking, and behavior. It is the fourth leading cause of death in adults, after heart disease, cancer, and stroke. According to the president of the National Alzheimer's Association, "We are at the threshold of a golden [age of] research of Alzheimer's disease at the present time" (Eastman, 1997).

The disease, first described by Alois Alzheimer in 1907, knows no social or economic boundaries and affects men and women almost equally. It is said that Alzheimer's is the disease of the 20th century and will be an epidemic of the 21st century. Ten percent of persons over the age of 65 and almost half of those over 85 will develop AD (Alzheimer's Association brochure, Ronald and Nancy Reagan Research Institute, A World Without Alzheimer's Disease: A Dream Within Reach, 1997). However, AD can strike in the 40s and 50s. Most AD victims are cared for at home, although many people in long-term care facilities have dementia (Alzheimer's Disease and Related Disorders Association [ADRDA], 1988).

Symptoms of AD include a gradual memory loss, decline in ability to perform routine tasks, impairment of judgment, disorientation, personality change, difficulty in learning, and loss of language skills. The disease eventually renders its victims totally incapable of caring for themselves (ADRDA, 1988).

There is no single clinical test to identify AD. Before diagnosis of the disease is made, other conditions must be excluded. These include potentially reversible conditions such as depression, adverse drug reactions, metabolic changes, nutritional deficiencies, head injuries, and stroke. Each person with possible AD symptoms should have a thorough evaluation. Recommended tests include physical, neurological, psychological, and psychiatric examinations and laboratory studies, including blood studies, computed tomography, electroencephalography, occasionally studies of the cerebrospinal fluid, and, in some instances, positron emission tomography. Whereas this evaluation may provide a clinical diagnosis, confirmation of AD requires examination of brain tissue, which can be performed only at autopsy.

Although no cure for AD is available at the present time, good planning and medical and psychosocial management can ease the burdens of the patient and the family. Appropriate medication can lessen agitation, anxiety, and

Box 23-2   ASSESSMENT FOR DEMENTIA

History (both client and family)

- Medical, past and present—emphasis on cardiovascular, neurological, endocrine (diabetes, thyroid) nutritional
- Medications—including over-the-counter drugs, alcohol
- Nutrition
- Onset of symptoms and rate of progression (critical to differentiate between delirium, depression, and irreversible dementias, esp. Alzheimer's disease)
- Psychological problems—depression, anxiety or agitation, paranoid ideations, psychosis
- Social—living arrangements, support systems, ADLs and IADLs
- Special problems—wandering, disruptive behavior, etc.

Physical Examination

Diagnostic Tests

- Complete blood cell count
- Glucose
- Blood urea nitrogen
- Electrolytes
- Liver function
- Thyroid (crucial)
- Vitamin B_{12} and folate (crucial)
- Calcium, phosphorus
- Human immunodeficiency virus—when indicated

Radiographic Studies (to rule out tumors, hemorrhage, fluid in the brain)

- Chest radiograph
- Computed tomography
- Magnetic resonance imaging—if indicated
- Positron emission tomography—to evaluate oxygen consumption and metabolic activity of nerve cells (in limited use because of high cost)

Other Diagnostic Studies

- Electrocardiogram
- Electroencephalogram—to rule out seizure problems
- Urinalysis—to rule out infection
- Lumbar puncture—to rule out syphilis (not routinely done)

Mental Status Evaluation

- The *Mini-Mental State Examination* (see Figure 23–2)
- The *Hachinski Ischemic Rating* scale (see Figure 23–3)
- The *Geriatric Depression Scale* questionnaire (see Figure 23–4)
- The Functional Assessment tool (see Figure 23–1)
- Neuropsychological tests (administered by specially trained psychologists).

unpredictable behavior; improve sleeping patterns; and treat depression. Physical exercise and social activity are important, as are proper nutrition and health maintenance. A calm and well-structured environment may help the afflicted person to maintain as much comfort and dignity as possible.

The course of AD in people who are afflicted has been described by various experts as ranging from three to seven or more phases or stages. We will look at four comprehensive stages here. Some of the symptoms may overlap the stages, or the same symptoms may become progressively worse. In each stage, there are cognitive, personality, behavioral, and functional changes. There are also severe deficits in language in both comprehension and expression as the disease progresses.

FIRST PHASE, OR EARLY PHASE (DURATION, 0–4 YEARS)

Early manifestations are insidious, subtle, and imperceptible, as a consequence of which the patient is usually brought in for diagnosis and treatment after having been afflicted for 2 or more years. Family members may have attributed the changes in behavior to normal aging. If the individual is young or middle-aged, both the family and the affected person may go through a stage of denial. Nonetheless, the early stage of AD impacts on the family and the patient.

> ### W e l l n e s s
>
> 66*Many older adults, both after retirement and in very advanced age, have discovered hidden talents in themselves, such as writing poetry or short stories, painting or sculpting, and other creative activities.*99

Cognitive Changes. In the early phase, the cardinal symptom in AD is the loss of short-term (recent) memory, while long-term memory may still be intact. People with early-stage AD may be keenly aware of what is happening and try to compensate for their deficiencies. They may go to work and perform routine chores without much difficulty and, by avoiding new situations, be able to use simple judgments to overcome memory loss. Individuals might find it difficult to find the right word—especially nouns. They may forget familiar names and telephone numbers, try to rely on reminder notes, and then forget where the notes are. (This is unlike age-associated memory impairment, wherein there is delayed recall.) One of the most common problems in early AD is that individuals who previously had meticulous accounting and numbers skills will begin to make blatant mistakes in their checkbook. This could be the first sign that alerts a family member to the change in the patient's cognitive impairment. The patient begins to prefer familiar surroundings and activities. Mental status evaluation may reveal some impairment in orientation and abstraction.

Personality and Behavioral Changes. Personality changes may be gradual—such as being less close to a loved one, exhibiting less spontaneity and laughter, losing interest in the environment, becoming indifferent to social life, and showing less initiative (although social graces are maintained). The family usually recognizes the changes in their loved one's behavior. Patients are aware that there is something wrong with their memory. The patient and the family may be in the denial stage and cover up these deficiencies. Some patients have expressed this stage as their brain having "cobwebs" or "being foggy."

Somatic Complaints. Somatic complaints may include constipation, insomnia, or change in sleeping patterns, and the patient may have decreased energy.

Functional Changes. Individuals are considered functionally competent when they are capable of taking care of activities of daily living (ADLs) (e.g., bathing, dressing, toileting) and IADLs (e.g., preparing meals, shopping, and independently making decisions concerning self). Although people with early AD may be capable of ADLs in the first phase of the illness, they are hesitant to enter unfamiliar surroundings. For people to be independent, they need to be confident about both ADLs and IADLs. The functional assessment scale of Figure 23–1 is self-explanatory. After using this tool, or a similar one, the nurse can determine what support services are needed and make decisions regarding the level of care and the options available. This functional assessment tool can be administered by any health care professional with proper instruction.

SECOND PHASE, OR MIDDLE PHASE, FULLY DEVELOPED DEMENTIA (DURATION, 4–10 YEARS)

Cognitive Changes. In this phase, there is obvious loss of recent memory, with a short attention span and more difficulty in word finding; the patient is unable to conceptualize, think

ADL SCALE

CLIENT _____   DATE _____

1. **BATHING:**
   - (2) NO, does by self. Can turn water on/off and get in and out of tub/shower by self (if tub/shower is usual means of bathing).
   - (1) YES, needs some physical help (e.g., getting in and out of tub, washing feet or back or other parts).
   - (0) YES, needs bedbaths or help with more than just one or two body parts.
2. **DRESSING/UNDRESSING:**
   - (2) NO, gets clothes and gets completely dressed without assistance.
   - (1) YES, needs some help.
   - (0) YES, someone must dress client or change.
3. **EATING:**
   - (2) NO, feeds self and eats without assistance.
   - (1) YES, feeds self, and requires some other assistance (e.g., cutting meat, buttering bread).
   - (0) YES, must be fed partly or completely by another or by intravenous or tube feeding.
4. **TOILETING:**
   - (2) NO, does by self and has control over bowels; no incontinence.
   - (1) YES, needs some help or has occasional incontinence. Supervision in the same room (or nearby room) for toileting

   should be counted as help/assistance.
   - (0) YES, completely unable.
5. **WALKING:**
   - (2) NO, does by self (may use cane).
   - (1) YES, requires help from a person or a walker.
   - (0) YES, completely unable to walk (bedridden, wheelchair-bound).
6. **TRANSFERRING IN AND OUT OF BED OR CHAIR:**
   - (2) NO, does by self without assistance from another person (may use object for support such as cane or walker).
   - (1) YES, requires assistance from another person.
   - (0) YES, has to be lifted.
7. **GROOMING:**
   - (2) NO, does by self.
   - (1) YES, needs some help with hair combing (brushing, hairwashing, shaving).
   - (0) YES, completely unable.
8. **CAN A PERSON NEGOTIATE STAIRS?**
   - (2) NO.
   - (1) YES, with assistance.
   - (0) YES, independently.
9. **DOES PERSON USE A WHEELCHAIR?**
   - (2) NO.
   - (1) YES, intermittently.
   - (0) YES, continuously.

Figure 23–1. Functional assessment tool.

abstractly, reason, or use sound judgment. Clients in this phase find it difficult to perform complex tasks on the job and are totally unable to handle finances and checkbooks. It becomes apparent that they tend to lose their train of thought. Individuals avoid situations that might lead to failure. Paranoia arises as the result of a decreased ability to remember, and the affected person blames others for stealing personal belongings. People at this stage tend to hide things and forget where they were hidden. They can still talk about familiar things but have difficulty in speech and comprehension. There is no "cognitive flexibility"; that is, the individual cannot do two things at a time. Visual and spatial abilities begin to deteriorate. The patient with AD could have a full-blown dementia at this stage but still experience lucid moments that last for a very short period of time.

Personality and Behavioral Changes. There is increased self-absorption and very little interest in others, even close family members. The AD patient gradually withdraws from people. However, social graces (e.g., saying thank you or please or smiling) may still be maintained, which often deceives other people (especially nonfamily members) about the person's condition. The person may begin manifesting symptoms of agitation, hallucinations, and delusions. Problems with speech become apparent.

Functional Changes. The person is unable to initiate ADLs and may have sleep disturbances. There is a significant problem with personal hygiene, and the individual may forget the sequence of events in a simple activity such as brushing the teeth.

IADL SCALE

1. PREPARING MEALS:
(2) NO, does by self.
(1) YES, needs some help, but can prepare selected foods.
(0) YES, completely unable to prepare any meals.

2. DOING HOUSEWORK:
(2) NO, does by self.
(1) YES, needs some help, but can do light chores (e.g., making a bed, and laundry).
(0) YES, completely unable to do even light chores (e.g., making a bed, and laundry).

3. PLANNING AND DECISION-MAKING:
(2) NO, capable of independent planning and decision-making.
(1) YES, occasional memory lapses but is oriented to time, person, place.
(0) YES, totally dependent on others for planning and decision-making.

4. SHOPPING:
(2) NO, does by self.
(1) YES, can shop if someone goes with client.
(0) YES, completely unable to do any shopping. Must send someone to shop for client.

5. TAKING MEDICINE:
(2) NO, takes medication by self in correct dosages at correct time.
(1) YES, needs help (i.e., is able to take medicine if someone prepares correct dosage).
(0) YES, completely unable to administer.

6. USING TRANSPORTATION:
(2) NO, travels independently on public transportation or drives own car.
(1) YES, needs some help (e.g., needs escort).
(0) YES, must rely on specialized vehicles such as van, ambulance.

7. MANAGING MONEY:
(2) NO, does by self (e.g., writes checks, pays rent and other bills, and keeps track of income).
(1) YES, needs some help (e.g., with managing checkbook) paying bills.
(0) YES, incapable of handling money.

8. USING TELEPHONE:
(2) NO, does by self. Operates telephone on own initiative, looks up and dials numbers, etc.
(1) YES, needs some help (e.g., can answer phone but needs assistance with dialing or getting a number).
(0) YES, completely unable to either make or receive telephone calls.

Total Scores = ADL + IADL _____

30	=	No disability
25–29	=	Mild disability
20–24	=	Moderate disability
0–19	=	Severe disability

Figure 23–1. (*Continued*)

THIRD PHASE, FULLY DEVELOPED DEMENTIA, REACHING CHRONICITY (DURATION, 3–5 YEARS)

Cognitive Changes. The individual uses maladaptive mechanisms to cover up intellectual deficits (e.g., denial, confabulation, perseveration, agitation, wandering). There is total disorientation to time and place and misidentification of individuals. When patients are tested for mental status, to cover up their deterioration they may avoid responding to a question

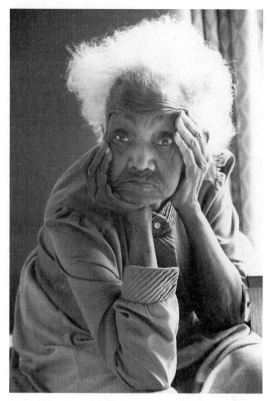

Alzheimer's disease deprives too many adults of cognition in their final years.

by saying that it is not worth answering. Directions or instructions have to be repeated often; the patient verbalizes in disjointed sentences or makes comments that have no relevance to the questions. In addition to complete loss of short-term memory, long-term memory deficits become obvious. The individual is unable to express or understand speech or writing, is very confused, and may employ uninhibited vocabulary that may be embarrassing to family and friends. The individual is unable to cope with the simplest problems and may react with violent behavior (catastrophic reaction). **Catastrophic reaction** is a response of violence that occurs when the AD patient is presented with a situation that overwhelms the coping mechanisms.

Personality and Behavioral Changes. The person is insensitive to other people and may be hostile, often has increased paranoia and becomes aggressive, does not initiate social contacts, and may sexually expose himself or her-

self in public (more common in men). On the other hand, the person may become very docile and dependent on the caregiver, who is either a family member or a health care professional. Patients may be fearful of being left alone and follow the caregiver everywhere. As a result, the family member may never have privacy or personal time unless respite care is provided.

Functional Changes. The person may have loss of control of bladder and bowel, be unable to perform ADLs, and walk with a shuffling gait (due to psychomotor changes). A supervised, safe environment is needed. There is marked loss of weight that is unrelated to caloric intake. In fact, the patient may have a voracious appetite because the sensory signals from the brain may be absent, which prevents the person from knowing the stomach is full. There is extreme psychomotor retardation, with little response to any kind of stimuli. As a result of increasing immobility, the person may become prone to infections (e.g., urinary tract infection or pneumonia).

FOURTH PHASE, OR TERMINAL PHASE (DURATION, 1–2 YEARS)

Cognitive Changes. In the terminal stage, the brain of the individual ceases to adapt to the intellectual deficits. There is severe deterioration in the person's intellectual function. The patient is typically described as a "shell of the former person." Speech becomes incoherent and unintelligible; in some cases, the person becomes mute. Individuals are unable to read and unable to recognize family and friends or even their own reflection in the mirror or recognize themselves in photographs.

Personality and Behavioral Changes. The person is totally confused and may either display aggression (with violent episodes that may harm caregivers and others) or completely withdraw. The person is disoriented to time, place, and person, usually in this order.

Functional Changes. Either the person forgets to eat and drink and becomes very weak and bedridden or the patient may try to eat everything in sight—including objects. There is a compulsion to touch everything in sight. There is total incontinence of bowel and bladder, either because the person is unable to locate the bathroom or because the brain does not signal when there is an urge to urinate or defecate. The person needs assistance in all activities.

Death is imminent owing to physiological complications that include cardiovascular, respiratory, and decubital problems. Frequently, there may be seizures and/or coma, followed by death. The most common cause of death is bronchopneumonia, usually due to aspiration, because the person is unable to chew and swallow food. The person is totally dependent on caregivers for all needs. The individual is totally uninhibited (will urinate, defecate, expose self, use inappropriate or obscene language). Family members are likely to be embarrassed at the person's behavior, although they are aware that the abnormal behavior is the direct result of pathology in the brain.

Caring

❝ *Health care professionals who are caregivers can be of great assistance to family caregivers through compassion and empathy.* **❞**

There is wide variation in the "typical stages" of AD and, also, not all affected individuals go through all the phases. The duration of each phase may vary from patient to patient, with deterioration occurring more quickly in some patients than others. However, it is useful to know the stages of the illness so that family members and health care professionals can more effectively anticipate the needs of an afflicted person and plan for his or her care. Health care professionals can also offer anticipatory guidance and counsel to family members who are the primary caregivers until the person is institutionalized.

Multi-infarct Dementia

The second most common irreversible dementia is multi-infarct dementia. This dementia arises from multiple occlusions of small arteries in the brain that result in infarction in many areas. Hypertension and diabetes mellitus may be predisposing causes. This dementia devel-

ops in a stepwise fashion, rather than by the gradual, steady decline typical of AD. There are focal neurological abnormalities. There may be mini-strokes, a condition that finally becomes dominant. The behavioral symptoms manifested depend on the location of the cerebral infarct (National Institute on Aging Task Force, 1980).

Nursing management will include interventions similar to those for a stroke patient (depending on the severity of the stroke and cognitive disability). Although the cognitive impairment may be mild to severe, depending on the extent and the location of the infarct, an attempt should be made to rehabilitate the patient physically and in language-deficient areas. The quicker and earlier the intervention, the more likely it is that the patient will regain some of the deficits.

The third most common irreversible dementia is the result of chronic alcoholism over a long period of time which has been untreated.

Delirium (Acute Confusional State)

Delirium is an acute confusional state with global cognitive impairment. It develops within a short period of time, usually over the course of a day, and is accompanied by the cardinal symptom of clouding of consciousness. Although it is rare for delirium to persist for more than a month, the memory impairment may last for a longer time. Acute confusional state is, for the most part, reversible with early intervention. Table 23–1 presents a comparison of the clinical features of acute confusional state and dementia.

The change in the mental status of a person with ACS generally occurs because of one or more organic factors (Morency, 1990; National Institute on Aging Task Force, 1980). These include:

- Endocrine and metabolic diseases (e.g., thyroid, diabetes, parathyroid)
- Systemic or local infection (e.g., urinary tract or lung infections or impaired kidney metabolism)
- Drug toxicity, interaction, or sudden withdrawal
- Nutritional deficits (dehydration, electrolyte imbalance)

TABLE 23–1. Clinical Comparison of Acute Confusional State (ACS) and Dementia

Feature	ACS	Dementia
Essential feature	A clouded state of consciousness	Not based on disordered consciousness; based on loss of intellectual functions of sufficient severity to interfere with social and occupational functioning
Associated features	Variable affective changes with fear, apprehension, and bewilderment predominating Symptoms of autonomic hyperarousal; some degree of disorientation	Affect tends to be superficial, inappropriate, and labile and includes apathy, depression, and euphoria with some degree of personality change; attempts to conceal deficits in intellect
Onset	Acute/subacute, depends on cause; abrupt	Chronic, generally insidious, depends on cause
Course	Short, diurnal fluctuations in symptoms, worse at night, in the dark and on awakening	Long, no diurnal effects; symptoms progressive yet relatively stable over time
Duration	Hours to less than 1 month	Months to years
Awareness	Fluctuates, generally impaired	Generally normal
Alertness	Fluctuates, reduced or increased	Generally normal
Orientation	Fluctuates in severity, generally impaired	May be impaired
Memory	Recent and immediate impaired, unable to register new-information or recall recent events	Recent and remote impaired; loss of recent first sign; some loss at a later stage of common knowledge
Thinking	Disorganized, distorted, fragmented, slow, or accelerated	Difficulty with abstraction
Perception	Distorted, based on state of arousal or mood, illusions, delusions, and hallucinations	Misperceptions often absent
Sleep-wake cycle	Disturbed, cycle reversed	Fragmented
Electroencephalogram	Predominance of slow or fast cycles related to state of arousal	Normal or slow

From Foreman MD. (1986). Clinical comparison of acute confusional state (ACS) and dementia. Nurs Res 35(1):35.

- Hypoxia due to respiratory or cardiac problems
- Excessive drinking or sudden withdrawal of alcohol
- Trauma, especially after surgery
- Sensory deficits (visual and hearing impairment)
- Sleep deprivation
- Fecal impaction
- Dehydration
- Relocation (e.g., hospitalization)

The symptoms of delirium (Hoch, Reynolds, and Houck, 1988) include

- Inattention and not being alert
- Disorganized thinking
- Perceptual disturbance
- Altered sleep/wake cycle
- Disorientation to time, place, and person
- Memory impairment

The problems of delirium may be reversible approximately 30% of the time. It is important to reorient the patient, provide a safe environment, and treat the cause of the confusion. Managing these patients may be very challenging to the nurse and other team members. The cause of delirium must be managed promptly and efficiently. The cognitive impairment is managed similarly to that of dementia.

Delirium Related to Acquired Immunodeficiency Syndrome

Although the prevalence and incidence of dementia increases in the older population, the incidence of dementia before age 65 could dramatically increase because of the acquired immunodeficiency syndrome. The majority of these patients will develop dementia when the virus infects the brain.

ASSESSING PATIENTS FOR SUSPECTED DEMENTIA

Comprehensive assessment of cognitively impaired patients is critical so as to identify and rule out all reversible conditions before labeling a patient as *demented*. This will relieve both the patient and family members of unnecessary fear.

Because some types of dementia are irreversible and some are reversible, it is crucial to differentiate between the two and to initiate treatment in a timely manner. In the past, many reversible dementias were diagnosed as irreversible (some of which eventually became irreversible because they were untreated) and the quality of life was devastating for both the patient and the family caregivers. But great strides were made in the 1990s, owing to advanced diagnostic technology. This is particularly important because dementias will become one of the most common health problems in the 21st century. Box 23–2 (p. 442) briefly outlines the assessment that should be performed on all older adults for early detection of dementias.

Assessment Tools

The *Mini-Mental State Examination* tool was developed by Folstein and Folstein in 1975, and variants of it are used widely (Figure 23–2). This 30-item questionnaire includes the topics of orientation, attention span, language, short- and long-term memory, and spatial perception, all of which are cognitive functions. This tool must be administered by health care profes-

sionals with proper training. With a total possible score of 30 points, a score below 24 indicates that cognitive disorder is present.

The *Hachinski Ischemic Rating* tool was developed to differentiate between degenerative dementia (e.g., Alzheimer's disease, Parkinson's disease) and arteriopathic dementia such as mini-strokes or transient ischemic attacks (TIAs) (Figure 23–3). It should be administered by a physician or a nurse. Each item (total = 13) is given a score of 0, 1, or 2. The higher the score, the greater the possibility of vascular pathology. Items include medical history, present illness, and psychological and neurological states (Hachinski, 1975).

> ### *W e l l n e s s*
> **❝***A calm and well-structured environment may help the person with dementia to maintain as much comfort and dignity as possible.***❞**

There is no one test that can be viewed in isolation when attempting to make a diagnosis, and there is no definitive test for diagnosing AD. At the present time a probable diagnosis can be made on the basis of the patient's medical history and results of a complete physical examination and diagnostic tests discussed in this chapter, especially those on cognitive ability. Blood and skin tests are in the experimental stages. However, a definitive diagnosis is currently based on the presence of plaques and tangles in the brain tissue, which are seen only on autopsy after the patient's death.

Functional Assessment

The nurse can be of significant help in assessing the patient's functional ability, either by observing the patient doing some ADL activities (e.g., undressing for the examination and dressing again) or by asking the patient to fill in some information on a form (IADL). In some clinics, the patient is presented with a tray of food and observed in handling the fork, knife, and spoon and managing the eating process. The nurse can also observe IADLs by asking the patient to dial a familiar phone number.

Patient's Name: _____   Social Sec. #: _____

Examiner's Name: _____   Date Administered: _____

Assess the patient's level of consciousness along this continuum

| Alert | Drowsy | Stupor | Coma |

Maximum Score	Patient Score	

Orientation

5 _____ What is the (year) (season) (date) (day) (month)?

5 _____ Where are we (state) (county) (town) (hospital) (floor)?

Registration

3 _____ Remember these three words: cup   pencil   airplane
Ask the patient to say all three. If the patient fails to say one or more of the words, repeat all three again up to a maximum of six repetitions.
Number of repetitions_____

Attention and Calculation

5 _____ I want you to count backwards from 100 by sevens.
Stop after five subtractions (93, 86, 79, 72, 65). Score one point for each correctly placed number.

If the patient refuses or will not attempt serial sevens, ask the patient to spell the word "WORLD" backwards (D-L-R-O-W).

Recall

3 _____ Please tell me the three words I gave you earlier.

Language

2 _____ *Naming*   Point to a pencil and a watch.
                              Have the patient name them as you point.

1 _____ *Repetition*   Ask the patient to repeat the following:
                              "No ifs, ands or buts"

3 _____ *Three-Stage Command*   Place a piece of paper in front of the
                              patient and say:
                              "Take the paper in your right hand, fold it in half, and put it on the table."

1 _____ *Reading*   Ask the patient to read and obey the following sentence.

"CLOSE YOUR EYES"

1 _____ *Writing*   On the following page, ask the patient to write a sentence.

1 _____ *Copying*   Ask the patient to copy the intersecting five-angle designs and give one point if all sides and angles are preserved and if the intersecting sides form a quadrangle.

30	_____	**Total Score**
Maximum Score	**Patient Score**	

Scoring: 0–12 (severe), 13–22 (moderate), 23–24 (mild), 25–30 (none). These ranges vary.

Figure 23–2. Folstein's Mini-Mental State Examination (MMSE). (From Folstein M, Folstein S, and McHugh, P (1975). Mini-mental state: A practical method of grading the cognitive state for the clinician. J Psychiat Res 12:189.

Nurses can also obtain the functional history from the family member. The health care professional or provider should be aware of the fact that there may be discrepancies between the patient's responses and the family member responses. It is likely that the caregiver lacks objectivity because of emotional involvement with the patient, and an exhausted caregiver may tend to exaggerate the patient's symptoms, especially regarding ADLs and IADLs. Conversely, the patient may try to hide and underestimate deficiencies or may not be cognizant of them.

Functional assessment is a very critical and reliable tool that will aid in assessing what stage of the illness the patient is in and in assisting caregivers in planning care (see Figure 23–1). Functional assessment will enable the nurse to select the appropriate referral agency for the type of care the patient needs—home health care, daycare center, or nursing home—depending on the severity of the functional deficits and the family situation.

Feature	Score
Abrupt onset	2
Stepwise deterioration	1
Fluctuating course	2
Nocturnal confusion	1
Relative preservation of personality	1
Depression	1
Somatic complaints	1
Emotional incontinence	1
History of strokes	2
Evidence of associated atherosclerosis	1
Focal neurological symptoms	2
Focal neurological signs	2
History of hypertension*	1

*Defined as either a history of present or previous hypertensive therapy or a current and consistent blood pressure of 170/110 or more.

Figure 23–3. Hachinski Ischemic Rating. (From Hachinski VC, Iliff LD, Zilka E, et al. (1975). Cerebral blood flow in dementia. Arch Neurol 32:632–663.)

MANAGEMENT OF PATIENTS WITH DEMENTIAS

When managing patients with AD (and other dementias), it should be remembered that there are individual differences in the loss of cognitive abilities and responses to interventions. It is essential to assess cognitive function with the utmost care and diligence. Because AD is the most predominant type of dementia, the discussion of management is addressed to the care of patients with AD; however, the same principles of management are applicable to other types of dementia. The philosophy of treatment for the patient with AD can be summarized as the highest degree of humaneness; it encompasses the care components of empathy, compassion, therapeutic touch, gentleness, tolerance, and patience. The main goals in caring for patients with AD (Philipose, 1988) are to

- Promote their high quality of life, with dignity.
- Maintain maximal levels of functional activities, to facilitate their independence as long as possible.
- Accept their intellectual level with grace.
- Individualize care, taking into consideration

the patient's pre-dementia personality and lifestyle.

Nursing interventions are similar for all patients who have dementia. There are activities that a memory-impaired older adult can do with assistance from either a health care professional such as a nurse or from a family caregiver. The following are some examples and specific suggestions:

1. *Build on preserved, well-learned skills.* If the individual was a painter or mechanic or cook, continue to engage him or her in these activities as long as it remains possible.
2. *Avoid teaching complicated new activities that the brain cells cannot process.* Attempts to learn new activities would only lead to frustration and anger and may trigger a catastrophic reaction.
3. *Keep activities very simple.* Repetitive acts often work best. Use simple language and short sentences, and repeat if necessary.
4. *Be flexible and adjust your expectations to fit the patient.* The patient's attention span is usually short, depending on the stage of the illness.
5. *Break down activities into separate steps as*

needed. For example, if you wish the patient to paint, you assemble all the necessary equipment. Then (a) ask the patient to sit in a chair, (b) tie on an apron, (c) open the paint book, (d) take the brush in hand, (e) begin. You will get more cooperation if instructions are short and simple. Show your appreciation by positive reinforcement.

6. *Play music chosen from the patient's era.* Almost all AD patients enjoy music that is familiar to them. Music should not be very loud. If patients find it jarring, they may leave, or it may trigger a catastrophic reaction.

7. *Observe facial expression and body movement for frustration.* If frustration is evident, discontinue the activity and distract patients by offering a snack or a drink, or by walking with them.

8. *Keep conversation at an adult level as much as possible.*

9. *Limit activities to 20 or 30 minutes at most.* This prevents fatigue and frustration as attention spans get shorter with progression of the disease.

10. *Choose meaningful activities.* It could be a brief news item, exercise, dance, or storytelling. Some patients could be taken for short tours to museums or exhibits.

11. *Choose enjoyable activities and encourage a sense of humor in patients.*

12. *Give a patient the option of leaving a group activity.*

There is a window of hope for patients with even the most advanced dementia when you touch them and show your compassion in some demonstrable way.

Facilitating Daily Care

Patients with cognitive impairment are coping with a bewildering array of emotional experiences. They are frightened of their decreasing cognitive abilities, they are depressed because of their helplessness and hopelessness, and they are frustrated because of their gradual loss of control of their lives. However, when they are at the end stage of the illness, many of them appear to live in a state of bliss most of the time.

Here are some therapeutic actions that may be taken to facilitate daily living:

1. As far as possible, *maintain a consistent daily routine* because of the patient's increasing inability to learn and remember new activities. Reinforce former strengths (from the patient's history) in planning ADLs. Patients will gradually lose the capacity to accomplish their previous IADL activities.

2. *Provide a safe environment* by maintaining uncluttered surroundings, with minimal furniture and other objects (especially if the patient paces or wanders). Remove any equipment that could be physically dangerous to the patients (e.g., knives, scissors, detergents, prescription and over-the-counter medications), especially in the advanced stage of the illness. Encourage patients in the beginning stage to perform simple routine chores they were formerly used to performing (e.g., setting the table, watering plants, collecting the trash, painting) so they will continue to feel useful and maintain their self-esteem.

3. It is important to *provide sensory stimulation* for the patient with AD. However, both understimulation (which might cause boredom) and overstimulation (which might cause agitation) can be detrimental to the patient. The nurse must assess the patient's level of tolerance for activities. A good example of an "overstimulation site" in a long-term care facility is the nurses' station, where patients often sit before and after meals. The constant ringing of the telephone, the intercom, and human traffic may be very confusing and disturbing to the patient.

W e l l n e s s

"Older adults who continue to use their cognitive abilities in occupations that require thinking and problem solving show less decline in cognitive tests than those who do not continue to work or otherwise remain mentally active."

4. *Provide regular periods of rest and exercise.* It is advisable to keep the patient active during the day to promote better sleep at night. Patients with AD have erratic sleep patterns; many of them suffer from insomnia and

keep their roommates (in nursing homes) or family caregiver (at home) awake. Encouraging ambulation prevents complications from immobility; however, some patients with AD are overactive and engage in constant pacing.

5. *Minimize disorientation* by having large clocks and calendars that are visible to the patient. Personal reminders for routine activities are helpful. Familiar objects and furniture brought from home when the patient relocated provide familiarity. In the early stages, family albums are helpful for reminiscing and identifying family members and friends. When the patient cannot read or write any longer, posters with symbols for restrooms and dining rooms provide guideposts. Patients' own photographs posted outside their rooms may be of help. In the terminal stage, however, these memory joggers may not be of much help. It is crucial to attend to visual and hearing problems, especially when the patient can still make sense out of environmental clues. Eyeglasses should be kept clean and handy, hearing aids should be in good working order, and the caregiver should remind the patient to use them.

6. Encourage the patient to get involved again in former hobbies and interests as long as abilities remain. Known as *reminiscence therapy,* this is highly recommended; it is used to revive interest that once existed, before the patient's illness (in many patients, long-term memory may remain intact until the second and third stages). Encourage patients to talk about early experiences in life; they can relate to those experiences much better than immediate ones. However, reminiscing may bring sad memories, so the caregiver must be mindful of individual reactions.

7. *Attend to medical problems as soon as they occur.* For instance, if patients exhibit increased confusion within a 24- or 48-hour period, it might be due to infection in the urinary, gastrointestinal, or respiratory systems, or retention of stool or urine, even fecal impaction. The patient may be unable to express the physical problem or may not be aware that there is a problem.

8. *Identify the ADL or IADL tasks with which the patient needs help,* to prevent anxiety and frustration. As dementia progresses, however, the patients' safety becomes critical. Boxes 23–3 and 23–4 give suggestions for those who can no longer cook or drive.

9. *Be judicious in administration of medications* for agitation, anxiety, depression, hallucinations, or any physical problems; this cannot be overemphasized. Medications may make the behavioral situation even worse, if given for a prolonged period of time without careful monitoring. For example, (a) haloperidol (Haldol), which is commonly prescribed for agitation, can have the severe side effect of tardive dyskinesia; (b) chlorpromazine (Thorazine) might make some patients even more agitated; and (c) hypnotics might cause more confusion. If carefully monitored, mild tranquilizers and antidepressive agents are generally effective and recommended (Table 23–2). Other agents under investigation as therapeutic for AD are prostigmine, choline, and lecithin. Some foods that contain lecithin include egg yolk, liver, haddock, soybeans, dried peas, and wheat germ. Because liver has large amounts of cholesterol, it must be

---

Box 23-3   SUGGESTIONS FOR THOSE WHO CAN NO LONGER DRIVE

Men are especially frustrated when they are not allowed to drive. This is an activity they have performed for years, which gave them independence and status. A few solutions for family caregivers:

- Ask the patient's physician to say that "health" does not permit driving.
- A written prescription *not* to drive is sometimes persuasive.
- Give the patient the wrong car keys. After trying to start the car with the wrong keys, the patient may become frustrated and give up.

Box 23-4   SUGGESTIONS FOR THOSE WHO CAN NO LONGER COOK

Cooking may be more difficult for a woman to give up. Safety in the kitchen is paramount, with burns and cuts being the most common hazards.

- The patient may be allowed to wash or cut vegetables under supervision only.
- Stirring ingredients may be done under supervision.
- Setting the table may be an acceptable substitution for some patients.
- Caregivers usually remove stove controls if it is necessary to leave the patient briefly.
- In general, the same rules apply as would apply for toddlers.

eaten judiciously. More recent drug therapy includes Aricept, Cognex, Metrifonate, and Exelon; others are still being tested. These drugs used as neurotransmitter-enhancers do not cure the disease but are likely to postpone the symptoms for 6 to 12 months. Small doses of antiinflammatory nonsteroidal drugs such as aspirin and Ibuprofen may also delay the onset of the disease. Neuroscientists now suggest that the brain cells in AD patients may be going through an inflammatory process. These drugs should be taken cautiously due to the irritation caused in the gastrointestinal tract. Es-

trogen is recommended for older women with AD to maintain verbal and visual memory. Vitamin E, an antioxidant, is said to improve the immune function and protect the brain cells from degenerating and slowing down the progression of AD (Springer and Gegax, 1998).

Preventive Interventions

Patients with dementia are commonly at risk for certain problems that require specialized interventions. Such problems include falls; hy-

TABLE 23–2. Current Pharmaceutical Therapy for Alzheimer's Disease

Medication	Other Uses	Probable Action in Alzheimer's Disease Patient
Estrogen (postmenopausal estrogen therapy)	Heart disease and osteoporosis in women	Delay the onset of Alzheimer's disease
Ibuprofen	Arthritis	May decrease the inflammation in the specific beta-amyloid plaques found in patients' brain tissue; might forestall the disease
Selegiline (Eldepryl)	Parkinson's disease	May delay decline of ADLs
Tacrine (Cognex)		Assist in behavioral changes, and improve ADLs for some time
Other drugs (prostigmine, choline, lecithin)		May produce healthy nerve cells (dead neurons cannot be returned to function)

ADLs, activities of daily living.

peractivity, sometimes with pacing and wandering; nutritional deficiencies and eating issues; incontinence of bowel and bladder; communication issues; aggressive behavior; and depression.

FALLS

Although falls are a problem for many older adults, dementia itself is a major risk factor for falling. These risk factors are both intrinsic and extrinsic. Intrinsic factors arise from patients' own characteristics, such as medical conditions (e.g., gait problems may be associated with dementia). Patients may be receiving medications for both the dementia and the associated gait problem. Extrinsic risk factors are environmental; for instance, admission to a nursing home or to an acute care setting for health problems may cause the patient to become increasingly confused. Other common risk factors both at home and in other settings are slippery floors, glare in hallways, throw rugs in patient rooms, cluttered and crowded rooms or hallways, and inadequate lighting. (It is imperative that the bathroom be lighted, especially at night.) It is essential to keep the environment simple and uncluttered.

Interventions/Management. Generally, the intrinsic factors cannot be altered in a patient with cognitive impairment, but the environmental risk factors can be minimized or eliminated. It is essential to identify a patient prone to falling, using the patient's history as a guide. Patients who are newly admitted should be given special attention by nursing and other staff. Initially, a close family member should be encouraged to stay with the patient as much as possible, to reduce the patient's anxiety and restlessness. If the patient falls, immediate postfall assessment and intervention must be implemented to minimize serious complications due to fractures and hospitalization.

The extrinsic factors are easier to address. Preventive measures include eliminating physical hazards such as cluttered floors and dim lighting. Hand rails and grab bars should be installed where necessary. Sun glare should be avoided. Cables and wires should be fastened down. The nurse should also evaluate the drug regimen and be responsible for seeing that the medications that are precipitating the falls be eliminated or decreased to the lowest therapeutic dose.

There is a steep deterioration in the patient's health status after a fall (most common fractures are in the hip, wrist, and shoulder). Cognitive impairment usually worsens.

HYPERACTIVITY, PACING, WANDERING

The patient with AD continues to be physically able and seems to have normal motor activity in the first stage of the illness; however, as the illness progresses, the continued destruction of cortical and other brain cells causes the patient to lose appropriate motor skills. Abnormal motor activities of pacing and wandering may occur because the patient may be seeking familiar surroundings and security. It is possible for an AD patient to walk for 9 to 12 hours a day, which is fatiguing for the patient and exasperating for the caregivers at home. Additionally, the patient is at a physical risk for injury or getting lost (Rader et al., 1985).

Interventions/Management. Goals for the care of the wandering patient are to provide safety and minimize exhaustion and debilitation.

1. Schedule adequate daily exercise for the patient. Walk with the patient once or twice a day. A family member can assist, which will reassure the patient and decrease agitation. The patient should be appropriately clothed for the weather if outdoor walking is chosen.
2. Seat the patient in a beanbag chair, which will limit activity. Although a beanbag is comfortable seating, it is difficult to get out of the chair without assistance.
3. Change the locks at home, and put latches and bolts at the bottom of the doors. Cover the door knobs with child-safe covers, which fit loosely over the knob (only the cover will turn). These are available in children's departments, along with an array of safety products designed originally for children.
4. Install a bell or other sound producer at front and back doors to alert family members if the patient tries to go out. Alarm systems designed for institutions can also be purchased for home use.

5. Curtains or portable screens placed at entrances and exits of facilities, along with STOP signs, have been very successful.
6. Fences and walls, along with chairs and rest areas, have proven effective in both homes and institutions.
7. If the patient wanders and gets lost, identification improvisations, such as Medic Alert, necklaces, bicycle reflectors, and bright-colored clothing, have been useful. A *recent* photograph of the patient is necessary when alerting police, because appearance changes drastically as the disease advances toward the terminal stage.
8. It is advisable to keep a piece of the patient's unwashed clothing handy. In the event that the patient gets lost, this will aid tracking dogs to locate and identify the patient.

Caring

66Volunteers and friends are also significant contributors in the care of patients with Alzheimer's disease. Residents look forward to these visitors, who provide nurturing and variety in their lives.99

NUTRITIONAL DEFICIENCIES, EATING ISSUES

The nutritional intake of patients with AD depends on the stage of the illness and the behavioral patterns that are manifested. Early in the disease, the person might have increased appetite, whereas in a later stage the person might lose interest in eating or even forget to eat entirely. The AD patient is then at risk for developing vitamin deficiencies, which affect tissue healing, skin integrity, and muscle atrophy. Other nutritional conditions that may mimic dementia include malnutrition, dehydration, electrolyte imbalance, alcoholism, anemia, and vitamin B_{12} and folic acid deficiencies. Other problems may include constipation, impacted stool, and hypoglycemia. (For reasons not well understood, hyperglycemia is not a common problem in patients with AD.)

Interventions/Management. By helping at mealtimes, the nursing staff can assist the AD patient with nutritional intake and prevent complications. The following tips have proven successful in most cases:

1. Follow the mealtime schedule, both at home and in health care settings.
2. Avoid serving foods or liquids at too high a temperature, because of the person's inability to perceive temperature.
3. Avoid hard foods and those that are difficult to chew (e.g., nuts, carrots, hard candy, popcorn) to prevent choking.
4. Offer only one or two choices on the menu, and also on the plate, because patients may get confused when given too many items.
5. Thick liquids or semisolids (e.g., gelatin, pudding) are better than thin liquids (e.g., soft drinks, fruit juices, coffee, tea). Patients have a tendency to choke on thin liquids, especially if a straw is used.
6. Whenever possible, encourage the patient to self-feed with supervision.
7. Add more finger foods to the menu, because patients manage these foods better.
8. Use utensils that were designed for patients with stroke, such as the ones in which a vacuum is used to stabilize utensils on the table.
9. Remind the patient how to use spoons and forks; avoid sharp knives. Cut meat into small pieces for the patient.
10. To prevent aspiration, which is a common cause of death, keep the patient in as upright a position as possible. Swallowing difficulties are associated with impaired ability to perform oral praxis (voluntary oral movements), and dysphagia also occurs in severely demented patients. After a meal, check to see if the patient has any food in the mouth, to prevent aspiration or choking later.
11. Prepare food with herbs and choose a variety of vegetables to stimulate the taste buds and olfactory sensory system.
12. Remind or offer the patient to drink fluids, to prevent dehydration.

A separate place in the dining room is better for patients who have problems with eating, and it is important that mealtime be carefully supervised, to prevent aspiration.

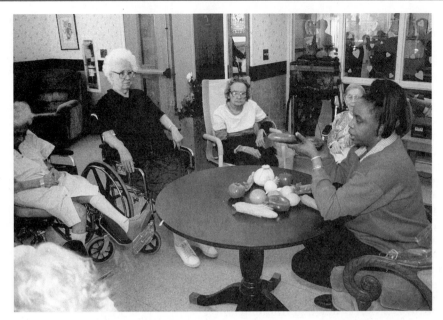

This nurse is helping patients with dementia to relearn the names for fruits and other common objects of their world.

INCONTINENCE

Because problems of bowel and bladder are discussed elsewhere in the text (see Chapters 21 and 22), interventions specific to dementia are addressed briefly here.

Interventions/Management. To have a baseline assessment, a written record of continent and incontinent voidings and bowel movements should be maintained. The person should be reminded to go to the bathroom every 3 to 4 hours or can be assisted to the bathroom. If the patient is unable to walk, a bedpan, urinal, or commode should be offered.

Patients with AD who are disoriented may be unable to locate the bathroom. Visual aids, such as big-lettered signs or a picture of the toilet, may assist those in early stages to locate the site. Bathrooms should be well lighted; bedside commodes are a convenience for some, especially at night.

Fluid intake during the day is encouraged, and fluid intake after dinner should be limited, to prevent nighttime incontinence. As far as possible, use of laxatives should be avoided. High-fiber foods can be added to the diet instead, and drinking plenty of fluids is encour-

aged. The patient may be unable to verbalize about constipation, which is a common problem, so caregivers must observe and assess indirect signs of constipation, such as loss of appetite, abdominal distention, more confusion in an already confused person, lethargy, or pacing.

COMMUNICATION—VERBAL, READING, AND WRITING

The patient with AD has serious problems with language and speech, which causes frustration both in the patient and in the family or staff who are providing care.

Interventions/Management. The following suggestions might help the patient and the caregiver:

1. *Use short sentences, and speak clearly.* The sentences may have to be repeated more than once.
2. *Use simple language.* It has been suggested that using different words that have the same meaning might assist the patient in understanding; others contend that it may confuse the patient even more. In this case, caregivers should use their own judgment.

The key is to familiarize oneself with the patient's specific mode of communication.

3. *Avoid saying things like "Don't you remember?" or "I told you already"* because if patients could remember they would not be asking the same question repeatedly.

4. *Always face the person while speaking.* Avoid startling the patient with loud noises or by coming up behind without any warning. Even a caretaker's minor actions, or something unusual in the environment, may initiate a catastrophic reaction.

5. *Treat the person with dignity and as an adult.* It is very important to praise the patient, to be encouraging and reassuring, especially in the early stages of the illness when the person may be depressed.

6. Many patients with AD still maintain a sense of humor and sometimes laugh at themselves. This may be one way a person copes and adapts to a progressively deteriorating situation.

It has been observed that, even when people have totally lost the ability to communicate verbally, they can still respond to the caretaker's nonverbal cues (e.g., eye contact, a genuine smile, gentle touch, and tone of voice), all of which are reassuring and comforting. As the patient's cognitive impairment worsens and speech becomes unintelligible, nonverbal cues may become even more distinct. Caregivers thus need to become even more cognizant of nonverbal communications. Staff in long-term care facilities need in-services to make them aware of the importance of nonverbal cues (e.g., facial expressions, withdrawal from activities) in these patients.

AGGRESSIVE BEHAVIOR

To understand disruptive behavior, it is necessary to understand the losses associated with dementia and the behavioral and functional changes that accompany these losses. There is a cause and a purpose for every behavior of the patient with AD. Some are due to internal factors and others are external. The internal factors include a sense of fear (there is invasion of personal space when the person gradually loses control of ADLs), frustration with tasks that exceed the person's present ability, impaired perception of the staff and other residents, fatigue, and the effects of medications. External

factors that may trigger aggressive behavior include unfamiliar physical environment, use of restraints, nature and degree of environmental stimulation, and interaction with staff and others in a long-term care facility.

Aggressive behavior can occur in the home of the patient with AD as well as in a health care setting. Such aggression is usually demonstrated by hitting, slapping, screaming, pacing, or verbal abuse of the caregiver. Patients with AD may themselves be victims of abuse by a family member or caregiver. Abuse may be overt, including hitting, slapping, denying food, or tying the patient to a chair or bed. The caregiver may lock up the patient or simply use abusive language. AD is called "the disease of two people, the patient and the caregiver"; each party is victimized by the other.

Interventions/Management.   Caregivers should anticipate some aggressive behavior when the patient with AD is fearful, anxious, or exposed to new stimuli; sometimes it can happen when the caregiver assists in personal care. The basic goals for managing aggressive behavior are to offer the patient with AD a non-threatening, safe environment. The person should be allowed to retain a sense of control, even in a small way, and the caregiver should enhance situations that will bring comfort and minimize stressful situations for the patient. It is important to approach the person with a calm voice and avoid confrontation, reasoning, or arguing with a cognitively impaired person. The stimulus for aggression can be removed by diverting and/or distracting the person, which is not very difficult to do. For instance, if the patient with AD is aggressive, divert attention by taking the person for a walk, or offer a snack, or play some music that is to the person's liking. It is amazing to observe the instant change in the patient's aggressive behavior when simple distraction is initiated.

DEPRESSION

Depression is a common symptom in patients with AD, especially in the early stage of the illness. Understandably, when the individual initially realizes that memory is impaired, depression often occurs as the person tries to hide the impairment from family and friends. The person with AD who has a superimposed depression is likely to be more cognitively impaired and functionally disabled than one who is not depressed.

In addition to the routine diagnostic tests discussed earlier, the Geriatric Depression Scale (GDS) of Yesavage et al., 1983) is often administered to patients suspected of early AD (Figure 23–4). This evaluation tool is only useful in the early stage of onset, before problems of comprehension begin to appear. Because depression is common among older adults, the GDS may be administered to all older adult patients as a routine screening tool. It consists of a 30-item scale and an abridged, 15-item scale, both of which have been tested for their reliability and validity and are available in Spanish also. They are administered by physician,

---

1. Are you basically satisfied with your life?	yes/no
2. Have you dropped many of your activities and interests?	yes/no
3. Do you feel that your life is empty?	yes/no
4. Do you often get bored?	yes/no
5. Are you hopeful about the future?	yes/no
6. Are you bothered by thoughts you can't get out of your head?	yes/no
7. Are you in good spirits most of the time?	yes/no
8. Are you afraid that something bad is going to happen to you?	yes/no
9. Do you feel happy most of the time?	yes/no
10. Do you often feel helpless?	yes/no
11. Do you often get restless and fidgety?	yes/no
12. Do you prefer to stay at home, rather than going out and doing new things?	yes/no
13. Do you frequently worry about the future?	yes/no
14. Do you feel you have more problems with memory than most?	yes/no
15. Do you think it is wonderful to be alive now?	yes/no
16. Do you often feel downhearted and blue?	yes/no
17. Do you feel pretty worthless the way you are now?	yes/no
18. Do you worry a lot about the past?	yes/no
19. Do you find life very exciting?	yes/no
20. Is it hard for you to get started on new projects?	yes/no
21. Do you feel full of energy?	yes/no
22. Do you feel that your situation is hopeless?	yes/no
23. Do you think that most people are better off than you are?	yes/no
24. Do you frequently get upset over little things?	yes/no
25. Do you frequently feel like crying?	yes/no
26. Do you have trouble concentrating?	yes/no
27. Do you enjoy getting up in the morning?	yes/no
28. Do you prefer to avoid social gatherings?	yes/no
29. Is it easy for you to make decisions?	yes/no
30. Is your mind as clear as it used to be?	yes/no

Copyright 1981, J. Yesavage, T. Brink

This is the scoring for the scale: One point for each of these answers.
Cutoff: normal– 0–9; mild depressives– 10–19; severe depressives– 20–30.

1. no	6. yes	11. yes	16. yes	21. no	26. yes
2. yes	7. no	12. yes	17. yes	22. yes	27. no
3. yes	8. yes	13. yes	18. yes	23. yes	28. yes
4. yes	9. no	14. yes	19. no	24. yes	29. no
5. no	10. yes	15. no	20. yes	25. yes	30. no

Yesavage JA, Brink TL, Rose TL, et al.: Development and validation of a geriatric depression screening scale: A preliminary report. *J Psychiat Res 17:* 37–49, 1983.

Figure 23–4. Geriatric depression scale.

nurses, and social workers. A score of 9 indicates depression on the 30-item scale, and a score over 5 indicates depression on the 15-item scale. If results indicate depression, the person with AD is treated with antidepressant drugs, which may improve mood and functional status in some depressed patients but do not improve or worsen cognition.

An older adult who becomes depressed may also appear intellectually impaired and confused, even though AD is not present. These individuals are concerned about their memory deficit and complain of decreased appetite and energy, apathy, and feelings of worthlessness. Such individuals are typically identified as having **pseudodementia,** so-called because the symptoms of depression may mimic dementia in the early stages (St. Pierre et al., 1986) (Table 23–3). Usually, these people respond to antidepressant drugs, psychotherapy, or counseling. Electroconvulsive therapy (ECT) is very effective in the treatment of depression. Pa-

TABLE 23–3. Main Clinical Manifestations in Dementia, Delirium, and Pseudodementia

Characteristics	Dementia	Delirium*	Pseudodementia (Depression)
Onset	Insidious	Acute/abrupt	Brief onset
Duration of symptoms	Lifelong, irreversible after onset	May be reversible, depending on etiology	Usually reversible
	0–15 years	Days to a month	Weeks/months
Consciousness	Clear/intact	Fluctuates, cloudy (cardinal symptom)	Clear
Attention span and concentration	Present in the initial stage of the illness	Severely decreased	May decrease temporarily
Orientation	Impaired as disease progresses	Impaired until cause is reversed	May appear to be disoriented
Cognition	Globally impaired and irreversible	Globally impaired, but may be reversible	May be selectively impaired and reversible
Affect	Labile in moderate to severe stages	Labile; anxiety, restlessness, irritability; reversible	Depressed; temporary unless history of psychiatric illness
Speech	Perseveration; dysphasia as disease progresses; aphasia	Incoherent	Normal, slow or rapid
Activities of daily living	Gradually impaired (irreversible)	Impaired (reversible)	Impaired (reversible)
Therapeutic	Palliative (not treatable)	Effective most of the time (if treatable)	Most often effective
Judgment	Severely impaired	Temporarily poor	Temporarily poor
Insight	Permanently impaired as the disease progresses	Temporarily impaired	May be temporarily impaired
Sleep	Day and night reversal of sleep in moderate-to-severe stages of the illness	Altered sleep and wake cycle	Insomnia or somnolescence

* Symptoms and their reversibility depend on the type of organic disease the patient has developed.
From Lipowiski, ZJ. (1982). Differentiating delirium from dementia in the elderly. Clin Gerontol 1(1):1–9.

tients treated in any of these modalities, singularly or in combination, may experience complete recovery (especially those who do not have a history of depression before the onset of AD) (St. Pierre et al., 1986).

The GDS is used as a routine evaluation in many geriatric centers to rule out depression. If a resident is diagnosed with depression, treatment with antidepressants is initiated for 3 to 6 months, or up to a year. After a year's treatment, if the resident's dementia symptoms are the same or worsening, the person's dementia is confirmed as dementia.

Special Units for Patients with Dementia

Increasingly, many nursing homes are assigning patients with AD and other dementias to special units. There is still controversy over the separation of these patients. Those who are in favor of "mixing" patients advocate that it will be beneficial to the patients with dementia to be exposed to "normal" older adults. Those who are opposed contend that it will be emotionally detrimental to the patients who are not cognitively impaired but who are physically vulnerable. Despite the controversy, many long-term facilities are assigning one or two units to patients with dementia, a trend that began in the 1970s. Many states are also building long-term care centers specifically modeled for residents with cognitive impairment.

Major issues to be considered when building special units are (1) creating a safe and spacious place for patients with AD to walk and pace and (2) simplicity of decor and furnishings. Long-term care facilities are often built attractively to have an appeal for family members rather than for the comfort of the patients. Furniture should be simple and uncluttered, so that residents can find their way easily. Built-in sound systems are useful in providing music that soothes residents who may be anxious or fearful. For the staff to maintain constant supervision, the nurses' station should be placed in such a manner that all the resident rooms are visible. Each unit should be limited to 8 to 10 patients, depending on the level of care they need.

Pastel or soft colors soothing to the patients' eyes should be used to differentiate each wing of the unit. Symbols and large-letter signs should be posted for special areas such as rest rooms, dining room, and recreation and physical therapy rooms. The temperature should be adjustable for the patients' comfort, because AD patients are unable to express problems of feeling hot or cold. There should be provision for family members to visit the patient at any time of the day or night. Live trees, plants, and flowers should be avoided, because patients with middle- to late-stage AD do not differentiate edible from nonedible things.

A "golden rule" is that the staff should take all safety precautions for these residents that they would normally take for a toddler. However, older adults should be treated with dignity despite all the restrictions placed on them. It is important to remember neither to overstimulate nor understimulate residents (which might cause even more sensory deprivation). Insofar as possible, the environment should be minimally threatening. To accomplish this, preadmission assessment is necessary. A description of the prospective resident's cognitive and physical function, previous interests, occupation, likes and dislikes, and communication skills will be helpful for proper placement.

Staff need to be psychologically prepared to work in the special units. Professional and other caregivers must be required to attend continuing education classes about dementia and the needs of those afflicted with it. This could be done within the facility if relieving the personnel for a full day is not possible.

CAREGIVING AND CAREGIVERS

A broad spectrum of categories of individuals are included as caregivers, all of whom make a concerted effort to enhance the quality of life for the patients in their care.

Formal Caregivers

Formal caregivers in many long-term care centers who, in one way or another, are contributing to the patients' care include nurses, physicians, social workers, speech pathologists, physical therapists, activities directors, nutritionists, pharmacists, nursing assistants, and kitchen and janitorial staff. In some facilities, musicologists and massage therapists are invited to work with the residents. A team approach should be the hallmark in the care of patients with AD, to avoid burnout in caregivers. Communication among the various staff members is critical. This can be achieved by case study conferences, in which every member's input is significant.

Often, patients confide in *janitorial and kitchen staff*. Unfortunately, these two groups of staff who come in contact with patients most are not included in the team conferences. Because of this exclusion, some important information about the residents may be overlooked (Philipose, 1983). One of the prominent psychiatrists of the 1970s, Elizabeth Kübler-Ross, did much of her research on terminal cancer patients. In her study, Kübler-Ross discovered that patients generally confided in the cleaning staff because these employees had time to listen to the patient and were nonthreatening (Kübler-Ross, 1974).

Another group of formal caregivers who are insufficiently recognized are the *nursing assistants*. These people have limited access to patients' records and are often not included in care planning conferences where their input would be valuable, sometimes even critical, for residents' care (Philipose, 1983).

Social workers assess the psychosocial needs of the patient and family and identify and locate available resources in the community. They can provide counseling for family members and support groups.

Speech pathologists evaluate the patient with AD for language and speech deficits. This assessment includes reading comprehension, information retrieval, auditory comprehension, oral expression, and writing skills. The deficiencies may not be evident in routine neurological tests, especially in the early stages of the illness. The speech pathologists may assist the patients and the caregivers in recognizing their problems in speech and language in many instances earlier than the other members of the diagnostic team.

The function of *pharmacists* is to monitor drug interactions, especially those that would contribute to more confusion in the patient—a most critical care component.

The *nutritionists* can plan the appropriate nutritional content for residents. Many patients with AD lose weight drastically. Those afflicted with AD are incapable, at the end stage, in the selection of foods and in eating unassisted.

The *activities directors* comprise one of the most significant groups of professionals in care of patients with AD. They spend a great deal of time with the patients, planning activities that are appropriate for the patients' functional abilities and for the stage of illness, and refer patients to speech pathologists, psychiatrists, podiatrists, and other specialists as necessary.

Volunteers and friends are also significant contributors in the care of patients with AD. Residents look forward to these visitors, who provide nurturing to their lives.

Informal Caregivers

PSYCHOSOCIAL ISSUES

It has been suggested that, in AD, two people suffer with the disease: the person with AD and the primary caregiver—who may be a spouse, an adult child (usually a daughter), a sibling, or occasionally a grandchild or a friend. No other disease is as devastating to a caregiver as AD, because there is no reciprocity of appreciation or love from the person cared for. There may come a time when the individual with AD does not even recognize the caregiver. This is often devastating for the person who continues to give care.

Caregivers experience many painful and conflicting emotions. Initially, there is a stage of denial wherein both the caregiver and the person with AD may be unwilling or unable to come to terms with the disease. After the denial stage, the caregiver experiences sadness that the past relationship has ended. Not only will it never be the same but it will also deteriorate progressively. (However, the most successful relationships are those that were healthy and loving before the illness.) The roles of the caregiver multiply in assisting the patient. Demands become excessive and frequently overwhelming. They are frustrated that nothing can be done for their loved one and experience feelings of helplessness and hopelessness.

Caregivers often feel guilty, believing that they have not done everything possible for their loved one. Sometimes the caregiver is angry with the patient and feels guilty about that, even though the caregiver knows that the person's actions are out of his or her control and may even be belligerent. Caregivers may also feel guilty that they long for the death of the person they are caring for.

Caregivers may lose their contact with friends and relatives, who are either uncomfortable about the situation or because the caregiver has no free time to socialize. The patient progressively depends on the caregiver for all ADLs and IADLs, which can be overwhelming. Caregivers come to feel they have lost a loved one who is still alive. Often they develop stress-related health problems. It is not uncommon for the caregiver to die before the patient dies, owing to the enormous physical and mental strain he or she has experienced.

Depression is very common among caregivers. In their despair, even the strongest among them at times may find it difficult to cope, since it is perceived as an enormous, unending burden.

Just as the patient grieves when each time another functioning ability is lost, the caregiver also grieves these losses and becomes overburdened with having to take on so many additional roles in the family (perhaps ones involving responsibilities for which the caregiver has no experience). The caregiver also mourns, long before the death of the patient, due to the loss of intimacy, which grows worse with time.

Another burden on the caregiver is loss of freedom, because caring for a patient with AD requires nearly 24 hours a day of vigilance in the moderate and severe stages of the illness. As a result, the caregiver may experience loss of friends and even contact with other family members.

The caregiver has many moments of despair and doubt about his or her ability to cope with the circumstances.

The caregiver becomes painfully embarrassed when the patient with AD eventually loses all social graces and/or becomes uninhibited in behavior (e.g., sexual exposure, using inappropriate language). Often, there is disagreement between the caregiver and other family members, who may be only occasional visitors but who nevertheless offer suggestions regarding the care of the patient. As a result, there may be conflict in the family until the patient's demise.

ECONOMIC DEPRIVATION

Either because of the caregiver's inability to generate income or owing to loss of the AD patient's former earning power (if the patient was previously the family's main provider) there may be a vast drop in the caregiver's standard of living. It is usually recommended that families read the classic *The 36-Hour Day* (Rabins and Mace, 1995) for help in coping with the day-to-day care.

STRATEGIES FOR COPING

If family relationships were loving and caring before the person's illness, the emotional hazards are usually bearable. The following suggestions might be helpful to the caregiver to cope with the overwhelming and devastating situation.

1. *Conserve physical and emotional energy* and "take it one day at a time" (although this is easier said than done). Because the patient's behavior is unpredictable, the caregiver should not worry about problems that may not happen. But the caregiver should be prepared to handle such challenges by reading the anticipatory guidance information available from local AD chapters or by attending support groups.
2. *Acknowledge anger and frustration,* which are likely to be frequent emotions for the caregiver as the AD patient's illness progresses. Acknowledging this and trying to do something constructive to control the anger is important because, if the anger is directed toward the person with AD, the situation becomes worse. There are numerous reports of physical abuse by caregivers toward people with AD; sometimes the situation is reversed, with the caretaker becoming the victim.
3. *Do not expect rewards from the person with AD.* The patient may have lost the art of appreciation. The caregiver must remember that these responses are due to the person's cognitive inability to express intellectual or emotional satisfaction. The caregiver also needs to understand that the AD person's "mean" behaviors are not deliberate.
4. *It is extremely important for the caregiver to take time off,* either by taking mini-vacations

(without feeling guilty) or by sending the patient to a daycare center for a few hours each day, regularly if possible. Many daycare facilities have fees based on a sliding scale; some are subsidized by local, state, or federal funds. Some home health agencies also offer respite care services. However, these services may be expensive and may not be accessible to some families with fixed incomes. These services not only offer respite to the caregiver but also forestall the AD patient's admission to a nursing home. Thus, the patient with AD is able to live at home for a longer time and thereby enjoy a better quality of life. The caregiver needs to spend time with other family member(s) and friends occasionally.

5. *The caregiver should try to cultivate a sense of humor.* This is an excellent coping mechanism. (Indeed, patients with AD often tend to use humor as their coping mechanism after their initial negative defense mechanism is no longer successful or effective.)

6. *Caregivers should seek professional counseling if needed.* Family members and friends try to be supportive, but they may be uncomfortable or not know what to say under the circumstances. Support groups, where one can meet with other families who are experiencing similar problems, can help a great deal and are available in most places. Caregivers can also seek help from their synagogues, churches or other religious or social organizations for respite care. Health care professionals who are caregivers can be of great assistance to family caregivers.

Caregivers' Bill of Rights

In 1986 the Alzheimer's Disease and Related Disorders Association published a caregivers' Bill of Rights. Following are its tenets:

- The right to live our own life to retain our dignity and sense of self.
- The right to choose a plan of caring that accommodates our needs and the needs of those we care about.
- The right to be recognized as a vital and stabilizing source within our families.
- The right to be free of guilt, anguish and doubt, knowing that the decisions we make

are appropriate for our own well-being and that of our loved one.

- The right to love ourselves enough to have the confidence to do the best that we are able.

When Ronald Reagan, former president of the United States, was diagnosed with AD in 1994, he made it known publicly to the nation. He realized the psychological burden his wife was experiencing. President Reagan said "Unfortunately, as Alzheimer's disease progresses, the family often bears a heavy burden. I wish there was some way Nancy's would be easier."

Summary

According to the National Alzheimer's Association, AD is the most expensive uninsured illness that threatens Americans as they move into their older years. There is no one who is immune to this illness. Everyone is at risk. It is a serious problem. The projection is that by the middle of the 21st century, there will be nearly 14 million persons who are victims of AD.

Nurses are in a strategic position to address Alzheimer's disease as caregivers and advocates. It is essential that nurses give humane and compassionate care to persons afflicted with AD and be their advocates. Nurses can teach and support the family members. With ongoing scientific research in the United States and all over the world, great strides have been made in this decade. There is hope that some day there will be "a world without Alzheimer's disease—which is a dream within reach" (Alzheimer's Association Ronald and Nancy Reagan Research Institute, 1997).

RESOURCES

Alzheimer's Association
The Alzheimer's Association, founded in 1980, is a privately funded national voluntary health organization. Headquartered in Chicago, the Alzheimer's Association has more than 1200 support groups and 188 chapters and affiliates nationwide.

The Alzheimer's Association has five major goals: (1) supporting research into causes, treatment, cures and prevention; (2) stimulating education and public awareness of both lay people and professionals on AD; (3) encouraging chapter formation for a nationwide family support network and implementation of programs at the local level; (4) advocating improved public policy and needed legislation at federal, state, and local levels; and (5) establishing patient and family services to aid present and future victims and caregivers.

The national office promotes public awareness; maintains liaisons with government agencies and national professional organizations; stimulates family support activities; administers a research grant program to initiate new investigations into the cause(s), prevention, and cure of AD; serves as a clearinghouse for information; and publishes a quarterly newsletter. The Alzheimer's Association sponsors a month-long public awareness campaign for National Alzheimer's Disease Awareness Month each November.

Information Line

A nationwide 24-hour information and referral line links families who need assistance with nearby chapters and affiliates. Those interested in help may call (800) 621-0379 (Illinois residents, call [800] 572-6037) or write to:

Alzheimer's Disease and Related Disorders Association, Inc.
70 East Lake Street
Chicago, IL 60601

Alzheimer's Association Brochure (1997) Ronald and Nancy Reagan Research Institute, A World Without Alzheimer's Disease, A Dream Within Reach.

Alzheimer's Disease Education and Referral (ADEAR) Center. Sponsored by the federal government's National Institution on Aging, Phone 1-800-438-4380

Web site at http://www.Alzheimer's org/adear
Ann Schimke

(The Washington Post "Health Section" July 14, 1998 pg. 28)

REFERENCES

Alzheimer's Disease and Related Disorders Association. (1988). Fact Sheet on Alzheimer's Disease. Chicago: ADRDA.

Butler RN, Gleason H. (1985). Productive Aging: Enhancing Vitality in Later Life. New York: Springer-Verlag.

Eastman P. (1997). Slowing down Alzheimer's: New drug treatments offer hope of delaying the disease progress. AARP Bull 38(9):1.

Folstein ME, Folstein SE, McHugh P. (1975). Mini-Mental State: A practical method for grading the cognitive state of patients for the clinician. J Psychiatr Res 12:189–195.

Foreman MD. (1986). Clinical comparison of acute confusional state (ACS) and dementia. Nurs Res 35(1):35.

Hachinski VC, Iliff LD, Zilka E, et al. (1975). Cerebral blood flow in dementia. Arch Neurol 32:632–637.

Heston LL. (1982). Alzheimer's dementia and Down's syndrome: Genetic evidence suggesting an association. Ann NY Acad Sci 396:29–38.

Hock CC, Reynolds CF, Houck PR. (1988). Sleep patterns in Alzheimer, depressed, and healthy elderly. West J Nurs Res 10(3):239–256.

Hooyman NR, Kiyak HA. (1991). Cognitive changes in aging. In Social Gerontology: A Multidisciplinary Perspective. 2nd ed. Boston: Allyn & Bacon.

Horn JL, Donaldson G. (1980). Cognitive development in adulthood. In Brim OG, Kagan J, eds. Constancy and Change in Human Development. Cambridge, MA: Harvard University Press.

Huyck M, Hoyer WJ. (1982). Adult Development and Aging. Belmont, CA: Wadsworth.

Jarvik LF, Falek A. (1963). Intellectual stability and survival in the aged. J Gerontol 18:173–176.

Katz R. (1991). What does education mean as a risk factor? Conference on Epidemiology of Alzheimer's Disease. The International Search for Environmental Risk Factors. Bethesda, MD, July 9–12, 1991. Sponsored by the National Institute on Aging and the World Health Organization.

Kubler-Ross E. (1974). On Death and Dying. Lecture at the University of Colorado, Health Sciences, Department of Psychiatry, Denver.

Lipowski ZJ. (1982). Differentiating delirium from dementia in the elderly. Clin Gerontologist 1(1):1–9.

Morency CR. (1990). Mental status changes in the elderly: Recognizing and treating delirium. J Prof Nurs 6(6):356–365.

Morris JC. (1994). What if it is not Alzheimer's disease? In Current Findings on Related Disorders. Presented at the Eighth Annual Joseph and Kathleen Bryan Alzheimer's Disease Research Center Conference, Duke University Medical Center, Durham, NC, February 10, 1994.

National Institute on Aging, National Institutes of Health. (1995). Progress report on Alzheimer's disease 1995. Bethesda, MD: National Institute on Aging.

National Institute on Aging Task Force. (1980). Senility reconsidered: Treatment possibilities for mental impairment in the elderly JAMA 244:259–263.

Philipose V. (1988). Medicine and Management for Alzheimer's disease patients. Presentation at Northern Colorado Medical Center, Grealey, CO. Sponsored by The Administration on Aging.

Philipose V. (1983). Developing a grounded communication theory: A comparative analysis of patterns of communication among institutionalized elderly residents. Unpublished dissertation. University of Denver, Co.

Rabins PV, Mace N. (1995). The 36-Hour Day. Baltimore: The Johns Hopkins University Press.

Rader J, Doan J, Schwab StM. (1985). How to decrease wandering, a form of agenda behavior. Geriatr Nurs (July/August):196–198.

St. Pierre J, Craven RF, Bruno P. (1986). Late life depression: A guide for assessment. J Gerontol Nurs 12(7):4–10.

Springer K, Gegax TT. (1998). Alzheimer's: Losing more than memory. Newsweek June 15:52–54.

Yesavage JA, Rose TL, Lum O. (1983). Development and validation of a geriatric depression screening scale. J Psychiatr Res 17(1):37–49.

CRITICAL THINKING EXERCISES

Blanca Flores, a 78-year-old woman, moved with her husband Pedro into a continuing care retirement community 2 years ago. Six months after they moved, her husband of 45 years had a fatal heart attack. Three months after Mrs. Flores' husband died, her primary care physician referred her to a psychiatrist for treatment of depression. She responded to the treatment.

Mrs. Flores has a daughter who has her own family but visits her mother frequently. Mrs. Flores' condition had deteriorated gradually over the past 9 months. She developed urinary incontinence and occasional bowel incontinence. One time she phoned her daughter at 3 in the morning to ask her to take Mrs. Flores to her "Mommy," who died more than a decade ago. Mrs. Flores is disoriented and is unable to buy her groceries or write checks.

Except for some mild hypertension, she is in relatively good health. Her daughter was overwhelmed when the physician told her that Mrs. Flores probably has Alzheimer's disease.

1. As a nurse on staff at the retirement community, what tests would help to determine the presence or absence of Alzheimer's disease in Mrs. Flores? What interventions would you take to address the possibility of Mrs. Flores' having Alzheimer's disease?
2. What data would you collect to assess whether Mrs. Flores can continue to live independently? Be specific and inclusive.
3. What strategies would you consider to assist the family in coping with Mrs. Flores' present health status?

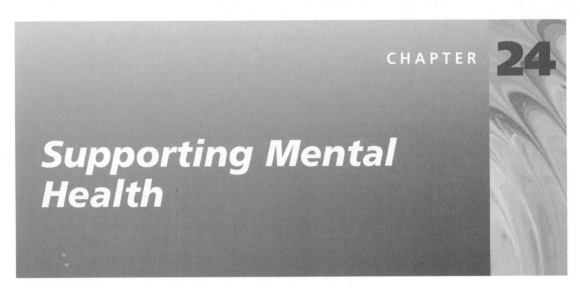

CHAPTER 24

Supporting Mental Health

Shirley Rose Tyson, RN, MA, EdD

OBJECTIVES

After completing this chapter, the reader should be able to:

1. Analyze the psychosocial and physiological changes of aging as they relate causally to mental health.
2. Compare and contrast the symptoms of physical illness and depression, and identify the assessment techniques that can be used to produce an accurate diagnosis.
3. Teach a client who is abusing one or more substances the facts about the substance and available resources for dealing with the abuse.
4. Differentiate among the types of mental illness presented in the chapter and identify the factors that may initiate or exacerbate symptoms in older adults.
5. Teach a classmate interventions to meet the needs of family caregivers of a mentally ill older adult.
6. Describe the nurses' responsibility in elder abuse and specify questions and observations that could be used to identify the problem.

KEY TERMS

caregiver
compulsions
delusions
depression
functional psychosis
generalized anxiety disorder
geropsychiatric nursing
hallucinations
obsessions
phobias
schizophrenia

As the survivors of many life experiences, mentally healthy older adults have developed the flexibility to adapt to daily stresses and challenges. Successful aging and ongoing mental health are achieved through positive interaction of the psychological, biological, sociological, and spiritual aspects of the person. The majority of older adults have successfully negotiated life crises and the aging process itself because they have learned to bring an array of life skills to bear in any situation that arises.

In a minority of older adults, this positive response to life challenges has proved to be beyond the person's capabilities. Mental illness represents a maladjustment to life and the inability to adapt to change. In some individuals, mental illness may have manifested early and repeatedly over the life span. In others, mental health problems arose in later years when the challenges of age proved too great. Older adults with mental health problems are in need of self-respect, friendship, mental stimulation, and a feeling of safety and security. Health care professionals, especially nurses, are often in a position to offer support to mentally ill older adults.

Older adults as a group are not likely to seek out mental health services. When they do, it becomes obvious that mental health services designed to assist this age group are inadequate. In addition, poverty, racism, sexism, and ageism profoundly affect access to and the delivery of services when they *are* available. As health care professionals, there is much we need to do to improve mental health services to the aging population of our society.

■ THE MENTALLY HEALTHY OLDER ADULT

Healthy living practices, positive social relationships, varied interests and activities, adequate personal income, mobility, and individual self-worth all contribute to successful aging. Mental health and mental illness are related to the individual's ability to function successfully within the environment, to communicate effectively, and to maintain optimal levels of physical health.

As people grow older, adaptability to changing needs and requirements is a primary characteristic of successful living. Mentally healthy people emphasize abilities over disabilities. They place a high value on autonomy and independence, which allows them to maintain control over their lives and personal decision-making. Mental health professionals need to look at the differences in the ways in which aging is experienced among diverse racial, ethnic, and cultural groups and identify the strengths (psychological, physiological, spiritual, genetic, and social) that contribute to longevity and mental health.

Wellness is a concept that has revolutionized care. Today's older adults are participating in health and wellness programs in unprecedented numbers. Nutrition, exercise, and recreational programs are responsible for positive lifestyle changes that enhance the mental health of older adults and help to eradicate the stereotypical picture held by our society. For many older adults, physical condition is not nearly as important as the ability to enjoy meaningful activity and to maintain control over their lives.

■ AGE-RELATED CHANGES

Continuing mental health requires that older adults become acquainted with the normal changes that occur with aging and understand that some adjustments may be required to meet these changes. Health teaching about possible sensory deficits or declining abilities can help older adults to prepare for losses without experiencing psychological pain. This teaching must be done with the knowledge that aging occurs at an individualized pace and in a unique manner for each person.

Physiological Changes

Many older adults appear younger than their chronological age, are physically active, exercise regularly, maintain social relationships, and eat properly—all of which promote physical and mental health and prevent illness. Yet the normal physiological changes of aging may be observed in cardiac output, peripheral resistance, pulmonary function, glomerular filtration rate, sensorimotor deficits, oral-digestive disturbances, and modified thermoregulatory function. Physiological changes of aging occur in virtually every body system, although some can be modified or delayed by careful attention to health maintenance practices.

Reduction in sensorimotor function, loss of strength, loss of hair, appearance of wrinkles, a slowing gait, and changes in posture are some of the more obvious changes with which older adults are confronted. Supportive devices may become necessary for the first time. These can include eyeglasses, hearing aids, dentures, walkers, canes, pacemakers, and wheelchairs. Older adults must be able to include such aids in their daily lives, as necessary, without impairing their self-image, and they may need support in doing so.

In a relatively stress-free environment, minimal impairment of any body system may not seriously interfere with a person's functional capacity; however, for some older adults the stress of a fall or an infection can disrupt homeostasis and may result in an inability to regain equilibrium. Frailty or chronic illness, associated with the loss of physical autonomy, self-mastery, and control of basic necessities of life, leads to dependence on others. Age-related memory deficiencies, particularly for recent events, may occur. Intellectual functioning does not decline with age, but the length of time required for learning increases.

The assessment process is important in identifying physiological changes. Physical assessment of the older adult should include mental and emotional health states, self-care, nutrition/hydration, mobility, sexuality, sensory function, and use of medications (see Chapter 2).

Psychosocial Aspects of Aging

Aging is a universal biological phenomenon, but it is experienced differently depending on

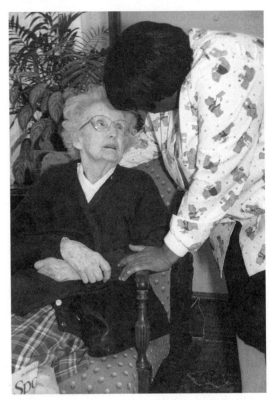

Touch is one of the most potent tools for helping a person who is depressed.

where you happen to be. The aging process involves physiological, psychological, and social factors that can bring about changes in an older adult's self-image and self-concept. In many cultures older adults are revered for their wisdom, but in our own culture older individuals depend on their own perceptions, and the responses of those with whom they associate, for a sense of belonging and worth. Thus, attention by health care professionals to the self-esteem needs of older adults is crucial at a time in life when limitation of mobility, chronic illnesses, and loss of significant others may be occurring.

Erikson's (1963) psychosocial theory has the greatest relevance for gerontological nurses and supports the positive mental health of older adults. Old age, according to Erikson, is the culmination of life—the point toward which all previous development has been evolving. Erikson's is a life-cycle theory that encourages older adults to work through difficult areas of their personalities.

There are a minority of older adults for whom aging is a negative event to themselves, their families, their supportive friends, and caregivers. There is also a correlation between low self-esteem, decreased life satisfaction, and negativity. A phenomenon that is common among older adults is *bereavement overload,* which occurs when many losses over a short period are experienced, and the individual is unable to resolve one before another is experienced.

A thorough mental health assessment includes the older adult's physical, psychosocial, cultural, functional, and behavioral status; it should be undertaken to assess for specific mental health problems or simply to promote and maintain a mentally healthy state. Psychosocial responses to aging, hospitalization, loss, physical or mental illness, or abuse, include but are not limited to

- Anxiety
- Disorientation or confusion
- Changes in self-concept
- Changes in role perception
- Perceived changes in sexuality
- Hostility
- Withdrawal
- Dependency

Cognitive changes can also occur and are manifested in

- Decreased motivation
- Decreased problem-solving ability
- Changes in perception and sensorium

The nurse should be able to recognize and assess psychosocial responses. Because these responses and changes often may be frightening to the older adult, the nurse should demonstrate a caring and supportive attitude in interactions with patients. Nursing diagnoses based on a psychosocial assessment would identify impaired physical and mental function, social isolation, and disturbances in self-concept, self-esteem, or body image.

Any psychosocial nursing assessment should focus on the strengths of the older adult (Box 24–1). It is important to ask how the individuals perceive themselves in coping with physiological and psychological changes occurring with aging, and what coping behaviors they utilize. Family members should be asked whether older adults consult with them or call on them for assistance.

The assessment interview should be conducted in a private area that is comfortable and free from interruptions. The nurse needs to be sensitive to the older adult client and explain that information will only be used to assist in treatment. Verbal and nonverbal expressions, changes in mood, and difficulties in answering questions should be given attention. Questions must be asked in a direct, simple, and concrete manner. It is necessary to follow all health care agency guidelines and protocols for documenting observations.

Health Maintenance

As a person ages, the goal is to preserve functional capacity, health, and well-being. To maintain physical and mental health, older adults should receive health education and guidelines for healthy lifestyles. This works to

---

Box 24-1   PSYCHOSOCIAL ASSESSMENT QUESTIONS FOR OLDER ADULT PATIENTS

1. Have there been recent changes in your life?
2. Describe what is a usual day for you.
3. What did you do yesterday?
4. How do you handle difficult situations?
5. Are there specific problems you are experiencing that are related to your aging?
6. Have you made any recent changes in social contacts with family members, friends, or others?
7. Do you have many friends? How do you get along with people?
8. Is your self-esteem affected by your health status? If so, in what way?

eliminate some unhealthful behaviors (e.g., smoking, excessive drinking of alcohol, overuse of over-the-counter drugs, dietary excesses, lack of exercise). Older adults should be made aware that physical inactivity is also a major threat to health.

It is important to remember that chronological age does not reveal much about a person but lifestyles do. Living conditions, socialization, adequate nutrition, physical exercise, and mental stimulation all contribute to an older adult's health status and health maintenance. The following are special considerations for health maintenance in older adults:

1. Over-the-counter drugs can interact with prescribed drugs, so the physician should be consulted to prevent polypharmacy.
2. Participation in some form of daily exercise (e.g., aerobics, swimming, gardening, walking) is highly beneficial.
3. Appropriate balanced diet with adequate roughage, fiber, and water is essential.
4. Adequate rest and sleep are needed for healthy functioning.
5. Social activity maintains healthful attitudes and vigor.
6. Mental stimulation is essential to maintaining mental function.
7. Regular visits to physician and dentist for preventive care are important.

■ THE MENTALLY ILL OLDER ADULT

Older adults, as a group, receive less support for mental health problems and less access to the mental health care system than individuals in all other age groups. Older individuals have a greater incidence of chronic illnesses and physical and mental disabilities; however, there are many barriers to mental health care for the older population.

Societal attitudes—including those of older individuals themselves—are deterrents to seeking care. Psychotherapy is viewed by many as time-consuming, expensive, and inappropriate for older adults. In spite of recent advances in mental health care the stigma associated with mental illness remains very real, and older adults rarely seek care for fear of being labeled or becoming institutionalized.

Mental health needs of the older adult population include both maladaptive patterns of adjustment and mental illness related to declining physical health. Services are required in diverse settings, including acute- and long-term care, home and community outreach, outpatient clinics, special care units in institutionalized settings, and accommodations for the homeless mentally ill.

Nurses can help to remove the stigma and allay the fears associated with mental illness by providing health education about mental disorders and mental health services. There are currently insufficient numbers of nurses and other health care professionals in the mental health system to adequately provide geriatric mental health services in a much-needed and rapidly growing subspecialty to an underserved group. Although more than half of all nursing home residents in the United States need mental health care, less than 20% receive it, even if they live in a facility that provides such care (News Watch, Geriatric Nursing, 1993).

Mental health assessment of older adults may be challenging because physical problems may mask mental illness. A comprehensive assessment should be performed. Older adults may have been diagnosed with mental illness since young adulthood or may experience a mental disorder in later life. Loneliness, isolation, substance abuse, depression, suicide, and paranoid reactions are among the most common mental health problems experienced by the older adult population.

Behavior Problems

Most cultures label behavior as mental illness on the basis of incomprehensibility and cultural relativity. When observers are unable to find meaning or comprehensibility in behavior, they are likely to label that behavior as mental illness. Individual cultures determine the meaning of behavior (Townsend, 1993).

Behaviors observed with chronic mental illness are

- Dependence
- Social incompetence
- Periodic hospitalizations
- Symptomatic behavior
- The sick role
- Label or stigma
- Low level of functioning

Dependence is the reliance on others. This is observed when the patient's needs are undertaken by the family caregiver. *Social incompetence* is the inability to perform basic skills necessary for activities of daily living. *Periodic hospitalizations* can be part of ongoing treatment and can benefit the individual in the therapeutic process. *Symptomatic behavior* includes delusions and hallucinations, which are symptoms of psychosis. *The sick role* is one that an individual adopts, when ill, and can lead to dependency on others including health care professionals. *Label or stigma* accompanies mental illness. The illness is seen as a disgrace, and the mentally ill person is deprived of multiple resources and a sense of belonging. A *low level of functioning* is manifested in self-care deficits, inability to support one's self financially, and the inability to live independently.

Loneliness and Social Isolation

Individuals, regardless of age or social position, experience loneliness at some point in their lives. The older adult has learned to adjust to many losses over a lifetime. Having survived to the sixth or seventh decade or older necessitates having encountered loss, loneliness, and social isolation on some level. Causes of loneliness are usually attributed to one or more of the following:

1. Death of a spouse, child, relative, friend, or pet
2. Children, family, friends moving away to new locations
3. Inability to communicate in the language of the environment
4. Experience of pain and no one to provide comfort

Loneliness is a common stressor for older adults as they adjust to recurrent losses. Social isolation is a manner of interacting that is manifested by an avoidance of interpersonal contact and a retreat into an individual's personal world. Characteristics include seclusiveness, expression of feelings of aloneness and rejection, preoccupied appearance, active avoidance of others, minimal participation in activities of daily living, and sleeping during the daytime. Reasons for social isolation include severe psychological stress, maturational or situational crisis, and illness. To increase the client's

interaction with others in the environment, the nurse needs to encourage group activity, give positive feedback when the older adult reaches out to others, request verbal communication, reduce tendency of staff and others to withdraw from the patient, and provide activities that will keep the older adult from isolation.

Anxiety and Anxiety Disorders

Anxiety is common in old age and is manifested in many ways, including tension, insomnia, difficulty concentrating, disturbance in focusing, trembling, hyperactivity, or impatience. Anxiety is considered a normal reaction to a perceived danger. When that danger is no longer seen as present, the anxiety will dissipate. Anxiety in the older adult is not well understood. Confinement in a nursing home, hospitalization for an illness, and the experienced losses of older adults perpetuate anxiety, which can lead to distortions in the way an individual thinks, feels, or acts. It is thought that anxiety, seen as feelings of apprehension, is often symptomatic of an underlying mental or physical disorder in older adults.

On a continuum, anxiety has pathological and maladaptive forms. Anxiety disorders are particularly severe and pervasive forms of maladaptive anxiety. The most common anxiety disorders found in older adults are obsessive-compulsive, phobic, and generalized anxiety disorders.

Obsessions are thoughts that recur and cause discomfort. They are often coupled with **compulsions,** which are acts or rituals that must be performed in order to lessen the anxiety, often causing embarrassment. **Phobias** are irrational fears. An example is *agoraphobia,* which is fear of being in a public place from which escape may be difficult or help might not be available (American Psychiatric Association, 1994). **Generalized anxiety disorder,** which tends to be chronic, is characterized by symptoms of tension, inability to relax, frequent urination, dizziness, or excessive worry about life.

Psychotherapeutic management should be instituted to help the anxious older adult explore the reasons for anxiety. In spite of attitudes by society, older adults *can* benefit from such intervention. Table 24–1 presents medications that are sometimes prescribed for anxiety, depression, and other symptoms; Table 24–2

TABLE 24–1. Commonly Used Psychoactive Drugs

Antianxiety Drugs (Anxiolytics)

BENZODIAZEPINES
Alprazolam (Xanax)
Clorazepate (Tranxene)
Chlordiazepoxide (Librium)
Diazepam (Valium)
Lorazepam (Ativan)
Oxazepam (Serax)
Prazepam (Centrax)

BARBITURATES
Amobarbital (Amytal)
Mephobarbital (Mebaral)
Phenobarbital

Antidepressant Drugs

TRICYCLIC COMPOUNDS
Amitriptyline (Amitril, Elavil)
Amoxapine (Asendin)
Desipramine (Norpramin)
Doxepin (Sinequan, Adapin)
Fluoxetine (Prozac)
Imipramine (Tofranil)
Maprotiline (Ludiomil)
Nortriptyline (Aventyl)

MONOAMINE OXIDASE INHIBITORS
Isocarboxazid (Marplan)
Phenelzine (Nardil)
Tranylcypromine (Parnate)

Antimanic Drug

LITHIUM CARBONATE
Lithium (Eskalith, Lithonate)

NURSING CONSIDERATIONS
1. Blood chemistry should be monitored regularly for lithium because dosage adjustment may be required.
2. Patients should be monitored for side effects of the prescribed medication.
3. The therapeutic effects of the antidepressant medication may take up to 4 weeks to bring about changes in the patient.
4. Patient teaching about the prescribed drug is important.

Major Tranquilizers (Antipsychotics, Neuroleptics)
Chlorpromazine (Thorazine)
Clozapine (Clozaril)
Fluphenazine (Prolixin)
Haloperidol (Haldol)
Loxapine (Loxitane)
Mesoridazine (Serentil)

TABLE 24–1. (*Continued*).

Molindone (Moban)
Perphenazine (Trilafon)
Thioridazine (Mellaril)
Thiothixene (Navane)
Trifluoperazine (Stelazine)

NURSING CONSIDERATIONS
1. Close monitoring of patients. Anything amiss must be reported.
2. Documentation of side effects and behaviors exhibited.
3. Instruct patients to be aware of urinary retention, constipation, and hypotensive effects.
4. Gradual weaning off the medication is required.
5. To prevent the incidence of tardive dyskinesia and other extrapyramidal symptoms, medications such as trihexyphenidyl (Artane) and benztropine (Cogentin) should be administered simultaneously with the antipsychotic medication.
6. Patient teaching about the prescribed drug is important.

summarizes patient teachings about psychoactive medications.

Substance Abuse (Alcohol)

Drinking of alcohol is abusive if it (1) occurs at regular daily intervals, on weekends, or on binges, and (2) disrupts routine patterns, with impaired social functioning and difficulty in stopping. There are warning signs of impending alcoholism, which can be identified through a thorough nursing assessment. The following questions may be asked:

1. How old were you when you first started drinking alcoholic beverages?
2. When was the first time you knew you had problems with alcohol?
3. Have there been problems on the job (if working)? At home? With family members? Any falls?
4. Have there been problems with the law? Auto accidents, arrests, altercations?
5. Do you have problems with appetite and intake of adequate nutrition?
6. Tell me how you view yourself at this time.

TABLE 24–2. Nursing Considerations and Patient Teachings for Older Adults Receiving Psychotropic Drugs

Antipsychotic Drugs: Neuroleptics

Some cause extrapyramidal symptoms. Examples are haloperidol (Haldol), thiothixene (Navane), and fluphenazine (Prolixin).

Because older adults are particularly susceptible to tardive dyskinesia, antiparkinsonian drugs such as trihexyphenidyl (Artane) and benztropine (Cogentin) are prescribed with the antipsychotic drugs.

Thioridazine (Mellaril) and clozapine (Clozaril) have a low incidence of extrapyramidal symptoms.

Agranulocytosis is most common in older women and is a risk factor when clozapine is prescribed.

Anticholinergic side effects are a problem with older adults.

Symptoms of tardive dyskinesia are abnormal movement of limbs; chewing movements and puckering; lip smacking; tongue thrusting; parkinsonism; shuffling gait; tremors; rigidity of muscles in neck, trunk, and limbs; and pinrolling tremors with fingers.

Antianxiety Agents: Benzodiazepines

Benzodiazepines with shorter half-lives prescribed for older patients include lorazepam (Ativan), oxazepam (Serax), and alprazolam (Xanax).

The half-lives of some benzodiazepines are made longer by age-related changes that prolong sedation, cause poor coordination and disorientation, and may lead to misdiagnosis.

Antidepressant Drugs: Tricyclic Antidepressants

Caution should be taken when tricyclics are administered to older adults with cardiovascular disease.

Amitriptyline (Elavil) produces the most anticholinergic side effects.

Nortriptyline (Aventyl) has little hypotensive effect.

Toxicity can be manifested in disorientation, confusion, memory loss.

Anticholinergic side effects are dry mouth, fever, blurred vision, urinary retention, insomnia, agitation, confusion, disorientation, and restlessness.

Other assessments include observation and history-taking to identify areas such as vision difficulties, tremors, seizures, delirium tremens, blackouts, hallucinations, or tingling and pain or numbness in extremities. It should also be determined whether the individual has been experiencing stressful problems that have led to drinking.

There is increasing evidence that older adults in our society today are abusing alcohol. The abuse leads to impairment in memory functioning and learning ability. Underlying causes are psychological, with manifestations of

- Desire to escape from personal problems, which may be health-related or associated with family and financial causes.
- Increased stress, which may be recent or prolonged
- Low self-esteem
- Disruptions in self-identity with aging
- Feelings of discomfort

There may be biological reasons (e.g., genetics, family history of alcoholism) as well as sociocultural reasons of permissiveness and easy availability of alcohol in our society. The interaction of alcoholism and aging affects mental health and mental illness in many ways. Psychological problems may mask, mimic, or appear as mental illness in behaviors such as depression, withdrawal, hostility, suspiciousness, hallucinations, delusions, and suicidal ideation, threats, or attempts.

Nursing interventions should focus on maintaining the self-esteem of the older adult who abuses alcohol:

- Show a caring attitude.
- Be nonjudgmental.
- Assist the patient with expression of feelings.
- Communicate positive outcomes and successes.
- Assign small tasks that can be accomplished.

All of the above help to establish a trusting nurse/client relationship. The nurse can work with family members and other caregivers in handling co-dependency and enabling behaviors. *Co-dependency* may be expressed by the family's helping to acquire the alcohol, and *enabling* gives the person "permission" to continue the maladaptive behavior. This aspect of care is extremely important if the older adult lives in the community and is receiving home health care, because alcohol is more accessible to the older adult who is living in the community. Alcohol-related disorders include

- Alcohol dependence
- Alcohol liver disease
- Alcohol gastritis
- Alcohol poisoning

Not included are hospitalizations due to alcohol-related falls, accidents, confusion, and malnutrition. It is of utmost importance that the gerontological nurse incorporate patient education in the treatment of substance abuse while caring for older adults with this diagnosis.

Substance Abuse (Drugs)

Frequent use of drugs that causes impairment in functioning for at least 1 month is considered substance abuse. Drug use includes prescribed drugs, addictive drugs, over-the-counter drugs, and home remedies. Because of declining health, older adults may require prescribed drugs that enable them to function, and they are also the most frequent users of over-the-counter drugs. A drug abuse problem exists when there is difficulty in reducing the amount of the drug or stopping the use of the drug.

Among medications frequently overused by older adults are hypnotics or sedatives for sleeping. Older individuals do experience disturbances in the sleep-wake cycle, which often leads to the use of drugs. Alternate methods should be explored before drugs are prescribed for sleep. Drugged sleep is not normal sleep and may further incapacitate the older adult.

Nursing assessment includes careful history, observation, and data collection. The following questions may be asked of the older adult:

1. What drugs are you taking more than prescribed? And how much more?
2. Can you describe why you decide to use more of this medication?
3. Does this medication disrupt your functioning? How does it disrupt your functioning?
4. Does your medication cause you to neglect caring for yourself?
5. Do you have problems with appetite and intake of adequate nutrition?
6. Are you having any financial problems?

7. Have you ever received treatment for drug misuse?
8. How do you view yourself at this time?

Maladaptive behaviors include depression, violence, labile moods, dependency needs, manipulation, withdrawal, mistrust, suspiciousness, and suicidal ideas, threats, or attempts. Older adults who have been misusing drugs for many years can be manipulative; they need professional help in reducing manipulation and drug misuse.

Nursing interventions include limit-setting, exploring alternative coping strategies, establishing positive nurse/patient relationships, involving the patient in activities, avoiding or lessening dependency, and fostering independence and autonomy. The nurse should be accepting of the patient, nonjudgmental, and consistent in therapeutic approaches.

W e l l n e s s

❝A mentally healthy older adult has learned to adapt to life changes and to utilize successful coping skills.❞

Older adults who abuse substances have the potential for trauma, injury, self-injury, altered thought processes, self-care deficits, sensory-perceptual alteration, self-esteem disturbance, ineffective individual coping, and caregiver role strain.

Older adults who are declining in physical health may, for financial or cultural reasons, fail to visit a physician but use over-the-counter drugs to care for themselves. There are many who self-medicate with drugs and alcohol to relieve psychological and physical pain. Loneliness in old age may lead to substance abuse and prevent its detection, whereas life changes in aging can lead to the use of alcohol and drugs as a means of coping with stress. The nurse should encourage patients to ask their pharmacist about potential drug interaction and misuse.

Aggressive Behaviors

Considering the rapid growth in the older adult population, a growing challenge facing staff of long-term care facilities is the management of aggressive behavior. Aggressive behavior is a problem for patients, staff, and the individual exhibiting the behavior. To deal with disruptive behavior effectively, the behavior must be understood. Aggressive behavior often arises out of a real need to gain attention; violence can be described as a powerful communication of need.

Burgio and associates (1988) define a behavior problem as a "diverse array of patient responses which are considered noxious" to those involved. When violent behavior occurs, a process is involved that can be described as follows:

1. An alteration of biopsychosocial need is expressed.
2. A threat to the self-esteem is posed.
3. A state of arousal occurs (feelings of stress and tension are present).
4. Severe anxiety emerges. (Perceptual field is narrowed with a tendency to perceive only details.)
5. Feelings of helplessness and entrapment arise.
6. The person is impelled to reduce anxiety and overcome feelings of helplessness and entrapment.
7. The person resorts to behaviors that have successfully given mastery and control in the past over intense feelings of anxiety, helplessness, and entrapment.

■ CASE STUDY

Mrs. J, age 80, paces the halls rapidly. She does not choose to discuss her concerns with the primary nurse, who has reviewed her assessment and the history provided by her family. In the assessment it was determined that Mrs. J is experiencing a high level of anxiety made worse by her recent admission to the facility. She is now loud and boisterous, shouting at everyone and being verbally abusive.

The nurse approaches Mrs. J in a calm manner. She does not touch Mrs. J but invites her over to a quiet corner, where she tells her she is going to administer her, as necessary, antianxiety medication. Mrs. J is agitated but nods affirmatively. The nurse does not argue or reason with the already aggressive patient.

The nurse later develops a care plan focused on Mrs. J's environment. Stimuli are to be decreased. Mrs. J is informed of expectations for her behavior. The care plan is made

with input from Mrs. J who states that she feels "locked up" and would like to be outside.

Mrs. J and her nurse meet in the mornings for a walk outside. Mrs. J also begins to participate in group activity. She rests in her room before lunch, listening to her favorite country-western music, which has a soothing effect on her. Mrs. J's aggressive behavior decreases, and she appears to be enjoying her morning walks and music therapy.

Other patients are allowed to ventilate their feelings about the incident. They are told that their safety is paramount.

Nursing interventions instituted for Mrs. J were to:

- Reduce stimuli in the environment
- Increase structured activities in order for patient to release energy
- Set limits on behavior by telling patient the expectations
- Encourage supportive relationships, group activities, and music therapy
- Include patient in plan of care
- Review plan of care with patient periodically
- Implement behavior modification
- Add social skills training

Aggressive behaviors can take various forms, including physical (striking out), verbal (swearing), subtle (breaking a promise made to another), or turning on oneself (self-mutilation or suicide). Aggressive behaviors may be directed at another person. The adverse effect of aggressive behavior on caregivers and others in the environment is of great concern and has implications of caring for large numbers of aggressive older adults in long-term care settings.

Factors contributing to aggressive behavior include fatigue, impaired perception (as hearing and visual deficits), pain, fear, a perceived threat to one's person, frustration, anger, or hostility. The lack of control the residents have over their lives in a nursing home environment is a constant source of frustration. The behavior of staff and other patients may be misinterpreted. Patients experience social isolation and lack of environmental stimulation and may react in an aggressive manner.

Nursing interventions should reflect whether the aggressive behavior was provoked, related to institutionalization, or associated with hallucinations, delusions, or cognitive deficits. Nonpharmacological methods are advantageous to the patient, and there are no associated side effects. When pharmacology is indicated, psychotic symptoms are usually treated by neuroleptics (see Table 24–1), which are the most widely prescribed drugs for aggression and agitation in older adults.

Vaccaro (1988) undertook a study in behavior modification in which basic rewards of juice and cookies reinforced positive behaviors and a verbal censure or removal from group activity was used to show disapproval of aggressive behavior. Social skills training can also be used with aggressive patients (Vaccaro, 1990). The nurse should offer reassurances during a task that appears threatening and tell patients that they are safe and that no one is going to hurt or harm them. Patients should be allowed their personal space. Diversion and distraction can be used. A calm environment can be provided. The nurse should interact with the patient in a caring manner.

Caring

"The nurse should be nonjudgmental and assist the alcoholic patient with expression of feelings."

Because of legal considerations, accurate observation and documentation are essential. Patients who are aggressive continue to have feelings, dignity, and both human and legal rights. The patient needs to be treated safely with the least amount of restriction, and the nurse should not overreact to the situation. Environmental stimuli should be decreased. The nurse should try to intervene before the aggressive behavior escalates. If the patient can verbalize feelings of hostility, this should be encouraged. The nurse should never strike the patient nor shout, touch, argue, or reason with an already aggressive patient. Any prn medications should be administered as ordered. If the nurse does not feel competent in handling the situation, assistance should be obtained as soon as possible. Other patients in the area must be protected. Patients can be allowed to ventilate their feelings, especially after the situation has been resolved.

Because other patients have their own needs and problems, the nurse must be careful not to give attention to the "sickest" patient only. The aggressive patient is helped to develop or increase feelings of self-worth. Expression of feelings in a nonaggressive manner should be encouraged. The patient can be taught how to deal with tension, about the illness, and about medication use, if applicable. Patient teaching can assist the patient in complying with treatment and medication regimens, increase awareness of feelings associated with aggressive behavior, and show how better to handle the situation, using the techniques taught by the nursing staff.

Geropsychiatric Disorders

SCHIZOPHRENIA

Comparatively little has been published on the characteristics of people with schizophrenia who grow old, either in a psychiatric facility or in the community. Elderly schizophrenic patients are those older than 65 years of age who have been in continual psychiatric contact for several years.

Of all the mental illnesses responsible for suffering in society, schizophrenia probably causes more lengthy hospitalizations and more chaos in family life than any other. **Schizophrenia** is a **functional** (not related to an organ) **psychosis** that involves a thought disorder characterized by altered concepts of reality, such as delusions and hallucinations. It is considered to be a serious psychiatric disorder that tends to be chronic and generally leads to severe disabilities. Other symptoms include loss of contact with reality, impaired communication, and deterioration from a previous level of functioning in self-care, work, and social relationships.

With schizophrenia there is a disturbance in thought process, perception, affect, or mood. The illness can occur at any age across the life span, although generally it presents during late adolescence or early adulthood. Older adults with schizophrenia have probably suffered from the illness for many years, with exacerbations experienced as the stresses of aging increase. Schizophrenia and delusional disorders may continue into old age or may manifest for the first time during senescence. After age 60, schizophrenia is not common; when it does occur, it is in the form of persecutory delusions or hallucinations.

Older adults with schizophrenia may be cared for in nursing homes, other residential settings, or at home; some are homeless. Some have been taking neuroleptic medications (see Tables 24–1 and 24–2) for many years and are at high risk for gastrointestinal, liver, kidney, or cardiovascular diseases, although older adults with schizophrenia tend to underreport medical symptoms and overrate their physical well-being. The course of the illness is chronic, and the treatment includes supportive psychotherapy and psychopharmacology (Townsend, 1993).

DELUSIONS

Delusions are false beliefs with no basis in reality. Delusions may be the primary symptom, as in a *delusional disorder*. They can be one of several symptoms manifested by the patient, as in schizophrenia, alcohol intoxication, or major affective disorder. Some people may have fixed delusions (especially those with paranoia) that persist throughout their lives. Most psychotic patients have transient delusions that appear after specific episodes but do not last over time.

Caring

❝*Offering hope for change in intolerable circumstances may deter a suicide attempt.***❞**

Delusions are often of a persecutory nature and can be traced over time, in some instances, from a gradually increasing sense of victimization to a full-fledged paranoid state. When anxiety is reduced, the need for the delusion is also reduced. Nursing interventions should focus on the content of the thoughts expressed and the process being used by the delusional older adult. The paranoid state in an older adult can be reflective of a functional disorder, an organic brain syndrome, or an abnormal personality.

Paranoia is an attempt to deal with the onset of memory loss in dementing illness. Sudden gaps in memory are frightening. Patients may rationalize losing things by claiming to be robbed by family members and others. Nursing interventions are to reassure and not argue

with patients. Belongings should be organized in a way to prevent loss. A safe environment and specific comfort measures are beneficial.

HALLUCINATIONS

Hallucinations are false sensory perceptions that are not associated with real external stimuli. Hallucinations are generally symptoms of schizophrenia or bipolar affective disorder and may also be seen in substance abuse and organic disease. They are associated with an increase in anxiety that, when reduced, will also reduce the need for the hallucination.

Nursing interventions should provide contact with reality, orientation to time, place, and person, and ways of dealing with anxiety. Also, the nurse needs to teach the patient that a hallucinatory experience may occur when there is a stressful situation or a change in routine activities.

■ CASE STUDY

Mr. M, who is 70 years old, has a diagnosis of chronic undifferentiated schizophrenia persisting for the past 45 years. Over the past several years he has had multiple hospitalizations, with great emotional upheaval to his family. Since the death of his parents 15 years ago, Mr. M has lived in a neighborhood residential care facility. His prescribed medication is 300 mg/d of chlorpromazine (Thorazine). Nursing staff observe that any increase in his medication produces side effects. Mr. M has been experiencing delusions and auditory hallucinations. Recent changes in the operation of the facility have precipitated some anxiety and psychotic behavior in Mr. M.

Nursing staff spend more time with Mr. M, offering support and safety. The extra time spent with him in group activities and nurse/patient activities has resulted in a decrease in his anxiety. Early identification of the cause of the behavior (instead of increase in medication dosage) has been of benefit. Nursing intervention of supportive therapy to alleviate anxiety resulted in disappearance of psychotic symptoms.

Mr. M is an example of an older adult with schizophrenia who has experienced many hospitalizations. He has been taking neuroleptic medications for many years. The course of his illness has been chronic, with supportive therapy and psychopharmacology as treatment modalities.

The nurse should

- Assess to determine the role of anxiety in increased symptoms.
- Administer prescribed psychopharmacological medication.
- Keep patient in contact with reality although hallucinations and delusions are present. Reality orientation is critical.
- Make a list of possible activities, inside and outside the residential care facility, that Mr. M can participate in.
- Encourage supportive relationships with staff and others.

DEPRESSION

Depression is an affective or mood disorder that can be preventable and reversible. Although it is a treatable illness, it can go unrecognized, untreated, and even ignored. Depression in the older adult population is not a normal part of aging but a serious mental health problem for this age group. It is the most prevalent of all psychiatric disorders in older adults. It can be associated with bipolar disorder with mania or be a major clinical depression. The diagnostic criteria for major depression are presented in Box 24–2.

Depressive disorders are characterized by exaggerated feelings of sadness, worthlessness, hopelessness, helplessness, emptiness, and dejection that do not disappear with logic, reasoning, or reality. Depression can occur secondarily to physical illness and may be masked by multiple somatic complaints or pain, usually of the back, neck, head, or abdomen. Fatigue and gastrointestinal complaints are particularly common.

Loneliness, unresolved grief, anger, and guilt can contribute to depression. Other factors contributing to depression include losses and aging changes. Some losses that may lead to depression are

- Loss of sight and/or hearing or other sensory deficits
- Loss of loved ones or significant others
- Loss of healthy status
- Loss in economic ability
- Loss of job and job activity due to retirement
- Loss of cognitive ability
- Loss of home, relocation, or change in environment

Medications prescribed for other illnesses may cause a depressive episode. Among these are

- Neuroleptics (major tranquilizers)
- Sedatives
- Antihypertensive agents
- Antihistamines
- Anticonvulsants
- Analgesics
- Barbiturates
- Cardiogenics
- Amphetamines
- Antibiotics

Medical conditions that can be associated with depression include

---

Box 24-2   SYMPTOMS OF DEPRESSION

The differential diagnosis of depressive symptoms in late life (DSM-IV) lists the following as diagnostic criteria for major depression.
Depressed mood and/or loss of interest or pleasure plus *four* of the following:

- Weight loss or gain
- Insomnia or hypersomnia
- Psychomotor agitation or retardation
- Loss of energy
- Feelings of worthlessness
- Difficulty in concentrating
- Recurrent thoughts of death or suicide

- Renal disease, uremia
- Endocrine disorders
- Some neoplasms
- Vitamin deficiency
- Infections
- Nutritional problems
- Parkinson's disease
- Cancer
- Arthritis
- Early stages of Alzheimer's disease

To accurately assess and treat depression, a comprehensive geriatric assessment should be done. Areas of concern are

- An accurate diagnosis
- Medications and treatments, prescribed and administered
- Nutrition
- Continence
- Defecation
- Cognition
- Emotional status
- Mobility
- Compliance with prescribed care
- Sleep

Bereavement often produces a form of depression that few older adults escape, and it may lead to suicidal thoughts and behavior. Bereavement is problematic if it

- Lasts longer than 1 year
- Is accompanied by deterioration of health
- Is characterized by extreme guilt and hopelessness
- Is accompanied by suicidal ideation

If bereavement becomes problematic, the older adult should receive medical care and bereavement counseling.

Suicide

Suicide is a form of violence to self. It remains one of the major causes of death among the fastest growing segment of the U.S. population—people aged 65 and older. Many older adults who commit suicide have been in recent contact with health care professionals and expressed symptoms of anxiety and depression. Risk factors include

- Age (increasing)
- Sex (male more successful, although females make more attempts of a nonlethal nature)

- Race (white)
- Presence of painful or disabling physical illness
- Previous history of suicidal behavior, frequency and intensity of suicidal ideation, or psychiatric illness
- Alcoholism
- Current stress factors
- Significant life events (e.g., bereavement overload)
- Solitary living conditions
- Depression, especially associated with agitation, excessive guilt, self-reproach, and insomnia

The primary cause of suicide is intolerable life circumstances. The cumulative effect of losses over time seems to increase the older adult's vulnerability to suicide. Depression should be assessed through the use of a standardized depression scale and treated. Undiagnosed and untreated depression can lead to poor patient outcomes. A psychosocial history should focus on past anxiety, depression, use of alcohol and drugs, paranoia, hallucinations, social skills, support system, and family history of anxiety and depression.

Suicidal ideation is defined as thoughts of committing suicide. *Suicidal gesture* is self-destructive behavior that is not lethal (e.g., taking 10 aspirin tablets). A *suicide attempt* is self-destructive behavior that is potentially lethal. Suicidal precautions are specific actions taken by the health care team to protect a patient from self-harm and necessitate close 24-hour observation of a suicidal patient.

A suicide prevention plan can be developed by the patient and the nurse. Emotional support should be available to the older adult. Staff must be available to listen, be empathetic, and encourage communication. Older adults need to acknowledge and work through depression and suicidal ideation. They need to have someone listen and respond, which is a difficult task for family and friends. If health care providers offer hope for change in intolerable circumstances, older adults reduce or abandon suicidal ideation. Helping to find solutions to even one problem may contribute to a sense of control and hope. Religious belief is a strong deterrent to committing suicide. The older adult patient can be asked to agree to a "no-suicide contract" drawn up with the nursing staff, who should monitor the patient's level of self-control. The patient must always be treated with dignity and appreciation of worth.

Because older adults are now encouraged by society to participate in end-of-life decisions through measures such as advance directives and living wills, the process of death and dying presents issues to be faced. Nursing staff who are willing to discuss these issues find that many older adults want to talk about the ending of their lives, and (1) they have given much thought to their own death, and (2) are grappling with the issues surrounding "natural death," euthanasia, passive suicide, actual suicide, and physician-assisted suicide.

While trying to dissuade terminally ill older adults who have talked about suicide, nurses can suggest the option of hospice. If an ethical dilemma occurs regarding the terminally ill patient's desire for assisted suicide, clergy or the Hemlock Society (see Resources) or an ethics committee should be contacted for assistance in conflict resolution (see Chapter 3). Knowledge of the availability of hospice service and of advance directives may assist the patient in deciding against contemplated suicide. The Dying Patients' Bill of Rights can be used by nurses as a guide to planning care, whether or not they are supportive of suicide. Nurses are in an excellent position to develop a preventive role with regard to suicide, because of their frequent, often prolonged therapeutic engagement with patients.

CHRONIC MENTAL ILLNESS IN OLDER ADULTS

Mental illness in older adults may move from the acute to chronic stage when additional stressors are confronted. Many of the stressors associated with aging can neither be eliminated nor ignored. Those most likely to exacerbate mental illness include bereavement, poverty, physical frailty, inadequate or absence of support systems, and inaccessible or nonexisting services.

With the aging of society, there are increasing numbers of older, at-risk individuals. Many have unrecognized physical disease, and their illnesses tend to be complicated by substance misuse or abuse. Enhancing social supports has been an alternative means of protecting older adults who are at risk for mental illness.

In 1963, when Congress passed the Community Mental Health Act, there was a mandate for deinstitutionalization. Mentally ill patients were discharged from psychiatric hospitals. Some reentered communities with support systems that included mental health centers and halfway houses, and others reentered communities with no available services. Many of these had families not able or unwilling to care for them. Thus, many older adults became homeless or lived a marginal existence in rooming houses or shelters. The process of deinstitutionalization has contributed to increasing numbers of untreated chronically mentally ill older adults over the last 35 years.

Screening of all nursing home admissions for mental illness was initiated with the Omnibus Reconciliation Act of 1987. For those already in the nursing home with a diagnosis of mental illness, discharge was recommended. Services for the chronically mentally ill older adult are sparse in many areas and nonexistent in others. Medicare, the primary health insurer for older adults, reimburses only limited and acute mental health needs.

Caring

"*It is important to tell aggressive patients that they are safe and no one is going to hurt them.***"**

Clearly, the chronically mentally ill older adult is found in the community. Assessment by community health care professionals should include patient's needs, available services, community supports, and appropriate housing. For those who live in shelters, mental health services should be made available. Food and housing are the greatest needs and should take precedence over outpatient treatment and short-term hospitalization. The lack of services necessary for basic survival makes it difficult for the chronically mentally ill older adult to receive adequate treatment.

The chronically mentally ill older adult usually has a diagnosis of depression (the most prevalent of all psychiatric disorders in older adults) or of a schizophrenic disorder. Older people with schizophrenia often have fewer and less severe symptoms, owing to the so-called burnout of schizophrenia. This patient population is usually found in residential settings and shelters or is undomiciled and presents a challenge to nurses. The nursing care is complex because of the chronicity of the illness and the years of treatment required.

THE NEEDS OF CAREGIVERS

Caring for the older adult has been and, it appears, will continue to be a family responsibility. The older adult population is rapidly becoming the largest sector of the American population, with the most rapidly growing age group older than 85. Population aging is the major driving force in the caregiving crisis in America.

Chronic poor physical or mental health of care recipients often affects the caregiver adversely. A **caregiver** can be defined as one who provides unpaid, informal care to an older adult who requires help with daily activities and personal needs.

Care of the older adult who is mentally ill is very stressful, and this can be compounded if it is accompanied by disruptive behavior. As deinstitutionalization of older adults with severe mental illness has proceeded since the 1960s, the families of these people have become the "institution of choice." Families have been forced to become caregivers, and they are unprepared for the job. Incapacitated families cannot assist their ill family member.

The burden of care can induce stress in the caregiver, causing chronic fatigue, anger, hostility, guilt, grief, powerlessness, and fear:

1. Chronic fatigue is experienced when the caregiver is tired and does not receive adequate rest, respite, or leisure time for self.
2. Anger is often felt toward the care recipient but can be directed at other family members or "the system."
3. Hostility is an emotion that carries guilt because the caregiver realizes the older adults cannot care for themselves but the caregiver still experiences and exhibits angry behavior toward the person in care.
4. Guilt is felt because the caregiver often dislikes the role and experiences ambivalence but is unable to bring about a change in the situation.
5. Grief is a prominent feature in the lives of families of older adults with severe mental illness. The cycle of recovery and relapse is painful.
6. Powerlessness is felt when services, help, and even a cure cannot be found.
7. Fear is felt for the older adult care recipient if the caregiver feels inadequate in caregiving. The caregiver can feel fearful if the patient is hospitalized, is physically or verbally abusive, or is threatening or assaultive toward the caregiver.

Informal caregivers need support and should be taught care management. The anguish inflicted on family caregivers must be corrected. Significant factors that impact family caregivers are

- Lack of help with caregiving responsibilities
- Disturbed sleep and sleep deprivation
- Physical and mental exhaustion
- Lack of opportunities to socialize and participate in hobbies or recreation
- Depression

These factors are often the cause of the family caregiver's inability to continue to function, and they contribute to a decline in the number of informal caregivers as well as a decrease in the tasks that need to be performed. Health care professionals should intervene whenever possible and work collaboratively with family caregivers. Combined intervention will maximize the older adult's mental health and minimize deterrents to positive health of both caregiver and care recipient.

Family caregivers do not have an easy task. The large majority of the care given to older adults is provided by family members, and family caregivers need help. The second most common reason for admission to nursing homes is "unmanageable" behavior such as agitation, assaultiveness, paranoid ideation, confusion, depression, wandering, and cognitive impairment (Harper, 1993). The stress experienced by family caregivers may be increased at the time of the older adult's admission to or discharge from a hospital or nursing home. Stress may be displaced as hostility to nursing personnel, who should take time to communicate meaningfully with family members in allaying their anxieties

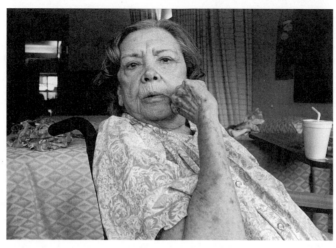

The anxious patient may be treated psychotherapeutically as well as with medication.

and offering assistance with coping skills. Knowledge of how family caregivers have approached, experienced, and managed other stressors is helpful to the nurse who is assessing the situation and developing an effective plan of care and intervention.

Needs of family caregivers include

1. Information regarding the availability of community resources
2. Support groups to provide emotional assistance and knowledge of how other families manage in similar situations
3. Respite services provided by hospitals, nursing homes, or in-home, where the older adult can receive care while the caregiver receives some time for self
4. Health care for the caregiver
5. Health promotion measures and techniques to keep the caregiver as healthy as possible for the task of caregiving
6. Education on how to deal with the stress of caregiving and on how to become better-prepared caregivers

ELDER ABUSE

In recent years the media have begun to spotlight issues of abuse. Child abuse, sexual abuse, and domestic abuse are still more generally recognized than abuse of older adults, which may be more readily concealed because of the limited mobility of many older adults—particularly those with disabilities or those in the old-old group. Elder abuse may take the form of physical, psychological, or verbal abuse. Types of abuse and neglect include

- Physical abuse
- Physical neglect
- Sexual abuse
- Emotional maltreatment

It appears that elder abuse is sufficiently extensive to merit public concern. Abuse is a reportable incident whether occurring in a nursing home, in the community, in the older adult's home, or wherever an older adult's rights are violated. The Nursing Home Reform Amendments (NHRA) have several provisions for the health and welfare of older adults, including the right to be free from abuse and neglect and adult protective services laws that monitor, report, and respond to abuse, neglect, and exploitation of vulnerable adults (Omnibus Reconciliation Act, 1987).

Elder abuse laws exist in almost every state, with mandatory reporting by health care professionals of suspected abuse of older adults. Elder abuse is a form of victimization that

W e l l n e s s

"Healthy living patterns, positive social relationships, interests, pleasures, economic status, and individual self-worth contribute to successful aging."

threatens the physical and psychological safety of many older adults. Neglect is failure to provide some degree of minimal care for a person. It can be deliberate or unintentional.

The abused-elder profile suggests a white woman older than age 75 years. There are reported incidents of abused men where the abuser was a spouse. Abuse may be inflicting pain or injury; stealing from the person; withholding food, care, or money; confining the person; or exploiting an older adult. Caregiver stress can lead to abuse.

Nurses have a legal and ethical responsibility to report and document abuse. They must be knowledgeable about the laws of the state in which they practice. Careful assessment is necessary in identifying abuse and/or neglect. Skills of observation and communication by a caring health care professional in a safe environment are necessary in eliciting the information required to make the diagnosis of elder abuse, neglect, or maltreatment.

■ NURSING MANAGEMENT AND INTERVENTIONS

The gerontological nurse must incorporate patient education into the assessment process, which is crucial to the treatment plan. Selection of the "right" assessment tool or instrument is important. The many available tools include

- FROMAJE: Functional, Reasoning, Orientation, Memory, Arithmetic, Judgment, and Emotion
- Mini-Mental State Examination
- Short Portable Mental Status Questionnaire (SPMSQ), geriatric
- Geriatric Depression Scale
- Older Americans Research Assessment Tool (OARS behavioral assessment)

Wellness

66 Wellness is a concept that has revolutionized care. Today's older adults are participating in health and wellness programs in unprecedented numbers. These positive lifestyle changes enhance the mental health of older adults. 99

- Older Americans Research Social Resource Scale
- Substance abuse assessment
- Caregivers assessment—safety and long-term considerations

Additional assessments include

- Mental and emotional health status
- Self-care and self-responsibility
- Nutrition/hydration
- Sexuality
- Caregiver stress and how it affects the patient
- Mobility/immobility status
- Personal and demographic data
- Resource allocation and availability
- Environmental and safety concerns
- Finances and effect on patient's well-being
- Relationships and social affiliations
- Medications being used
- Specific physical and emotional patterns/lifestyle

A social history should be taken that provides data on cultural background, family composition, education, employment, retirement, language, and social relationships, including marital situation, social contacts, and household composition. Religious activities of interest, frequency, and limitation should also be assessed.

The most important therapeutic approach in working with a geropsychiatric patient is to build a trusting relationship as soon as possible. Verbal communication and a caring manner are used to provide a nonthreatening, therapeutic environment. An outlet is provided for the patient's feelings, tension, and agitation to decrease psychotic symptoms. There should be an adequate balance of rest, sleep, and activity.

In specific areas of anxious behavior, delusions, or hallucinations, the nurse should remain with the patient and move to a quiet area with minimal or decreased stimuli. Self-esteem is promoted and the steps of decision-making are facilitated. The patient should be prevented from harming self, others, or property. The nurse should interrupt the patient's pattern of hallucinations and should not argue about delusions (false beliefs). The patient can be taught therapeutic communication and social skills, and practice of those skills can be encouraged through feedback, behavior modification, and reinforcement.

Counseling and psychotherapy (individual,

group, and family) are interventions used in the care and treatment of geropsychiatric patients. Group psychotherapy is an important and valid treatment modality for the psychiatrically impaired elderly (Pearlman, 1993). The group format offers a reality-based social context in which patients may explore their concerns. The therapist should be sensitive to issues such as sensory loss and debilitating illness while leading geriatric psychotherapy groups.

Psychopharmacology, with patient education of drug interactions and side effects, is a potent treatment modality. Pharmacological management of a major depressive disorder receives emphasis as the mainstay of treatment. Antidepressants, psychosocial and cognitive nursing, and clinical interventions and outcomes are utilized. Neuroleptics are used in the treatment of acute and chronic psychosis. Anxiolytic (antianxiety) drugs are minor tranquilizers used in the treatment of anxiety disorders, anxiety symptoms, acute alcohol withdrawal, preoperative sedation, and relief of anxiety (see Tables 24–1 and 24–2).

The legal implications associated with the administration of psychotropic medications must be understood by the nurse. Laws differ from state to state; most adhere to the patient's rights to refuse treatment. Exceptions exist, however, in emergency situations when it is believed that patients are harmful to themselves or others. When psychoactive drugs are prescribed for this age group, it should be in amounts that are one half or one third the amount prescribed for younger adults of comparable weight, in doses divided over the course of day (see Table 24–2).

Other therapeutic interventions for the geropsychiatric client include electroconvulsive therapy, which is used in the treatment of severe depression, especially in those patients experiencing psychotic symptoms, psychomotor retardation, and disturbance in sleep, appetite, and energy. Electroconvulsive therapy is especially beneficial for older adults who experience insomnia and anorexia. Institutional procedures should be followed in the administration of this therapy.

Milieu therapy structures the environment in such a way as to improve the individual's mental health and functioning. The environment *is* the therapy, and activities within the environment are designed to be therapeutic. Structured activities teach the patient new coping strategies, social skills, and healthy behavior. In a therapeutic community can be found occupational, recreational, art, and music therapy; psychodrama; and the interdisciplinary treatment team, presenting several therapeutic modalities, approaches and interventions.

Reminiscence and life review are modes of interaction in which older adults share their memories by telling stories about themselves. The content is based on the individual's strengths and is informative. Nursing staff become knowledgeable about their patients as they relate more positively to them, thus increasing their patients' self-esteem, sense of belonging, and identity. The natural tendency of the patient to talk about life experiences can be facilitated by even an inexperienced group leader. Reviewing life events is a means of focusing attention, exercising the mind, and stimulating memories that have lain dormant, thus enabling a psychotherapeutic process. The nurse/group leader should always work toward increasing the patient's self-esteem.

C a r i n g

"*Abilities must always be emphasized over disabilities.***"**

Geropsychiatric nurses require special preparation and expertise in several areas of nursing (gerontological, psychiatric, mental health, community health, medical, and surgical) to intervene with a holistic approach when caring for geropsychiatric clients. **Geropsychiatric nursing,** a fairly new subspecialty of psychiatric nursing, is a caring interactive process that maximizes independence and autonomy of older adults in the activities of daily living. It promotes, maintains, and restores mental health while assessing, planning, implementing, and evaluating care of older adults.

Summary

The older population is increasing at a faster rate than the general population. Most older adults remain relatively healthy, mentally and physically, into later life. Mental health in later life is closely related to intrapersonal, interpersonal, and environmental interactive processes.

The most underserved segment of the population in need of mental health services is the older adult age group. Inaccessibility of care and stigmatization are some deterrents. Common mental illnesses are depression, suicidal behavior, substance abuse, and cognitive impairment. Dysfunctional bereavement, multiple losses, isolation, and loneliness are risk factors that contribute to the mental illness of older adults.

Mentally ill older adults are cared for in psychiatric hospitals, nursing homes, and at home with their families as caregivers. Family caregivers need much emotional support and assistance in caregiving.

Therapeutic interventions, including psychotherapy, should be explored and implemented. Medications are not a substitute for other therapies and need to be carefully monitored because older adults excrete medications less efficiently and are at risk for drug toxicity.

RESOURCES

Alcoholics Anonymous
15 East 26th Street, Room 1817
New York, NY 10010
(212) 683-3900

Al-Anon Family Group Headquarters
1372 Broadway
New York, NY 10018
(212) 302-7240

The Hemlock Society
PO Box 11830
Eugene, OR 97440
(503) 342-5748
This group provides information regarding advance directives and assisted suicide.

The Right to Die Society
250 West 57th Street
New York, NY 10107
(212) 246-6973
This organization merged with Concern for Dying in 1991, creating Choice in Dying. These organizations champion the rights of patients to refuse unwanted life support.

REFERENCES

American Psychiatric Association. (1994). Diagnostic and Statistical Manual of Mental Disorders. 4th ed, revised. Washington, DC: American Psychiatric Association.

Burgio L, Jones L, Butler F, Engel B. (1988). Behavior problems in an urban nursing home. J Gerontol Nurs 14(1):31–34.

Erikson EH. (1963). Childhood and Society. New York: WW Norton.

Harper M. (1993). Career profiles in psychiatric—mental health nursing. In Johnson B, ed. Adaptation and Growth: Psychiatric—Mental Health Nursing. Philadelphia: JB Lippincott.

News Watch. (1993). Geriatr Nurs 14(4):177.

Pearlman I. (1993). Group psychotherapy with the elderly. J Psychosoc Nurs Ment Health Serv 31(7):7–10.

Townsend M. (1993). Psychiatric Mental Health Nursing: Concepts of Care. Philadelphia: FA Davis.

Vaccaro FJ. (1988). Successful operant conditioning procedures with an institutionalized aggressive geriatric patient. Int J Aging Hum Dev 26(1):71–79.

Vaccaro FJ. (1990). An application of social skills training in a group of institutionalized aggressive elderly subjects. Psychol Aging 5(3):389–398.

CRITICAL THINKING EXERCISES

1. Have three students role play a nurse, an older adult client, and the client's caregiver, in the following situations:
   a. The nurse suspects the caregiver has been abusing the client.
   b. The client is behaving aggressively toward the nurse.
   c. The client caregiver appears to be "high" on something.
2. Canvass your community and find how many and what kind of mental health programs are available to older adults. How many are outpatient facilities? Residential? Serve the undomiciled?
3. Use the Internet to research one of the following:
   a. Homelessness related to mental illness
   b. Substance abuse in older adults
   c. New psychoactive drugs
   d. Remedies for elder abuse
   e. Suicide, prevention of, or assisted

CHAPTER 25

Death and Dying

Shirley Rose Tyson, RN, MA, EdD

CHAPTER OUTLINE

OBJECTIVES

After completing this chapter, the reader should be able to:

1. Construct a teaching plan to provide support for the family, caregivers, and friends of a dying person.
2. Teach a classmate how to identify the physical, affective, and behavioral expressions of grief.
3. Formulate a plan of care that will provide comfort measures to a dying older adult.
4. Apply the concepts of loss, bereavement, and grief to the particular needs of the older adult population.

bereavement
grief
hospice
mourning
palliative care
thanatologists

Dying is a part of life, just as birth is. It is a normal process, the culmination of the entire life span, and represents the end of the aging process.

Many people are unwilling, and perhaps afraid, to deal with the fact that death is inevitable. Fear of the unknown is often associated with ideas of death. Working with older adult patients and families necessitates that nurses have a pragmatic knowledge of dying and an understanding of loss. Nurses are called on to provide emotional support to patients and families, teaching and utilizing coping strategies, because dying and death occur mostly in facilities where care is provided by nurses.

CARE OF THE DYING PERSON

The needs of the dying person are physical, emotional, psychological, and spiritual. Care of the dying person is called **palliative care.** Psychiatrist Elisabeth Kübler-Ross (1969) worked with dying patients and wrote that the dying process extends throughout life and that all of us go repeatedly through the stages of this process as we examine significant changes in our lives. In her book on death and dying, Kübler-Ross (1969) described a five-stage process of dying:

1. *Denial and isolation.* Regarded as healthy, denial can function as a buffer after unexpected news; it allows people to collect themselves and mobilize other defenses.
2. *Anger.* Patients ask "Why me?" Anger may be displaced and projected toward the people around them.
3. *Bargaining.* People may bargain with God to gain more time. Usually family events or projects are mentioned.
4. *Depression.* Increasingly severe evidence of disease may manifest as pain and weight loss; anger and rage are replaced by feelings of depression and profound loss.
5. *Acceptance.* Negotiation of the above stages enables the patient to reach a place where dying can be accepted. In this phase, patients may turn inward with their thoughts and feelings and their worldly interests diminish. During this phase, families may need more help, support, and understanding than the dying person does.

The research of Kübler-Ross led health care professionals to a better understanding of the needs of dying patients and their families. Some attitudes related to the dying process, as experienced by the older adult, are now found to be in opposition to those previously described by Kübler-Ross. Emotions such as anger, denial, and hopelessness are not necessarily felt as these patients face their final hour (Voss-Morice, 1996). However, dying patients often feel despair and loneliness and need the emotional support of the caring nurse.

W e l l n e s s

"Examining the nurse's own feelings and attitudes about death can be therapeutic for the nurse and helpful in the care of dying patients.**"**

Older adults who are dying may find comfort by expressing their feelings and talking openly with family and friends. Many times, patients seek this comfort from their nurse. Even if the nurse feels uncertain as to what should be said, just sitting quietly beside the patient is supportive. The patient needs respect and companionship at this time and will usually set the tone of the interaction. By being sensitive to the expressed and nonverbal needs of the patient, both the nurse and family members can help the person experience a peaceful death.

Emotional needs are met when patients are encouraged to verbalize their feelings and nurses listen. It is essential that nurses be truthful in their responses. Backer, Hannon, and

Russell (1994) state that people deserve thorough assessments of their needs and of their abilities to cope with the knowledge of dying; they do not allow themselves to hear more than they are ready to accept at that moment. The dying person can withdraw in despair to repress negative emotions or can reach out to others. Dying can be seen as a growth process, in that emotional growth requires commitment to experiencing self, to becoming aware of one's own identity, to communicating that experience to others, and to accepting that one's life has purpose and meaning. Nursing interventions linked to these concepts can be viewed as promoting wellness and supporting healthy introspective practices.

Physical needs pertaining to symptom-specific care must be met. In addition, some physical changes that generally occur during the dying process (Voss-Morice, 1996) include

1. Cardiovascular changes, with decreased peripheral circulation resulting in skin-color changes, mottling, coolness, and cyanosis.
2. Respiratory alterations, with decreased ability of the lungs to ventilate adequately, resulting in increased accumulation of fluid in the bronchioles. Dyspnea occurs in conjunction with cardiovascular decline, resulting in prolonged periods of apnea and Cheyne-Stokes breathing patterns.
3. Gastrointestinal changes, with decreased appetite, anorexia, intestinal blockage, and bloating. Dysphasia occurs as the involuntary swallowing musculature loses tone.
4. Diminished blood flow to the kidneys means decreased elevated blood urea nitrogen levels and urosepsis.
5. Neurological changes, with poor oxygenation, decreased cerebral blood flow, and synaptic alterations. Disorientation, lethargy, and delirium occur as levels of consciousness decrease.
6. Vision and hearing changes.

Offering pastoral support is an intervention that can help to meet spiritual needs if the patient desires it. Often, the patient may not previously have expressed the need for religion or pastoral support and may need prompting. Death evokes a feeling of ultimate powerlessness because, for most people, the time and cause of death are unpredictable. Perception of death may be influenced by religion, culture, and social status.

Near-death experiences have been described by many people. Decreased death-anxiety, life review, and a sense of self-transcendence seem to be part of the near-death

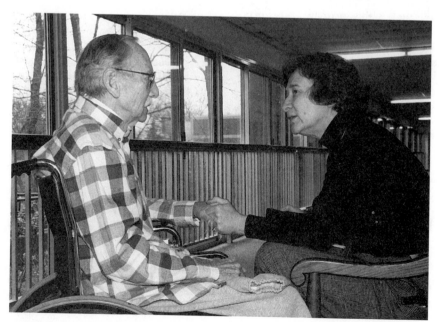

Hospice care is offered to a dying patient who has elected to have no further treatment.

experience. These experiences have been described as "out-of-body" phenomena and appear to be a reaction to the perception of imminent death.

A philosophical attitude tends to accept what life offers, including death. Each culture has both individual and institutional means of coping with the universal human experience of death and bereavement. In Western cultures, religion is involved to varying degrees with the traditions surrounding death. Cultural supports of ritualized patterns of dress, behavior, and religious expression facilitate the process of dying, death, and mourning.

Assisting the dying patient to recognize and verbalize spiritual needs, and meeting the spiritual needs of the dying patient, should be of utmost concern to the nurse, other health care team members, and the family. The nurse is in an excellent position to encourage an openness on the subject of dying and death, so that both the dying person and the family may have the opportunity to complete any unfinished business.

Palliative Care

The caring nurse recognizes anxiety about death and empowers patients and their families to cope (see Supporting Family, Caregivers, and Friends in this chapter). Death awareness needs to be handled with sensitivity and should be part of staff training.

Advance directives can guide family and significant others in decisions consistent with the patient's wishes and personal values. Living wills are signed and witnessed documents directing the extent of care the patient wishes to receive. A durable power of attorney is appointed to represent the patient should he or she become unable to represent himself or herself. Living wills and durable powers of attorney for health care vary from state to state. Each state attorney general's office will have available that state's version of living will laws (Carney and Morrison, 1997). (See Chapters 3 and 4.)

Nursing interventions for palliative care include the following comfort measures for the dying patient:

- Provide an environment that enables the dying patient to die with dignity.
- Provide companionship, especially if family

and friends are not available. Reassure the patient that you will be there.
- Provide pain relief, as directed by physician's orders.
- Provide for hydration and elimination.
- Provide repositioning frequently; gently massage bony areas of body surface.
- Keep the environment quiet and comfortable for the patient.
- Provide comforting conversation. Use good communication skills.
- Listen carefully. Patients give cues to feelings and anxieties.
- Serve as the patient's advocate in decisions about dying and death.
- Permit family and friends to visit and remain nearby.
- Provide holistic, individualized care.
- Deliver excellent physical care, including skin and mouth care.
- Conduct life review; some people request it.
- Support and educate family members and caregivers.
- Respond to requests for prayers, rituals, a religious reading or service from the patient or family. Contact the hospital or nursing home's chaplain or the patient's spiritual advisor.
- Be aware that hearing and vision may decrease and plan interventions accordingly.

Pain Management

Older adults will perceive and express pain differently according to culture, status, gender, medical diagnosis, emotional state, and cognitive function. Some patients will verbalize that they have pain and discomfort, whereas others will use nonverbal responses. Because a patient does not verbalize that there is pain, it should not be assumed to be absent. The nurse can use observational skills to assess the presence and level of pain.

Pain can escalate over time; therefore, patients should be taught to report pain as soon as possible. The goal of pain management for the dying patient is to manage the pain so that it is prevented from occurring. There are many kinds of interventions—pharmacological and nonpharmacological—to help the dying patient. Box 25–1 presents nonpharmacological interventions.

Pharmacological interventions are usually

analgesics. Many are available for use in pain management. The route of administration can vary from oral to intravenous drip to a "patch" containing medication that is worn on the body. Pain management is an area that is rapidly expanding. Many patients are given control of their medications, which can be self-administered in the home or hospital setting, because they are the ones who know when they need the therapy and how much they need. Patients should be encouraged to inform the health care team when their medication is ineffective.

Medication for pain administered to an elderly dying patient should be assessed frequently. The age of the patient, the type of medication, and the dosage affect the outcome for which it was prescribed and administered. The potency of the drug and the age of the patient dictate close monitoring for safety.

Because research has shown that many people die in pain, attached to machines, with their wishes to stop treatment ignored, a consortium of major medical and consumer groups has launched a national campaign to improve care of the dying. The effort, called "Last Acts," brings together the American Medical Association, the American Hospital Association, nurses, medical schools, hospice organizations, and the American Association of Retired Persons in the ongoing debate over how best to care for people who are terminally ill (Montgomery, 1997).

The group's purpose is to push for changes

in the medical profession, the insurance industry, and public attitudes, to make pain control and home care for the dying more widely available. Last Acts believes that beginning to talk about the end of life is important.

Medical schools are increasingly introducing their students to ideas about dying through special courses. Death education is a part of the curriculum. Continuing education courses are offered for practicing physicians. The federal government has approved a diagnostic code for "palliative care," so that reimbursement can take place when trying to cure is displaced by trying to alleviate symptoms (Montgomery, 1997).

Steps aimed at improving care of the dying, proposed by Last Acts (Montgomery, 1997), are to

- Provide comprehensive insurance for hospice care and pain management
- Specify professional standards for physicians, nurses, lawyers, and financial planners on counseling clients about dying
- Set stronger hospital accreditation standards for end-of-life care
- Require hospice experience for medical residents and nursing students

Box 25-1 NONPHARMACOLOGIC PAIN MANAGEMENT THERAPIES

- Relaxation exercises
- Counseling
- Acupuncture
- Acupressure
- Hypnosis
- Guided imagery
- Massage
- Reflexology
- Herbal medicines and teas
- Soothing baths
- Application of heat and cold
- Therapeutic touch
- Alcohol back rubs

- Use medical tests that depict death as a part of life
- Establish workplace programs to help employees plan for terminal illness and care for a dying loved one
- Provide notices on driver's licenses to indicate whether the holder has a living will

Groups such as Choice in Dying advocate for assisted suicide. Advocates for patients' rights are looking at the problem. Many agree that there is a need to improve care of the dying. It is hoped that the campaign effort initiated by Last Acts will bring about changes in the medical profession and other groups that will make assisted suicide unnecessary (Montgomery, 1997). The group hopes to accelerate the movement within the medical profession and bring sharper focus to other issues such as increased access to and insurance coverage for hospice care. These are some of the social issues surrounding care of the dying person. Care of the dying should be made an available resource for all.

Hospice Care

Hospice is defined as a palliative and supportive service that provides physical, psychological, social, and spiritual care for dying people and their families (Bohannan, 1994). The purpose of hospice is to provide support and care for people who are in the last phase of terminal illness so that they may live as fully and comfortably as possible.

Hospice care is concerned with both the care-giver and the dying patient. Care is provided in the home; if home care is no longer feasible, the person may be admitted to a hospice center, if one is available. Curative medical

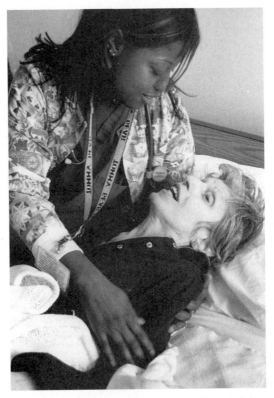

Nurses who work with the dying must address their own personal issues to be effective in the care they give to patients who are facing death.

treatment is not attempted. The person receives individualized nursing care and medications, mainly to control pain. Local community service agencies provide support for hospices. Hospice staff can serve in an important way by keeping the caregiver healthy. Hospice staff can listen to and support the caregiver in mobilizing effective coping strategies. Prebereavement counseling can reassure caregivers that reactions to loss are normal and anticipated.

Hospice nursing is fairly new. In 1974 there was one hospice in the United States. Today there are thousands, ranging from small volunteer groups to larger institutions that care for hundreds of dying patients and their families (Bohannan, 1994). Increased attention to dying and death has resulted in several trends that include the hospice movement, preparation of personnel to provide counseling for dying patients, and living will legislation. The right to die with dignity is inherent in the philosophy of hospice (Milliken, 1993).

Inherent in the concept of dying with dignity is the freedom allowed dying individuals to choose the style of dying; to retain some measure of control; to prepare for dying in their own way, maintaining quality of life; and to be allowed to discuss death openly. Many patients in hospice care request to spend their final days at home in familiar surroundings, with family and friends and (sometimes) pets. This is an attractive alternative to dying in an institution, which is allowed by the hospice movement.

The nurse can

- Instruct family members and caregivers on the stages of dying and the physiological changes that accompany dying.
- Use hospice care to help homebound older adults live as fully as possible on a day-to-day basis.
- Assist the homebound older adult in completing the dying phase if hospice care is not available.
- Provide symptom control.
- Address psychological needs of older adults.
- Assist with spiritual concerns.
- Handle environmental problems as they occur.

Hospice nursing requires intensive care in the home. Most of the care is provided by family members and volunteers. The role of the hospice nurse is to educate, supervise, and support family caregivers.

Bohannan (1994) states that the hospice physician must assume medical responsibility. The patient must sign an informed consent form clearly stating that the patient is revoking curative treatment. This decision is often frightening, and many physicians and patients do not want to make this transition. Critically ill older adults who have no primary caregiver might require inpatient services and may not be as readily accepted by hospice organizations.

Medicare reimbursement benefits for hospice services provided by certified programs was made possible by the National Hospice Reimbursement Statute passed by Congress in 1983 (Bohannan, 1994). Older patients who are eligible for Medicare Part A may elect hospice care if they are certified by their physician to be terminally ill with a life expectancy of 6 months or less.

The hospice nurse must be an expert practitioner, teacher, and counselor and must be able to work closely with other members of the hospice team. The nurse who is counseling the terminally ill older patient and family must consider many social and financial variables to direct the patient to the best resource and the most effective intervention for that specific person.

Supporting the Family, Caregivers, and Friends

The family, caregiver, and friends may be hesitant to talk with the older adult about death. They think, sometimes erroneously, that this could be upsetting to the older adult.

■ CASE STUDY

The nurse, Ms. Adams, visited a terminally ill older patient, Mrs. Bundy, in her home as part of hospice service. Ms. Adams was greeted at the door by Mrs. Bundy's son Jim. Jim said to the nurse, "Do not discuss my mother's condition with her because she does not know her diagnosis nor how ill she is." As Ms. Adams entered the patient's room and greeted her, Mrs. Bundy said "I'm dying, you know, but my family is not able to accept it. Let's work together with them to help them deal with my dying."

The interaction between the nurse and the patient reveals that the older adult is often accepting of the condition and does not find it upsetting. A family conference may need to be arranged. Each family member and caregiver can approach this experience differently. As family members and the older adult discuss feelings, the nurse offers support to help them through this stage in preparation for the death. They can grow, adjust, accept each day, and allow the older adult to move on to complete life's tasks and life review, until death.

Patients and their families are often stronger and more powerful than they appear. The nurse must not underestimate the patient's and family's abilities and strengths. Nurses can invite patients and their families to reveal their strengths. They can help them to recognize their emotional and spiritual power. Nurses can empower dying patients and their loved ones by strengthening their self-confidence and feelings of control over their situation. Dying patients should be informed of the right to self-determination and other rights (see Chapters 3 and 4).

Supporting the Staff

Caring for a terminally ill patient can be extremely demanding on one's psyche and one's body. Providing palliative care to dying patients can be a traumatic experience. Staff need to be able to assess their own feelings about dying and death. Death education is important. If it is not part of the nursing and medical curriculum, there are many conferences and continuing education classes that health care professionals can attend.

Because health care professionals usually practice within a context of "curing," they are often very reluctant to adjust to dying and death. However, nurses have always provided "care" when "cure" was no longer achievable. Palliative care has always been provided by nurses and has been the domain of the nurse.

On occasion, some nurses have been known to avoid the dying patient and family. This could indicate that the staff member has difficulty working with dying and death and needs emotional support. Support should be provided by colleagues, educational director, hospice staff, **thanatologists** (individuals who study death), and others. Staff should be encouraged to verbalize their feelings and express them through crying, if the need arises, or any other form of expression. Nurses who work most closely with patients should ask for and receive all the support they need, including relief as they work to help patients through the dying process and death. This is very important. This time can be a growth-promoting experience for the nurse.

Nurses can also empower themselves to cope with and intervene in the dying process

and death. They can seek out ways to relieve their anxieties and to resolve issues concerning death. Because nurses coordinate the care and decisions made by various people involved in caring for the dying person, their emotional health is important to them and their patients and patients' families. Milliken (1993) suggests that until nurses accept their own mortality and complete their own "unfinished business" of grieving related to past losses and their own fears related to death, they cannot be fully effective in helping others to cope with dying and death.

The Meaning of Death

What is death? Death may be viewed as a part of the process of living. Some beliefs support fear of death, whereas others reflect acceptance of death as natural or see it as a transition. Perception of death is strongly influenced by cultural, religious, and social factors. With a growing older population and an increase in chronic illnesses, nurses will be caring for more dying older patients into the future. It is important to understand the array of attitudes toward death and to be sensitive to those of the dying patient.

What indicates that a person is dead? In some situations, brain death is used as the primary criterion. Others may use cardiopulmonary function, with cessation of respiratory and circulatory functions, as the indication of death. Most people die old, in a hospital, and in conscious awareness.

Death is the termination of life and the culmination of all work, play, successes, achievements, and accomplishments. Because death is inevitable, one may ask why it is so often feared. It evokes a feeling of ultimate powerlessness. Thanatologists have called the United States a "death-denying" society, possibly because the culture focuses on youth and beauty (Backer et al., 1994).

The meaning of death for each person is closely related to life experiences. The way in which a person reacts to death depends on the meaning that death has for that person. Recently, there has been increasing awareness of a need to examine societal attitudes toward death and care of the dying. More families now participate in the dying process as recent societal changes recognize and respect the dying person (Milliken, 1993).

COPING WITH LOSS

Older adults may experience an array of personal, social, and economic losses, but the most difficult and significant losses are personal. Because losses may be multiple over time, and may occur suddenly, the older adult's mental health can be compromised. Causes of psychic pain experienced by older adults include losses of significant others, illnesses, interpersonal difficulties, and situational losses, including economic hardship. The older adult experiencing loss should receive a thorough assessment. Part of this assessment includes a careful history to ascertain the following (Nauss, 1993):

- Previous experiences with significant losses
- Coping methods
- Recent losses (financial, role changes)
- Spirituality, a belief in a power greater than oneself
- Religious affiliation and attendance

Family and friends should be asked to identify inappropriate behavior, ability to discuss loss, and any new plans, habits, or relationships. Family and friends can intervene in helping the older adult adjust to loss. Support groups can also be of help.

One major loss is death of a spouse, resulting in widowhood. Women naturally live longer than men, which means that more women than men are faced with the problems of widowhood. Perhaps because of this, women are frequently more familiar with the tasks necessary to survive and continue life. Widowhood may bring about changes in living arrangements, financial status, and interactions with social groups. Some of these changes may lead to isolation. Loss of a spouse requires the remaining person to assume both roles, in the way they were defined in the marriage, immediately. This can seem overwhelming to someone who is in the midst of grieving.

Staff can be supportive to older adults who are experiencing loss by being resource persons, identifying support groups, and being knowledgeable about volunteer activities, senior centers, and church and other community activities. Coping strategies must be developed for the older adult to survive (see Chapter 6). Staff may themselves be in need of support when they lose a patient through death (see Supporting the Staff in this chapter). Loss requires saying good-bye to some aspect of one's life, but loss can also mean a new beginning.

GRIEF AND MOURNING

Grief is the normal emotional state that accompanies a personal, biological, or social loss. Grief may be defined as the ultimate price of loving, of attachment, and of meaningful relationships with the object of grief (Backer et al., 1994). Thus, we find grief in a person who has lost a spouse, family member, or friend, but we may also find it in a person who has been diagnosed with a chronic illness and is grieving the loss of health and vigor. A disability may trigger grieving, as may any perceived loss associated with a medical condition. Finally, grief may follow the loss of a role or position in business or in the community. *Anticipatory grieving,* in which the grieving process begins before the loss is experienced, often facilitates adjustment when the loss actually occurs (e.g, the loss of a spouse). Milliken (1993) states that spending quality time with the dying person (e.g., touching, holding, expressing feelings, sharing memories) facilitates anticipatory grieving and eases the dying process. Although anticipatory grieving may not diminish the pain of loss, it assists in accomplishing adaptation to it.

Any person experiencing a loss has the right to grieve. The ways people grieve tend to be consistent with their personality and their usual coping styles. In the past, in our society, grief was considered a private matter, and even ritualized by temporary retirement from social settings and the wearing of special clothes. Today, those who are grieving may continue to carry on ordinary daily responsibilities, but attention must be paid to the tasks of grieving for recovery to occur. Friends and family need to grant each survivor the right to grieve in the way that the person chooses. Grief has specific physical and psychological effects, which are noted in Table 25–1.

Caring

"The nurse can encourage an openness on the subject of dying and death, so that both the dying person and the family may have the opportunity to complete any unfinished business."

TABLE 25–1. Expressions of Grief

Physical	Affective	Behavioral
Palpitations	Confusion	Crying
Shortness of breath	Disbelief	Social withdrawal
Choking sensation	Sadness, sorrow	Sleep disturbances
Empty feeling in stomach	Depression (mild to moderate)	Absentminded behavior
Tension	Anger	Inability to concentrate
Lack of muscular power	Guilt	Restlessness or overactivity
Numbness	Relief if deceased was ill for a long period	Sighing
Dry mouth	of time	Aloneness
Hypersensitivity to noise	Separation anxiety	Irritability
Decreased appetite	Mental pain	
Somatic problems		

Adapted from Browning M. (1995). Depression, suicide, and bereavement. In Hogstel M, ed. Geropsychiatric Nursing. 2nd ed, St. Louis: CV Mosby.

There is no best way to grieve, to cope, to love, or to despair. Learning to cope with the pain of loss is a skill learned throughout life and is essential to emotional and mental health. Uncompleted grief is harmful to mental and physical health. Grief work cannot begin until the physical effects of the initial shock have subsided. If a year has passed, the grieving person may need professional counseling to facilitate the completion of grief work (Milliken, 1993).

After the initial shock and the response of intense feelings, a restructuring or recovery takes place so that normal function can resume. Resolution of grief occurs when the person experiencing the grief begins to reach out to others, makes new friends, sets goals, joins groups, learns new skills, maintains contact with family and friends, and helps others. Older adults with support systems will recover and cope better (Nauss, 1993).

Mourning is the normal psychological process that follows the death of a loved one. The period of mourning is a time for healing and adaptation to the loss. In some cultures there is a designated period of mourning that is accompanied by prescribed mourning rituals. Mourning is a time for healing, adaptation to the loss, and growth as a result of the experience (Backer et al., 1994). This period is an "acceptable" time for grieving. In the United States, mourning practices vary among the many subcultures represented. Regardless of the outward manifestation, emotional support at this time should come from those with whom the bereaved must restructure life, resuming daily routines of old responsibilities, assuming new responsibilities, and restructuring relationships that no longer include the deceased (Milliken, 1993). Eventually, the bereaved reaches a stage of adjustment and begins "getting on" with life.

BEREAVEMENT

Bereavement is the reaction of the survivor to the death of a family member or close friend. Deep sorrow is frequently experienced in the process of mourning this profound crisis. Backer and colleagues (1994) state that bereavement is the actual state of deprivation caused by a loss. In late life, the deprivational aspects of bereavement may be particularly emphasized, leading to loneliness and insecurity. Nurses must be aware that the stress of bereavement may have adverse effects on health. It is the task of the nurse to determine the needs of the bereaved older adult and address them.

The bereaved should be encouraged to (1) talk about the death, (2) understand that his or her feelings are normal, (3) allow sufficient time for the expression of grief, and (4) solve immediate, practical problems but postpone long-term decisions such as place of residence or change of job. Bereaved people should participate in some social activity to prevent emotional withdrawal, but it may be wise to avoid initiating deep emotional relationships for a time. The bereaved should be provided with intermittent but continuing support for at least a year, be monitored for abnormal coping styles, and avoid substance abuse. Interventions are needed when the acute phase of grieving appears unduly prolonged, when coping style is abnormal, or when physical illness supervenes or is exacerbated.

Spousal bereavement is a time that is dreaded but inevitable. It is a process that occurs at its own pace, in its own time. Successful bereavement outcomes are influenced by adequate income coupled with the ability to manage finances and by whether the bereaved person has been employed, has social interaction skills, and is immersed in a close-knit world of family, neighbors, and friends after the spouse's death (Browning, 1995).

Bereavement overload is experienced when the older adult experiences multiple losses within a short period of time. These losses may include deaths of friends and family and loss of job or financial security, of health, of status, of role function, or even of a body part. Nursing intervention includes the following (Browning, 1995):

- Teach that bereavement symptoms are a normal part of grieving and will abate with time.

- Allow the bereaved person expression of feelings.
- Assist the person to distinguish normal from abnormal feelings.
- Give positive feedback to successes in lifestyle changes achieved by the bereaved.
- Provide a list of available community resources.
- Provide referrals to appropriate agencies, with request for follow-up notification, to be informed of the bereaved's progress.

Multiple losses can be damaging to the adaptation capacity of most older adults. As soon as they begin to recuperate from one loss, another loss occurs. The onset, process, interventions, and outcomes of bereavement are presented in Figure 25–1. There may be successful bereavement over time, with adaptation, healing, and renewal, or there may be no change or movement toward healing. The process of grieving, mourning, and healing is a highly individualized one. There is no set time frame for adaptation to death, and throughout the process of grieving the bereaved may suffer various physical symptoms.

Sometimes people assume that the bereaved will "get over it." More programs of support are needed to help older bereaved adults through this difficult period. Death of a spouse is often

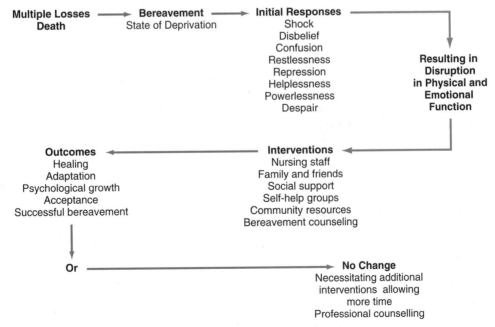

Figure 25–1. Loss, bereavement, and outcomes.

Wellness

"Nurses can intervene by inviting patients and their families to assess their strengths and recognize their emotional and spiritual power."

the most devastating loss, representing both loss of companionship and destruction of the hopes and dreams that the couple shared. Loss of a spouse can leave the remaining older adult emotionally depleted, often with no support system if significant others have preceded the bereaved person in death.

It is of great importance that the health care team and the community facilitate grief work and provide support so that bereaved individuals are able to move toward continued growth and development. The bereaved person can accomplish successful outcomes through nursing intervention, support groups (such as groups for widows and widowers), involvement in meaningful activities, and professional counseling (Fig. 25–1).

Summary

With the growth of the aged segment of the population, gerontological nurses will be caring for an increasing number of older patients at the time of their death. Societal advances and legislative interventions dictate attitudinal changes surrounding issues of dying and death. It is important that nurses become familiar with contemporary issues concerning the patients for whom they care. Even more important, nurses should first examine their own feelings related to dying and death and receive help, if indicated, in resolving those issues.

This chapter addressed dying, death, loss, grief, mourning, and bereavement. Nurses need to develop awareness of and sensitivity toward these areas to meet the needs of their older adult patients through effective practice. Caring for the dying is a privilege, and members of the health care team are usually the last people to minister to their needs.

RESOURCES

Last Acts
Call: Robert Wood Johnson Foundation
(609) 452-8701

Choice in Dying
(800) 989-WILL

National Hospice Organization
1901 North Fort Meyer Drive, Suite 402
Arlington, VA 22209
(703) 243-5900

REFERENCES

Backer B, Hannon N, Russell N. (1994). *Death and Dying: Understanding and Care.* 2nd ed. New York: Delmar.

Bohannan P. (1994). Death: The end of the aging process. In Hogstel M, ed. *Nursing Care for the Older Adult.* 3rd ed. New York: Delmar.

Browning M. (1995). Depression, suicide and bereavement. In Hogstel M, ed. Geropsychiatric Nursing. 2nd ed. St. Louis: CV Mosby.

Carney M, Morrison R. (1997). Advance directives: When, why and how to start talking. *Geriatrics 52*(4):65–73.

Kübler-Ross E. (1969). *On Death and Dying.* New York: Macmillan.

Milliken M. (1993). *Understanding Human Behavior: A Guide for Health Care Providers.* New York: Delmar.

Montgomery L. (1997). Groups launch campaign to improve care of the dying. *The New Mexican Knight-Ridder Tribune,* Feb. 16, 1997.

Nauss B. (1993). Losses and grief. In Loftis P, Glover T, eds. *Decision Making in Gerontological Nursing.* St. Louis: CV Mosby.

Voss-Morice S. (1996). Geriatric Nursing. *The Skidmore-Roth Publishing Series, Outline Series 169.* Aurora, CO: Skidmore-Roth Publishing.

CRITICAL THINKING EXERCISES

1. Would you prefer to die before your spouse? Explain your answer.
2. In assessing your community, make a survey of services for the bereaved. What do your findings indicate about treatment of the bereaved?
3. Imagine that a family member or a close friend has just died. How would you like to be notified of this person's death? Who would you like to tell you? Who would you like to be with you when you are notified, and why?
4. Write your own eulogy.

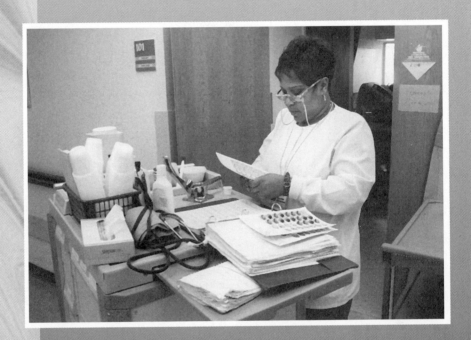

The Professional Gerontological Nurse

CHAPTER 26

Choices in Gerontological Nursing

Clari Gilbert, RN, MA

CHAPTER OUTLINE

OBJECTIVES

After completing this chapter, the reader should be able to:

1. Analyze the impact of gerontological needs on nursing as a profession.
2. Differentiate the roles of the gerontological nurse in both clinical and educational settings.
3. Specify the functions of a nurse supervisor and discuss the attributes of good leadership in a nursing facility.
4. Teach a classmate about subacute care. Be able to define it, explain the reasons for its emergence, and place it within the health care continuum.
5. Give at least three reasons for the importance of the education and practice alliance.

KEY TERMS

capitation
role
span of control

The increasing numbers of older adults affected by long-term illness have caused a renewed interest in the practice of gerontological nursing. Professionals who were looked on negatively for working in geriatric facilities are now being consulted to assist in policy and procedure development. Older adults in geriatric settings have been a nursing responsibility for decades, primarily by default. However, the profession has recently begun to appreciate and assume accountability for providing quality care for the older adult.

During the 1960s, social policy for older adults emerged in the form of the Older Americans Act, along with a variety of other services. A 1971 study of nursing homes conducted by the U.S. Department of Health, Education, and Welfare revealed poor medical and nursing care. Programs were developed to prepare nurses as gerontological specialists and geriatric nurse practitioners to assist other nurses in improving the care of the older adult. In 1975, the American Nurses' Association (ANA) changed the term used from *geriatric nursing* to *gerontological nursing*. It implies that care and treatment are given from a holistic approach rather than focusing on diseases.

The division of geriatric nursing practice was the first ANA specialty to establish standards. The standards issued in 1969 addressed the following areas:

- The nursing process
- Involvement of older adults in decision-making and goal setting
- Nursing functions, which must include teaching and supervising health maintenance
- Maximizing the older adult's biological, psychological, and social resources

The revisions in 1987 included educational requirements for nurse executives in long-term care.

IMPACT OF SOCIAL CHANGES ON NURSING SERVICE

The projections of an aging population, in addition to the increase in the number of disabled older adults, have led to an imposing challenge in the need for gerontological services. It is estimated that by 2030 there will be 2.6 million adults in nursing facilities, more than 100% of the current nursing home population. Older adults occupy more than one half of all hospital beds and use approximately 60% of all health services (Kelly and Maas, 1993).

Wellness

"*High-quality health care for older adults is a growing demand. Innovative practice models are continually emerging.***"**

The prospective payment system implemented in 1983 has resulted in early hospital discharges of a sicker population to both the community and nursing homes. The complexity of care that is now needed has forced nurse administrators to develop subacute and managed-care programs in areas such as respiratory disorders, head injury, and peritoneal dialysis, along with specialty units to improve care, services, and quality of life.

The creative, innovative gerontological nurse must seize these opportunities to improve clinical skills by attending in-service educational programs and seminars and by reading nursing journals. On the other hand, gerontological nurses are due a broader acceptance from their professional counterparts in acute-care settings.

DIVERSE CLINICAL ENVIRONMENTS

Nursing Homes

The Omnibus Reconciliation Act (OBRA) of 1987, which included the Nursing Home Reform Act, has had an impact on the practice of nursing in long-term care. The law, although providing only minimum standards, has created employment opportunities for registered nurses. It legalizes good nursing care and supports the nurse practice act, in that it requires care planning be based on resident assessment. It requires a registered professional nurse be on duty at least 8 hours a day; in addition, there must be a full-time registered nurse as the director of nursing who may no longer assume unit responsibilities. However, staffing inadequacies remain in many facilities because the law did not dictate a nurse:patient staffing ratio. In June 1994, the U.S. Congress authorized the Institute of Medicine to convene a nursing commission to study the relationship of nursing staff levels to patient care. The nursing commission is to determine the extent of the need for nurses in hospitals and nursing homes to promote quality of patient care. The commission will analyze existing data on staffing levels and patient outcomes and hold public hearings before issuing a report to Congress.

The Subacute-Care Environment

Subacute care is comprehensive, goal-oriented, coordinated, inpatient care designed for an individual who has had an acute illness, injury, or exacerbation of a disease process. It is rendered immediately after, or instead of, acute hospitalization to treat medically complex problems. Subacute care requires the coordinated services of an interdisciplinary team who are knowledgeable and trained to assess and manage these specific conditions. Subacute care is more intensive than traditional nursing home care and less intensive than acute inpatient care.

Subacute care can be provided in multiple settings (e.g., long-term care hospitals, rehabilitative hospitals, free-standing nursing facilities, or hospital-based nursing facilities) (Table 26–1). The trend, however, is moving toward low-cost providers or nursing facilities. The challenges of providing subacute care in a nursing facility are numerous and complex. Individuals requiring subacute care are different from traditional nursing home residents. They enter into an OBRA "resident" environment while they remain patients (short term). Subacute-care units must comply with long-term care standards. Patients at times refuse to commingle with residents, which creates redesigning challenges. The goal is to provide a homelike environment.

The U.S. Department of Health and Human Services has announced funding of the first na-

TABLE 26–1. Categories of Subacute Care			
	Transitional	**General**	**Chronic**
Length of Stay	5–30 days	10–40 days	60–90 days
Nursing Care Hours	5.5–7.0 PPD*	3.5–5.0 PPD	3.0–5.0 PPD
Case Mix and Services	Highly skilled Intensive nursing care Integrated rehabilitation Substitute for patient hospitalization 24-hour respiratory therapy 7 day/week therapies Variety of physician specialists Daily physician visits	Less-acute level of care Subacute care rehabilitation Intravenous therapies Goal: discharge home or lower level of care Dedicated unit or scattered beds Physician visits biweekly or monthly	Little hope of recovery Comatose Progressive neurological disorders Therapies to stabilize Discharge home or long-term care unit Physician visits monthly

*PPD, per patient day.

tional policy to review subacute services. The focus will be on definition, growth, implications, characteristics of users and providers, physical structures, staffing patterns, quality, and cost of care. The demand for nurses in nursing facilities will increase as subacute-care units are developed (Table 26–2). Learning new skills will be crucial for nurses in nursing facilities. Nurses can also play a significant part in subacute-care design and construction.

The Managed-Care Environment

Managed care is a concept of grouping individuals into a health care delivery system that offers comprehensive benefits, with an emphasis on primary and preventive care. The shift toward managed care is accelerating the use of new payment patterns. Health maintenance organizations (HMOs), hospitals, and large businesses are now contracting with nursing facilities for transitional care of patients who need rehabilitation, infusion therapy, antibiotic ther-

apy, pain control, and other clinical interventions before discharge.

Capitation, the payment source that is driving managed care, is a single payment per patient that is meant to cover the complete care of either transitional or long-term care. This fee covers services that may be required during the patient's stay. Capitation is also the force behind case management. Case management involves the monitoring of the members of a health plan to anticipate their needs and direct them to the most cost-effective services and settings. The concept of case management was introduced to long-term care in the 1970s to address the problem of inappropriate placement in nursing homes. During the 1980s, the focus of case management shifted to a mechanism for controlling costs. Now, in the 1990s, the emphasis is on managing services, the precursor to controlling cost (Coile, 1993). The primary activities of case managers include

- Case selection
- Preadmission screening
- Patient assessment
- Discharge planning
- Information and referral
- Patient/family counseling
- Postcare coordination

There are challenges and opportunities that exist within the managed-care environment. The professional nurse, however, must be able to carve out a niche within the system.

The Community

The demographics on aging present new challenges to the gerontological nurse involved in community health services. The age group of adults older than 80 years is the fastest growing of our population. It is projected that by 2020 that segment of the population will have increased by approximately 90% from 1987.

Medicare, Medicaid, and other third-party payers have supported and encouraged ambulatory care services in an effort to reduce costs. However, many older adults lack appropriate posthospitalized care owing to inappropriate referrals and absence of family members in the home. Gerontological nurses working in community settings must be educated about the continuum of services that exist to be better able to offer appropriate choices to the older adult to ensure psychosocial and physical well-

TABLE 26–2. Comparative Subacute Staffing Levels	
Traditional Nursing Facility	**Subacute Care Facility**
2.5–3.5 NCHPPD* *PT/OT/ST contact staff	4.0–7.0 NCHPPD On-staff therapists
25%–30% RNs/LPNs	60%–65% RNs/LPNs
70% certified nurse aides	40% certified nurse aides
Physician visits once per month	Physician visits three to five times per week
	Added nursing supervision
	Documentation need to support increased nursing hours and other unit costs
	More one-to-one recreation therapy
	Increased social work staff
	Psychiatric staff

*NCHPPD, nursing care hours per patient day; *PT/OT/ST, physical/occupational/speech therapy.

being. Table 26–3 provides a summary of the home care services that are provided in just one community—New York City.

Corporations are now employing geronto-logical nurses to assist employees to cope with the responsibility of balancing their lives between the job and caring for an older parent or spouse. Research has shown that this will be the

TABLE 26–3. Sample of Home Care Services

Features	Long-term home health care program: "nursing home without walls"	Certified home health agency	Home attendant program/personal care program
Certification and/or Licensure	Certified by HCFA*; licensed by New York State Department of Health	Certified by HCFA*; licensed by New York State Department of Health	Noncertified
Client's Eligibility Criteria	Medicaid eligibility (some clients are also Medicare eligible) Chronically ill that are eligible for nursing home placement	Medicare, Medicaid, or private insurance, eligible, or self pay Acute episode of illness, injury, surgery	Medicaid eligibility Frail, elderly or disabled Needs assistance with one or two activities of daily living
Services	Skilled nursing Rehabilitative therapies Physical therapy Occupational therapy Speech therapy Respiratory therapy Social work Nutrition Durable medical equipment and supplies Home health aide Personal care aide Transportation	Skilled nursing Rehabilitative therapies Physical therapy Occupational therapy Speech therapy Home health aide Durable medical equipment	Home attendant and/ or personal care aide
Case Management	24-hour availability Services coordinated by a registered nurse	24-hour availability Services coordinated by a registered nurse	Services administered by Human Resources Administration
Quality Assurance	Plan of care ordered by a physician Orders are renewed every 62 days	Plan of care ordered by a physician Orders are renewed every 62 days	Plan of care ordered by patient's physician
Duration of Services	120 days to several years	Two weeks to 2 months	Renewed every 6 months
Cost	Cost of care cannot exceed 75% of cost of nursing home care	Cost as per insurance companies' coverage	No cost control

*HCFA, Health Care Financing Administration.

trend as we move into the 21st century. Family caregivers of older adults are experiencing stress-related disorders that result in absenteeism and low productivity on the job. (For more about caregiver burnout, see Chapter 23.) Some gerontological nurse experts are now developing teaching programs and referral aids while working with corporate executives to assist employees with the knowledge and resources needed to deal with this problem.

Acute-Care Settings

The increased numbers of older adults in acute-care settings are presenting many challenges for nurse managers and opportunities for gerontological nurses. Owing to variations in length of stay since the implementation of diagnosis-related groups, different classification systems were designed. Nurses are now faced with patients requiring longer lengths of stay and a geriatric population that has multiple chronic health problems. A project funded by the federal government through the Stanford University Hospital was conducted by geriatric nurse specialists from July 1990 through June 1993. Its purpose was to prepare nurses to care for geriatric patients in acute-care hospitals. Evaluation of the project found that nurses who participated had more positive attitudes toward older adults, as well as improved knowledge and skills in caring for them.

Acute-care settings have a growing need for gerontological nurses. Older adults manifest problems due to confusion, separation anxiety, loneliness, and life-threatening diseases. Although acute-care nurses are well prepared in disease prevention and health promotion, they often lack the skills needed to care for that unique population appropriately.

▉ ROLE OF THE REGISTERED NURSE

A **role** can be defined as a set of related activities carried out by an individual or ascribed to a position or job title. A role can be actual or perceived. A perceived role can sometimes create conflict between the individual performing the activities of the role and other individuals of a particular group. Therefore, it is essential

that activities that determine a particular role should be stated verbally or, better, in writing. Most institutions require that role expectations be stated in the form of job descriptions, policies, rules, and regulations.

With the many changes in the health care delivery system and the impact of gerontological care on nursing, roles are constantly changing at every level of nursing. Nurses who are entering the clinical practice of gerontological nursing must be flexible and innovative, and they need to be proponents of change.

Caring

❝Students develop positive attitudes toward aging individuals by observing their educators responding in a nurturing, caring, health-promoting manner to the needs of both well and frail older adults.❞

A registered nurse is an individual who has completed 2 or more years of nursing education in an academic setting. The individual must complete the requirements of a particular state in which practice is desired and then be licensed by that state. A license permits an individual to utilize the skills and knowledge obtained and also protects the public from incompetence. Individual states have developed nurse practice acts that serve as guidelines for practice. Registered nurses may assume different roles in the health care continuum, based on knowledge and experience.

Staff Nurse

The entry-level position in most geriatric facilities is that of a staff nurse. This nurse is a graduate of a nursing program, who may or may not have experience beyond the academic setting.

The staff nurse may assume multiple roles depending on the setting, work assignments, and availability of support staff. Staff nurses in geriatric settings have been taking care of a sicker population since the implementation of a prospective payment system; therefore, it is necessary that the staff nurse attend ongoing in-service training to upgrade knowledge and skills. The staff nurse must stay abreast of the legal aspects of gerontological nursing practice. OBRA 1987 brought revolutionary changes in the areas of resident rights, assessment, care planning, and restraints that impact directly on the staff nurse's role.

To provide care effectively in a geriatric setting, the staff nurse must be knowledgeable in group process, be creative, and have good communication skills. Care planning is no longer the sole responsibility of the nurse. It is an interdisciplinary process, and the client or designated representative now has a legal right to participate.

Nurse Supervisor

The registered nurse may assume the role of a supervisor or nurse manager and the responsibility for the coordination of care on several nursing units. The supervisor is expected to have a thorough knowledge of the job responsibilities and be technically and clinically competent. The scope of supervision or management varies, depending on the structure of the nursing department and the health care facility. However, some basic principles apply.

First, the supervisor must assume the responsibility for those within the span of control. **Span of control** refers to the number of employees an individual supervises. Training, experience, and knowledge are factors that influence the decision as to the span of control. The individual characteristics of nurses are also of vital importance; if nurses are self-directed and competent, the span of control can be broadened.

Second, the supervisor must act as a connecting link between the employees and nursing administration. Interpersonal relations are paramount in a supervisor's role, partly because of the complexities of personnel, patients, and family members. The supervisor must encourage open communication and be a good listener.

Seven nurse supervisory roles identified through research are planning, organizing, staffing, leading, communicating, decision-making, and controlling. Although definitions vary with time and research, the basic requirements exist for each function:

- *Planning* is intellectual; it determines in advance what should be done and is a function that cannot be delegated. An effective supervisor uses this function as a continuous process; however, planning must coincide with the overall philosophy and objectives of the nursing department.
- *Organizing* determines how the work is to be accomplished. It requires the supervisor to structure and design work assignments and responsibilities.
- *Staffing* involves the recruitment, training, and appraisal of employees. A supervisor may not necessarily participate in all aspects of staffing.
- *Leading* involves being familiar with the department's philosophy and goals and having the professional knowledge to provide advice and counsel.
- *Communicating* is a linking managerial function and is important in maintaining effective vertical and horizontal relationships.
- *Decision-making* is a process that links all managerial functions. Conclusions must be reached by managers before implementation, and they require sound judgment.
- *Controlling* is a process that checks performance against standards and is closely related to the planning function.

The supervisory role of a registered nurse is diverse and complex and is constantly changing to meet the needs of the health community. However, the success of a supervisor is dependent on effective utilization of the basic functions.

Nurse Clinician

A gerontological nurse practitioner (GNP) is a clinician with advanced skills in health assessment, physical examination, disease management, health promotion, and maintenance. The GNP has knowledge about the aging process, along with both chronic and acute illnesses of the older adult. The first nurse practitioner program was initiated in 1965 at the University of Colorado. Its purpose was to offer a new educational experience and prepare nurses to assume an expanded role in pediatrics. After decades of debate and political maneuvering, there are now about a dozen nurse practitioner specialties, including GNPs.

Nurse practitioner roles were developed in response to a need to advance the nursing profession. The GNP is qualified to receive direct reimbursement under the Medicare regulations; however, payment structure varies according to the clinical setting and state laws. The federal payment guidelines require nurse practitioners to be reimbursed at 85% of Medicare fee schedule for physicians. A GNP functions in a variety of settings across the health care continuum. The primary role of a GNP is accountability to the client while expanding nursing practice.

The ANA has defined the nurse practitioner as an individual who has completed a program of study leading to competence as a registered nurse in an expanded role. The educational trend is to make the entry level for practice at the master's level. However, in some states the preparation is on a continuing-education basis. The basic qualification for ANA certification is a baccalaureate degree in nursing. The GNP certification was established in 1981, and by 1992 there were 1232 GNPs.

A report generated by the U.S. Congress, Office of Technology Assessment, in 1986 stated that nurse practitioners appear to give better care than physicians to patients with chronic health problems (Aaronson, 1991). In 1988, the W. K. Kellogg Foundation funded a GNP project that surveyed graduates of four universities to evaluate the effectiveness of the GNP in providing cost-effective, alternative models of care in various settings. The results suggest that the GNP is able to function all along the health care continuum. The New York State Department of Health, with grant support from the Robert Wood Johnson Foundation, is implementing a research project with several nursing homes investigating the cost-effectiveness of different models of care, including care given by the nurse practitioner.

ROLE OF THE LICENSED PRACTICAL (VOCATIONAL) NURSE

The practical nurse is an individual who has completed at least 1 year of training after high school or graduated from a high school practical nurse program. On completion of the program, graduates are eligible to take the National Council Licensure Examination (NCLEX-PN). According to the U.S. Department of Labor, nearly 20% of all practical nurses work in nursing homes and other geri-

atric settings (Occupational Outlook Handbook 1994–1995). They are valued members of the health care team. They work under the supervision of registered nurses and provide bedside care, administer medications, evaluate residents' needs, and develop care plans.

Economic trends have shifted the nursing staffing ratio from registered nurses to practical nurses in most nursing facilities. In addition, the growth of the aging population and capitation have also increased the demand for this level of nursing. On the evening and night tours, practical nurses are usually in charge of a unit. In states where the law allows, they may start and administer intravenous fluids; however, in many states this is prohibited.

The Intravenous Nurses Society (INS) stated in a position paper that they believe practical nurses can aid in the delivery of some aspects of intravenous therapy under the supervision of a registered nurse (Position Paper, 1997). If their position is adopted by state nurse practice acts, it will assist nursing facilities in improving the quality of life for subacute care residents. Practical nurses can then be responsible for all aspects of resident care, including intravenous therapy under the supervision of the registered nurse.

ROLE OF THE CERTIFIED NURSE AIDE

Nurse aides are the primary caregivers in most geriatric settings. They perform care and services to patients who do not require the skills of a licensed practical nurse or a registered nurse.

In 1986, a position statement was issued by the ANA concerning mandatory training for nurse assistants. This statement supported the recommendations of the Institute of Medicine that a federal standard be established requiring all nurse aides to complete a preservice, state-approved training program. The purpose of the standard would be for all nurse aides to demonstrate competency in basic nursing tasks, interpersonal communication skills, and knowledge of patient rights.

Included in the OBRA 1987 regulations were nurse aide training and competency evaluation requirements that were mandated to be met by all states. Nurse aide programs were mandated to provide at least 75 hours of education and practical training. The minimum curriculum would include

1. At least 16 hours of training, before any direct contact with a resident, in:
   - Communication and interpersonal skills
   - Infection control
   - Safety/emergency procedures
   - Providing resident's independence
   - Respecting residents rights
2. Basic nursing skills
3. Personal care skills
4. Mental health and social service needs
5. Care of cognitively impaired residents
6. Basic restorative services

Included in the regulations were exemptions that "grandfathered" nurse aides who completed 75 hours of nurse aide training before July 1, 1989, and had at least 24 consecutive months of employment in a nursing facility before December 19, 1989. In some states, nurse aides who were exempt from the 75-hour course work were still required to demonstrate competency in basic nursing tasks. Each state must develop and maintain a registry of all nurse aides who have successfully completed competency examinations. Before employment, the employer must validate the nurse aide's certification status with the state's registry. Although OBRA's intent was to improve quality, costs have increased as the result of ongoing training requirements and recordkeeping. Recertification is biannual, with the completion of 12 hours of in-service training annually.

▮ ROLE OF THE NURSE EDUCATOR

The importance of gerontological nursing continues to grow because of the ever-expanding number of older adults with concomitant health care needs. This phenomenon creates the demand for nurses to be educated in gerontological nursing. As trends, issues, and societal changes emerge, nurse educators are creatively challenged to respond, investigate, assess, analyze, and design programs with the gathered data. Motivating students for active involvement in the process of learning about age and aging requires that nurse educators become knowledgeable in gerontological nursing.

Nurse educators function as role models for students. Observing their educators responding in a nurturing, caring, health-promoting manner to the needs of both well and frail older adults helps students develop positive attitudes toward aging individuals. The nurse educator also assists students in applying the components of gerontological nursing in such clinical settings as the home, hospital, adult daycare center, or long-term care facility.

The practice of gerontological nursing mandates the use of a nursing model of care. Nursing home care has been organized for too long around a medical model, which is based on medical diagnosis and disability, with overwhelming emphasis on illness rather than the individual and the individual's needs. Because the chronically ill individual will not be cured, models of care that promote autonomy and independence with an emphasis on health promotion and prevention of illness can maximize the individual's quality of life. These nursing models of care must be taught in schools and practiced in gerontological settings.

The nursing home can provide role models and quality clinical experience for nursing students through observation of nursing staff who are knowledgeable about caring for older adults. Nurses in academic and practice settings can form alliances to work together through sharing, learning, and caring. These alliances have positive effects on staff, nurse educators, students, and other health care professionals, as well as the quality of care given to older adults (Tyson, 1992).

Time spent in the nursing home clinical setting allows the nurse educator to observe the role of the gerontological nurse and participate whenever possible in the following:

- Case presentations, team conferences, and geriatric care

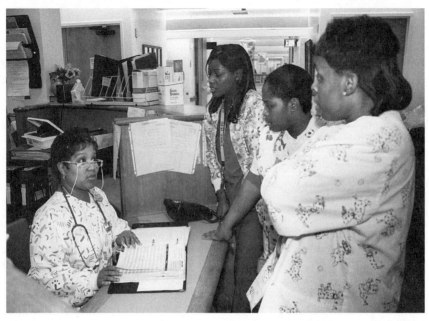

In the years ahead, gerontological nursing will offer even more opportunities for service and professional fulfillment.

- Development of gerontological nursing activities
- Gerontological nursing research activities
- Development of geriatric educational programs
- Fostering an educational environment among staff

Nurse educators improve the image of the facility by their very presence, and the college of nursing confers status on the long-term care nurse by establishing the practice of long-term care nursing in the curriculum. The facility staff assists the student in recognizing the knowledge and creativity required to meet the challenge of the nursing specialty. Staff identify the independent nature of their practice, their ability to provide continuity of care, and the appreciation of the residents and families (Cobe and Eisenhart, 1988).

The education and practice alliance permits the input of long-term care providers in assessing curriculum changes, while confirming that educators must be responsive to the needs of the health care system. Selection of clinical sites that provide positive experiences is crucial. Hartley and Dietsch (1988) stated that the clinical learning environment should provide

1. A director of nursing and an administrator who are committed to the educational process and to promoting gerontological nursing as a career option
2. Registered nurses who are positive role models, knowledgeable in gerontological nursing, and able to promote positive attitudes about working with long-term residents
3. Healthy nursing staff to resident ratios
4. A holistic model of care in which residents' psychosocial, spiritual, and physical dimensions are addressed through multidisciplinary care planning
5. Emphasis on restorative nursing that maximizes functional abilities in activities of daily living and minimizes dependency
6. A variety of social and recreational programming and opportunities to exercise accustomed roles
7. A caring, friendly environment in which residents' dignity, individuality, and right to

W e l l n e s s

“Nursing has recently begun to appreciate and assume accountability for providing quality care for the older adult.”

make choices are respected and valued above institutional routines

A number of faculties have already selected clinical learning environments that are considered "ideal" and that meet the just listed criteria. Clinical faculty and nursing staff know the importance of role modeling positive attitudes and behaviors. Knowledge and skills learned in gerontological nursing can prepare students for extended roles in health care practice.

■ THE FUTURE OF GERONTOLOGICAL NURSING

An increased demand for nursing care will continue to occur, particularly in the community, nursing homes, other long-term care facilities, and home health care arenas. In view of the projections of dramatically increasing numbers of older adults into the next century, gerontological nursing will hold a critical position in the health of the nation and the world.

There are four groups of older adults who will require nursing care in varying degrees:

1. Older adults who do not have a chronic illness but require education and health promotion/protection strategies (e.g., a gerontological nurse meets with older adults in a senior center twice monthly, providing education and literature while teaching a wellness promotion class)
2. Independent older adults who are self-sufficient in functional abilities and have adapted to their chronic illnesses (e.g., a 79-year-old client with diabetes and hypertension who complies with the medical and nursing regimen of medications, diet, and exercise). Nurses working with this group should empower these older adults to practice self-care behaviors in maximizing and maintaining their health status.
3. Caregiver-supported older adults with mild to moderate deficits who are living within the community and who derive support from family members and local senior care organizations (e.g., an older adult with Alzheimer's disease who can perform activities of daily living with family prompting)
4. Frail older adults who rely on others for their functional and health care needs (e.g.,

nursing-home residents and home health care patients)

Some community health agencies such as senior centers, geriatric day treatment centers, and home health care programs help moderately ill older adults remain in the community and receive the nursing care and supportive assistance they require.

The future of gerontological nursing is dependent on the following (Gueldner and Brent, 1995):

1. Creative teaching and role modeling that generate positive feelings toward older adults
2. Shaping scholarship in areas of research, publication, presentation, utilization, and social policy
3. Clinical practice that incorporates the expectation of wellness, even in the presence of chronic illness and substantive impairment
4. National health care insurance, with need for growth in services such as mental health, counseling, and health education, as the old-old population grows
5. Innovative, creative forms and models of care designed to intervene therapeutically in an aging society where dwindling resources are a reality

The GNP of the future will work at the forefront of challenging and exciting changes in the health care system, while influencing future developments. As gerontological nursing becomes part of the undergraduate curriculum, and as graduate and postgraduate nursing students embrace gerontological nursing as a specialty, nurses educated in research methodology will conduct research that will enhance and improve the quality of care and quality of life for older adults.

An increasing number of nurses are becoming certified in gerontological nursing each year through the ANA. Several professional nursing journals afford practicing nurses the opportunity to update skills and learn about emerging trends through home study by reading articles and answering accompanying questions. Continuing-education programs, conferences, and the print literature provide many opportunities for nurses to share learning as they practice gerontological nursing.

Caring

"We need to emphasize restorative nursing that maximizes functional abilities in activities of daily living and minimizes dependency."

Summary

The clinical practice of gerontological nursing is becoming more challenging. The complex needs of older adults are creating shifts in the care delivery system in every aspect from institutional to ambulatory care. Diagnostic and treatment centers, adult daycare centers, and outpatient rehabilitation centers are on the increase. Nursing facilities, on the other hand, are creating subacute-care and short-term rehabilitation units while developing contracts with managed-care companies.

Nurses must be prepared to adapt to these changes in the provisions of care to the older adult. They must be proficient in their area of practice by way of certification or continuing education. Nurse educators and service providers must collaborate to achieve positive outcomes for both the student and the nursing staff. An affiliation solely with a college or university is becoming outdated; academia and service providers need to start discussions on new dimensions of partnerships as the 21st century approaches.

Gerontological nurses are practicing nursing in a very exciting era. High-quality health care for older adults is in growing demand. Innovative practice models continually emerge. As educators, researchers, and practitioners working together, we can determine the shape of gerontological nursing for the future.

REFERENCES

Aaronson WE. (Winter 1991). The use of physician extenders in nursing homes: A review. Med Care Rev 48(4): 39–41.

Cobe G, Eisenhart L. (1988). The nursing home and the ADN curriculum: Employer-educator issues. In Associate-Degree Nursing and the Nursing Home. Publication #15-2241. New York: National League for Nursing.

Coile RC. (1993). Transitional care: Redefining long-term care for a managed-care marketplace. Hosp Strategy Rep 5(6): 13–14.

Gueldner S, Brent B. (1995). Gerontological nursing issues and demands beyond the year 2005 (guest editorial). J Gerontol Nurs 21(6): 1–2.

Hartley C, Dietsch K. (1988). Clinical learning environments in long-term care today and tomorrow. In Associate-Degree Nursing and the Nursing Home. Publication #15-2241. New York: National League for Nursing.

Kelly K, Maas M. (1993). Managing nursing care. St. Louis: CV Mosby.

Position Paper. (1997). The role of LPN, LVN in the clinical practice of intravenous therapy. J Intravenous Nurs 20(2):75–76.

Tyson S. (1992). The design, implementation, and evaluation of a faculty development program in gerontological nursing. Doctoral dissertation, Nova Southeastern University, Ft. Lauderdale, Florida (unpublished).

Occupational Outlook Handbook 1994–1995. US Department of Labor, Statistics Bulletin 2450–1. Washington, DC: US Government Printing Office.

CRITICAL THINKING EXERCISES

1. Describe your own socio/political/economic health plan for aging adults as we approach the new millennium. How would you prioritize?
2. Organize a group of gerontological nurses to network together. As organizer, identify some topics that could be used to initiate discussion.
3. You are currently near completion of an advanced degree in gerontological nursing. As an upcoming professional gerontological nurse, where would you like to position yourself for the 21st century?
   a. Clinician—on the cutting edge of new health trends
   b. Educator—designing innovative curricula
   c. Administrator—organizing, administering, and guiding creative professionals
   d. A new job title that you have created and for which you will write the job description
4. Give reasons for your career decision.

Achalasia. Failure of the esophageal sphincter to relax while swallowing, causing the esophagus to become dilated and to trap air, fluid, saliva, and food.

Acquired immunity. Antibodies and activated lymphocytes attack and destroy specific organisms or toxins.

Activities of daily living (ADLs). Ordinary self-care activities such as bathing, eating, and toileting.

Activity theory. To age successfully, an individual must retain active roles in life or find suitable replacement for roles that must be abandoned.

Advance directives. Legal documents that specify the individual's wishes for treatment before a crisis occurs.

Advocacy. The art of working with or on behalf of an individual or system to bring about positive change. Advocacy is a vital function of the gerontological nurse.

Ageism. Discrimination based on a person's age.

Aging. A reduced capacity to replace worn-out cells that manifests as the body grows older. The process begins at conception and is a normal part of growth and development. Aging involves many factors and occurs across the life span.

Alterations. Limitations, changes, or modifications in health and lifestyle and organs.

Angina. Chest pain generated when arterial occlusion deprives the tissues of life-sustaining blood (*ischemia*).

Angiodysplasias. Small vascular abnormalities of the gastrointestinal tract.

Antibody (immunoglobulin). A protein molecule that is produced by immune system plasma cells, adheres to antigens, and assists in combating antigens; a serum agent that inactivates a foreign substance in the body.

Antigen. A foreign substance that causes an immune response.

Anxiety. A normal reaction to that which is threatening to one's body, lifestyle, values, or loved ones. A feeling of apprehension, worry, uneasiness, or dread.

Aphasia. Loss of the power of expression through words or symbols.

Assisted living. Any group residential program that is *not* licensed as a nursing home, that provides personal care to people with need for assistance in the activities of daily living, and that can respond to unscheduled needs for assistance that might arise.

Assistive device. A machine, apparatus or object constructed to perform a specific function.

Audiometry. Technology for testing hearing acuity.

Auscultation. The process of listening to sounds within the body to determine if there are alterations to what would normally be expected.

Autoantibody. An antibody that can act against a native body material.

Autoimmune reaction. An immune response against a normal body part.

Azotemia. An excess of urea in the blood.

Beneficence. Acting for the benefit of patients. Health care professionals must actively pursue good and benefit the patients in their care.

Bereavement. The reaction of the survivor to the death of a family member or close friend; the state of deprivation caused by such a loss.

Bioethics. The study of ethical problems arising from scientific advances in biology and medicine.

Block nursing. Nursing care given to people by a nurse who lives on the same block, according to their need rather than their ability to pay. It allows older adults to remain in their homes even though they are not totally independent.

Bradykinesia. The inability to initiate movements or to change direction easily.

Capitation. The term used to describe a way of allocating medical costs by number of patients cared for, so that costs are controlled, in managed-care systems.

Caregiver. One who provides unpaid, informal care to an older adult who requires help with daily activities and personal needs.

Caregiver stress. Physical and psychological forces experienced by the caregiver that disrupt equilibrium or produce strain.

Caring. An attitude of genuine concern for another; a fundamental value of nursing.

Cataracts. A natural, painless, age-related clouding of the transparent lens of the human eye.

Catastrophic reaction. A response of violence that occurs when the patient with dementia is presented with a situation that overwhelms the coping mechanisms.

Cerebrovascular accident (CVA). The formation of an embolism, thromboembolism, or hemorrhages within the intracerebral or subarachnoid areas of the brain that deprive the brain of oxygen. Neuromuscular deficiencies become apparent when certain divisions of the brain become ischemic. Also known as stroke.

Chemical dependency. A prolonged, habitual reliance or dependence on a substance that has a negative impact on physical and mental health and may also mask symptoms of other serious diseases.

Chyme. The mixture of partly digested food and digestive secretions found in the stomach and small intestine during digestion of a meal.

Circadian rhythm. Pertaining to repetitions that follow the 24-hour day.

Cochlear implant. A device for individuals with severe hearing loss. It is implanted into the cochlea, located in the middle ear.

Cognition. Mental function, which includes intelligence, learning, and memory.

Cohorts. Groups having common characteristics that are being observed scientifically.

Competency. The capacity of ability to perform the task at hand and the ability to handle one's affairs in an adequate manner.

Compulsions. Acts or rituals that must be performed to lessen anxiety, often causing embarrassment to the person carrying out the ritual.

Continuing care retirement communities (CCRCs). This living arrangement integrates three levels of housing: independent living, assisted living, and skilled nursing facilities. A CCRC may be purchased or rented, guaranteeing shelter and full services.

Continuity of care. Coordination of community services before discharge is necessary for continuity of care, especially because many patients are now discharged with complex equipment and materials that require complicated procedures to care for them.

Continuity theory. The idea that individuals try to sustain personal patterns of activity and interaction as they age; adjustment to aging is optimized by maintaining the level of social activity achieved in younger adulthood. Basic personality traits are said to remain unchanged as one ages.

Coping. To contend or strive, especially successfully.

Crackles. Crackling sounds in the bases of the lungs. They may be a normal finding in the older adult or bedridden patient and usually clear with deep breathing or with the use of an incentive spirometer.

Crisis. An unstable period in a person's life characterized by inability to adapt to a change resulting from a precipitating event.

Culture. The totality of socially transmitted behaviors, art, beliefs, and other products of human work and thought; a style of social and artistic expression peculiar to a society or class; a way of life belonging to a designated group of people.

Delirium. An acute, reversible, organic mental disorder characterized by reduced ability to maintain attention to external stimuli and disorganized thinking (as manifested by rambling, irrelevant, or incoherent speech), reduced level of consciousness, disorientation to time and place, and memory impairment.

Delusions. False beliefs with no basis in reality.

Dementia. An organic mental disorder characterized by a general loss of intellectual abilities involving impairment of memory, judgment, and abstract thinking, as well as changes in personality. It does not include loss of intellectual functioning caused by clouding of consciousness, as in delirium, nor that caused by depression or other functional mental disorder.

Deontology. The belief that the highest good is to fulfill obligations. Deontologists believe that duty, laws, and rules are based on prior agreements and fundamental or essential facts. Without concern for outcome, ethical decisions are to be made out of respect for what one *ought* to do.

Depression. An affective (mood) disorder that is preventable and reversible. It is characterized by exaggerated feelings of sadness, worthlessness, hopelessness, helplessness, emptiness, and dejection that do not disappear with logic, reasoning, or reality.

Discharge planning. A schedule initiated as soon as possible in preparation for the patient's release from a facility.

Disengagement theory. The idea of a gradual, mutual withdrawal between the older adult and society. This mutual separation benefits both—freeing the older adult from constraining roles and expectations and providing younger people with the opportunity to take their place in society.

Diverticulum. A sac created by herniation of the mucous membrane through a defect in the muscular wall of a tubular organ such as the intestine.

Do-not-resuscitate (DNR) order. An order stating that the individual does not want to be revived by cardiopulmonary resuscitation (CPR), should breathing cease and the heart stop beating.

Durable power of attorney for health care (DPAHC). A written document (or the person designated by it) that authorizes one person to act in the place of, or on behalf of, another person. It specifically applies to situations in which the person who conferred the power has become incapacitated or disabled, and in many states it is applicable to health treatment decisions.

Duty. The moral or legal obligation to follow a certain line of conduct.

Dyspareunia. Painful coitus, usually resulting from a disparity in size of sexual organs or vaginal dryness due to lack of estrogen.

Dyspepsia. Indigestion occurring after meals.

Dysphagia. Difficulty in swallowing.

Dysphrasia. Impairment of speech wherein words are arranged out of sequence arising from a central nervous system lesion.

Dysrhythmias. Irregular heart rhythms.

Elder abuse. An act of omission or commission that leads to harm or threatened harm to the health and welfare of an older person. Elder abuse may be physical, psychological, verbal or sexual, and can include neglect.

Elder cottage housing opportunity (ECHO). ECHO housing is a small, freestanding, factory-built temporary housing unit that is often erected next to the home of an adult child.

Empathy. A feeling of compassion; important when communicating with a client.

Erythema. Redness of the skin produced by congestion of the capillaries that may be due to a variety of conditions.

Eschar. A slough on the surface of the body produced by necrotic material (e.g., from a pressure ulcer or burn).

Ethical dilemma. A perplexing situation necessitating a choice between unpleasant alternatives.

Ethical egoism. The belief that whatever is best for the individual making the decision is morally "good" or "right." Thoreau was an ethical egoist.

Ethics. Codes of conduct adopted by a group of people relating to the rightness or wrongness of certain actions or behaviors.

Ethnic. Pertaining to a religious, national, racial, or cultural group.

Ethnicity. A social differentiation based on such cultural criteria as a sense of peoplehood, shared history, a common place of origin, language, dress, food preferences, club participation, and so on.

Ethnocentric. Pertaining to the belief in the superiority of one's own ethnic group.

Euthanasia. The deliberate ending of the life of a person suffering from an incurable and painful disease.

Fear. An unpleasant emotional state that arises from a specific external threat or danger.

Functional psychosis. A psychosis that is not due to an organic disease.

Gait. Manner of walking.

Generalized anxiety disorder. An illness that tends to be chronic and is characterized by symptoms of tension, inability to relax, frequent urination, dizziness, or excessive worry about life.

Gerontological nursing. The aspect of nursing that is concerned with caring for the population age 65 and older.

Geropsychiatric nursing. Subspecialty of psychiatric nursing that serves older adults and is a caring interactive process that maximizes independence and autonomy of older adults in the activities of daily living.

Grief. The normal emotional state that accompanies a personal, biological, or social loss (i.e., the loss of a family member or friend).

Hallucinations. False sensory perceptions that are not associated with real external stimuli.

Health. A condition in which all functions of body and mind are normally active.

Hematopoiesis. Blood cell function.

Hemianesthesia. Anesthesia of half of the body.

Hemiparesis. Paralysis affecting only one side of the body.

Holistic. Pertaining to the theory that reality is made of organic or unified wholes that are greater than the sum of it parts; anthropologists have stressed the interrelationship of all aspects of culture, the biocultural totality of the human experience.

Hormone. A chemical transmitter with a specific regulatory function in the body.

Hospice. A place and a philosophy of care designed to give palliative care to terminally ill clients and their families; focuses on the psychological, social, and spiritual needs of the client and families, helping the client to die with dignity and assisting the family with the grieving process.

Hyperventilation. An increase in the amount of air entering the alveoli of the lungs.

Iatrogenesis, adj. **iatrogenic.** The creation of additional problems or complications resulting from treatment by a health care professional.

Immobility. The state or quality of being immobile; preventing movement; keeping in place.

Immune response. The activities of the immune system in combating an antigen.

Immunity. The ability to resist most types of organisms or toxins that damage the tissues and organs.

Incidence. The rate at which new cases appear.

Incontinence. Inability to control urinary or bowel function, a primary reason for the institutionalizing of older adults.

Informed consent. A principle that requires a physician or other health care provider to disclose to patients the information necessary for them to make informed choices about their own health care. Based on the autonomy of the individual, it means that, as long as the patient is able to comprehend information given, all procedures must be completely explained and cannot be implemented without the patient's expressed or written consent.

Innate immunity. A generalized process that includes phagocytosis of bacteria or other invaders by white blood cells, destruction by acid secretions of the stomach and digestive enzymes, resistance of the skin to organism invasion, and presence of certain compounds in the blood that attack foreign organisms or toxins and destroy them.

Instrumental activities of daily living (IADLs). Ordinary functional activities that include meal preparation, doing laundry, using transportation, housekeeping, financial man-agement, medication management, grocery shopping, and the ability to use a telephone.

Integrated community living. The practice of dwelling independently in one's own home within the greater community.

Ischemia. Insufficient blood in the tissues.

Koebner's phenomenon. A cutaneous response seen in psoriasis and other dermatoses wherein skin lesions typical of the disease appear on a newly traumatized area of skin, on scars, or at points where clothing presses on the skin.

Leukocytes (white blood cells). Cells formed partly in the bone marrow and partly in the lymph tissue, specifically transported to areas of serious inflammation, providing a rapid and strong defense against an infectious agent.

Lichenification. Cutaneous thickening and hardening from continued irritation to the skin.

Lifecare. Lifecare facilities are similar to CCRCs except that the older adult enters by purchasing a unit (paying an entrance fee), then paying a monthly service charge that never varies whatever the level of care required by the resident. With lifecare, the resident is able to age in place and have peace of mind, knowing that monthly fees will not vary with the level of care needed. The main disadvantage of lifecare is cost; entrance fees are very high.

Life review (reminiscence). An intervention often used in the treatment of older adults; its purpose is to provide for the successful integration of experiences that offer new significance to an individual's life. Reminiscence is a reassessment of life that can bring forth depression, acceptance, or satisfaction in final years.

Living will. A legal document that spells out the patient's right to a natural death.

Long-term care. The care of the older adult (or the disabled younger adult) individual through a continuum of services over months to years.

Macular degeneration. A progressive deterioration of retinal cells in the macula, due to aging.

Menopausal osteoporosis. Reduction in the amount of bone mass, particularly to the trabecular bone, occurring in some women after menopause.

Middle old. Refers to people 75 to 84 years of age.

Minimum data set (MDS). A core set of screening and assessment elements that forms the foundation of the comprehensive assessment.

Morals. Established rules that provide standards of behavior and guide the behavior of an individual or social group.

Motility. Ability to move spontaneously.

Mourning. The normal psychological processes that follow the death of a loved one. The period of mourning is a time for healing and adaptation to the loss. In some cultures there is a designated period of mourning that is accompanied by prescribed mourning rituals.

Myocardial infarction (MI). Death of the heart muscle owing to lack of oxygen and nutrients.

Myxedema coma. A condition caused by prolonged, untreated, acute hypothyroidism that can be fatal.

Natural law. The belief that there is a law of nature that humans are born with the ability to reason and to choose good over evil, and

evil acts are never condoned, even in the most unusual situations.

Nonmaleficence. Abstaining from doing any harm to others.

Nosocomial infections. Infections that were contracted in the health care setting that were not present at the time of admission of the patient—infections the patient acquired from health care providers or staff, other patients, or possibly visitors.

Nursing process. The organizing framework through which nurses determine the care needed to manage health problems and how necessary care can best be implemented. Steps include assessment, diagnosis, planning, implementation, and evaluation.

Obsessions. Thoughts that recur and cause discomfort. They are often coupled with compulsions, which are acts or rituals that must be performed to lessen the anxiety, often causing embarrassment.

Odynophagia. Pain in swallowing.

Old old. Refers to people who are 85 years of age and older.

Oliguria. Diminished urine production in relation to the amount of fluid ingested.

Omnibus Budget Reconciliation Act of 1987. Public Law 100–23 enacted in December 1987. It contains three main elements: (1) conditions of participation related to resident care, (2) survey and certification, and (3) enforcement remedies and sanctions to ensure that residents in long-term care facilities receive satisfactory care.

Osteopenia. Reduced bone mass due to a decrease in the rate of osteoid synthesis below that necessary to compensate for normal bone lysis.

Otosclerosis. The condition characterized by chronic progressive deafness, especially for low tones.

Palliative care. Care of the dying person; it replaces curative care.

Palpation. An assessment technique accomplished by using the fingers or hands to feel for abnormalities or evidence of disease.

Papillae. Many and variously shaped elevations on the surface of the tongue.

Papule. A small, circumscribed, superficial solid elevation of the skin.

Parish nursing. Nursing care that is provided to members by a church or other religious organization.

Perception. The evaluation of information gathered by the senses and the interaction or meaning attached to it.

Percussion. A technique in which the fingers of one hand are placed on an external surface of the body and the fingers of the other hand, lightly but sharply, tap the fingers placed on the body. Abnormalities are determined by feeling for alterations in vibrations and listening for alterations in the pitch and resonance of the sound emitted.

Phagocytosis. The envelopment and digestion of bacteria or other foreign bodies by cells (e.g., leukocytes).

Phimosis. Constriction of the orifice so that the prepuce cannot be retracted back over the glans of the penis.

Phobias. Irrational fears, often intense.

Pica. Bizarre eating compulsion, often of non-nutritive items such as dirt or laundry starch.

Plaque. Any patch or perceptible flat area of the skin.

Polypharmacy. The administration of many medications (prescription and over-the-counter) concurrently, creating a danger of unforeseen interactions.

Presbycusis. A progressive hearing loss affecting both ears that may come about rapidly over a short time or slowly over a period of 5 to 10 years.

Prevalence. The percentage of the entire population with a disease at any given time.

Primary, secondary, and tertiary sources. The primary source of information is provided by the person who is being assessed. Secondary sources include information from medical and nursing records, significant others, and multidisciplinary health care professionals knowledgeable about the individual. Tertiary source information is obtained from literary sources, professional journals, or textbooks.

Pruritus. The sensation of itching.

Pseudodementia. A tentative diagnosis made when an individual may appear intellectually impaired and confused, complaining of memory deficit, decreased appetite and energy, apathy, and feelings of worthlessness. If the patient responds to antidepressant drug therapy, true dementia is not present.

Psychosocial. Related to both psychological and social factors.

Pustule. A visible collection of pus in or under the epidermis.

Qigong. A practice that combines movement, meditation, and breath regulation to enhance the flow of vital energy in the body.

Recommended dietary allowances (RDAs). A set of nutrient intake requirements recommended for "healthy" individuals.

Recovery. Recovery from chemical dependency can occur only when chemical use is discontinued; it is an active developmental process with predictable stages.

Religion. A belief system with concepts that relate to something greater than the self. Common elements of religions include rituals that reflect feelings of awe, adoration, and reverence. Every religion includes such themes as a world view and the purpose of human existence; a belief in a supernatural being(s) or power(s); a moral system or code; and social organization.

Resident assessment protocols (RAPs). Tools that provide structured, problem-oriented frameworks for organizing the MDS information about a resident's health problems or functional status.

Residential care facilities (RCFs). Housing run by homeowners who provide meals, laundry, and housekeeping for older adults. Quality varies from appalling to excellent.

Resource utilization groups (RUGs). A classification system that groups patients based on activities of daily living (ADLs).

Rhonchi. Gurgling sounds heard during inspiration and expiration that are produced by secretions in the trachea and large bronchi. They may be heard in patients with pulmonary edema or in patients who are unable to cough up their secretions and usually clear on coughing.

Rights. Those things to which an individual is entitled by society and formalized into law.

Role. A set of related activities carried out by an individual or ascribed to a position or job title. A role can be actual or perceived.

Rugae. Wrinkles or folds of mucous membrane, as found in the vagina.

Schizophrenia. A functional psychosis that involves a thought disorder characterized by altered concepts of reality, such as delusions and hallucinations.

Self-image. Concept of oneself or of one's role.

Sensation. An awareness made possible by one of the five senses.

Sexuality. The collection of characteristics that mark the differences between male and female.

Sleep apnea. A condition wherein breathing temporarily ceases during sleep.

Span of control. The power indicated by the number of people supervised by an individual.

Spiritual distress. A nursing diagnosis that can be defined as the state in which the individual or group experiences, or is at risk of experiencing, a disturbance in the belief or value system that provides strength, hope, and meaning to life.

Spiritual needs. The needs for connectedness to self, others, and a higher being; or the need for an ability to transcend the self, space, and time.

Spirituality. A basic or inherent quality in all humans that involves a belief in something greater than the self and a faith that positively affirms life.

Single-room occupancy (SRO) housing. Single-room occupancy housing is offered at the low end of the economic spectrum and is often located in undesirable areas.

Stress. A force or influence that tends to alter an existing equilibrium and causes mental strain or pressure.

Stressors. Agents or conditions capable of producing stress.

Stroke. The formation of an embolism, thromboembolism, or hemorrhages within the intracerebral or subarachnoid areas of the brain that deprive the brain of oxygen. Neuromuscular deficiencies become apparent when certain divisions of the brain become ischemic. Also known as cerebrovascular accident (CVA).

Subacute care. Comprehensive, goal-oriented, team-coordinated, inpatient care designed for an individual who has had an acute illness, injury, or exacerbation of a disease process. It is rendered immediately after, or instead of, acute hospitalization to treat medically complex problems. Subacute care is more intensive than traditional nursing home care and less intensive than acute inpatient care.

Subluxation. An incomplete or partial dislocation.

Substance abuse. The continued use of substances despite persistent or recurrent social, occupational, psychological, or physical problems.

Substance dependence. A prolonged, habitual reliance on a substance that has a negative impact on physical health and may also mask symptoms of other serious diseases.

Synovial joint. A joint that is lubricated by synovial fluid, a transparent alkaline viscid fluid resembling the white of an egg that is secreted by the synovial membrane.

T cell. A type of immune-system cell formed from an unspecialized lymphocyte because of the influence of the thymus on the lymphocyte; T lymphocyte.

Thanatologists. Individuals who study death.

Thermal sensitivity. An assessment, through a test, of heat and cold in older adults. Temperature regulation and thermal sensitivity alterations occur with aging.

Thyroid storm. The life-threatening emergency that results from acute, untreated hyperthyroidism.

Tinea. A fungal infection of plantlike organisms that consume organic matter.

Tissue load. Distribution of pressure, friction, and shear on the tissues.

Trabeculae. Anchoring strands of connective tissue.

Utilitarianism. The belief that the greatest human thought, action, and happiness should be achieved in each situation. Benefits should be maximized and harm or danger minimized; "the greatest good for the greatest number."

Values. Personal beliefs used as criteria for justification of action taken.

Vesicle. A small, circumscribed epidermal elevation usually containing a clear fluid.

Volvulus. Knotting or twisting of an organ (e.g., stomach, intestine).

Wellness. A feeling of satisfaction or well-being about one's health or physical condition; involves a balance between internal and external environments and the physical, emotional, spiritual, social, and cultural processes of life.

Wheezes. Continuous musical, high-pitched sounds in the lungs. They have a whistle or squeak and are usually heard on expiration, but they may also be heard on inspiration.

Wisdom. A combination of experience, introspection, reflection, intuition, and empathy, all of which are integrated into a person's interaction with the environment. Simply put, the combination of knowledge and experience.

Xerosis. Dry skin.

Xerostomia. Dry mouth.

Young old. Refers to individuals between the ages of 65 and 74.

Index

Note: Page numbers in *italics* refer to figures; page numbers followed by t refer to tabular materials.

A

Depression (*Continued*)
in dementia, 458–461, *459*
in independently living older adults, 226–227
major, diagnostic criteria for, 250
vs. dementia, 251
Dermatitis, eczematous, 352–354
seborrheic, 354–355
Detached retina, 164
DETERMINE nutritional screening tool, 146
Diabetes, 373–379
and malnutrition, 142–143
clinical manifestations of, 373–374, 374t
complications of, acute, 377–378
chronic, 378–379
diagnosis of, 374
management of, 374–376, 376t
monitoring blood glucose in, 376–377
resources for, 381–382
Diabetic ketoacidosis, 377–378
Diabetic retinopathy, 164
Diarrhea, 413
assessment of, 404
Diet. See also *Nutrition.*
and blood lipids, 143–144
and hypertension, 143–144
fat in, in healthy older adults, 224
for client with dysphagia, 140
for diabetes, 142–143, 375
for diverticulosis, 413
for gastric ulcers, 410
for gastroesophageal reflux disease, 407
for gluten enteropathy, 411
for iron deficiency anemia, 139
general guidelines for, 146–148, *147*
in African-American culture, 98
kosher, 103
Dietitian(s), role of in nutrition education, 149
Digestion, aging and, 402–403
Digitalis, toxicity of, 202
Dignity, preservation of, as ethical issue, 55t
Discharge planning, in acute care setting, 252–253
Disease-modifying antirheumatic drug(s) (DMARDs), 325
Disengagement theory of aging, 15
Distributive justice, 61
Diverticulosis, 412–413
DMARD(s) (disease-modifying antirheumatic drugs), 325
Do Not Resuscitate (DNR) order(s), 78t, 80–81
Documentation, of use of restraints, 207–208
Down syndrome, and Alzheimer's disease, 441
Driving, aging and, 203–205, *205*
dementia and, 453t
Drug(s). See *Medication(s).*
Dry eye(s), 165
"Dry" macular degeneration, 163
Dual-energy x-ray absorptiometry, 313
Durable power of attorney for health care, 78t, 80–81
Duty, definition of, 60t
Dying person(s), care of, 488–494
assessment in, 489
hospice, *489,* 492, 492–493
pain management in, 490–492, 491t
palliative, *489,* 490
physical needs in, 489
spiritual, 489
staff support in, 494

Dying person(s) (*Continued*)
caregivers of, support for, 493–494
rights of, 491
Dysgeusia, 171–172
Dysphagia, 284, 406
and malnutrition, 140–141
Dysphasia, 284
Dyspnea, assessment of, 294

E

Ear(s), anatomy of, *167*
ECG (electrocardiography), 280t, 2890
ECHO housing, 239–240
Echocardiography, 280
Economic issue(s), aging and, 17
Eczema, 352–354
Edema, in cardiovascular disease, 277
Education, continuing, as ethical issue, 58t
patient/family. See *Patient/family education.*
role of gerontological nurses in, 8, 509–510
Egoism, ethical, 53
Eldepryl (selegiline), 343t
Elder abuse, 83–86, 84t, 215–216, 483–484
clinical manifestations of, 215
definition of, 84, 84t
detection of, 84–85
incidence of, 83
nursing interventions for, 215
prevention of, 85
reporting of, 86
Elders Health Program, 212–213
Electrocardiography (ECG), 280, 280t
Electrostimulation, for urinary incontinence, 430
Emergency(ies), informed consent in, 75
Emergency care, 253
Empathy, 28
Emphysema, 300
Empowerment, and wellness, 6–7
Endocrine function, aging and, 372t
Endocrine theory of aging, 14
Enteral nutrition, complications of, 133t
Enteropathy, gluten-induced, 411
Environment, safety of, for patient with dementia, 452
Environmental aging theory, 15
Environmental assessment, for fall risk, 186–187, 206
impaired mobility and, 184
in sleep disorders, 195t
Enzyme(s), in brain, aging and, 337
Erectile dysfunction, 124, 125t
Error catastrophe theory of aging, 14
Esophageal motility, aging and, 402
Esophagus, dilatation of, 407
disorders of, 405–409
squamous cell carcinoma of, 408–409
Essential pruritus, 355–356
Essential tremor, 337–338
Estrogen replacement therapy, for osteoporosis, 314
Ethical decision-making, 69
Ethical dilemma(s), 66–68
Ethical egoism, 53
Ethical issue(s), 50–71
access to health care as, 55t
access to medical records as, 57t

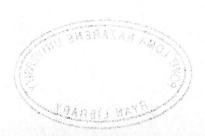